Treatment of Voice Disorders

About the Author

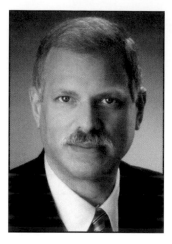

Robert Thayer Sataloff, MD, DMA, who has organized this volume especially for speech-language pathology students and clinicians who are new to the field of voice care, is Chairman of the Department of Otolaryngology-Head and Neck Surgery at the Graduate Hospital in Philadelphia and Professor of Otolaryngology-Head and Neck Surgery at Jefferson Medical College, Thomas Jefferson University. He is President-Elect of the American Laryngeal Association; Chairman of the Speech, Voice and Swallowing Committee of the American Academy of Otolaryngology-Head and Neck Surgery; and Chairman of Board of Directors of the Voice Foundation and the American Institute for Voice and Ear Research. A prolific author, Dr. Sataloff has contributed to more than 500 publications, including 23 textbooks. Dr. Sataloff is also Editor-in-Chief of the *Journal of Voice* and the *Ear, Nose and Throat Journal*.

Treatment of Voice Disorders

Robert Thayer Sataloff, MD, DMA

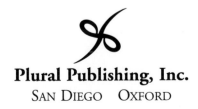

Plural Publishing, Inc.
SAN DIEGO   OXFORD

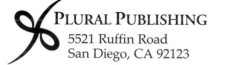

PLURAL PUBLISHING

5521 Ruffin Road
San Diego, CA 92123

e-mail: info@pluralpublishing.com
Web site: http://www.pluralpublishing.com

49 Bath Street
Abingdon, Oxfordshire OX14 1EA
United Kingdom

Treatment of Voice Disorders is one of three student editions prepared for speech-language pathology students and clinicians who are new to the field of voice care from selected chapters of the third edition of *Professional Voice: The Science and Art of Clinical Care* to provide relevant information in an affordable format.

Care has been taken to confirm the accuracy of the information presented in this book and to describe generally accepted practices. However, the authors, editors, and publisher are not responsible for errors or omissions or for any consequences from application of the information in this book and make no warranty, expressed or implied, with respect to the currency, completeness, or accuracy of the contents of the publication. Application of this information in a particular situation remains the professional responsibility of the practitioner

ISBN 1-59756-040-5

Library of Congress Control Number: 2005905964

Contents

Foreword

Robert T. Sataloff's *Treatment of Voice Disorders* covers its subject with exceptional breadth and clarity. This book, consisting of 26 chapters, is the essential compendium of information on treating voice disorders. As suggested in the opening chapter ("Voice Care Professionals"), the contemporary treatment of voice disorders draws on interdisciplinary expertise, and the book is true to that perspective. The team approach to voice treatment is realized through the contributions of laryngologists, speech-language pathologists, singing voice specialists, nurses, physiotherapists, acting voice trainers, and others. The reader will find discussion of various treatment procedures, including surgical, pharmacological, and behavioral. It should be emphasized that this volume presents essential information that allows for the effective interaction of various specialties. For example, behavioral specialists can draw on the excellent information that is given on surgery, trauma and injury, and medications. This book is at once a template for team-based treatment and a deep informational resource for treatment alternatives. Its scope and depth make it a book that the voice specialist will want to keep close at hand.

This impressive book draws on Dr. Sataloff's substantial experience as a clinician, researcher, and scholar. He has ably recruited a cadre of related professionals to achieve an interdisciplinary view that is unified and collective, overcoming the risk of fragmentation that often characterizes interdisciplinary efforts. The information is current, and it is presented lucidly yet concisely. Surely, *Treatment of Voice Disorders* is an essential volume for anyone concerned with voice disorders. It is a landmark publication in the field of voice.

Raymond D. Kent, Ph.D.
Madison, Wisconsin

Preface

Treatment of Voice Disorders is part of a five-book student edition of selected chapters from the third edition of *Professional Voice: The Science and Art of Clinical Care*. That compendium fills nearly 2000 pages, including 160 chapters and numerous appendices, and it is not practical for routine use by students. However, *Professional Voice* was intended to be valuable to not only laryngologists, but also to speech-language pathologists, voice teachers, performers, students, and anyone else interested in the human voice. *Treatment of Voice Disorders* and the other volumes of the student editions were prepared to make relevant information available to students in a convenient and affordable form, suitable for classroom use as well as for reference.

Chapter 1 introduces the many professionals who may be involved in voice care and explains their roles. Chapter 2 introduces the basic concepts of treating voice abuse. In chapter 3, the late Carol Wilder provides still current perspective on the role of the speech-language pathologist in caring for professional voice users. Chapter 4 is a comprehensive chapter on voice therapy directed primarily at management of professional voice users. Chapter 5 discusses what little is known about voice rest and concepts of management following vocal fold trauma or surgery. Chapter 6 provides guidelines on effective vocal presentation (speaking), which may be useful for patients as well as for students and teachers. In chapter 7, Richard Miller reviews the important interactions of voice science and voice teaching. Chapter 8 presents an invaluable historical overview of voice pedagogy. This information is useful not only useful for singers, but also for laryngologists and speech-language pathologists who may need to understand the basis and thinking of various schools of voice training through which their patients may have been influenced by their teachers. Chapter 9 on the singing voice specialist includes techniques for management of the singing voice and for using singing techniques to help nonsingers. Chapter 10, The Use of Instrumentation in the Singing Studio, was added to help train singers. Chapter 11, Choral Pedagogy, introduces the complex nature of choral singing particularly fashion. Chapter 12 defines the role of the acting voice training in medical management of the professional voice user. Chapter 13 on laryngeal manipulation is written by an osteopathic physician and two laryngologists. This topic was added because of their unusual experience and success and because laryngeal manipulation has been used for decades by voice therapists and for centuries by singing teachers. This chapter is intended to provide an introductory medical perspective on the subject. Chapter 14 reviews important information on postural analysis, a subject more familiar to other medical specialties (such as physiatry) than to otolaryngology. Chapter 15 summarizes basic concepts of exercise physiology and its applications for vocal exercise. Chapter 16 reviews common medications and their effects on the voice. Chapter 17 discusses the use of botulinum toxin in detail. Chapter 18 provides an extensive review of voice surgery. This chapter is important not only for surgeons, but also for speech-language pathologists and acting voice professionals. All voice care professionals are prepared better to work with a patient who has undergone surgery if they understand the nature of the individual procedures. Vocal fold scar is one of the most common challenging problems following vocal fold surgery or phonotrauma, and this topic is reviewed in chapter 19. Chapters 20 and 21 provide detailed information on evaluation and treatment of trauma to the lungs, trachea, and laryngeal joints. Chapter 22 reviews therapeutic and surgical aspects of treating transgender/transsexual patients. Chapter 23 summarizes treatment and provides the most current management approaches to laryngeal cancer. Chapter 24 describes nursing considerations in the management of voice users. Chapters 25 and 26 describe controversies in the management of professional voice users and speculate about future developments in and understanding of diagnosis and the prospective on near-future horizons in laryngology and voice research.

Robert Thayer Sataloff, MD, DMA

Contributors

Timothy D. Anderson, MD
Senior Staff, Otolaryngologist
Lahey Clinic Voice and Swallowing Center
Department of Otolaryngology-Head and Neck
Surgery
Burlington, Massachusetts

Joseph Anticaglia, MD
Ear, Nose, and Throat Associates of New York
Flushing, New York

Margaret M. Baroody, M.M.
Singing Voice Specialist
Voice Technology
American Institute for Voice and Ear Research
Philadelphia, Pennsylvania

Ed Blake, MSc (Phty), MCST, SRP
Physiatrist
Specialist in Dance and Vocal Medicine
Physio-Ed Medical
London, England

Linda M. Carroll, PhD, CCC-SLP
Voice Consultant
The Eugene Grabscheid, MD, Voice Center
Department of Otolaryngology
Mount Sinai Medical Center
New York New York

Susan E. Cline, MS, CCC-SLP
Clinical Voice Specialist
The Voice Care Center at
Presbyterian Hospital
Charlotte, North Carolina

Carolyn A. Dennehy, PhD
Biological Sciences in the College of Arts and
Sciences
University of Northern Colorado
Greeley, Colorado

Kate A. Emerich, BM, MS, CCC-SLP
Voice Pathologist/Vocologist
Singing Voice Specialist
Gould Voice Center
Denver Center for the Performing Arts
National Center for Voice and Speech
Denver, Colorado

Adrian J. Fourcin, Ph.D.
Professor of Experimental Phonetics, Phonetics, and
Linguistics
University College London
London, United Kingdom

Sharon L. Freed, BA, MFA
Acting-Voice Trainer
American Institute for Voice and Ear Research
Philadelphia, Pennsylvania

Thomas M. Harris, MA, FRCS
Consultant ENT Surgeon
University Hospital Lewisham
Director, The Voice Clinic
Queen Mary's Hospital
Honorary Senior Lecturer, Guy's King's St. Thomas'
Medical Schools
London, United Kingdom

Mary J. Hawkshaw, RN, BSN, CORLN
Otolaryngologic Nurse Clinician
Executive Director
American Institute for Voice and Ear Research
Philadelphia, Pennsylvania

Yolanda D. Heman-Ackah, MD
Assistant Professor, Department of Otolaryngology-
Head and Neck Surgery
Jefferson Medical College
Thomas Jefferson University
Philadelphia, Pennsylvania

Reinhardt J. Heuer, PhD
Professor, Department of Communication Sciences
and Disorders
College of Allied Health Professionals
Temple University
Consultant Scientist
American Institute for Voice and Ear Research
Philadelphia, Pennsylvania

Michelle Horman, MA, CCC-SLP
Voice Pathologist
American Institute for Voice and Ear Research
Philadelphia, Pennsylvania

Jacob Lieberman, DO, MA
Osteopathic Physician and Psychotherapist
London, United Kingdom

Karen M. Lyons, MD
Clinical Assistant Professor of Otolaryngology
Thomas Jefferson University
Philadelphia, Pennsylvania

Lesley Mathieson, DipCST, FRCSLT
Visiting Lecturer in Voice Pathology
The University of Reading
Reading, United Kingdom

Richard Miller, DHL
Professor of Singing
Director, Otto B. Schoepfle Vocal Arts Laboratory
Oberlin College, Conservatory of Music
Oberlin, Ohio

Michael C. Neuenschwander, MD
Director and Facial Plastic Consultant
Skin and Body Rejuvenation Center
ENT of Georgia
Riverdale, Georgia

Kathe S. Perez, MA, CCC-SLP
Doctoral Student
Department of Communication Disorders and
Speech Sciences
University of Colorado Health Sciences Center
University of Colorado-Boulder
Boulder, Colorado

Edmund A. Pribitkin, MD
Associate Professor of Otolaryngology-Head and
Neck Surgery
Thomas Jefferson University
Philadelphia, Pennsylvania

Bonnie N. Raphael, PhD
Professor and Head of the Professional Actor
Training Program
Center of Dramatic Art
University of North Carolina at Chapel Hill
Chapel Hill, North Carolina

Clark A. Rosen, MD
Director, University of Pittsburgh Voice Center
Associate Professor, Department of Otolaryngology
University of Pittsburgh School of Medicine
Pittsburgh, Pennsylvania

Adam D. Rubin, MD
Department of Otolaryngology-Head and Neck Surgery
Lake Shore ENT
St. Clear Shores, Michigan

John S. Rubin, MD, FRCS, FACS
Consultant ENT Surgeon
Lead Clinician Voice Disorders Group
Clinical Head of Service
Royal National Throat Nose and Ear Division
Royal Free Hospital NHS Trust
Honorary Consultant ENT Surgeon

St Bartholomews Hospital
Honorary Senior Lecturer
Institute of Laryngology and Otology
University of College London
Visiting Associate Professor
Department of Otolaryngology
Albert Einstein College of Medicine
Bronx, New York

Rhonda K. Rulnick, MS, CCC-SLP
Speech-Language Pathologist
Princeton Speech-Language and Learning Center
Princeton, New Jersey

Robert Thayer Sataloff, MD, DMA
Professor
Department of Otolaryngology-Head and Neck
Surgery
Thomas Jefferson University
Chairman, Department of Otolaryngology-Head
and Neck Surgery
The Graduate Hospital
Chairman, Board of Directors
The Voice Foundation
Faculty, Academy of Vocal Arts
Faculty, The Curtis Institute of Music
Chairman, American Institute for Voice and Ear
Research
Philadelphia, Pennsylvania

Keith G. Saxon, MD
Visiting Professor
Department of Otolaryngology
Albert Einstein College of Medicine
New York, New York

Carole M. Schneider, PhD
School of Kinesiology and Physical Education
University of Northern Colorado
Greeley, Colorado

Brenda J. Smith, DMA
Assistant Professor of Music (Voice)
School of Music
University of Florida
Gainesville, Florida

Kimberly M. Steinhauer, PhD
University of Pittsburgh Voice Center
Department of Communication Science and Disorders
University of Pittsburgh School of Health and
Rehabilitation Sciences
Pittsburgh, Pennsylvania

Carol N. Wilder, PhD (deceased)
Former Professor of Speech Science
Teachers College
Columbia University
New York, New York

Acknowledgments

I am indebted to the many distinguished colleagues who collaborated in writing this book. Their friendship and wisdom are appreciated greatly. I also remain indebted to the many friends and colleagues who have helped develop the field of voice over the last few decades, particularly the late Wilbur James Gould.

As always, I cannot express sufficient thanks to Mary J. Hawkshaw, RN, BSN for her tireless editorial assistance, proofreading, and scholarly contributions. Without her help, many of my books would still be unfinished. I am also indebted to Helen Caputo and Beth V. Luby for their tireless, painstaking preparation of the manuscript and for the many errors they found and corrected and to my associates Joseph Sataloff, MD, DSc, Karen M. Lyons, MD, and Yolanda D. Heman-Ackah, MD. Without their collaboration, excellent patient care, and tolerance of my many academic distractions and absences, writing would be much more difficult. In addition, I am indebted to Sandy Doyle from Plural Publishing Company, Inc. who has done a truly superb job editing this book and preparing it for publication.

My greatest gratitude goes to my wife Dahlia M. Sataloff, MD, and sons Ben and John who patiently allow me to spend so many of my evenings, weekends, and vacations writing.

Dedication

*To my wife Dahlia Sataloff, MD, my sons Benjamin Harmon Sataloff and Johnathan Brandon Sataloff,
my parents Joseph Sataloff, MD and Ruth Sataloff, and my friend and editorial assistant
Mary J. Hawkshaw RN, BSN, for their unfailing patience and support*

and

*To Wilbur James Gould, MD, friend, scholar, educator, and founder of the Voice Foundation,
who devoted his life to improving, understanding, and caring for the human voice.*

and

To Howell S. Zulick, my voice teacher for twenty-nine years and an inspiration for life.

and

*To Walter P. Work, Charles J. Krause, and Malcolm D. Graham, the professors who trained me and
cultivated the love for academic medicine inspired by my father and for which he wisely sent me to Ann Arbor.*

1

Voice Care Professionals: A Guide to Voice Care Providers

Robert Thayer Sataloff, Yolanda D. Heman-Ackah, and Mary J. Hawkshaw

Optimal voice care is delivered by an interdisciplinary team consisting of physicians and nonphysicians. The physician may be an otolaryngologist (a specialist who practices all aspects of ear, nose and throat medicine) or a laryngologist, who specializes in voice disorders. The physician commonly collaborates with other professionals, such as a speech-language pathologist, singing voice specialist, acting-voice specialist, and others who constitute the voice care team. Under the best of circumstances, all of the members of the team have received special training in not just the general aspects of their disciplines but also additional training in care of the voice. Although even the best training does not guarantee clinical excellence, it does improve the probability that a practitioner will provide superior, modern voice care. This chapter reviews the typical training and qualifications of the professionals associated most commonly with voice care teams.

The Voice Care Team

A voice care team is ordinarily under the direction of a physician who is usually an otolaryngologist or laryngologist. In addition to the physician who diagnoses and provides medical treatment for voice disorders, the team includes the speech-language pathologist, who provides voice therapy and attends to problems that affect the speaking voice; a phoniatrist in countries without speech-language pathologists; a singing voice specialist; an acting-voice specialist; a nurse and/or a physician's assistant; and consultant physicians in other specialties. It is helpful for patients

to understand the background and role of each member of the voice team, as discussed below.

Otolaryngologist/Laryngologist

The leader of the voice care team is ordinarily a physician (otolaryngologist). Otolaryngologists are physicians (surgeons) who specialize in problems of the ears, nose, and throat (ENT). Laryngologists are otolaryngologists who specialize in care of disorders of the larynx and, in some cases, related problems such as swallowing. To practice laryngology, one must first complete training as an otolaryngologist. To become an otolaryngologist, a person completes college, 4 years of medical school, 1 or 2 years of training in general surgery, and 4 years of residency in otolaryngology—head and neck surgery. In the year following completion of residency, the physician takes a national, standardized board examination given in two parts (written and oral) to become a "board certified" otolaryngologist. Certification by the American Board of Otolaryngology, or the equivalent organization in other countries, is an important indicator of mastery of basic knowledge in otolaryngology and is considered a basic, minimum qualification. The only exception is "board eligibility" in the case of a physician who has finished residency but has not yet successfully passed the board examinations. Board certification is not granted until a physician has had 1 year of clinical experience following residency and demonstrated competency on the oral and written board examinations.

Most otolaryngologists' clinical practices include many or all components of the specialty, such as otology (disorders of the ear and related structures), laryngology (disorders of the voice and upper airway structures such as the throat and trachea), head and neck cancer, head and neck neoplasms (masses including benign or malignant lesions), facial plastic and reconstructive surgery, allergy and immunology, bronchoesophagology (lower airway and swallowing disorders), rhinology (nose, sinus, taste, and smell disorders), and pediatric otolaryngology (ear, nose, and throat disorders of children). Most otolaryngologists and laryngologists care for patients of all ages from early childhood through advanced years. Some otolaryngologists subspecialize, in caring for disorders in just one or two areas of otolaryngology, as described above. This subspecialization can either be a keen interest in a specific area while still providing a broad range of ear, nose, and throat care or the focused practice of only one or two of the subcomponents of otolaryngology. Laryngology is one such subspecialty.

Most of the physicians specializing in laryngology today did not receive laryngology fellowship training. That is always the case as a new field develops. Modern laryngology evolved out of an interest in caring for professional voice users, especially singers. The first comprehensive article guiding otolaryngologists on care of professional singers was published in 1981[1]; the first major modern American otolaryngology textbook with a chapter on care of the professional voice was published in 1986[2]; and the first comprehensive book on care of the professional voice was published in 1991.[3] So, most of the senior laryngologists practicing at the turn of the 21st century were involved in the evolution of the field before fellowships were developed. Most fellowship training programs started in the 1990s, although a few informal fellowship programs existed in the1980s and earlier. It is reasonable to expect most voice specialists who finished residency training in the 1990s or later to have completed a fellowship in laryngology. There are approximately a dozen laryngology fellowship-training programs in the United States, and they are highly competitive. At present, completion of a fellowship is a reasonably good indicator of superior knowledge and clinical training in laryngology. Most laryngology fellowships include training in the diagnosis and treatment of voice disorders in adults and children, neurolaryngology (neurological problems that affect the voice and larynx), swallowing disorders, airway reconstruction, and laryngeal cancer. The training includes both medical diagnosis and treatment, and sophisticated laryngeal surgery. Typically, laryngologists care for both routine and complex problems that affect the voice. Such problems include voice dysfunction associated with something as simple as a common cold,

especially when it affects the voice of a professional singer or actor. However, laryngologists also are called on to diagnose and treat structural lesions such as nodules or polyps, prolonged infections of the vocal folds, cancer, traumatic injury from fracture or internal trauma (intubation injuries from anesthesia, vocal fold injuries from previous surgery), neurological disorders, and other voice problems. The laryngologist is responsible for establishing a medical diagnosis and implementing or coordinating treatment for the patient. The laryngologist may prescribe medication, inject botulinum toxin, perform delicate microsurgery on the vocal folds, or operate through the neck on the laryngeal skeleton. He or she is also usually responsible for initiating evaluation by other members of the voice team and for generating referrals to other specialists as needed.

Laryngologists may practice in university medical centers or private offices; and in major cities in the United States, they are usually affiliated with a voice team including at least a speech-language pathologist, a singing voice specialist, and sometimes an acting-voice specialist. Laryngologists should also have, or have access to, a clinical voice laboratory with equipment to analyze the voice objectively and a stroboscope to visualize the vocal folds in slow motion. They also should be familiar with physicians in other specialties who have an understanding and interest in arts-medicine. Even for patients with a voice disorder who are not singers and actors, such knowledge and sensitivity is important. Just as nonathletes benefit from the orthopedic expertise of a sports-medicine specialist, voice patients receive more expert care from physicians trained to treat singers, the "Olympic" athletes of the voice world.

Currently, there is no official additional certification for those who have completed a laryngology fellowship. However, there are organizations (medical societies) with which many of the leading laryngologists are affiliated. Essentially all laryngologists in the United States are fellows of the American Academy of Otolaryngology—Head and Neck Surgery (http://www.entnet.org), and laryngologists in other countries are members of their nations' analogous organizations. A few are also members of the American Laryngological Association (ALA), the most senior otolaryngology society in the United States (http://www.alahns.org). The ALA also accepts "associate members" from other countries. Some laryngologists belong to the American Bronchoesophagological Association (http://www.abea.net), and the Voice Foundation (http://www.voicefoundation.org). The Voice Foundation was founded in 1969 and is the oldest organization dedicated to voice education and research. It provides seed grants for research, sponsors an annual symposium on care of the professional voice that started in 1972, and fosters voice education through conferences, educational videotapes, books, and publications such as the *Journal of Voice* and the *Voice Foundation Newsletter*. In recent years, several countries have developed organizations similar to the Voice Foundation, such as the British, Canadian, and Australian Voice Foundations. Laryngologists in such countries are usually members of their national organization, and many are also members of the Voice Foundation (Philadelphia, Pa). Although membership in these organizations is not a guarantee of excellence in practice, it suggests interest and knowledge in laryngology, particularly voice disorders.

Speech-Language Pathologist

The speech-language pathologist is a certified, licensed health care professional, ordinarily with either a master's degree (MA or MS) or doctorate (PhD). After college, speech-language pathologists generally complete a 1- or 2-year master's degree program, followed by a 9-month, supervised "clinical fellowship," which is similar to a medical internship. At the conclusion of the clinical fellowship year, speech-language pathologists in the United States are certified by the American Speech-Language-Hearing Association, and use the letters "CCC-SLP" after their names to indicate that they are certified. Like otolaryngology, speech-language pathology is a broad field that includes care of patients who have had strokes or other neurological problems affecting speech and swallowing, undergone laryngectomy (removal of the larynx), have swallowing disorders, have articulation or stuttering problems, have craniofacial disorders, or have other related fluency disorders of speech. Some speech-language pathologists subspecialize in voice, which includes the care of voice disorders and swallowing disorders. The speech-language pathologist affiliated with a voice team is usually such a subspecialist and may call him- or herself a "voice pathologist" rather than a speech-language pathologist, although "voice pathologist" is not a term recognized officially by the American Speech-Language-Hearing Association, yet. Relatively few speech-language pathology training programs provide extensive education in voice, and there are virtually no voice fellowships for speech-language pathologists. Many speech-language pathology training programs do not require even a single course on voice disorders. Thus, it cannot be assumed that all speech-language pathologists are trained in or comfortable with caring for individuals with voice problems. Most acquire the subspeciality training they need through apprenticeships, extra courses, and symposia or by obtaining doctoral degrees that include voice-related research.

Speech-language pathologists are responsible for voice therapy and rehabilitation, which is analogous to physical therapy. The speech-language pathologist analyzes voice use and teaches proper voice support, relaxation, and voice placement to optimize use of the voice during speaking. A variety of techniques are utilized to accomplish this goal. Speech-language pathologists do not ordinarily work with the singing voice, although they are involved in the treatment of speaking voices of singers.

Speech-language pathologists may be found in universities, private offices, or freestanding speech and hearing centers. In the United States, most are members of ASHA (the American Speech-Language-Hearing Association), and its voice-related special interest division (SID-3), which can be accessed on the Internet. Many speech-language pathologists with special interest in voice in the United States and elsewhere are also members of the Voice Foundation. Like otolaryngologists, speech-language pathologists who subspecialize in voice provide more incisive, state-of-the-art treatment for voice disorders than most general speech-language pathologists who care for patients with various problems encompassing the entire field. So, it is worthwhile for patients with voice disorders to seek out a subspecialist to improve the likelihood of a rapid, excellent treatment result. Referrals to speech-language pathologists specializing in voice are usually obtained through a laryngologist or otolaryngologist.

Phoniatrists

Phoniatrists do not exist in the United States, but they provide voice care in many European countries. The phoniatrist is a physician who is in some ways a hybrid of the laryngologist and speech-language pathologist. Phoniatrists receive medical training in diagnosis and treatment of voice, swallowing, and language disorders, including voice therapy; but they do not perform surgery. In countries with phoniatrists, surgery is performed by otolaryngologists. In many cases, the phoniatrist and otolaryngologist collaborate as a team, just as otolaryngologists and speech-language pathologists do in the United States and elsewhere. A physician who has completed training in phoniatry is generally well qualified to diagnose voice disorders and provide nonsurgical medical care, as well as voice therapy.

Singing Voice Specialist

The singing voice specialist is a singing teacher with special training equipping him or her to practice in a medical environment with patients who have sustained vocal injury. Most singing voice specialists have a degree in voice performance or pedagogy, although some have only extensive performing and teaching experience without a formal academic degree. Nearly all have professional performance experience, as well as extra training in laryngeal anatomy and physiology of phonation, training in the rehabilitation of injured voices, and other special education. The singing voice specialist must acquire knowledge of anatomy and physiology of the normal and disordered voice, a basic understanding of the principles of laryngology and medications, and a fundamental knowledge of the principles and practices of speech-language pathology. This information is not part of the traditional training of singing teachers. Moreover, so far there are no formal training or fellowship programs that assist singing teachers in becoming a singing voice specialist. Their training is acquired by apprenticeship and observation. Many take courses in speech-language pathology programs, but usually not as part of a formal degree or certification program[4]; because there is no certification of singing voice specialists. A few of the best singing voice specialists are also certified, licensed speech-language pathologists. This combination is optimal, provided the speech-language pathologist has sufficient experience and training not only as a performing artist but also as a teacher of singing. In patients with vocal injuries or problems, the fundamental approach to training the singing voice is different in important ways from that usually used with healthy students in a singing studio. Hence, even an excellent and experienced voice teacher may harm an injured voice if he or she is not familiar with the special considerations for this population. In addition, most voice teachers do not feel comfortable working with a singer who has had a vocal injury or surgery.

Virtually all singing voice specialists are affiliated with voice care teams. Most are members of the National Association of Teachers of Singing (NATS), or the equivalent organization in another country, and of the Voice Foundation. In many cases, their practices are limited to work with injured voices. They work not only with singers, but also with other patients with voice disorders. As a member of the voice treatment team working with nonsingers, they help teach speakers the "athletic" techniques utilized by singers for voice production. Singing is to speaking as running is to walking. When rehabilitating someone who has difficulty walking, if the person can be helped to jog or run, leg strength and endurance improve and walking rehabilitation is expedited. The singing voice specialist applies similar principles to voice rehabilitation in collaboration with the speech-language pathologist and other voice care team members.

Acting-Voice Specialist

Acting-voice trainers are also called voice coaches, drama voice teachers, and voice consultants. Traditionally, these professionals have been associated closely with the theater. Their skills have been utilized as part of a medical voice team only since the mid-1990s.[5] Consequently, few acting-voice trainers have any medical experience; but their contributions have proven invaluable.

Acting-voice trainers use a variety of behavior modification techniques designed to enhance vocal communication, quality, projection, and endurance in theatrical settings. They train actors to speak or scream through eight shows a week, and/or theatrical runs that may last years, without tiring or causing injury to their voices. They also teach techniques for adding emotional expression to vocal delivery, and they work with body language and posture to optimize vocal delivery and communication of information. They may be a great asset to the voice team in teaching people how to apply the many skills learned through the speech-language pathologist and singing voice specialist to their everyday lives. Acting-voice trainers are especially valuable for people who speak professionally such as teachers, lecturers, politicians, clergy, sales personnel, and others concerned with effective vocal delivery and with vocal endurance.

There are no formal programs to prepare voice coaches to work in a medical milieu. Those who do receive training generally do so through apprenticeships and collaboration with medical voice care teams under the direction of a laryngologist.

Acting-voice trainers interested in working with voice patients are generally members of the Voice and Speech Trainers Association (VASTA) and the Voice Foundation.

Nurse

Nurses are indispensable assets in medical offices, and they are important members of the voice team in many centers. Nurses who work closely with a laryngologist generally have vast experience in the diagnosis and treatment of voice disorders. They are wonderful information resources for patients and frequently provide much of the patient education in busy clinical settings. These nurses are usually members of the Society of Otolaryngology—Head and Neck Nurses (SOHN). Nurses with advanced knowledge and skills may be certified (by SOHN) as otolaryngology nurses and are identified as such by the initials "CORLN" (certified otolaryngologic nurse) after their names.

Nurse practitioners are advanced practice nurses with master's degrees, who are licensed to provide independent care for patients with selected medical problems. They are identified by the initials "CRNP" (certified registered nurse practitioner). They work in conjunction with a physician; but they can examine, diagnose, and treat selected problems relatively independently. A few nurse practitioners specialize in otolaryngology and work with voice teams. They ordinarily receive special training "on the job" from the otolaryngologist, and they provide care within their scope of practice. Nurse practitioners can also become members of SOHN, become certified through examination by SOHN, and on certification will also use the certification CORLN after their names.

Physician Assistants and Medical Assistants

Physician assistants, like nurse practitioners discussed above, function in association with a physician. Physician assistants graduate from a training program that usually lasts 4 years and teaches them various aspects of medical diagnosis and physical examination. They use the initials "PA" (physician assistant) after their names. They practice in conjunction with physicians but can perform examinations and treat patients independently. They are licensed in many states to write prescriptions. A few physician assistants specialize in otolaryngology, and a smaller number have had extensive training and experience in voice care. In collaboration with a laryngologist and voice teams, they are qualified to evaluate and treat patients with voice disorders.

Physician assistants should be distinguished from "medical assistants" who have less training and are qualified to assist in medical care and patient education but generally not to diagnose and treat patients independently. Medical assistants generally are trained to perform tasks such as phlebotomy (drawing blood) and perform electrocardiograms. In a laryngology office, a good medical assistant can be trained to perform many other tasks, such as taking histories, assisting with strobovideolaryngoscopy, and assisting during the performance of surgical procedures in the office, participating in research, and other tasks.

Consultant Medical Professionals

Otolaryngologists often refer voice patients for consultation with other medical professionals. Other specialists consulted commonly include neurologists, pulmonologists (lungs), gastroenterologists (stomach and intestinal system), psychologists, and psychiatrists. However, physicians in virtually any medical specialty may be called on to care for voice patients. Traditional and nontraditional ancillary medical personnel may also be involved in voice care, including nutritionists, physical therapists, chiropractors, osteopaths (for manipulation), acupuncturists, and others. Within virtually all of these fields, there are a select few professionals who have an interest in and an understanding of arts-medicine. Just as caring for voice professionals (especially singers) involves special considerations and challenges for the otolaryngologist, caring for hand problems in a pianist or ankle problems in dancers also poses challenges for the orthopedic surgeon. Orthopedic surgeons, neurologists, pulmonologists, and others who are accustomed to working with performing artists (dancers, wind instrumentalists, etc) are most likely to have the insight, sensitivities, skills, and state-of-the-art information needed to provide optimal care to voice professionals. Many such physicians tend to be associated with arts-medicine centers or are performers themselves. There is no certification or broad-based national or international organization that helps to identify such physicians, although some are members of the Performing Arts Medicine Association (PAMA). In most fields, there are no formal arts-medicine training programs or associations. Physicians acquire such training through their own interests and initiative and through apprenticeship or observation with colleagues. If there is no arts-medicine center in the area in which a patient is seeking care, arts-medicine physicians are identified best by word-of-mouth or through arts-medicine-related Web sites. Referrals can be obtained through the local laryngologist or voice specialist or by consulting with eminent performing arts teachers in the community. For example, the leading private university and conservatory violin and piano teachers often know who the best hand specialists are; the wind instrument teachers know whom to see for neurological and pulmonary problems that affect musicians; and dance teachers know the best foot-and-ankle physicians.

Conclusion

Voice care has evolved into a sophisticated, well-organized medical science. Patients with voice disorders are served best by a comprehensive voice team that coordinates the skills of professionals trained in various disciplines. It is important for health care professionals to assemble interdisciplinary teams and to affiliate with arts-medicine specialists and other disciplines in order to provide comprehensive care for voice patients. It is also important for patients to be educated about the kind of health care that is now available for voice disorders and how to evaluate and select health care providers.

References

1. Sataloff RT. Professional singers: the science and art of clinical care. *Am J Otolaryngol.* 1981;2(3):251–266.

2. Sataloff RT. The professional voice. In: Cummings CW, Frederickson JM, Harker LA, et al, eds. *Otolaryngology—Head and Neck Surgery.* Vol 3. St Louis, Mo: CV Mosby; 1986:2029–2056.

3. Sataloff RT. *Professional Voice: The Science and Art of Clinical Care.* New York, NY: Raven Press; 1991:1–542.

4. Emerich KA, Baroody MM, Carroll LM, Sataloff RT. The singing voice specialist. In: Sataloff RT. *Professional Voice: The Science and Art of Clinical Care.* 2nd ed. San Diego, Calif: Singular Publishing Group; 1997:735–753.

5. Freed SL, Raphael BN, Sataloff RT. The role of the acting-voice trainer in medical care of professional voice users. In: Sataloff RT. *Professional Voice: The Science and Art of Clinical Care.* 2nd ed. San Diego, Calif: Singular Publishing Group; 1997:765–774.

2

Introduction to Treating Voice Abuse

Robert Thayer Sataloff

Abnormalities Associated with Voice Dysfunction

A great number of physical and psychological problems may be responsible for voice dysfunction. These include derangements in virtually any body system. Most of the organic, psychological, and technical problems that may be related to voice complaints are discussed in detail in other chapters. It is important for the physician to identify and sort out dysfunction in each category (organic, psychological, and technical); abnormalities in all three categories are frequently present simultaneously. For example, if the initial problem is an abnormality on the vocal fold, fear and psychological stress are normal reactions, and the performer frequently changes his or her technique (often unconsciously) in an effort to compensate for vocal impairment. Alternatively, technical dysfunction (such as hyperfunctional voice abuse or muscular tension dysphonia) may have been the initiating factor. This may have produced vocal fold pathology (such as nodules) and subsequent psychological reaction. In contrast, extreme, poorly compensated anxiety may have been the original culprit and caused laryngeal and technical problems. For each scenario, the treatment approach is different, and all appropriate members of the voice care team must understand the pathogenesis in order to design a treatment program that addresses not only immediate performance crises, but, long-term solutions to the principal problem. It is usually best to address all existing problems through a team approach. The team should include consultants in various specialties with special interest in and knowledge of professional voice users. Because of the frequency and importance of voice abuse problems, the otolaryngologist must acquire extra training in technical aspects of voice production for speech and singing and should work closely with a speech-language pathologist and singing voice specialist, acting voice specialist, and other professionals.

Voice Abuse

Vocal complaints are often due to abusive speaking or singing habits, especially hyperfunctional techniques. These problems and therapeutic approaches to them are discussed in detail later in this book. Laryngologists must be familiar with the specific techniques used by speech-language pathologists, singing voice specialists, and acting-voice specialists to diagnose and modify vocal abuses.

Physicians must be careful not to exceed the limits of their expertise or responsibility in applying this knowledge in the office. However, if the physician is trained in singing and notices a minor technical error such as isolated excess muscle tension in the tongue, this may be pointed out. Nevertheless, the singer should be referred back to his or her voice teacher or to a competent singing-voice specialist for management of these problems. Abdominal muscle problems should be noted and should also be referred back to the vocal teacher. Of course, any medical cause must be corrected.

Most of the important historical aspects and many treatment suggestions regarding voice abuse in speaking and singing are covered in chapters 4 and 9, although these chapters concentrate on the responsibilities of the team members other than the laryngologists.

When voice abuse is due to extracurricular activities such as conducting, screaming during athletic events, or shouting at children, the physician should advise the patient about measures to protect the speaking voice and, consequently, the singing voice. However, if it is a matter of strain in the singing or speaking voice under ordinary circumstances, treatment should be deferred to a voice teacher or speech-language pathologist. In many instances, training the speaking voice will benefit the singer greatly, and physicians should not hesitate to recommend such training. Similarly, most singers benefit from formal training of the speaking voice. Surprisingly, most singers have not had such training, and they often speak much more abusively than they sing. The specially trained speech-language pathologist can be of great value to these singers, and usually only a few sessions are required. Subsequently, work with an acting-voice trainer is often invaluable.

Speech-Language Pathologists

An excellent speech-language pathologist is an invaluable asset in caring for professional voice users. However, laryngologists should recognize that, like physicians, speech-language pathologists have varied backgrounds and experience in treatment of voice disorders. In fact, most speech-language pathology programs teach relatively little about caring for professional speakers and nothing about professional singers. Moreover, there are few speech-language pathologists with vast experience in this specialized area. Speech-language pathologists often subspecialize. A person who expertly treats patients who have had strokes, stutter, have undergone laryngectomy, or have swallowing disorders will not necessarily know how to manage professional voice users optimally. The laryngologist must learn the strengths and weaknesses of the speech-language pathologist with whom he or she works. After identifying a speech-language pathologist who is interested in treating professional voice users, the laryngologist and speech-language pathologist should work together closely in developing the necessary expertise. Assistance may be found through laryngologists who treat large numbers of singers or educational programs such as the Voice Foundation's annual Symposium on Care of the Professional Voice. In general, therapy should be directed toward relaxation techniques, breath control, and abdominal support.

Speech-language pathology may be helpful, even when a singer has no obvious problem in his or her speaking voice but has significant technical problems singing. Once a person has been singing for several years, it is often very difficult for a singing teacher to convince him or her to correct certain technical errors. Singers are much less protective of their speaking voices. Therefore, a speech-language pathologist may be able rapidly to teach proper support, relaxation, and voice placement in speaking. Once mastered, these techniques can be carried over fairly easily into singing through cooperation between the speech-language pathologist and voice teacher. This "back door" approach has proven extremely useful in the author's experience. For the actor, it is often helpful to coordinate speech-language pathology sessions with acting lessons, especially with the training of the speaking voice provided by the actor's voice teacher or coach. Information provided by the speech-language pathologist, acting teacher, and singing teacher should be symbiotic and should not conflict. If there are major discrepancies, bad training from one of the team members should be suspected, and changes should be made.

Singing Teachers

In selected cases, singing lessons may also be extremely helpful for nonsingers with voice problems. The techniques used to develop abdominothoracic strength, breath control, laryngeal and neck muscle strength, and relaxation are very similar to those used in speech therapy. Singing lessons often expedite therapy and appear to improve the result in some patients.

Laryngologists who frequently care for singers often are asked to recommend a voice teacher. This may put the laryngologist in an uncomfortable position, particularly if the singer is already studying with someone in the community. Most physicians do not have sufficient expertise to criticize a voice teacher, and we must be extremely cautious about recommending that a singer change teachers. However, there is no certifying agency that standardizes or assures the quality of a singing teacher. Although one may be slightly more confident of a teacher associated with a major conservatory or music school or one who is a member of the National Association of Teachers of Singing, neither of these credentials assures excellence, and many expert teachers hold neither position. However, with experience, a laryngologist ordinarily develops valid impressions.

The physician should record the name of the voice teacher of each of his or her patients and should observe whether the same kinds of voice abuse problems occur with disproportionate frequency in the pupils of any given teacher. He or she should also observe whose pupils usually have few technical problems and are seen only for organic disease such as colds. Technical problems can cause organic pathology such as nodules. So, any teacher who has a high incidence of nodules among his or her students should be viewed with careful concern. The physician should be particularly wary of teachers who are reluctant to allow their students to consult a doctor. The best voice teachers usually have a very low threshold for referral to a laryngologist if they hear anything disturbing in a student's voice. It is proper for the laryngologist to write a letter to the voice teacher (with the patient's permission) describing the findings and recommendations as he or she would to a physician, speech-language pathologist, or any other referring professional. A laryngologist seriously interested in caring for singers should take the trouble to talk with and meet local singing teachers. Taking a lesson or two with each teacher provides enormous insight, as well. Taking voice lessons regularly is even more helpful. In practice, the laryngologist will usually identify a few teachers in whom he or she has particular confidence, especially for patients with voice disorders. He or she should not hesitate to refer singers to these colleagues, especially those singers who are not already in training.

Pop singers may be particularly resistant to the suggestion of voice lessons. Yet, they are in great need of training. It should be pointed out that a good voice teacher can teach a pop singer how to protect and expand his or her voice without changing its quality or making it sound "trained" or "operatic." The author finds it helpful to point out that singing, like other athletic activities, requires exercise, warm-up, and coaching for anyone planning to enter the "big league" and stay there. Just as no major league baseball pitcher would go without a pitching coach and warm-up time in the bullpen, no singer should try to build a career without a singing teacher and appropriate strength and agility exercises. This approach has proved palatable and effective.

Physicians should also be aware of the difference between a voice teacher and a voice coach. A voice teacher trains a singer in singing technique and is essential. A voice coach is responsible for teaching songs, language, diction, style, operatic roles, and so on, but is not responsible for exercises and basic technical development of the voice. More specific details of evaluation and treatment are included in chapters 7, 9, and 10.

Voice Trainers

Drama voice trainers and coaches are the newest professionals on the voice care team. Ordinarily, they work in theaters, being responsible for training, polishing, and preserving the voices of actors. Like singing teachers, they may work with naive students, or world-renowned thespians. Also like singing teachers, they have no formal licensing or certification body.

However, they do have a national organization called the Voice and Speech Trainers Association (VASTA). Membership in this organization is at least encouraging evidence of serious study and exposure, although it certainly does not assure expertise. In recent years, a few distinguished voice coaches such as Bonnie Raphael, Lucille Rubin, and Sharon Freed have acquired experience working with patients with vocal fold injury, referred to them by laryngologists such as Dr. Wilbur James Gould and myself. To the best of our knowledge, the addition of Sharon Freed to our team in 1994 marked the first time a voice trainer was employed in a medical office for the purpose of collaborating with speech-language pathologists and singing voice specialists in the rehabilitation of injured voices. Our care experience has left us convinced that this is an extremely valuable addition to the voice care team, and is long overdue. Unfortunately, as with singing teachers, obtaining training in pathologic voice care is extremely difficult for voice trainers, as discussed in a subsequent chapter. We are currently working on solutions to this problem.

Voice Maintenance

Prevention of vocal dysfunction should be the goal of all professionals involved in the care of vocalists. Good vocal health habits should be encouraged in childhood. Screaming, particularly outdoors during athletic events, should be discouraged. Promising young singers who join choirs should be educated to compensate for the Lombard effect. The youngster interested in singing or acting should receive enough training to avoid voice abuse and should receive enthusiastic support for singing works suitable for his or her age and voice. Singing advanced pieces and playing Metropolitan Opera star should be actively discouraged. Training should be continued during or after puberty, and the voice should be allowed to develop naturally without pressure to perform operatic roles prematurely. Excellent regular training and practice are essential, and avoidance of irritants, particularly smoke, should be stressed early. Educating the singer with regard to hormonal and anatomic alterations that may influence the voice allows him or her to recognize and analyze vocal dysfunction and to compensate for it intelligently when it occurs. Cooperation among the laryngologist, speech-language pathologist, acting teacher, and singing teacher provides an optimal environment for cultivation and protection of the vocal artist.

3

Speech-Language Pathology and the Professional Voice User: An Overview

Carol N. Wilder

The practice of speech-language pathology means the application of principles, methods, and procedures for measurement, testing, identification, prediction, counseling, or instruction related to development and disorders of speech, voice, and language. It may be used for identifying, preventing, managing, habilitating or rehabilitating, ameliorating, or modifying such disorders in individuals or groups of individuals.[1] Although speech-language pathologists work with individuals with voice disorders, we do not diagnose or treat laryngeal disease or other physiological disorders, as does the laryngologist. Rather, speech-language pathologists are concerned with understanding, analyzing, and modifying vocal function, that is, with changing vocal behaviors. If the voice is within normal limits perceptually, and if it is being produced in a reasonably efficient, nonabusive manner, the speech-language pathologist does not seek to provide the special training that will develop the range, power, control, stamina, and esthetic quality of voice that are required for artistic expression, as does the singing or acting teacher. We are concerned primarily with the voice that presents a current problem or signs of a potential problem in one or more physical, perceptual, or behavioral dimensions. What happens when such a problem occurs in a professional voice user?

For the purposes of this chapter, the term professional voice user will be arbitrarily limited to individuals who use the voice extensively for some form of artistic expression, in other words, to performers. The definition includes professional singers and actors (eg, those who earn their living by performing), those seeking to become professional singers or actors, and those for whom skilled amateur performance is a major, personally important activity. Excluded for the purposes of this chapter are those individuals who indeed rely heavily on their speaking voices in their professional activities, but who do not use their voices for artistic purposes (eg, the classroom teacher, the trial lawyer, the clergyman, etc).

Having said what speech-language pathologists do *not* do, let me give the briefest possible summary of what we *do* do. First, we analyze, systematically and sensitively, the presenting vocal behaviors, both perceptually and with such objective measures as are clinically appropriate. Second, we analyze vocational, educational, and psychosocial factors that may interact with vocal behaviors to precipitate, maintain, or exacerbate the voice problem. Finally, we design and implement an individualized program for modifying vocal behaviors and, insofar as is possible, any contributing factors. I stress the terms systematically and sensitively, because both need to be equally emphasized when we work with voice disorders. This is both a science and an art.

With this summary in mind, let us consider two questions: (1) When compared with voice disorders in a nonperformer, will the speech-language pathologist find that there is anything significantly different about evaluating and remediating voice problems in the performer? (2) Is any special knowledge needed in order to do so? The answer to both these questions is affirmative, because of the complexity of vocational, environmental, and psychosocial factors that are unique to this population. These factors are so complex and interactive and beyond the scope of any single chapter, or even book. Nevertheless, I should like to highlight just a few of them that can be expected to have an impact on the activities of the speech-language pathologist.

The obvious factor that is special to this population is the way the voice is used. On the one hand, the range of vocal activities extends beyond the functional parameters we are used to dealing with in the nonprofessional voice patient, with respect to such things as pitch range, loudness extreme, control, and endurance. On the other hand, voice problems in the professional may be signaled by decrements in quality, sensation, or control, which are much more subtle than those we are used to working with. We cannot just sit back and be dazzled by the vocal displays in the cadenza or soliloquy, or be puzzled by the performer's intense concern about what might seem (in the nonprofessional) like a clinically insignificant change in voice control. It is our task to attempt to understand the physical processes that underlie both and to determine whether they relate to the presenting disorder. We must develop reasonable hypotheses about what is going on with respect to chest wall and laryngeal and supralaryngeal behaviors as they relate to lung volumes, pressure differentials, and the like, keeping firmly in mind the relationship of these hypotheses to our clinical purposes. Having made the hypotheses, we must test them. For these reasons, speech-language pathologists who want to work with the voice problems of the performer will find it useful to expand their knowledge of voice and speech science beyond the level that suffices for work with the nonperformer and to make a determined effort to keep abreast of the rapidly accumulating research on voice production.

To achieve a better understanding of the demands on the vocal mechanism of the performer, it is also useful to know something about music, if you are working with singers, or about the theater, if you are working with actors. One should develop an appreciation of the styles and vocal characteristics called for by different schools of performance or vocal training, or by specific composers and dramatists, because they may each call for very different kinds of vocal behaviors. Not only does this help us better understand the physical demands that may have contributed to the disorder, but it also helps us appreciate what kinds of vocal activities comprise the patient's hoped-for goals of therapy, to determine stepwise approximations toward the goals, and to better estimate whether these hoped-for goals are realistic.

The goals of therapy are another feature that distinguishes our work with the performer from our work with the nonperformer. With performers, there are no degrees of freedom with respect to the desired outcome, whereas, with our other voice patients, there is much more latitude in the range of vocal behaviors that constitute an acceptable outcome.

For better understanding of and more effective communication with both the patient and the voice teacher or coach (with whom we want to cooperate closely), speech-language pathologists should also try to become familiar with some of the technical rudiments of these disciplines and with their terms of imagery and their technical vocabulary. For example, if a singer mentions problems with *tessitura* or *leggiero* passages, or with vibrato, it is helpful if the speech-language pathologist can appreciate the physical implications of these terms, which are not a part of our general professional lexicon. If an actor complains about being upstaged, the speech-language pathologist should be aware that the term is not a cliché, but that it describes a specific physical situation that could be contributing to vocal stress.

Speech-language pathologists are always concerned about environmental contributors to voice disorders. However, there are a number of special environmental factors in the performer's world with which many speech-language pathologists (or any other nonperformers, for that matter) may be unfamiliar. To get a better appreciation about conditions that may affect performers' vocal behaviors, it is a good idea for the speech-language pathologist to visit a variety of performance environments (not just theaters and concert halls, but studios, rehearsal halls, and practice rooms) to experience first-hand the dust, fumes, temperature differentials, and ambient noise levels, as well as the general "feel" of the acoustic environment. The conditions are often far from ideal from the standpoint of what is good for the voice. See if you can arrange to visit when you can have the place to yourself as well. Go ahead and sing a song or recite a speech; the insights you get from those few moments may be better than those you get from hours of watching someone else do it.

When trying to delineate all the factors that may contribute to the voice problem, such things as stage direction, set design, and costume design should also be considered. Even an otherwise excellent vocal technique may be put under stress when the performer is in a situation that is physically awkward, uncomfortable, or even precarious. This is not at all uncommon. When some directors or designers are in hot pursuit of a particular artistic vision, concern about vocal stress is not exactly at the top of their priority list. A few years ago, I saw a Royal Shakespeare Company production in which a leading actor was required to deliver a long speech while hanging by his knees, upside down, from the top of a tall ladder. Fortunately, both his knees and his aplomb were equal to the task; but, not surprisingly, one heard signs of vocal tension that were never apparent when he was right-side up. In a memory that remains vivid after many years, I recall the awkwardness and discomfort I felt singing while wearing a costume that included a heavy pointed hat 3 feet long. It was the designer's idea of a medieval effect. I remember complaining that I had to tighten all the muscles of my neck in order to balance the hat to keep it from falling off. Looking back on it from my present perspective as a speech-language pathologist, it seems reasonable to assume that this feeling of tension reflected a degree of strap muscle tension that might well have contributed to vocal stress.

The voice may also be stressed if the performer gets so "carried away" by the emotional sweep of the performance that vocal techniques go by the boards, as it were. Muscles tighten; postures change subtly. These behaviors may not occur in any other vocal situation, making it useful for the speech-language pathologist to observe the patient in an actual performance situation whenever possible.

The essential point is that the performance environment is liberally endowed with "vocal ill-health potential." Some potential stressors are less obvious than others; some the performer may not be aware of and hence may not volunteer when you are taking a case history. If the speech-language pathologist is to understand what areas need to be explored as factors potentially contributing to the voice disorder, he or she must become familiar with the full range of vocal stressors that may be found in the performance environment.

Now, back to that pointed hat. It might be asked why I simply did not refuse to wear it. It is in the answer to that question that the speech-language pathologist begins to encounter the unique psychosocial pressures experienced by vocal professionals, pressures that, indeed, make working with professionals different from working with other voice patients, pressures that may contribute to the development and maintenance of a voice disorder, pressures that can negatively influence the course of therapy if they are not taken into account by the speech-language pathologist.

A major and continuing source of pressure is the intense competition in the performing environment, the extent of which is sometimes difficult to appreciate unless you have experienced it. I did not refuse to wear the hat, because I was just beginning to develop as a performer and I did not want to make waves. I knew full well that many competent replacements were waiting in the wings, any one of whom would have been only too happy to have a chance to sing the role—hat and all. Star level performers may be able to insist on certain performance conditions, but the great majority of performers cannot afford this luxury. Moreover, there is ample evidence in revealing remarks, publicized feuds, and sensitivity over prerogatives that even superstars are not immune to the pressures of competition. Having got to the top, there is pressure to stay there. The reality of this pressure

must be acknowledged by the speech-language pathologist. There are times when a performer simply cannot follow your suggestions; cannot cancel a performance, audition, or competition; or cannot follow a therapeutic regimen that would change performance frequency, conditions, or style. It is up to us to understand and to adapt our therapeutic programs to this reality.

Another source of pressure is that the professional voice user is constantly on the line, with his or her performance judged not only by the audience, but by critics, conductors, managers, directors, producers, agents, teachers, and coaches. Most of us are not subject to such constant external scrutiny of our endeavors. The professional voice user lives with the realization that, if he or she makes even a minor goof during a performance, it will very likely be noticed, perhaps even pounced on. As if this were not a sufficient source of pressure, the standards of judgment to which the voice professional is held are frequently subjective, variable, and situation-bound. For example, two critics turn in such disparate reviews that you wonder if they went to the same concert, or contest judges disagree on a winner. After an audition, the performer may never find out *why* he or she did not get the contract or the part. Yet all these subjective, variable, and situation-bound judgments play major roles in determining the performer's career opportunities. No wonder there is performance anxiety; no wonder there are displays of insecurity or bravado. Clearly, this constellation of psychosocial pressures is also shared by instrumental musicians. However, the effect on vocal professionals may be even more profound because, for them, the instrument itself, the vocal mechanism, is known to be sensitive not only to stress-related muscle tension, but also to stress-related responses to the autonomic nervous system.

If there are all these pressures, if the rules of the game are so difficult, why is there so much competition? Why are so many people out there doing everything they can to become professional users of the voice? What possesses them? I am not sure there is any better answer to these questions than to say that they do, in fact, seem to be possessed (in some cases almost obsessed) by some sort of drive toward artistic vocal expression; and that brings me to the final area I would like to highlight that distinguishes our practice with this population.

If one is possessed by a drive toward artistic vocal expression, how devastating it is to develop any sort of a problem in the vocal mechanism, which is the foundation of one's endeavors? How frustrating it is if the problem develops at a pivotal or critical point in career development. How threatening for the established performer whose financial well-being rests on the condition of his or her vocal mechanism. As a consequence, speech-language pathologists who regularly work with professional voice users find that the response to the voice disorder is usually different from what we find with other types of voice patients—different not only in degree, but in kind. This response is a major consideration that must be factored into the management program. An experienced speech-language pathologist who has only relatively recently begun to work with the professional voice said to me that he had not entirely anticipated the intensity of the emotional reactions he has encountered with his professional voice patients. He described how one young woman's responses had ranged from shock at learning that she had a mass lesion of the vocal folds, to hope that it might be resolved through therapy, to tearful despair when she learned that, although the lesion was much smaller, it had not completely disappeared. This speech-language pathologist said that he had found the counseling of professional voice users to be a very heavy issue. Indeed, the ongoing education and counseling that are a part of our program with any voice patient must be handled with special thoroughness and exquisite sensitivity in the professional voice user.

These general highlights are intended for speech-language pathologists who have not yet had much clinical contact with professional voice users. Details of practice are discussed in chapter 68. An active effort to become further acquainted with special vocational, environmental, and psychosocial factors performers experience will help you to incorporate them—systematically and sensitively—into your evaluation and therapeutic procedures. Working with professional voice users is stimulating and enjoyable. Moreover, speech-language pathologists are not alone in their need to explore areas that were not included in their professional training curriculum. Currently, no single discipline adequately addresses the totality of skills needed in the care of the professional voice in its training program. Therefore, all of us with a special interest in this area can profit from learning from each other in a spirit that maximizes cooperative efforts and optimizes patient care.

Reference

1. California Speech Pathologists and Audiologists Licensure Act, Chapter 5.3, Division 2 of the Business and Professions Code, as cited in Flower R. *Delivery of Speech-Language Pathology and Audiology Services.* Baltimore, Md: Williams & Wilkins; 1984:6.

4

Voice Therapy

*Reinhardt J. Heuer, Rhonda K. Rulnick,
Michelle Horman, Kathe S. Perez, Kate A. Emerich,
and Robert Thayer Sataloff*

Professional voice users who need voice therapy require special diagnostic and intervention strategies. Each of these individuals has a vested interest in preserving and protecting the voice. They differ from the general voice population because of the unusual demands placed on their voices, especially singers, teachers, and actors. These demands are greater in both quantity and quality. In addition, professional voice users differ in many instances by requesting therapy for voices that might generally be regarded as "normal." However, since they may be required to perform in the supernormal range of voice production, speech-language pathologists must learn to recognize and help restore optimal, not merely normal, voice.

The focus of this chapter is on the unique requirements of the behavioral treatment of professional speakers whose careers have been disrupted by voice rest, surgery, or diminished vocal power associated with a disordered or diseased larynx. The following eight skills are required of speech-language pathologists when dealing with voice-disordered professional speakers. They are in no particular order, but all are equally important in the success of treating these special patients.

1. The clinician needs to be supersensitive to superspeaking. The goal in treating professional speakers is not just adequate speech and voice but excellent speech and voice. This patient may complain of problems that may seem insignificant to a clinician who does not have this supersensitivity, and that clinician may lose the respect and cooperation of the patient for minimizing such subtleties. Correction of minor technical faults is required to enable a pa-

tient who has already experienced voice difficulties to compete again in the professional arena.

2. The clinician needs to be skilled in counseling and in critiquing, in a positive manner, professional speakers who may perceive their current abilities as excellent. Professional speakers who have suffered vocal injury may be traumatized psychologically as well as physically. Most professional speakers believe they are proficient voice users. It may be difficult for them to admit that they have technical problems. Tactful handling, including gentle objective proof of the vocal faults related to the voice disorder, is necessary if the clinician wishes to gain the patient's confidence and cooperation. The patient may be unable to modify his or her vocal behavior easily, until emotional reactions to the voice disorder and its effects on the professional speaker's career have been discussed and resolved. The clinician should be ready to make appropriate referrals for psychological assessment or counseling, if warranted.

3. The clinician needs to concentrate on enhancing the professional speaker's vocal repertoire rather than teaching new skills. Rarely are appropriate behaviors missing from the professional speaker's repertoire; rather, faulty techniques have become preferred, either because of inappropriate training or because of the professional speaker's frantic struggle to *sound normal* in the presence of laryngeal change. Such an approach saves the patient from guilt and embarrassment about his or her skills and abilities. It also provides the patient with confidence that he or she still retains the ability to perform.

4. The clinician needs to focus on rebalancing the three-part system (respiration/phonation/reso-

nance) rather than isolated skill drills. The clinician needs to remember that, in treating voice-disordered individuals, changes in one function will produce subtle, or not so subtle, changes in the rest of the system. The patient needs to learn to hear and feel the results of each modification in all aspects of the speaking mechanism. We believe in a holistic approach to the treatment of voice disorders.

5. The clinician needs to explicitly describe the need, purpose, and function of each therapeutic activity. The complaint we hear most from professional speakers who have had previous therapy is that they did what was asked of them, but had no idea why they were doing it. Obviously, on occasion, the patient's memory may be faulty, but we need to continually remember that, although the rationales for our therapeutic tasks are obvious to us, they may not be so obvious to our patients. Most professional voice users are eager to broaden their understanding of vocal technique and are more motivated to refine skills when their impact on overall voice production is clear.

6. The clinician needs to emphasize carryover into everyday speech and professional activities rather than to assign practice periods only. Especially singers, but also trained speakers, tend to believe that dutifully practicing exercises will automatically make their voices better. They need to be reminded that the exercises are only practice for what they should be doing all the time. Patients will often ask, "I practiced the exercises regularly, why isn't my voice better?" unless they have been indoctrinated into the philosophy that the exercises are a skill builder and a reminder of what the professional speaker should be attempting to do whenever speaking.

7. The clinician needs to be prepared for rapid changes and have appropriate materials ready and available. Professional speakers are skilled at modifying vocal behaviors. Once a concept is grasped and a skill developed, that behavior must be generalized immediately into usage. A patient's progress should not be impeded because the clinician is not prepared to shift to a new and more difficult level. Voice therapy with professional speakers should not take a long time. If it does, the therapy goals may be inappropriate or the patient may not resolve his or her anxiety about the vocal disorder or speaking abilities.

8. The clinician may need to help the patient establish a good voice in spite of, or in the presence of, vocal pathology if approved by the otolaryngologist. The psychological, monetary, or career needs of a professional voice-disordered person may require the development of safe voice/speech skills prior to the completion of medical/surgical treatment. Often, by focusing on compensation by the respiratory and resonatory systems and reducing the patient's effortful use of the larynx, adequate, nondamaging voice can be achieved to allow the professional to continue performing during the treatment and hearing process.

In this chapter, we will often refer to the singer. The singer's need for flawless vocal technique is paramount, and singers are particularly capable of detailed vocal self-analysis and critical assessment of therapy. The voice mechanism of the professional speaker needs the same specialized care and training as the voice of the singer. Our approach to evaluating and treating singers is applicable to all professional voice users.

Classically trained singers are aware of the deleterious consequences of poor singing technique on the delicate tissues of the vocal folds. Even though they are usually conscientious in caring for their voices during singing, they often give little thought to how they use the same anatomy in speech, even though they may spend more time speaking than singing. Appropriate speaking technique is just as important for singers as for other professional voice users. They have much to gain from voice therapy. The elimination of vocal abuse during speaking can have a dramatic and positive effect on the singing voice. The process of acquiring good speaking technique often facilitates better singing, as well.

Many voice professionals, in particular teachers, have never received formal speech training. Hence, it is not surprising that vocal dysfunction occurs. This chapter outlines our approach to preventing voice problems and to treating injured voices. The approach is primarily behavioral. Voice problems are not solely mechanical in nature. Voices are produced by human beings. Therefore, a myriad of personal factors, stresses, and other mitigating circumstances can drastically affect a patient's voice, the therapy program devised, and the person's ability to benefit from therapeutic intervention. When the need arises, we solicit the assistance of other professionals (team members) so that each patient may be treated holistically.

We address the unique considerations of the voice professional as a team. The primary interdisciplinary team consists of:

- the *laryngologist*, whose primary responsibility is diagnosing and restoring the structure of the larynx through medical/surgical means

- the *speech-language pathologist*, whose responsibility is evaluating and treating specific abusive/misusive behaviors of the speaking voice
- the *singing-voice specialist/vocal teacher*, whose province is singing technique and voice production during singing
- the *stress manager/speaking coach* whose expertise lies in overall body response to the speaking act.
- the *acting-voice specialist* who works with high performance, projected speech, and related communication skills

Additional adjunct team members include:

- *voice researcher* or voice scientist
- *singing coach* (involved primarily with repertoire and style)
- *psychologist, hypnotherapist,* and *physicians* in different specialties (especially pulmonology, allergy, and neurology).

It is important for all team members to understand the principles and approach employed in voice therapy, and for the voice therapist to understand the expertise of each of the other members of the team.

Ideally the members of the primary team should be housed in the same facility to provide for direct and immediate interaction for the benefit of the professional voice user.

Evaluation

When working with singers and other voice professionals, our expectations of *normal* must be heightened, and stricter criteria must be used to assess these patients. State-of-the-art equipment and advanced techniques in voice analysis are incorporated routinely into the voice evaluation and are described in *Clinical Assessment of Voice*.[1] This provides extremely valuable baseline information and documentation that help to quantify and qualify the patient's voice problem. These instruments are important, but clearly our best clinical tools remain our own eyes and ears. With a few exceptions, this is especially true in recognizing degrees of supernormal function. Most of the commonly used instrumentation is better at distinguishing *abnormal* from *normal* than at identifying differences between "excellent" and "great" voices. The voice therapist may acquire the necessary skills to make these distinctions by learning to use adjunct instrumentation; by studying singing, acting, and public speaking; by observing as many singing and acting teachers as possible so as to refine their listening skills; and through experience working with a team, exchanging judgments after listening to the singing and speaking voice.

The voice evaluation is divided into five parts: case history, objective evaluation, subjective evaluation, trial therapy, and impressions/recommendations. This chapter includes a brief overview of our evaluation procedures.

Case History

A careful case history involves a description of the circumstances leading to the development and maintenance of the present vocal problem. In a medical setting, where the patient is seen by all team members during the initial visit, the laryngologist and speech language pathologist cooperate in gathering the background information. The information required is discussed in *Clinical Assessment of Voice*.[2] Additional history obtained by the speech-language pathologist explores how vocal abuses and vocal misuse affect the patient's voice on a daily basis. The focus is on the nature of the disorder, activities in daily professional or social life that may cause or aggravate vocal problems, voice patterns of other family members that may reinforce undesirable vocal behavior, daily vocal usage patterns, and details of previous voice therapy. For patients who have had previous voice therapy, asking the patient to demonstrate techniques and exercises used may provide valuable insight that can affect the current therapy plan. A complete inventory is made of vocal abuse factors that may have contributed to the present voice problems, with special attention paid to smoking, passive smoking, caffeine consumption, alcohol consumption, poor rest and sleep patterns, environmental factors (dryness, chemicals), excessive talking, yelling, loud talking, throat clearing, coughing, whispering, poor hydration, and stress and tension.

Singers are asked additional questions regarding the type of music they sing (rock, popular, classical, show/night club, gospel, jazz/blues), the extent of their training, their present singing difficulties, and their professional career goals. This case history information is obtained in cooperation with the singing specialist. All singers also complete a written questionnaire (Appendix Ia) and teachers are requested to complete a vocal abuse checklist (Appendix II). In addition to inquiries regarding duration of training, the patient's current goals with his or her singing teacher are explored in detail.

Although this section on history is covered only briefly in this chapter (because relevant areas of inquiry are discussed elsewhere in this book), it should be emphasized that a thorough history is of paramount importance. The speech-language pathologist must do more than merely ask the usual questions and add special questions relevant to performers and their specialized settings. The voice therapist must also pay attention not merely to the content of the history, but also to the voice used by the patient in reporting it. In addition, the clinician should explore in greater detail any discrepancies between the history given to the otolaryngologist and that given to the speech-language pathologist. Occasionally, patients will reveal information to one team member that they are reluctant to reveal to another. Questions to which answers change from one team member to another are often closely related to the patient's underlying problem and deserve delicate but diligent scrutiny.

Objective Evaluation

Data collection and its subsequent analysis furnish a detailed objective description of the voice. An audio recording is obtained using a high-quality analog tape recorder or a DAT recorder. As much vocal analysis as possible is done on line or with digitized samples. The protocol for the objective voice tasks is provided in appendix IV, and details of the voice laboratory and therapeutic uses of laboratory equipment are discussed in *Clinical Assessment of Voice*.[1] Briefly, a sample of sustained spoken and sung vowels, conversational speaking, and reading is analyzed. The acoustic voicing parameters that are measured include: speaking fundamental frequency (for conversation and reading), multiple estimates of pitch and intensity, perturbation, harmonics/noise ratios, percent voicing (for a reading sample), and physiological and musical frequency range. Aerodynamic measures include maximum exhalation or phonation times for /a/, /i/, /u/, and /s/, and /z/, s/z ratio, mean flow rates, and inverse filtered estimates of minimal and AC glottal flow. Respiration is measured by pulmonary function testing. Pulmonary function testing of all voice patients has proven beneficial in identifying singing-related respiratory dysfunction (ie, exercise-induced asthma). Measures are compared to normative data and judgments regarding the patient's phonatory ability are made. Aerodynamic measures are particularly useful in determining how the patient is using respiratory/vocal control in producing vocalization. Further information about the clinical usefulness of instrumentation is discussed in *Clinical Assessment of Voice*.[1]

Subjective Evaluation

Respiration

Many vocal problems are the result of improper breathing technique. When evaluating respiration, the volume of air is important, but more important is the manner in which the patient takes in the air (inhalation), and how the air is used to produce the voice (exhalation).

Abdominal/diaphragmatic breath control and support are desirable and the most efficient manner of providing the power source for the voice. The patient's respiration is observed in conversational speech and in reading. The following observations are made:

1. The pattern of breath support:
   ☐ Abdominal/diaphragmatic
   ☐ Upper thoracic
   ☐ Clavicular
   ☐ Combined or Mixed (thoracic and abdominal)
2. Improper body posture or head/neck alignment that may affect respiration adversely
3. Phrasing—Are the phrases too long or too short? Are pauses taken at appropriate places during ongoing speech?
4. Audible inspiration, forced exhalation or, labored breathing

Phonation

Phonation refers to the production of sound at the level of the vocal folds. Judgments about the voice quality (hoarseness, breathiness), loudness (appropriate, too loud, too soft), and pitch are made during conversational speech and reading (Appendix III). The following characteristics are particularly important:

☐ Hoarseness	☐ Diplophonia
☐ Breathiness	☐ Phonation breaks
☐ Glottal fry	☐ Harsh glottal attacks

Harsh glottal attacks are counted during a standard reading passage and a percentage is calculated.

Measures of respiratory and phonatory efficiency are obtained using measurements of maximum exhalation or phonation for the following sounds:

$$/a/\underline{\quad} \quad /i/\underline{\quad} \quad /u/\underline{\quad} \quad /s/\underline{\quad} \quad /z/\underline{\quad}$$

An s/z ratio[3] is obtained, which provides a quick comparison of the patient's ability to control airflow for these two speech sounds (voiceless and voiced). Although an s/z ratio is not necessarily a reliable assessment of phonatory ability or an indicator of laryngeal pathology, it provides useful information about the patient's ability to control exhalation in the presence or absence of voicing. That is, it is an indicator of laryngeal efficiency.

General observations are made regarding the patient's habitual speaking pitch. It is important to note whether the patient speaks too high (falsetto) or too low (glottal fry). The concept of *optimal pitch* is controversial, as *optimal* may not exist. More accurately there is an *optimal* manner of laryngeal function that yields an appropriate pitch level. Generally, an inappropriate pitch level can be the effect of a mass lesion, which may lower the pitch, or be symptomatic of muscular tension, which may raise the pitch. However, muscular tension dysphonia may also be present in association with low pitch, especially in a patient who forces his or her voice down near the lower end of the physiological frequency range.

Resonance

Resonance refers to the concentration of specific acoustic frequencies or harmonics within the cavities of the vocal tract (oral cavity, oropharynx, nasopharynx, hypopharynx). Clinically, certain resonant patterns have been labeled as being associated with specific anatomic areas. The terminology is useful, even if not completely accurate. Excessive pharyngeal or "throaty" resonance is a common characteristic and can be associated with physical discomfort in speaking. Oral resonance is desirable and is affected by the size and shape of the oral cavity. Many patients exhibit mandibular restriction while speaking, which diminishes the effectiveness of the oral cavity as a resonator. The presence of hypernasal or hyponasal speech is carefully assessed to rule out velopharyngeal incompetence. Functional or regional resonance deviations can be assessed using selected reading passages.

Tongue retraction occurs when the anterior portion of the tongue is pulled back from the lower incisors. The result is tongue muscle tension and a change in vocal tract shape that affects the resonance of the voice. Tongue position is observed during sustained production of /ɑ/. Posterior tongue tension often cannot be directly observed without instruments during speech and may be present even if the anterior tongue is relaxed. Posterior tongue tension is often responsible for a pharyngeal resonance quality.

Articulation

A judgment is made regarding the patient's general ability to precisely produce the sounds of the English language. If English is not the patient's native language, comparisons are made between speech in English and the mother tongue if the person is actively communicating in English. The ability of the articulators (tongue, lips, teeth, jaw, and velum) to function in a smooth and coordinated manner is determined. Although articulation disorders are rare in this population, occasionally a lisp has been identified. Particular attention is paid to any "hyperfunctional" articulation or tension sites in the articulators themselves. While tongue tension is common, it is addressed as a resonance imbalance or compensatory behavior and not an articulation problem.

Prosody

The prosodic features of speech (rhythm, fluency, timing, rate, pauses, and intonation or inflection patterns) are assessed very generally. These features often subtly affect the voice. The patient who demonstrates excessive laryngeal and strap muscle tension will often demonstrate faulty flow and blending of words in connected speech. A voice/speech pattern that lacks the normal prosodic features may be perceived as monotonous, and reduced variability of pitch or volume may result in vocal fatigue. Further, a voice that lacks vocal variety may indicate that a patient is not gaining maximum flexibility from the voice, either physically or artistically.

Sites of Muscular Tension

Poor respiratory control and support can lead to muscle tension in specific muscle groups. While this tension is observed in association with poor breath control, it can be created for a variety of reasons. We observe these tension sites as we examine the levels of speech production, and have found a checklist helpful.

☐ Tongue	☐ Anterior or posterior neck
☐ Laryngeal rise or fall	☐ Shoulders
☐ Jaw or masseter muscle	☐ Upper chest wall

Oral/Facial

A screening of the oral/facial mechanism should be included to rule out any abnormalities in the structure, symmetry, strength, range of motion, or coordination that might impact on normal vocal function. This includes neurological problems.

Singing

The speech-language pathologist (unless specifically trained) is not qualified to evaluate the singer's technique in detail. However, observations are made that are extremely useful in determining the constancy of technique from one modality (singing) to another (speech). A checklist for observing the singer's technical misuses includes:

- ☐ Sites of tension: face, neck, tongue, jaw, shoulders, forehead
- ☐ Poor breath support

- ☐ Tongue retraction
- ☐ Hoarseness following singing

- ☐ Tone focus
- ☐ Difficulties through the passagio

- ☐ Vocal placement
- ☐ Loss of upper/lower range

Trial Therapy

Various facilitating techniques are introduced on a trial basis during the evaluation. This gives the examiner an opportunity to observe how these changes affect vocal quality and whether the patient can feel and hear differences in vocal production. Further, it enables the examiner to make inferences about the patient's learning ability and prognosis for remediation through therapy.

Impression and Recommendations

The voice evaluation, in addition to establishing baseline measures, affords the speech-language pathologist the opportunity to observe the patient and to formulate an impression of the factors that may have contributed to the voice problem. Techniques to facilitate improved vocal production were introduced during the *trial therapy* portion of the evaluation. The speech-language pathologist assesses which modifications resulted in an immediate change in vocal quality or ease of production, and a starting point for therapy is established.

The interpretation of what was observed is discussed with the patient. Providing a thorough explanation of which factors have been most contributory to the voice problem is essential. The goals of therapy are enumerated along with the procedures and their rationales. There is no clear delineation between where evaluation ends and therapy begins. Evaluation occurs throughout the therapy process as the speech-language pathologist continually monitors the efficacy of treatment.

At the conclusion of the evaluation, recommendations are made regarding whether voice therapy is indicated. Goals are defined. Often other referrals are made, such as specialized singing instruction. Occasionally other testing is needed (ie, articulation or mo-

tor speech). The recommendations, including the anticipated length of time (in weeks or months), approximate number of sessions, and how often the sessions are to be scheduled (weekly, biweekly, monthly) are reviewed. The patient is informed of the need for home practice and active participation, so that the goals can be met.

Approaches to Therapy: An Overview

Various approaches to voice therapy are in use. Most of them involve techniques to optimize the efficiency of respiration, and economy of muscle activity. There is considerable overlap among voice therapy techniques; and, in our opinion, speech-language pathologists should combine aspects of various regimens in an individualized program, designed for each patient. Although most of the this chapter is devoted to describing the approaches we have found helpful in a majority of professional voice users, it is helpful to be familiar with many of the well-recognized approaches to voice intervention.

Confidential Voice Therapy

Confidential voice therapy involves use of a breathy, soft, gentle technique of speech. It should not be a whisper, but rather approximate the voice used when communicating confidential information to an individual in a room with other potential listeners. This technique helps prevent forceful vocal fold contact. It may be useful following cessation of post-operative voice rest, in the presence of serious vocal fold injury, or in patients with severe muscle tension dysphonia who do not respond promptly to other relaxation techniques and must continue communicating during the early therapy period. Patients must be trained well and supervised so that confidential voice does not deteriorate into a forced whisper. Confidential voice is rarely used for more than a few weeks, after which other techniques (eg, resonant voice therapy) may be utilized for long-term voice modification.

Resonant Voice Therapy

Resonant voice therapy is a technique or construct used by speech-language pathologists. Resonant voice involves gentle vocal fold contact (flow phonation), which differs from the forceful vocal fold approximation typical of muscle tension dysphonia (pressed phonation). Resonant voice therapy strives for a "forward focus" that makes the voice resonate within the facial bones and allows the patient to feel phonatory vibrations in his or her lips, tongue, and nasal bridge. Resonant voice therapy is a mainstay of vocal rehabilitation in professional voice users and others and is widely used for patients with muscle tension dysphonia and related structural lesions such as nodules.

Optimal Pitch

Optimal pitch therapy is a generally discredited technique that focuses on modifying the patient's habitual pitch. Although it is true that many patients with muscle tension dysphonia speak with an habitual pitch that is excessively low, an increase in pitch should be achieved through techniques that eliminate hyperfunction through muscle relaxation and proper breath support rather than directly. Therapeutic approaches that utilize pitch elevation as a primary technique do not educate patients consistently in the technical modifications necessary to achieve healthy phonation.

The Accent Method

In the accent method, therapists teach patients to use accented and rhythmic alterations in pronunciation and in related body movements. In theory, synchronizing voice production with a recognizable rhythm produced in another part of the body should help relax laryngeal muscles. The accent method may be helpful in modifying the timing and rhythm of breathing and inflection as therapy progresses. Progressively longer phrases are used, and external stimuli (body movements, percussion instruments) are eliminated. The accent method is an accepted approach to improve breathing technique and vocal clarity. It is used in Europe much more extensively than it is in the United States, although therapists in the US more commonly incorporate some accent methodology within a broader therapy regimen.

The Lee Silverman Technique

Dysarthria is a common manifestation of Parkinson's disease that increases in frequency and intensity with the progress of the disease. Typically, the voices of these patients include reduced intensity, monoloudness, monopitch, and short rushes of articulation that affect intelligibility and precision. Incomplete glottal closure, vocal fold bowing, and a reduction in respiratory support are commonly present and cause abnormal characteristics.

Traditional voice therapy for patients with Parkinson's disease has been provided for many years with variable success. Therapy has focused on a general treatment hierarchy of the subsystems of speech, respiration, phonation articulation, and resonation. In the last few decades, several researchers have reported therapeutic success by focusing on phonatory features alone.[4,5] Embellishing on the phonatory aspect of therapy, Ramig and her colleagues developed and documented the efficacy of very specific therapy protocol called the Lee Silverman Voice Treatment Program (LSVT).[6-8] This program seeks to modify the respiratory laryngeal and resonance subsystems of speech by targeting phonatory "effort." Ample evidence indicates that patients can improve their speech and voice characteristics, or maintain them as the disease progresses, by being stimulated to increase their phonatory effort. LSVT programs are based on an intensive regime of 4 individual sessions per week for 1 month during which loudness, maximum phonatory effort, high therapeutic effort, and voice awareness are targeted. Patients are encouraged in practice to go "longer and louder" and "higher and lower." The methods used include maximum duration sustained loud phonation, maximum frequency range (sustained highest and lowest pitches), posture, and maximal loudness. The simplicity of the program allows for home practice and successful carryover. Patients are encouraged to "think loud" and "think shout." It should be noted that this technique was designed for patients with a hypofunctional voice disorder. Even in these patients, it should be used only by specially trained voice therapists and with careful patient supervision. The therapist must be careful to avoid voice abuse while demonstrating the LSVT exercises. LSVT should be used rarely, if ever, in patients with normal neurological function or hyperfunctional voice disorders (ie, muscle tension dysphonia). If used in inappropriate patients or by a therapist with insufficient training, the technique may be harmful.

Circumlaryngeal Massage

In circumlaryngeal massage, therapists try to relax laryngeal and neck muscles and decrease odynophonia (pain while speaking) by teaching patients to massage the muscles of their neck. The therapist trains patients in the appropriate level, direction, and intensity of massage. Massage usually begins in the region of the hyoid bone and involves strap muscles. The technique may be useful in some patients with substantial tension in the neck and upper body and those who complain of pain or neck tenderness associated with vocal symptoms. It may also be helpful in patients with muscle tension dysphonia who have particularly rigid posture. Issues of posture and laryngeal manipulation are discussed in greater detail in chapters 13 and 14.

The Alexander Technique

The Alexander technique is a method of instruction developed by F. Matthias Alexander and designed to promote ease and freedom of movement, balance, support, flexibility, and coordination.[9,10] Teachers of the Alexander technique seek to help their students find greater functionality in all of their physical pursuits through the establishment of an efficient and dynamic alignment of the head, neck, and torso. Most voice therapists and professional voice users are aware that misalignment of the head and neck can result in increased tension in the muscles that stabilize the larynx and that vocal injury results often in maladaptive compensations in vocal technique, posture, and support. Although not defined as a therapeutic technique by its practitioners, the Alexander technique can be helpful in eliminating harmful habits that may develop in response to vocal injury. It also may benefit healthy voice users through the development of increased kinesthetic awareness and the elimination of tensions that can inhibit resonance, agility, and respiration.

Feldenkrais Technique

The Feldenkrais method was developed by Moshe Feldenkrais, who lived from 1904 until 1984.[11-14] The method was developed not only for performing artists and athletes, but also to assist patients with neurological and psychological disorders, chronic pain, and restricted movement. The Feldenkrais method combines martial arts (Dr. Feldenkrais was a Judo instructor and wrote books on Judo), psychology, biomechanics, and principles derived from motor development. Through movement, the technique strives to improve not only posture, movement, flexibility, and coordination, but also self-image. The Feldenkrais method uses movement and sensory differentiation to disrupt restrictive or undesirable habitual movement and behavior patterns and to access new patterns not only of movement, but also of thinking and feeling. It utilizes two approaches, awareness through movement (ATM) and functional integration (FI). Awareness through movement uses complex movement sequences delivered through verbally directed, gentle exercises. Lessons focus on virtually every joint and muscle group in the body and attempt to access sensory, motor, and psychological functions. Functional integration utilizes manipulation and passive movement to affect change and develop new body usage patterns. FI is applied particularly for patients with neurologic problems and substantial musculoskeletal dysfunction. The Feldenkrais method is somewhat more psychologically based than the Alexander method. Feldenkrais training may be helpful for selected singers and actors, particularly those who have had injuries, especially when aspects of Feldenkrais techniques are incorporated into a broader training and therapeutic approach.

Inhalational Phonation

Selected patients with severe dysphonia, particularly patients with adductor spasmodic dysphonia, may be able to speak fluently on inhalation, even though they cannot eliminate spasmodic activity when phonating during exhalation. In some cases, when patients have acquired the ability to speak on inhalation, they can carry over fluent speech into exhalation. This is more likely to be successful in patients with severe muscle tension dysphonia than in patients with spasmodic dysphonia.

Vegetative and Reflexive Techniques

In patients with psychogenic aphonia, normal voice is often revealed during coughing, laughing, throat clearing, and occasionally humming. These activities may be used to facilitate restoration of normal voice. For example, aphonic patients may be asked to cough and to sustain the sound produced at the end of the cough. If this can be accomplished as a coughed /a/, the /a/ can then be carried over into counting and running speech. Gargling, chewing, sighing, yawning, and other maneuvers also have been used similarly as facilitators.

Singing Voice Therapy and Acting-Voice Therapy

Singing voice therapy and acting voice therapy are discussed in chapters 9 and 12, respectively.

Voice Therapy for Transsexual Patients

This complex subject is discussed in chapter 22.

Therapy

In this chapter, detailed discussion of therapy will be limited to that appropriate for professional speakers/singers with behavioral voice problems, whether or not structural changes such as vocal nodules, cysts, or inflammation have developed. Therapy for organic problems such as vocal fold paralysis, central neurogenic dysphonias, cancer, or congenital problems will not be discussed.

Initially, the goals of therapy must be set. Goals may include establishing an excellent speaking voice of professional quality; developing a temporarily breathy or soft speaking voice to allow healing after vocal surgery or to allow nodules to be reduced; or establishing an easy, efficient speaking voice that does not cause fatigue or strain, and preserves the voice for singing or formal speaking situations. Ideally the goal is to produce an excellent speaker; realistically, the goal may be to develop a more efficient, less abusive speaker.

Level-One Therapy

Therapy for behavioral voice problems can be organized into several levels although this classificiation is not intended to imply that they must be stratified or done sequentially. In this chapter *Level-One Therapy* refers to an educational level, utilizing instruction, discussion, and modeling as its primary therapeutic tools. The patient and therapist talk about various vocal misuse or abuse patterns, make decisions about which can be deleted from the patients usual lifestyle and which must be retained to allow the patient to feel like him- or herself. Often singers, especially older ones, may object to modifying their breathing, voicing, or resonance patterns because such patterns have been effective in a long and successful career. Attempts to begin learning and practicing a new method are met with resistance, whereas discussion of what can or cannot be changed may be a gentler way to convince the more resistant patient that other changes may also be appropriate. Often modeling, without overt suggestions for change, may result in modification of the patient's behavior sufficiently to improve the speaking voice. The clinician continues to model easy, relaxed voicing. Frequently the patient begins to use the same type of voice within the context of the session and begins to carry over this behavior outside the session. This level of intervention is frequently effective and may be all that is needed for professional singers who are attuned to their bodies and in touch with the need to modify their lifestyle in order to maintain vocal health.

Voice professionals, singers and nonsingers, come to speech-language pathologists with varying degrees of knowledge about the factors that are responsible for their current problems. Positive alternatives to their vocally abusive behaviors are developed through a vocal hygiene program. A discussion of vocal hygiene is important at Level-One Therapy.

1. Throat Clearing
   In some cases, excessive mucus is a problem (associated with gastric reflux, postnasal drip, and allergies). More often, patients clear their throats out of habit, rather than need. This behavior, because it is traumatic to the vocal folds, should be eliminated. The following alternatives are useful:
   a. Dry swallow: Swallowing closes the vocal folds and can help rid them of mucus. The action of swallowing (in the post-abduction phase) can also relax the larynx, helping to alleviate the perceived need to clear the throat.
   b. Take small sips of water.
   c. Use a "silent cough." This is achieved by using abdominal support to push air through the folds (as if producing an /h/ sound). The strong airflow blows mucus off the vocal folds.
   d. Pant lightly, then swallow.
   e. Hum lightly.
   f. Laugh gently or giggle lightly, then swallow.
   g. Talk through the mucus without straining for vocal clarity. The natural vibration of the vocal folds may rid the vocal folds of secretions.
   h. For singers, vocalize lightly on five note scales in a comfortable range on /ɑ/, or slide up an octave softly on /ɑ/, and crescendo (get louder).

2. Whispering
   Many patients, especially singers, are aware that whispering should be avoided. During whispering in many instances, the anterior two thirds of the vocal folds approximate. Forced or loud whispering appears most harmful. The adverse effects of whispering have not been fully documented, but ample clinical experience supports the proscription. Although extremely soft whispering without vocal contact may be safe, few patients maintain this technique, and most resort to using forced whispering to be heard without even realizing it. Therefore, patients are cautioned that all whispering should be avoided. However, actors may need to make use of this type of vocal production in their work. In this case, specialized training is indicated.

3. Grunting/Noisy Vocalization
   Grunting when lifting or exercising creates forceful, traumatic adduction of the folds. Instead:
   a. Exhale slowly on the exertion phase of any exercise (preferred method), or
   b. Adduct the vocal folds gently, prior to initiating each exercise event (such as a sit-up or weight lift) and release (abduct) after each event.

4. Yelling/Screaming or Loud Talking
   Many performers and singers have gregarious, outgoing personalities. They commonly yell or scream as an expression of anger, frustration, elation, or joy. We advise them to save their voice for the performance and instead:

a. Use a whistle or bell.

b. Educate friends and family members about the harmful effects of yelling or screaming.

c. Engage the help of others for monitoring.

d. Use facial and other physical gestures to express emotions.

e. Use hissing as another nonvoiced outlet to express anger or frustration.

f. Know the limits of your vocal abilities. Be aware of how much loud talking can be tolerated before fatigue is experienced.

g. Cultivate the dramatic power of soft, articulated speech, which is often more effective than yelling.

5. Noisy Environments

Certain environments are inherently noisy (cars, airplanes, restaurants, social gatherings, night clubs). Special care should be taken not to speak over the noise level for long periods of time. Alternatives include:

a. Face the listener.

b. Gently overarticulate rather than increase loudness.

c. Speak at a slow rate to avoid the need for repetition.

d. Speak at normal pitch. There is a tendency to raise pitch and loudness in background noise. The normal, lower pitch often cuts through the ambient noise, decreasing the need to speak more loudly.

6. Excessive Talking

Gregarious patients find this a difficult habit to break. Modification can be facilitated using the following:

a. Schedule vocal naps. Observe 20 minutes of silence, 2 to 3 times a day. Wear an alarm watch as a reminder. In addition, inexpensive digital watches are available with time-elapsed functions that beep every 10 minutes or every hour. This signal can be used early in retraining as a reminder to check vocal behavior.

b. Limit the amount of time on the telephone.

c. Limit interrupting others in conversation. Be a good listener.

d. Ask questions to prompt others to do most of the talking.

7. Caffeine Consumption

Excessive caffeine intake has a diuretic effect and depletes the vocal fold tissues of needed hydration. The patient should:

a. Avoid caffeinated beverages (coffee, soda, tea) especially before heavy voice use, dress rehearsals, performances, lectures, trials, sermons, or teaching

b. Switch to decaffeinated beverages (water is the best substitute).

c. Drink a glass of water for every cup of coffee or soda, and follow the recommendations below for systemic dryness.

8. Systemic Dryness

Good systemic hydration is necessary for all patients. They are instructed to:

a. "Sing wet—pee pale" (in the words of Dr Van Lawrence). We have adapted this to: "Speak wet—pee pale."

b. Drink water every time they eat.

c. Keep water at hand at all times.

d. If a patient absolutely cannot tolerate water, try bottled spring water or tap water with a mild citrus twist.

9. Environmental Dryness

Environmental factors can create a drying effect on the vocal mechanism. If the patient is singing or performing in geographical regions where relative humidity is low, special attention to improving environmental hydration is needed. The best way to humidify room air is controversial at present. There is no convincing evidence for or against the use of hot or cold steam, or ultrasonic mist. Research is needed to determine which is best. The relative humidity on airplanes is initially about 5%, as discussed in *Clinical Assessment of Voice*,[2] and special precautions must be taken.

a. Superhydrate prior to and during air travel.

b. Use a humidifier and travel with it if possible.

c. Minimize talking on the airplane.

d. Provide a moist environment in hotel rooms by running the hot water in the shower.

e. Use steam inhalation to provide temporary relief.

10. Inadequate Rest and Sleep Patterns

General body fatigue is reflected in the voice. Optimal vocal efficiency may not be achieved when the performer or speaker is tired.

a. Get more rest and sleep prior to heavy voice use.

b. Be particularly careful when traveling (jet lag).

c. Allow time for a short nap before important speaking commitments whenever possible.

Additional vocal abuse and misuse problems typically exhibited by teachers and singers are enumerated in Appendixes Ia and IIb.

Level-Two Therapy

Level-Two Therapy involves the careful modification of inappropriate breathing, voicing, or resonance behaviors that do not resolve through Level-One discussions. The primary therapeutic tools are those of behavior modification, including drills, practice material, and small step changes in current behavior to extinguish inappropriate behavior and reinforce more natural and correct behaviors. During the evaluation and trial therapy, the clinician has had the opportunity to determine if a client needs to begin at Level One or Level Two. It is our experience that school teachers, lawyers, and other professional speakers who have not had singing training, often need to begin at Level Two.

Breath Control and Support

We are born with an innate ability to breathe healthfully and appropriately for the production of normal speech. Watch a newborn during quiet (tidal) breathing. The abdomen expands during inhalation. During vocalizations such as screaming or crying (exhalation), the abdominal muscles contract. Most adults have lost this natural habit of effortless breathing and support.

In the initial stages of therapy, difficulty arises when attention is called to breathing. Observe what happens when a patient is asked to take a nice deep breath. The abdomen is sucked in, the chest and shoulders rise, and the breath is held with the vocal folds tightly adducted. These are not the desired behaviors.

There are certain maladaptive behaviors that are automatically exhibited in response to certain words (eg, "breathe," "inhale," and "exhale"). Using appropriate vocabulary early in therapy facilitates the training of correct speech breathing. *Abdominal breathing* is referred to as *abdominal support*. The terms *expansion,* or *softening the belly,* are used for the inhalation phase, and *pulling* in is used cautiously (to avoid tension) for the exhalation phase.

Abdominal/diaphragmatic breathing should be explained to the patient in simple terms. During inspiration, the diaphragm moves inferiorly, enlarging the chest and compressing the contents of the abdomen. The abdomen must relax to make room for the stomach, intestines, and other structures that have been pushed downward by the diaphragm. As the abdominal muscles relax and the abdominal contents shift, the belly protrudes. During expiration, the diaphragm relaxes, and the muscles of the abdominal and back contract. As they do, the abdominal contents are squeezed upwards toward the chest, decreasing the size of the chest cavity and increasing the pressure of the air in the lungs. This is similar to squeezing a balloon. This sequence of activities during expiration constitutes abdominal "support"; but it cannot occur efficiently without appropriate, coordinated relaxation during inspiration.

Experience has shown that it is easier to teach a patient to pull in the abdominal muscles than to expand or soften the belly. Therefore, we begin the process of training appropriate speech breathing from the exhalation phase. The patient uses his or her expiratory reserve volume to begin speaking.[13] When the air is expelled, it triggers a spontaneous inhalation, a concomitant softening of the belly.

We provide an appropriate rhythm for this abdominal motion, which will be used extensively in later sessions. We explain that the rhythm is similar to a 3/4 time signature or slow waltz (58 or 62 bpm on a metronome). We count out the pace "1-2-3" as the patient pulls in the abdominal muscles, and "1-2-3" as they expand.

A discussion of the differences between support for speaking and support for singing is provided. Classically trained singers especially need the experience of adjusting the inspiratory phase of breathing. The respiratory needs for conversational speaking are considerably less than for singing. Although the basic principles are the same in both voice modes, by taking the focus off *breathing* and providing experience in the abdominal *pump* using the 3/4 rhythm, the singer learns how to feel appropriate speaking support and avoids exerting so much muscular tension that his or her support efforts become counterproductive.

The beginning steps in establishing breath control are incorporated into the warm-up and cool-down routines discussed in a later section. For convenience, a step-by-step approach is presented. However, it must be emphasized that, although this outlines our customary therapeutic direction, it is not a "cookbook" of techniques that can be applied indiscriminately without considerable clinical judgment and modification. This caveat applies not only to teaching breath control and support, but to all of the other topics covered in this chapter.

Step 1

We begin by introducing the concept of appropriate speech breathing for nonspeech tasks and isolated speech sounds.

Exercise 1: The patient is asked to pull in his or her abdominal muscles while blowing, as if blowing out a candle. Once the air has been fully expelled, the abdominal muscles expand naturally and the patient inhales spontaneously. This is repeated several times until it can be accomplished easily. During the process, the patient learns to sense and use abdominal and back muscles efficiently to support phonation.

Exercise 2: An alternative initial approach breaks down the abdominal breathing into muscular and respiratory components. The patient is asked to pull in his or her abdominal muscles and then to expand the abdomen as described above. However, an abdominal pump, with special attention to rhythm, is introduced. It is the rhythmic pattern and visual cuing that provide the patient with the appropriate mechanics of abdominal breath control and support. Once the rhythm of the pump is established, breath is added. The patient is instructed not to concentrate on inhaling, but instead to focus on blowing out. Once he or she is comfortable with the pump and blowing out, his or her attention is focused on the smooth and easy exchange of air. We describe this as a "cycle of breathing" and encourage the patient to feel breathing as a continuous action and motion. If the patient has difficulty exhaling a steady stream of air, it may be necessary to modify the exercise. The production of a sustained /s/ during exhalation provides increased auditory feedback and facilitates the monitoring of any constrictions of the vocal tract. It is important to establish early in therapy that the breath should neither be held nor restricted. Breathing techniques established through either initial approach are gradually shaped into speech for support through a series of steps.

Step 2

Quiet Breathing. The patient is asked to pay attention to his or her quiet or tidal breathing.

Exercise 1: The patient is asked to begin the exercise with active breathing for the "candle blowing" task using good abdominal support. The clinician provides the visual prompt to slow the breath, and the patient gradually changes the candle blowing to quiet breathing. He or she is asked to practice this exercise 10 times each day until a natural carryover of abdominal breathing for all quiet (nonspeech) breathing is established. The patient is also reminded to practice breath support while working on all other aspects of voice such as easy onset, decreased volume, or relaxation. Breathing exercises should be done in a sitting or standing position, the way most speaking is done. On occasion a patient may require early practice in more facilitating positions. Have the patient stand, bend at the waist and extend his or her arms to the arms of an armchair, positioning the feet in such a fashion that the patient's back is parallel with the floor. In this position the patient cannot lift his or her chest or shoulders and gravity assists the patient in being able to feel belly softening/expansion during inhalation exercises, and belly contraction during speech production.

Step 3

The transition from nonspeech tasks to speech tasks is accomplished systematically.

Exercise 1: The patient is asked to gradually pull in and to count from 1 to 50, with five numbers to a support group (eg, "1-2-3-4-5," expand, "6-7-8-9-10," expand).

Exercise 2: The patient is asked to count again from 1 to 50, this time varying the breath support group. For example, the patient may choose to inhale after the fifth number or whatever feels comfortable. The goal of this exercise is to achieve a flow and rhythm of the breath for simple ongoing speech tasks. Negative practice may be helpful at this stage. Have the patient count aloud at length, postponing the replenishing breath to experience the increased adduction that usually accompanies phonation on residual air. Explain that the patient should try to avoid this feeling of constriction by replenishing his or her breath before it occurs in speech.

Step 4

Phrasing is an important component of using appropriate breath control and support in ongoing speech.

Exercise 1: The patient is provided with a list of phrases from which to read (Appendix III). The phrases vary from 3 to 12 syllables per phrase. Onset and maintenance of breath control and support are monitored closely. The concepts of rhythm and of pacing the breath are of paramount importance. Imagery is helpful in establishing a relaxed, easy speech-breathing rhythm.

Exercise 2: The patient is provided with longer sentences that he or she is asked to phrase appropriately. At this time, the patient begins to exercise spontaneity and freedom of where to plan the breath. If need be, visual cues can be provided such as breath marks identified on the written page.

Exercise 3: Paragraphs are introduced. Phrases may be marked, or the patient may be asked to read the paragraph "cold," while it is audiotaped. This allows the patient and clinician to critique the paragraph together, then mark phrases and repeat the reading. Additional markings may include cues for easy onset of troublesome words and for attention to oral resonance or any other aspect that has been trained.

Exercise 4: The patient is provided with additional unmarked paragraphs for practice in breath control and support and phrasing.

Step 5

The transition from structured tasks to conversation is highly individualized. Some patients require very few techniques or strategies, whereas others need very organized exercises.

Exercise 1: Initially, the patient is asked to describe three things he or she will do during the rest of the day. Cues and prompts are provided as needed.

Exercise 2: Additional practice is gained by asking the patient to discuss specific topics, and to read aloud on a daily basis from a newspaper or magazine. It may be helpful for the patient to tape-record these practice sessions at home for review with the voice therapist in a subsequent therapy session.

Reducing Harsh Glottal Attacks

The term *harsh* or *hard glottal attacks* refers to the forceful or abrupt approximation of the vocal folds on words that begin with vowels. The acoustic result is a sudden, sharp, or explosive sound often called a *glottal click* or *glottal stroke*. The onset of voicing or phonation for vowels should be initiated gradually and easily. The key to easing harsh glottal attacks lies in the timing of the airflow with phonation.

Easy Onset Exercise 1: Negative Practice

The clinician demonstrates contrasts for the patient, using an abrupt initiation of the vowel sound in single words. These same words are then produced with an easy onset. Discrimination of easy versus hard onset can be provided for home practice. This is especially useful for adolescents or children. This negative practice is limited to only a few trials. After the clinician demonstrates, the patient is asked to say a word hard, then say it easy. Instructions to produce the word easily may include initiating the word with an /h/ sound, or feeling the air first.

Easy Onset Exercise 2: Minimal Pairs

A list of minimal-paired words (hate/ate, high/I, etc) is provided. The patient is directed to feel the openness of the glottis on the /h/ and the gentle closure on the vowel-initiated cognate.

Easy Onset Exercise 3: Single Words

Air naturally precedes vocal fold adduction when producing h-initiated words; therefore, easy vowel initiation can be shaped from such words. The word list (appendix V) is used as stimulus material in a variety of ways. One alternative is asking the patient to produce a light /h/ sound before each word. It is discussed that using the /h/ to slide into the word helps to initiate an easy onset. In some cases, the patient is asked to produce a breathy quality to ensure an easy onset. It is also useful to encourage a slide into the word with a slight elongation of the initial vowel.

A second method is to focus on the relationships between the initiation of exhalation and sound. Instruct the patient to "know what you are going to say before you take in air to say it." Begin by simply breathing in and breathing out in a regular cycle. Then try vowel-initiated words, making sure the patient is into the exhalation phase before attempting voicing. Cues of "Don't stop at the end of exhalation" and "Begin to voice just after you have begun to breath out" are helpful. Voice users with extensive prior voice training may find cuing to elevate the soft palate prior to voice onset helpful, as well.

Easy Onset Exercise 4: Long Versus Short Vowels

It is helpful to begin with single words initiated with the long vowels in English (eg, *eat, ice*) (Appendix III). The practice material is structured such that words beginning with the same vowel shape are rehearsed in a string (eg, *are, art, arm*). Minimizing the changes in oral cavity shape helps the patient focus his or her attention on the details of appropriate breathing, which assists in decreasing laryngeal tension. The task hierarchy proceeds from single words containing the long vowels to words beginning with short vowels (eg, *ill, it, is*). Once easy onset is established, a hierarchical approach is employed, moving from vowel-initiated words to vowel-initiated phrases to monitored reading to conversational speech.

Easy Onset Exercise 5: Delay Approach

Timing the onset of breath support is the key to a soft onset for words that begin with vowels. Singers are asked to imagine a score of music that begins with an eighth-note rest. Visual cuing is provided to help with the slow onset time. The patient is asked to posture his or her mouth for the word that will be produced, but delay the onset of phonation until the air, which is achieved with good abdominal/diaphragmatic support, has reached the level of the vocal folds. Additional suggestions include "breathe space between the vocal folds," "imagine that you are exhaling on the sound /h/" (an audible /h/ should not be produced for this exercise), "wait for the air to reach the folds, then produce the word" (eg, *are*).

Easy Onset Exercise 6: Downward Slide

Using a downward slide on the vowel sound that begins the word is another technique to reduce harsh glottal attacks. The patient is asked to expand the abdomen (to ensure a good supply of air), then slide down from a high pitch to a lower pitch on the vowel sound. Modeling is provided. It is important that the patient not think of this as singing.

Easy Onset Exercise 7: Key Word Approach

A key word carryover approach is used, with "I," "and," and other frequently occurring words in English. The patient may generate a list of vowel-initiated words (names of family members and friends) and practice using any of the other techniques described in this section.

Easy Onset Exercise 8: Blending

The above techniques pertain to vowel-initiated words that begin a breath group (words which are said on one breath). For vowel-initiated words that do not begin a breath group, a "linking" technique is used. Vowel-initiated words are linked to the word that precedes them. Connecting vowel-initiated words in ongoing speech is generally an easy task for singers. They are reminded that the same connected (legato) line and rules of phrasing in song apply to speech as well. A short list (Appendix III) of two-word combinations is used in which the first word is linked or blended to the second word.

Easy Onset Exercise 9: Conversation or Monologue

Conversation or a monologue is elicited. The patient's attention is directed to blending words and easing the onset of vowel-initial words as he or she begins a breath group. This should be tape-recorded and reviewed with the patient.

Oral Resonance

The distinction between *oral resonance* and *tone focus* is subtle. Speech-language pathologists use concepts of oral resonance as they are reported in therapy texts for the profession. Vocabulary such as *vocal placement* or *tone focus* is borrowed from the singing literature. There are numerous techniques to improve the resonance quality of the voice. We use exercises to increase oral cavity space. These include palatal, pharyngeal, and tongue exercises. The goal is to increase the oral cavity space anteriorly and posteriorly. We generally begin with awareness exercises that are especially important for the nonsinger or others who have not had any formal voice or speech training. Many speakers tend to keep the jaw closed and open it only when necessary on low vowels. A more appropriate resonance

pattern is to keep the jaw relaxed and open, and to only close when necessary on such sounds as /s/, /z/, /tʃ/, /dʒ/, /ʃ/ and /ʒ/. This necessitates increased activity of the anterior part of the tongue, in disassociation with jaw movements and may require additional practice, particularly with individuals with myofacial imbalance syndrome.

Jaw and facial tension are commonly observed in hyperfunctional voice users. Tension is often expressed as a "clenched teeth" posture, with little excursion of the jaw while speaking. By maintaining the jaw in a relatively fixed position, the tongue, pharynx, and other structures are forced to work harder to make the necessary adjustment for vowel differentiation. Further, the diminished space within the oral cavity compromises its effectiveness as a resonator.

In discussing the concept of jaw relaxation, it is preferable to use words such as "creating space" rather then "opening the mouth." "Opening" can be accomplished rather easily, but not necessarily in a relaxed position. Instructing the patient to feel space between the back teeth seems to achieve openness without tension.

Oral Resonance Exercise 1: Palatal Awareness

This exercise is useful for patients with functional or regional nasality and is often used to shape resonance for nonsingers. The patient is asked to stand and suggestions regarding appropriate head and neck position are provided. The patient is asked to sustain an /ŋ/ using good abdominal/diaphragmatic breath support. Cues are provided to facilitate self-monitoring and to direct the patient's attention to the soft palate. Visual monitoring (using a hand mirror) is especially useful. The /ŋ/ is repeated at least 10 times. While continuing to use the mirror, the patient is asked to change the sustained /ŋ/ to /ɑ/, and is guided to observe the movement of the soft palate and the tongue. The mirror is taken away, and the patient is asked to feel this action. The /ŋ/ to /ɑ/ is repeated 10 times while sustaining one tone. Changing the tone by using an upward or downward slide is an option. However, this should be incorporated only after the patient has acquired good soft palate movement.

Oral Resonance Exercise 2: Pharyngeal "Surprise"

This uses imagery to create an open pharynx and high soft palate position. The patient is asked to imagine walking into a freezer and being surprised by the coldness. A gentle gasp is produced. We take care to instruct that the gasp be produced softly, without tension. This is incorporated into the cycle of breathing for the inspiratory phase. The candle blowing maneuver or any isolated speech sound may be used. As the patient exhales (which we sometimes continue to use as the first step in the breathing cycle) the patient is asked to express the surprise upon inhaling. The patient is asked to observe the feeling of cold air as it touches the pharynx ("back of the throat") and soft palate. We ask the patient to imagine that the cold air lifts the palate.

Oral Resonance Exercise 3: Tongue Protrusion

Hyperextending the position of the tongue for a simple task such as counting or reading short phrases is an extremely useful technique for finding immediate relief to tongue tension. This technique is often used when the patient feels vocally fatigued or in physical discomfort from speaking. The patient is asked to protrude the tongue so that it rests lightly on the lower lip (but not beyond the lip). Instructions are provided to ensure good speech breathing. The patient repeats one number per breath up to the number 10, then repeat the sequence. This sequence (counting from 1 to 10) is repeated three times to ensure that the posterior tongue muscles have stretched and relaxed. Essentially, the posterior tongue fatigues during this exercise, making hyperfunction more difficult, while it increases patient awareness. When the tongue is placed back in the mouth, it is easier to maintain a comfortable, more forward tongue placement, and the tone quality produced is often strikingly free and clear.

Additional tongue protrusion exercises may be useful in some cases. After the sequence of counting from 1 to 10 is completed, the patient may be asked to count in groups of three (eg, 1-2-3) and to breathe after every third number. When using short phrases for this task, the patient is instructed to repeat the phrase three times, and to attempt to produce clearly identifiable words, using appropriate articulation especially of difficult consonants (/t/, /d/, /p/, /b/, etc).

Oral Resonance Exercise 4: Natural Open Vowels

Certain vowels and diphthongs have an inherent "openness" to them (eg, /ɑ/, /ɑi/, /æ/, /ɑu/) and naturally facilitate more vertical space within the oral cavity. The patient is provided with a practice list of words containing these vowels (Appendix III). These words are used as targets in phrases to enable the patient to experience this openness in connected speech. The patient is then asked to identify such words in longer phrases, paragraphs, and conversational speech.

Oral Resonance Exercise 5: Lowered Posterior Tongue

This exercise increases the posterior dimension of the mouth space. Back vowel sounds such as /u/, /o/, and /ɔ/ are used in conjunction with a downward slide to increase posterior oral dimension. The series of slides is practiced in consonant-vowel-consonant combinations. It is easier for a nonsinger to begin with a continuous consonant sound such as /ʃ/, /s/, /m/, and /l/. The combinations of sounds include /ʃ-u-t/; /s-u-t/, and the like. A series of downward slides is used. The pharyngeal surprise can be incorporated into this exercise to maximize the space in the pharynx.

Tone Focus/Vocal Placement in Speech

Incorrect vocal placement or tone focus is a common speaking error. The tendency to overuse the muscles of the pharynx and posterior tongue creates a distinct resonance quality. The terms used to describe this quality include: "throaty," "muffled," "swallowing the words," "heavy," "guttural," and "pressed." This excessive muscular tension can lead to physical discomfort and vocal fatigue.

The concept of "vocal placement" is a distinct entity and not synonymous with "pitch," even though changes in placement may concomitantly affect pitch. We usually avoid the use of the word pitch in therapeutic directions as it carries with it certain preconceived ideas that can interfere with desirable behavioral change.

Vocal placement can be conceptualized as occurring along two axes: up/down and front/back. Therapy begins with a discussion of this "two-axis theory," the difference between pitch and placement, and a heightening of awareness of articulatory placement within the oral cavity. We begin with consonants because they are easier to conceptualize, having a definite point of contact or placement. Any sound articulated on the alveolar ridge or anterior to that point is considered a "front" sound, including /t/, /d/, /n/, /l/, /s/, /z/, /ʃ/, /tʃ/, /dʒ/, /θ/ (voiced and voiceless), /f/, /v/, /p/, /b/, and /m/. "Middle" sounds include /r/ and /j/. Back sounds are represented by /k/ and /g/. Once frontal consonant placement is established, an attempt is made to create the image of vowels being carried forward with the consonants. A tape recorder is useful so that the patient can hear, as well as feel, the difference in production.

Vocal Placement Exercise

We begin by having the patient contrast naturally front words (eg, *neat*) with naturally back words (eg, *clock*) to heighten the patient's awareness. A list of the front-placed words is provided to reinforce the feeling of the voice buzzing in the front of the mouth (Appendix III). The patient then produces these words, following them with a phrase ending in that target word. If good placement is achieved at the beginning and the end of the utterance, it can hopefully be maintained in between (eg, *neat—please be neat*). The patient is then instructed to repeat and read sentences and short paragraphs, concentrating on the placement of the articulators and the focus of the voice. Conversational speech and short monologues are practiced in order to make more spontaneous use of this technique.

Glottal Fry

Glottal fry (also called *pulse register*) occurs in the voice in the lowest frequency (24 Hz to 44 Hz). The tone that is produced in this range is perceived as rough or gravelly. Glottal fry often occurs in association with inadequate breath support and/or pharyngeal vocal placement. Techniques to improve breath support, enhance appropriate vocal placement, negative practice, and attention to auditory feedback are particularly useful in eliminating this tonal quality.

Loudness versus Projection

The difference between *loudness* and *projection* is reviewed with each patient. We discuss the idea of frivolous loudness, which is most loud talking, yelling, or screaming. Projection is defined as maximizing listener intelligibility with minimal speaker effort. Projection techniques are preferable to loud talking or yelling. While adjustments in breath support provide the foundation, making changes in the production of speech can enhance the perception of increased loudness. We suggest gentle overarticulation, which helps to maximize the production of words. These projection exercises are intended for conversational settings in the presence of loud background noise, for the telephone, for classroom teaching, and for some public-speaking situations. They are not intended for the stage. Many years of training are required for stage projection. The patient's skills are developed using a hierarchy that begins with breath support tasks.

Projection Exercise 1: Single Words

Word lists (see Appendix III) are presented which contain tongue-tip and other frontal consonant sounds, and we introduce a game of "baseball." *Game rules:* The therapist "pitches" (by swinging an arm toward

the patient) a word. A small arm swing indicates that the word is to be spoken at a comfortable loudness. Very gradually, the therapist increases the excursion of the arm swing, which is the patient's cue to use more breath support (by pulling in the abdominal muscles with more energy). The result is a naturally louder production of the word. It usually takes 10 trials for the patient to reach maximum loudness for a given word. Tactile-kinesthetic monitoring of the strap muscles and posterior tongue ensures relaxation of these muscles.

Projection Exercise 2: Using Speech Sounds in Phrasing

Often the perception of loudness is related to the clarity of the tone, word, or phrase. We use diction exercises to enhance the speaker's understandability and refer back to our lists of words and phrases. The patient is instructed to produce ending consonants sounds precisely. Care is taken to insure that hyperfunctional overarticulation does not result.

Projection Exercise 3: Combination

After the patient has had experience with the baseball game and improving diction for selected phrases, two exercises are combined: The therapist pitches specific phrases to the patient. The phrases are usually kept short (three, four, five, or six syllables per phrase) for this exercise. Again, the patient is instructed to use breath support more efficiently and not to focus on merely getting louder.

Projection Exercise 4: Prosody

Prosody exercises also enhance loudness and projection in longer phrases. Patients are asked to decide which word or words carry the meaning of a phrase and are then asked to accent that word by raising the intonation slightly and adding more breath support. If the selected word begins with a vowel, care is taken to ensure an easy onset.

Oral Resonance Exercise 4 is also useful in enhancing vocal projection.

Prosody

Major prosodic disturbances are not commonly observed in the professional voice population. However, a loss of vocal variety may occur during therapy as other aspects of speech/voice production are changed. In some cases prosody exercises may be necessary.

Prosody Exercise 1: Polysyllabic words

Polysyllabic words are used and the patient is instructed to exaggerate an upward inflection on the accented syllable (eg, *ed-u-ca-tion-al*). (Not only *educational* but *beautifully*.) The patient is taken through a hierarchy of tasks to establish this technique. The patient's conversational speech is taped. On playback, the patient and clinician mutually critique the patient's success in implementing this strategy. Improper responses are repeated in corrected form.

Prosody Exercise 2: Homographs

A list of words that differ in meaning depending on how they are accented is provided (*content-content*). A slightly exaggerated rising intonation for the accented syllable is demonstrated. These words are produced in a string of pairs. The patient's attention is oriented directly to the intonation variation (Appendix III).

Prosody Exercise 3: Phrases

The patient is asked to use polysyllabic words in self-generated phrases while still using the exaggerated intonation.

Prosody Exercise 4: Reading

The patient is asked to identify the polysyllabic words in a reading paragraph. These words are used as the basis for the exaggerated intonation as the patient reads.

Prosody Exercise 5: Conversation

The patient's conversational speech is audiotaped. On playback, the therapist and patient mutually critique the patient's use of this exaggerated technique. Error responses are repeated in the correct form.

Pitch

Specific methods for changing pitch will not be addressed in this chapter. Inappropriate pitch is rarely the cause of a patient's vocal dysfunction. Rather, inappropriate vocal usage may cause deviant pitch. When proper breath support and vocal placement are established, appropriate pitch usually follows.

Bridging Exercises

Bridging exercises are used with all patients (singers and nonsingers) who receive joint specialized singing instruction. These exercises are designed to bridge the gap (when one exists) between singing and speaking technique. The patient is provided with experience in maintaining appropriate tonal balance with breath control and support when the task changes from singing to speaking exercises. These techniques are especially useful for experienced singers who have not applied their trained vocal production and technique to speaking. They are also valuable for non-singers who have worked successfully with the singing-voice specialist.

Bridging Exercise 1: Descending Slide on /m/

The patient is instructed to start in a high falsetto range and very slowly slide down on the /m/ sound. Care is taken to ensure good abdominal support, appropriate head/neck position, and appropriate tongue placement. This same slide is repeated five times and the starting pitch is slightly lowered each time.

Bridging Exercise 2: Descending Slide for /m/ and /a/.

The patient is asked to slide down on the /m/. About halfway down the slide the patient is instructed to open his or her mouth. The resulting sound is an /a/. The important aspect of this exercise is the careful transition from the /m/ to the /a/. The patient is directed to feel the slow, gradual change to the /a/.

Bridging Exercise 3: Sustained /m/ to Counting

The patient is asked to sustain an /m/ at a comfortable pitch and loudness. Cues are provided to help the patient focus on the sensory aspects that had been previously trained (eg, open/relaxed pharynx, relaxed tongue position). The patient is asked to change from the /m/ to counting. The /m/ serves to bridge from a tone that sounds like light humming to speech.

Bridging Exercise 4: Lip Trills

The singing-voice specialist and the speech-language pathologist incorporate the use of lip trills. For singers, this is often a familiar task, but nonsingers require careful instruction. Tactile monitoring of the strap muscles is needed to ensure that tension is not created as this task is learned. We begin with a silent lip trill that sounds much like the neigh of a horse, sometimes referred to as a "flub." Visual prompts are provided, which help pace the timing the breath. After several trials with the flub, voicing is added. It is helpful to have the patient initiate the flub first, then add phonation. Lip trills are used on ascending and descending slides. It is important for the patient to produce a tone that is smooth and free of tension.

Bridging Exercise 5: /ŋ/ to /ɑ/

Palatal awareness exercises are routinely incorporated into voice training. When used as a bridging exercise, the /ŋ/ to /ɑ/ is used during the production of ascending and descending slides.

Bridging Exercise 6: Ascending-Descending Slide on /m/

The patient is asked to slowly slide up, then down in pitch on one breath for /m/. Modeling is provided so that the higher pitch is not too high. Occasionally, a replenishing breath needs to be taken before the descending slide.

Bridging Exercise 7: Siren

The circular sound an emergency vehicle makes is used with isolated sounds such as /m/, /l/, /v/, and lip trills. The number of repetitions per breath depends on the patient's speech-breathing ability. This is also an excellent warm-up exercise for the morning.

Recitative

Classical singers are generally trained in *recitative,* a cross between singing and speaking that occurs between arias in opera and oratorio. Singers who have mastered recitative can carry over good vocal technique by gradually dropping pitch specificity during recitative passages, letting them gradually convert to spoken dialogue. Similarly, singers may read passages as recitative on improvised notes, learning how to apply their musically trained breathing, support, and placement techniques to conversational speech. For singers who do not have an operatic background, patter songs (eg, Gilbert and Sullivan) and rap are of similar value as bridging exercises.

Level-Three Therapy

Level-Three Therapy involves the management of emotional stress. Some professional voice users react strongly to voice change. Voice therapy is designed to help the patient feel better and sound better. Most patients come to therapy with somatic complaints such as pain, tension, and vocal fatigue. Therefore, it is im-

portant that they begin to find relief quickly. This helps to elicit their cooperation and motivation early in the training process.

In addition, management of the stresses of everyday living, performing, or teaching is essential in the overall management of the injured speaker or singer. Many voice patients experience tremendous stress and tension in their daily lives. Decisions as to whether these stresses may be managed by the speech-language pathologist or are deep-seated enough to require the expertise of the psychological professional need to be made during the initial evaluation session and reevaluated as therapy progresses. Often the tension associated with deep-seated stress interferes with the patient's ability to respond to Level-Two or Level-One therapeutic techniques, and it should be addressed first.

Simple stress management techniques can be applied by the speech-language pathologist. More deep-seated stress and reaction to emotions or environmental influences will require the special skills of a psychologist or psychiatrist.

Relaxation

Many voice therapy programs incorporate relaxation techniques. While this is useful for stress management, progressive or deep relaxation is not necessarily an integral part of voice therapy for all patients. We use relaxation techniques to reduce muscular tension and to energize those muscle systems used in voice production. We routinely use range of motion, muscle stretch, and physical energizing tasks. There are many popular techniques used to facilitate relaxation. Jacobson's Progressive Relaxation[16] allows the patient to contrast muscular tension with relaxation. We have found it useful with muscular tension dysphonia and for some hyperfunctional voice users. However, carryover of this relaxed state to voice production is often difficult to achieve, and we find additional techniques desirable for most patients.

The yawn-sigh technique has traditionally been a part of voice therapy and speech training.[15] Although it benefits some patients, it is not a technique that should be used indiscriminately. The initial inspiratory phase of a yawn creates a high soft palate position, a lowered vertical laryngeal position, and an open pharynx. However, once the yawn reflex is triggered, the same structures and muscles become tense. Phonating with this degree of tension is not desirable. The natural yawn may have some benefit in voice retraining, but the artificial yawn used as a therapy technique has many potential pitfalls. The yawn-sigh technique may be appropriate for:

1. Improving the patient's sensory awareness of the soft palate, muscles of the pharynx, and tongue.
2. Creating an open, relaxed pharynx.
3. Establishing a high soft palate position, useful for oral resonance improvement.

For relieving specific sites of muscular tension: Excessive muscular tension is observed in association with almost all voice problems. Developing tactile awareness of the muscle movements of voice and speech production is a supplemental goal of voice therapy and is facilitated through the muscle stretch exercises. Even if minimal muscular tension is observed, range of motion and self-massage exercises are often helpful. Patients with a history of head/neck injuries or cervical arthritis are not candidates for these exercises.

Range of Motion

We recommend these exercises only for patients who do not have a history of head or neck injuries, back pain, spinal cord problems, or cervical arthritis. This exercise is designed to provide a complete stretch to isolated muscles of the neck. The instructions are routinely put on an audiotape, which allows for correct home practice. Specific instructions are provided to the patient to stretch the trapezius muscle and the anterior and lateral strap muscles. During all range of motion and stretching exercises, the patient should be instructed to breathe normally and to avoid holding the breath. The following outline is provided:

1. *Head Forward and Backward:* The head comes forward and is held in that position for a count of 10. Slowly the patient rotates the head from side to side as if watching a ball roll back and forth in his lap. The patient is then asked to tip the head backward while gently opening the mouth, look at the ceiling, and hold that position for a count of 5. These steps are usually repeated twice, but more repetitions may be indicated for some patients.
2. *Head Side-to-Side:* The head rocks toward the right shoulder, as if the patient were trying to touch the right shoulder with the right ear. Instructions are provided to ensure that only the head moves and not the entire torso. While leaning toward the right, the head rocks forward and backward in one sweeping nod (as if nodding "yes"). The patient is asked to focus on the muscles on the left side of the neck as they stretch and elongate. The instructions are repeated with the head leaning to the left.
3. *Looking Over Each Shoulder:* The patient is reinstructed regarding appropriate head and shoulder alignment. The patient is then asked to look over the right shoulder as if something were behind him. This position is held for a count of 10, and the patient is instructed to feel the stretch of the sternocleidomastoid muscle. The same instructions are repeated for the left side.
4. *Shoulder Rolls:* The shoulders are rolled forward and backward, in isolation, and then together. Specific instructions are provided to help the patient attend to the muscles he or she is stretching.
5. *Shoulder Shrugs:* The patient is asked to raise the shoulders, hold for a count of three, and then allow the shoulders to drop. Attention is directed to the contrast between tension and relaxation. As the shoulders drop, the patient is asked to feel the tension leave the shoulders through the fingertips.
6. *Jaw Relaxation:* The patient is asked to let the jaw drop open or down to create space between the back teeth. The clinician observes that the jaw is comfortably open and gently hyperextended or "unhinged." This position is held for 3 seconds, then the jaw is closed. These steps are repeated five times.
7. *Tongue Stretch:* Posterior tongue tension is usually observed in association with pharyngeal or "throaty" resonance. The patient is asked to rest the tongue lightly against the bottom teeth or inside the lower lip. The patient is prompted to hyperextend the base of the tongue. This is repeated at least 10 times; 30 times is preferred. This repetition tires the posterior portion of the tongue and often has an immediate effect of producing a clearer resonant quality. Another approach consists of rapid repetitions of the same stretch. The patient is provided with the identical prompts, but using a double-time pace. The clinician counts the rhythm (eg, "one-two; one-two; one-two") to help the patient maintain this pace.
8. *Tongue Tension in Speech:* Ongoing observations of the patient's performance and reaction to the suggestions provided by the clinician is very important. During the warm-up/cool-down routine, watch the neck just under the chin for signs of tongue movement. Posterior tongue tension is especially obvious during production of /s/. To insure good tactile monitoring, the patient is instructed to observe the difference in the tongue for /s/, then /ʃ/. If need be, a sloppy /s/ production will minimize tongue tension. Using a staccato rhythm challenges the patient and should be employed after success is achieved for the prolonged /s/.
9. *Strap Muscle Hyperfunction:* The use of voiced/voiceless cognate pairs (eg, f/v, s/z, ʃ/ʒ, θ/ð) facilitates relaxed/easy voicing. In making the transition

from voiceless to voiced speech sounds, we often see the vertical laryngeal position shift upward, which squeezes the strap muscles and muscles of the pharynx. The result is a tight or pressed resonant quality. Occasionally, a downward shift of the larynx is observed. The patient is instructed to monitor neck tension (tactile-kinesthetic monitoring) and observe the transition from the voiceless sound to the voiced sound. The patient learns how to add voicing without the tension.

10. *Chewing:* A modified "chewing approach" is used to promote mobility and stretch of the muscles of the face, lips, jaw, and tongue.[17] The patient is instructed to chew slowly, with his mouth open, and to make smacking noises "like a cow on a lazy summer afternoon." The patient is encouraged to use all the muscles of the lips, tongue, face, and jaw. When phonation is superimposed on the relaxed muscular complex the result should be a clearer sound with more oral resonance.

This technique should not be applied indiscriminately. The chewing exercise is not a relaxing activity for all patients. Some patients are uncomfortable with the crudeness of chewing in such a socially unacceptable manner and therefore cannot relax with it. Chewing exercises may also be contraindicated for patients with temporomandibular joint syndrome.

Self-Massage

The face, temporal muscles, posterior neck, shoulders, and occasionally the anterior strap muscles are massaged by the patient.

1. *Facial Massage:* The masseter muscle is identified. The patient is asked to press in firmly with the fingertips under the zygoma bones, and to hold the pressure for a count of 10. The patient is always reminded to continue to breathe at this point. Holding the breath can reinforce muscle tension. The fingertips are then released, and the patient is asked to go to the same spot and massage this muscle using a firm, slow circular motion. These same instructions are repeated on the jaw line, where the masseter muscle finishes its course. Massaging the temporal muscles (on both sides of the forehead) is extremely beneficial for relieving jaw tension. The same instructions of pressing, then massaging are provided.

2. *Posterior Neck and Shoulder Massage:* Excessive posterior neck muscle tension is often created by inappropriate head/neck alignment. To massage the right side, the patient is asked to take the left hand, cross over to the right side, and press in on the trapezius muscle. The press is held for a count of 10, and is then released. The patient is instructed to keep breathing. Next, the instruction is given to go back to the same spot, press in firmly, then let the hand slide forward and down. These steps are repeated for two other places in the posterior neck and then two places on the shoulders. Both sides are massaged equally. The right hand is used to massage the left posterior neck and shoulder.

Body Posture and Head/Neck Alignment

Appropriate head and neck alignment and body posture are essential to developing efficient vocal production. Excessive anterior strap muscle and posterior neck tension is created when the head is tilted backward or the chin is jutted forward. Suggestions and prompts are provided in conjunction with the other therapy techniques including generalized overall body relaxation techniques.

The following exercises have been helpful for refocusing the patients' general overall stress reaction. The exercises can be practiced routinely each day or used in times of high stress. Each of these exercises can be put on an audiotape for playback at a later time. Many of our patients find it helpful to hear the therapist's voice guide them through the relaxation protocol.

Two-Minute Spot Check: This short exercise is practical and easy. It is also extremely useful in reinforcing self-monitoring skills, and facilitating the carryover phase of therapy. We tell the patient to:

1. Interrupt your thoughts—switch your thoughts to your breathing. Begin with the candle blowing, taking time to inhale and exhale fully. Take several cleansing breaths (quicker fuller breaths), which requires a more active exchange of air.
2. Scan your body for specific sites of tension (forehead, jaw, shoulders, neck, or tongue). Attempt to loosen this area (move gently, use the range of motion exercises, or self-massage).
3. Take two more cleansing breaths, then return to easy candle blowing, and return to your activity.

Range of Motion for Stress Management: This is similar to the range of motion provided as a daily warm-up exercise. For this purpose, more time is taken and more breathing is incorporated. On an audiotape, the patient is provided with instructions beginning with: "Find yourself sitting in a comfortable chair. Let your head come forward as if you wanted to place your chin on your chest. Let it remain there for a moment. The muscle you are now stretching is called your trapezius. Can you imagine the point where it begins at the base of your skull, and feel where it ends in the middle of your back?" The patient is led on tape through a brief muscle relaxation program that helps dissipate stress.

The Quieting Response: This takes less than one minute to complete. It can be done in the midst of chaos, panic, or stage fright.

1. Pant quickly using a forced expiration, gradually slow down your breathing, turn it into the candle blowing, then gradually return to quiet breathing.
2. Smile outwardly and inwardly. Suggest to yourself (silently or aloud) that you will be accepted and successful in what you are about to do. Imagine a positive outcome. Picture yourself being in a relaxed controlled state 5 minutes from now. Enjoy the feeling of accomplishment.
3. Resume your activity.

A Short Meditation: The patient is provided with a tape of this relaxation exercise which lasts 5 to 10 minutes. The therapist guides the patient through each step, then finishes with the guided imagery. The patient is instructed to:

1. Spot check the body for muscular tension. Release specific areas of tension with the stretch and/or range of motion exercises. Focus on a warm, glowing feeling sweeping throughout your body.
2. Warm your hands by rubbing them together vigorously. Visualize the sun's warmth on your hands. Place them gently on your face and sweep downward and outward.
3. Focus now on your thoughts. Imagine a panel of switches. As your turn off each switch (one by one) your breathing slows and becomes very regular.
4. In your mind, travel to a place that's warm and safe, and brings a smile to your face—the seashore, the country, your home, a good friend. Stay with this pleasant feeling.

Guided Imagery: Guided imagery works best once the patient is in a quiet and calm state with very slow, regular breathing. The patient is led through individualized images. For example:

Imagine yourself lying on a carpet of soft grass in a shaded forest. It is a warm, pleasant day. The sky is a bright clear blue. Sun rays filter through the leaves of the forest canopy above. The tree branches seem to embrace and protect this spot where you lie. A gentle breeze sings through the green grass and tickles the skin of your face. Imagine that there is a clearing in the branches and a shaft of yellow light is descending on you. Feel the warmth. Feel the warmth seeping onto your forehead, your cheek bones, your mouth, your chin. Feel the warmth flowing down your neck and into your chest. Take a deep breath . . . Smell the fragrant air . . . Hold the breath . . . Then, slowly let it go as you feel the tightness flow from your chest on down your arms, and out your finger tips. Let the sun's rays warm your chest, your abdomen. Take a deep breath . . . Hold the warmth in your torso, then slowly let it drift slowly down your legs, and out your toes. You may stay in this moment and enjoy this perfect summer day and a feeling of deep contentment.

The patient is cued that the clinician will stop talking for a moment so he or she can enjoy the feeling. The patient is cued that he or she is brought back to that moment in time by counting from 1 to 10. Once the patient is accustomed to this technique, it can be used essentially as a form of self-hypnosis in times of stress (such as immediately before a performance).

Warm-up and Cool-down Exercises: The warm-up and cool-down routine is important in training the voice. Singers appreciate the need to exercise the voice before singing. Speaking exercises provide the patient with the equivalent of vocalises (singing scales) for the speaking voice. Consistent practice each morning prepares the vocal folds and muscles of the vocal mechanism for the demands of the day. The evening cool-down regimen is similar to the athlete stretching and cooling down after running. An outline of the daily practice exercises (Appendix III) is provided on each visit. The routine includes a muscular stretch and range of motion exercises, which are useful for relaxation, but are specifically used to heighten the patient's tactile feedback system. The patient is then asked to vocalize (singing scales), which have been provided by the singing specialist and provide "aerobic" conditioning. If the patient does not receive concurrent singing instruction, this step is omitted. The speech-language pathologist does not provide instruction in this area. The final step in the daily routine is the speaking exercises. These usually include a variety of nonspeech tasks, voiceless speech, and voiced speech sounds, and bridging exercises. The therapist reviews each exercise and provides new tasks as the need arises. Any of the techniques described in this chapter may be suitable as a warm-up or cool-down exercise.

Level-Four Therapy

Preparation for Referral to Mental Health Specialists

Occasionally a professional speaker will demonstrate stress and emotional reactions that are not directly related to performance and are pervasive in his or her personality and reaction to the world. These patients are often unable to respond to the educational processes at Level One, are intermittently and inconsistently successful in changing vocal behaviors at Level Two, and are unable to carry over stress management techniques beyond the actual performance of the relaxation exercises.

The therapy process can be disrupted by the patient's need to talk about unrelated problems and incidents. Often patients with mental health problems may be able to admit to a voice disorder but are unable to acknowledge emotional issues that may be interfering with their ability to cope with their relationships or environment. Making a referral to a mental health professional may not be sufficient when the patient denies the need for such a referral.

Referral Technique 1

The patient may need to experience the supportive, noncritical one-on-one therapeutic relationship. The process of participating in a caring therapeutic environment may be sufficient to improve the patient's likelihood of following through on a referral to a mental health specialist. Deferring the referral until the patient has been in voice therapy for a period of time may be helpful in achieving compliance with such a referral.

Referral Technique 2

If the therapeutic process continues to be interrupted by the patient, stop and listen sympathetically to the problems the patient wishes to discuss. If the patient has developed trust in you, he or she may begin to vent emotional stress related to verbal and physical abuse, feelings of entrapment, signs of depression, or other pervasive emotional problems. Vocalize your concerns about such problems and admit that you are not trained sufficiently to deal with or provide advice about such matters. Provide an immediate referral source to someone who may be better able to help with such problems and difficulties.

Where to Begin

Organizing therapy strategies into levels may assist the speech-language pathologist in determining, on the basis of the initial evaluation, where to begin with therapy and, if therapy is unsuccessful, what to try next. The ideal and easy patient with the best prognosis is the patient who with Level-One educational techniques and information is able to say "Oh, I can do

that" and proceeds to modify both life-style and vocal behavior. Often patients are unable to alter their speaking or singing requirements and are not trained well enough to be aware of what they are doing physically when speaking or singing. For these patients, Level-Two strategies and direct behavioral change of vocalization is required and may be most effective. Others may present with stress and tension levels so high that they are unable to respond to direct behavioral change and require the use of Level-Three techniques to condition patients to a level of relaxation that will permit them to respond to Level-Two vocal exercises and Level-One education. Finally, there are patients whose mental energy is so absorbed in day-to-day coping that they must deal with these mental problems before they can focus on the vocal problems manifested from their emotional problems.

Carryover Strategies

All the therapy techniques and exercises we have to offer are essentially worthless if the patient does not use them in his or her daily life. *Carryover* is the term used to describe the process of extending the use of new skills outside the speech-language pathologist's office. Traditionally, carryover occurs toward the end of therapy and is accomplished by gradually changing the contexts in which desired behaviors are enacted. This is accomplished by changing the physical environment (eg, moving from the therapy office to the waiting room and beyond) and expanding the social contexts in which the new behaviors are to be demonstrated (eg, bringing significant others into the therapy office). However, we believe that carryover should begin in the early stages of therapy. Consistent practice on the patient's part may be the best way to facilitate this.

Beyond the carryover that occurs spontaneously with practice, there are other ways to encourage the use of newly learned behaviors in the patient's daily conversation. A key word/key phrase approach has been used successfully in facilitating the transfer of new skills. Patients tend to use certain words or phrases frequently in the course of their daily interactions and they are encouraged to employ specific strategies on those specific words or phrases. For example, when working toward the elimination of hard glottal attacks, ascertain the names of important people in the patient's environment that may be vowel-initiated. *I* and *and* are very frequently occurring words in the English language and are good key words for most patients.

Utilize environmental cues to signal the use of certain desired behaviors. For example, when trying to facilitate the carryover of breath support, the patient is instructed to "support" every time he or she answers the telephone. The telephone receiver becomes an external reminder of what the individual should be doing.

Choose particular time periods or situations when the patient is to consciously use a particular technique. "Every lunch hour, while conversing with your colleagues, make an effort to use your frontal consonant focus;" or "At every red light, check to see that you have space between your back teeth."

Carryover Exercise 1: Greetings as Reminders

The patient is instructed to use all greetings and departures (hello, goodbye, etc) as reminders to use appropriate support. These greeting words should be practiced in the office, and then serve to trigger the patient's awareness of speaking technique in person and during telephone conversations.

Carryover Exercise 2: Telephone Strategies

Most professional voice users report some degree of vocal fatigue if extended telephone use is required. We routinely provide details in how to "survive" with the telephone. These suggestions include:

1. Observe appropriate head and neck position.
2. Slow speaking rate.
3. Make more effective use of pauses by stopping before or after important content words.
4. Hold each pause slightly longer than usual. This helps to give your listener more processing time.
5. Use projection techniques to get volume with ease.
6. Use projection techniques to maximize diction.
7. Switch which hand you typically use to hold the receiver. This adds a novelty to the situation and helps to focus on the voice.

Carryover Exercise 3: People and Places/Situations

The patient is asked to identify three situations and persons with whom he or she will practice the speaking techniques. The three people consist of a personal relationship (spouse, child, parent); a social acquaintance (work colleague, neighbor); and a stranger (grocery clerk, bank teller). A hierarchy is developed depending on the patient's feelings of comfort in each of these situations. Some patients report that it is easier to practice with a stranger. Others report that the techniques work best at work. This carryover strategy is highly individualized. The patient makes these active choices and the therapist helps guide his or her perceptions and practice.

Carryover Exercise 4: Reminders

The patient is asked to describe his or her activities during the course of a typical day from the time the alarm clock rings until it is reset at night. A few events are selected as reminders to check vocal technique. These may include activities such as walking through the office door, taking a coffee break, coming through the door at home, and so on. The effectiveness of each of these activities as a vocal "reminder" is checked during subsequent therapy sessions.

Carryover Exercise 5: Communicative Stress

Since the general approach is geared toward relaxation, specific practice in dealing with pressured situations is beneficial. The clinician will provide a series of rapid questions. These questions vary in the complexity of answers they require. A sample of questions includes:

1. What's your birthday?
2. What's your spouse's birthday?
3. What's your telephone number?
4. Why do we use napkins?
5. Why do we have traffic lights?
6. Why do we have income tax?
7. How do you make a bed?
8. Describe how to make your favorite meal.
9. What if a child was left unattended?

The clinician helps the patient identify vocal stress that develops in response to these questions, and instructions are given for identifying and ameliorating vocally abusive behavior in daily situations.

Carryover Exercise 6: Habituation and Maintenance

The patient is instructed to read aloud at least 3 to 4 times weekly.

Carryover Exercise 7: Professional Feedback

The patient is instructed to converse with the voice therapist or a similarly skilled listener periodically (timing depends upon the stage of therapy). While this is not exactly an exercise, the importance of skilled feedback cannot be underestimated.

Concurrent Specialized Singing Lessons

Most patients (singers and nonsingers) are routinely evaluated by the singing voice specialist. Singing provides the nonsinger with exercises and training that greatly enhance the speaking voice. Professional voice users find that the demands of speaking seem less when they have had the "aerobic" workout that singing provides, and the symbiotic techniques of the singing teacher enhance the teaching of breathing, support, placement and other speaking techniques.

Interrelation of Voice Functions

Although a number of common vocal misuses have been identified and their remediation discussed individually, deviant vocal behaviors do not occur in isolation. Therapy for one behavior may obviate the need for specific, intensive work on another. For example, patients who speak too rapidly usually exhibit jaw tension. The reason for the association between the two is that in order to speak at a rapid rate, the speaker cannot afford the time needed for the mandible to make the necessary excursion consistent with jaw relaxation. Breath support and vocal placement are similarly related. When a patient successfully achieves good abdominal breath support, the voice is naturally carried to a more frontal placement, on the well-sustained airflow. The importance of these examples is to emphasize the dynamic nature of vocal production.

Value of Instrumentation in Voice Therapy

Use of instrumentation for voice therapy will not be discussed in detail in this chapter. However, under special conditions voice therapy techniques in combination with instrumentation such as the Kay CSL programs, Visi-Pitch, Sona-Graph, Laryngograph, PM-Pitch Analyzer, flexible fiberoptic scope, or rigid endoscope can be helpful. For example, the laryngograph in combination with the Sona-Graph has served as useful biofeedback for such disorders as spasmodic dysphonia or muscle tension dysphonia. After brief training and orientation, the patient can visually monitor correct versus incorrect productions for specific tasks. The PM-Pitch Analyzer has a built-in program designed for use in direct therapy. Since it can interpret longer speech samples, it is ideal for monitoring speaking misuses such as harsh glottal attacks in ongoing speech.

Conclusion

The speech-language pathologist is an essential component of the voice care team for professional voice users, regardless of whether the primary voice problem occurred during speech or singing. Close collaboration among the voice therapist, laryngologist, singing teacher, and other members of the voice care team facilitates the development of optimal speaking technique in these patients. To many speech-language pathologists beginning therapy with professional voice users, the voices will initially sound normal. However, with increasing experience, one develops a great appreciation for the voice disruption that may be caused by even minor misuses and abuses in voice professionals. Recognizing their need for near-perfection in vocal quality and endurance, and understanding the unusual stresses to which performers and their voices are routinely exposed, the speech-language pathologist will find exceptional gratification in working with this challenging group of patients. Professional voice users demand our most critical assessment acuity and therapeutic skills, excite our clinical imaginations, and achieve highly gratifying (and much appreciated) results.

References

1. Heuer RJ, Hawkshaw MJ, Sataloff RT. The clinical voice laboratory. In: Sataloff RT. *Clinical Assessment of Voice.* San Diego, Calif: Plural Publishing Inc; 2005:33–81.
2. Sataloff RT, Anticaglia J, Hawkshaw MJ, Patient history. In: Sataloff RT. *Clinical Assessment of Voice.* San Diego, Calif: Plural Publishing Inc. 2005:1–16.
3. Eckel FC, Boone DR. The S/Z ratio as an indication of laryngeal pathology. *J Speech Hear Disord.* 1981;46:147–149.
4. Johnson JA, Pring TR. Speech therapy and Parkinson's disease: a review and further data. *Br J Disord Commun.* 1990;25:183–194.
5. Ramig LO, Mead C, Scherer RC, Horii Y, Larson K, Kholer D. Voice therapy and Parkinson's disease: a longitudinal study of efficacy. Paper presented at the Clinical Dysarthria Conference; 1988; San Diego, Calif.
6. Ramig LO. Speech therapy for Parkinson's disease. In: Koller WC, Paulson G. eds. *Therapy of Parkinson's Disease.* New York, NY: Marcel Dekker; 1995:539–550.
7. Ramig LO Bonitati CM, Lemke JH, Horii Y. Voice treatment for patients with Parkinson's disease: development of an approach and preliminary efficacy data. *J Med Speech Lang Pathol.* 1994;2:191–209.
8. Ramig LO, Scherer RC. Speech therapy for neurologic disorders of the larynx. In: Blitzer A, Brin MF, Saski CT, Fahn S, Harris KH, eds. *Neurologic Disorders of the Larynx.* New York, NY: Thieme; 1992:163–181.
9. Alexander FM, McGowen D, eds. *Alexander Technique: Original Writings of FM Alexander: Constructive Conscious Control.* New York, NY: Larson Publications; 1997.
10. Conable B, Conable W. *How to Learn the Alexander Technique: A Manual for Students.* Columbus, Ohio: Andover Road Press; 1992.

11. Feldenkrais M. *Body and Mature Behavior: A Study of Anxiety, Sex, Gravitation and Learning.* New York, NY: International Universities Press 1950; 1980.
12. Feldenkrais M. *Awareness Through Movement: Health Exercises for Personal Growth.* New York, NY: Harper & Row; 1972.
13. Feldenkrais M. *The Elusive Obvious.* Cupertino, Calif: Meta Publications; 1981.
14. Feldenkrais M. *The Potent Self: A Guide to Spontaneity.* New York, NY: Harper & Row; 1985.
15. Boone D. *The Voice and Voice Therapy.* Englewood Cliffs, NJ: Prentice-Hall; 1983.
16. Jacobson E. *You Must Relax.* New York, NY: McGraw-Hill Books; 1957.
17. Froeschels E. Chewing method as therapy. *Arch Otolaryngol.* 1952;56:427–434.

Suggested Reading List

1. Andrews M. *Manual of Voice Treatment: Pediatrics through Geriatrics.* San Diego, Calif: Singular Publishing Group, Inc; 1999.
2. Aronson A. *Clinical Voice Disorders: An Interdisciplinary Approach.* 3rd ed. New York, NY: Thieme, Inc; 1990.
3. Boone DR, McFarlane SC. *The Voice and Voice Therapy.* 6th ed. Boston, Mass: Allyn & Bacon; 1999.
4. Brown WS, Vinson BP, Crary MA. *Organic Voice Disorders: Assessment and Treatment.* San Diego, Calif: Singular Publishing Group; 1996.
5. Colton R. Casper J. *Understanding Voice Problems.* Baltimore, Md: Williams & Wilkins; 1990.
6. Keith RL, Thomas JE. *Speech Practice Manual for Dysarthria, Apraxia, and Other Disorders of Articulation: Compare and Contrast.* Toronto, Canada: BC Decker Inc; 1989.
7. Kent RD. *Reference Manual for Communicative Sciences and Disorders: Speech and Language.* Austin, Tex: Pro-Ed, Inc; 1994.
8. Linklater K. *Freeing the Natural Voice.* New York, NY: Drama Book Publishers; 1976.
9. Mathieson L, Baken RJ. *Greene & Mathieson's The Voice and Its Disorders.* 6th ed. London, UK: Whurr Publishers, Ltd; 2001.
10. Richards KB, Fallow MO. *Workbook for the Verbally Apraxic Adult: Reproducibles for Therapy and Home Practice.* Tucson, Ariz: Communication Skill Builders; 1987.
11. Rodenburg P. *The Actor Speaks: Voice and the Performer.* New York, NY: St. Martin's Press; 2000.
12. Smith MC. *The Phonemic Speech Workbook for Dysarthria Therapy.* Tucson, Ariz: Communication Skill Builders; 1986.
13. Stemple JC, Gerdeman BK, Glaze L. *Clinical Voice Pathology: Therapy and Management.* 3rd ed. San Diego, Calif: Singular Publishing Group; 2000.

5

Voice Rest

Robert Thayer Sataloff, Susan E. Cline, Karen M. Lyons, and Adam D. Rubin

All too often, "don't sing" is the unnecessary prescription given to patients for various vocal maladies. "Don't speak" is a less common recommendation, and it is justified even more rarely. Certainly, in many circumstances, voice rest for short periods of time is safe, conservative, and helpful to an ailing performer. Because one can be fairly certain that a prescription of voice rest will not result in injury to the voice, it may also be a comforting course for the laryngologist who is not intimately familiar with the techniques and latitudes of vocal performance demands. It is true that improper voice use under adverse circumstances may result in injury to the vocal folds. However, while canceling concert commitments may not damage a larynx, cancellations may damage seriously a performer's career, especially in the early years of an artist's professional exposure. Consequently, it is helpful for the laryngologist, performer, and teacher to understand various forms of voice rest, as well as the circumstances under which their prescription is reasonable.

Absolute Voice Rest

Absolute voice rest is silence. The singer, actor, or other voice patient is instructed to communicate only with a writing pad or computer. In selected cases in which verbal communication seems essential (eg, a person at home with small children), the use of an electrolarynx may be helpful. Alternatively, common phrases may be recorded and played back as needed. In the past, absolute voice rest was prescribed for conditions ranging from vocal nodules to acute laryngitis. Sometimes it was enforced for 6 weeks or more. This is never appropriate and may cause muscle atrophy and further vocal injury. A recommendation of total silence is

virtually never required for more than approximately 1 week. In fact, some laryngologists no longer require absolute voice rest even after vocal fold surgery. However, following acute vocal fold injury such as a mucosal tear, or a mucosal incision from vocal fold surgery, a short course of absolute voice rest is reasonable to minimize trauma while the mucosa repairs itself.[1] This suggestion is supported further by canine research examining the effects of absolute voice rest (resected recurrent laryngeal nerve) after phonomicrosurgery.[2] Phonomicrosurgery was performed on 20 adult dogs. The recurrent laryngeal nerves of 10 of these dogs were divided simulating iatrogenic voice rest. The remaining 10 dogs were allowed to phonate normally after surgery. The healing process of each group was monitored weekly for the next 12 weeks. The dogs that were forced to rest their voices healed more quickly, with complete reformation of the basement membrane of the vocal folds noted 2 weeks postsurgically and complete rearrangement of the mucosal cover by 8 weeks. Based on these findings, the researchers recommended a 2-week voice rest period following phonomicrosurgery.[2] This somewhat conservative recommendation could be attributed to the fact that the dogs' healing vocal folds were examined only once weekly.

We recommend absolute voice rest until the mucosa has healed. This may take anywhere from 2 days to 7 days. Absolute voice rest is also reasonable following acute vocal fold hemorrhage to minimize local trauma and the chances of recurrent bleeding or unfavorable scarring. These are the only medical conditions that generally call for absolute voice rest; and even in these conditions, its efficacy has not been proven convincingly. Nevertheless, extensive anecdotal experience supports the use of voice rest under these circumstances.

Other possible indications for absolute voice rest exist. Research has shown that a short period of absolute voice rest may help achieve and sustain a longer period of voice improvement for spasmodic dysphonia (SD) patients following Botulinum toxin injection.[3] As outlined in this research, these findings may be linked to the vascular, biomechanical, or biochemical effects of phonation. In other research involving in vivo canine subjects, an increase in blood flow to the muscularis layer of the vocal folds was found during phonation.[4] This vascular change may diminish the effects of Botulinum toxin on the voice of the patient with SD, because it may promote removal of the toxin from the injection site. Further, the muscular contractions associated with phonatory activity may physically redistribute the substance from the target site to surrounding areas. Additionally, the molecular structure of Botulinum toxin (which is affected adversely by shaking and heating) may be physically changed by the vibration and heat associated with vocal fold movement.[3] Often other injections or implantations, such as collagen or fat, are introduced into the lateral aspects of the vocal folds to compensate for nerve paresis or weakness. It is possible that the vascular, biomechanical, and biochemical phonatory effects described above may affect the outcome of these procedures. Hence, the above research suggests that a short voice rest period might also be advisable for these cases.

Patients on absolute voice rest should be aware that whispering may result in vocal fold contact and is not an acceptable alternative to silence or soft verbal communication. A 1989 study examined laryngeal configuration during quiet whispering and stage whispering.[5] During performance of the "low-effort whisper," no subjects exhibited vocal fold contact; whereas 3 of 5 subjects exhibited vocal fold contact during "high-effort whisper" or "stage whisper." The authors noted that subjects intermittently switched between the two modes of whispering without being conscious of their behavior. Additionally, in some cases, the glottis was actually larger during production of the high-effort whisper.

Traditionally, we have not condoned the use of whisper as a form of voice rest due to the probability of excess tension in the extrinsic laryngeal musculature during high-effort whispering, the possibility of patients unknowingly switching whispering "modes," and the likelihood of patients not performing the low-effort whisper in the proper manner.[6] However, we have reexamined this belief recently and are reconsidering the appropriateness of whispering for voice rest in selected patients.[7]

Although otolaryngologists, voice therapists, and singing teachers for years have warned patients that whispering is more traumatic to the vocal folds than normal speech, no sizable series of patients had been examined fiberoptically to test this hypothesis. We evaluated 100 patients during flexible fiberoptic examination. The basic paradigm used to evaluate laryngeal hyperfunction was to look for compression of the supraglottic structures during phonation. If whispering is more harmful to the vocal folds than normal speaking, it seemed reasonable to assume that patients should demonstrate evidence of increased supraglottic hyperfunction and the true vocal fold should make firm contact during whispering. Whispering involves increased airflow in addition to a change in laryngeal resistance. An open channel through the larynx for air escape is necessary to produce a whisper. However, it is conceivable that the glottic opening might be wider during whisper than during normal speech; and despite an apparently unfavorable supraglottic configuration, the true vocal folds still might not touch during whispered speech (although it is not always possible to assess this by fiberoptic examination from above). In the majority of cases, we found that whispering appeared to result in laryngeal configurations that are probably more traumatic to the vocal folds than normal speech. However, in some patients, whispering did not appear to be more traumatic. In fact, in some patients, whispering appeared healthier for the true vocal folds than normal speech. Fourteen of our patients had no true vocal fold contact during whispered speech, and 5 of the 14 showed improved supraglottic configuration (reduced hyperfunction during whispering, compared with habitual speech). An additional 5 patients showed no change in supraglottic appearance. Comparisons with soft speech and "confidential voice" have not been made but are planned for future study. Although we consider our study inconclusive, and we recognize that absence of vocal fold contact does not necessarily ensure absence of vibratory margin trauma (from aerodynamic forces), we are less certain than we used to be that whispering is contraindicated for all patients on voice rest. Further study is recommended.

In addition, playing certain wind instruments is accompanied by significant vocal fold contact. If the patient is a brass or woodwind player, it is best to use a flexible fiberoptic laryngoscope to observe the patient playing the instrument. If vocal fold contact occurs frequently, playing should be restricted during the period of absolute voice rest.

Absolute voice rest also may be used for people who find moderation difficult and are unable to comply with recommendations for relative voice rest. Some people find it easier not to speak at all than to speak infrequently and softly. If a singer is psychologically unable to comply with recommendations for voice conservation, not speaking at all is better than not resting at all.

Relative Voice Rest

Relative voice rest means using the voice only when absolutely necessary and phonating technically well while singing or speaking. In its most restrictive form, it is best summarized by Dr. Norman Punt's admonition: "Don't say a single word for which you are not being paid." Throughout the rest of this chapter, "voice rest" will mean relative voice rest or voice conservation unless "absolute voice rest" is stated specifically.

Voice rest is often a helpful adjunct in the treatment of many voice problems. For example, acute inflammatory or infectious laryngitis involves inflammation of the vocal folds. The redness seen by the laryngologist in examining the larynx is caused by dilated blood vessels. Laryngitis also involves other changes in the mucosal cover layer of the vocal folds and their lubrication. Singing or speaking in the presence of these alterations is accompanied by an increased risk of further injury. Decisions on how much to speak and sing with laryngitis depend on the severity of the illness, the importance and difficulty of vocal commitments, and the experience and proficiency of the vocalist. However, although absolute voice rest is generally not necessary, relative voice rest (to avoid further injury and facilitate healing) is always beneficial. Absolute voice rest is also not the proper treatment for vocal nodules, which are products of voice abuse and misuse. Although silence minimizes abuse temporarily, it is unnecessary; and lesions will return if absolute voice rest is used alone without addressing underlying, causal behaviors. Vocal nodules resolve with proper voice use and should be treated with voice modification and relative voice rest, including avoidance of vocally abusive activities.

Between the extremes of absolute silence and unrestricted voice use, many modifications of vocal behavior are possible. Some techniques are practiced routinely by voice professionals, such as singers; others are utilized less frequently. The few suggestions for relative voice rest presented below should provide the laryngologist with practical and helpful guidelines for his or her professional vocalist patients.

Minimize Voice Use

Although this seems obvious, the importance of speaking or singing only when absolutely necessary cannot be overstressed. This is especially true for the singer or actor with laryngitis who is trying to get through a series of performances. He or she should avoid lengthy telephone conversations. It does not help to call all your friends on the telephone to tell them you have laryngitis! Staying away from school or work environments is helpful occasionally in avoiding the temptation—or necessity, depending on job requirements—to talk in these familiar surroundings. However, in most cases, this activity restriction should not be necessary for a disciplined, committed professional. It is reasonable for the singer or other voice professional to carry a note for his or her friends stating "I have laryngitis," even though the singer knows that limited speech is permissible. We sometimes even suggest wearing a small sign pinned to a lapel (Fig 5–1).

Warm-up Before Voice Use

Even during periods of voice rest, if the voice is used at all for speaking or for singing, a short period of controlled, soft vocal exercises first thing in the morning is invaluable. Even 5 minutes of gentle scales will allow a singer or other professional voice user to analyze, place, and control the voice before using it for speech. Besides improving vocal awareness, the physical benefits of such exercises are analogous to those experienced by runners and other athletes who stretch before exercising.

Avoid Abusive Environments

In addition to staying away from places filled with friends with whom one is tempted to converse, the

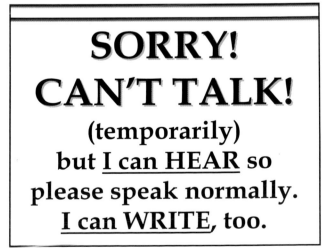

SORRY! CAN'T TALK! (temporarily) but I can HEAR so please speak normally. I can WRITE, too.

Fig 5–1. The authors suggest that voice professionals who are prescribed voice rest wear this sign.

sick voice professional should also try to avoid talking or singing in noisy situations. Cars, airplanes, choirs, parties, bars, and other areas with excessive background noise lead a performer to speak or sing more loudly than desirable. Vocalists should also avoid, as much as possible, environmental irritants such as dry heat, air conditioning, dusty areas (eg, rehearsal rooms undergoing construction), and similarly abusive atmospheres.

Optimize General Health

Dehydration, fatigue, and other general medical conditions may affect the mucosal covering of the vocal folds, alter lubrication, and decrease vocal efficiency. Optimizing the physical conditions that are under the individual's control, such as sleep, hydration, and nutrition, is an important part of any voice conservation regimen.

Do Not Cancel Voice Lessons

The injured voice benefits greatly from supervision. Voice lessons for a person on relative voice rest may consist of only 10 to 15 minutes of supervised vocal exercise, but they help ensure proper placement and vocal technique. This may be especially useful if the vocal malady is associated with an upper respiratory infection and "stuffy ears." Such illnesses impair the performer's ability to hear him- or herself, and feedback from a teacher familiar with the individual's voice may be invaluable. Many singing teachers are also sensitive to their students' use of a speaking voice. An alert teacher may detect deficits in support, breath control, pitch, or other speaking habits that may produce voice fatigue and aggravate laryngeal injury.

In all circumstances singers should speak with the same control and awareness they use in singing; but this is particularly important during periods of illness. When performers must speak during an illness, the assistance of a speech-language pathologist who specializes in voice can be invaluable. An appropriately trained speech-language pathologist can provide information on vocal hygiene, voice conservation, and ways to identify voice abuse/misuse and eliminate them to prevent fatigue or injury, and can help teach singers to apply the same techniques of vocal efficiency in speech that they have learned in singing lessons.

Learn to Mark and Beware of Occult Voice Abuse

Clinical Assessment of Voice[8] discusses various common forms of vocal abuse that accompany choral conducting, cheerleading, voice teaching, singing with electric instruments, singing inappropriate or unfa-

miliar repertoires, and other conditions. Performers also often strain their voices unnecessarily even when they are trying consciously to protect them. "Marking," or modifying a rehearsal to conserve the voice, is a skill that is frequently neglected in routine voice teaching. A few particularly common errors are worth stressing. Many singers are under the mistaken impression that learning music (or "marking a rehearsal") by whistling is restful to the larynx. In fact, whistling is accompanied by vocal fold abduction and adduction and may include vocal fold contact. It is not a good form of voice rest. Furthermore, unconscious of his or her vocal activity while whistling, a singer is likely not to support the activity as he or she would while singing.

Even merely listening or silently reading along with one's vocal lines during a rehearsal can be abusive in some people. Subvocalizing is common among readers, especially when they are reading musical vocal lines. Subvocalization may also occur when reading novels and even when listening to emotionally charged dramatic material, such as at movies or theatrical productions. There are several ways a singer can determine whether he or she subvocalizes. Subvocalization can be observed in some people with a fiberoptic laryngoscope, but a visit to one's laryngologist for this diagnosis is usually not necessary. If a singer finds that his or her neck muscles are tight and the throat is tired at the end of a session of silent reading or listening, or if his or her reading speed decreases when he or she tries to read and hum a steady tone simultaneously, subvocalization should be suspected. Activities associated with this occult and unsupervised vocal activity should be avoided, especially during periods of voice rest.

In a well-trained singer, marking is often accomplished best simply by singing reasonably softly in his or her normal voice, avoiding notes at both extremes of vocal range, and singing only essential portions of a rehearsal. Special care should be taken to practice good support technique, even when singing softly and low in the singer's vocal range. Because singers mark in the "easy" part of their voices, and because they are singing softly and trying to rest, there is a great temptation to rest abdominal and thoracic muscles as well. This is dangerous to vocal health. Proper marking requires technique as meticulously good as that practiced during unrestricted singing.

Cancel Nonessential Commitments

Singers and actors are steeped in the "show must go on" philosophy. However, when a vocal illness requires voice rest, the performer must exercise professional judgment in evaluating the risks and benefits of any commitment. Frequently, canceling rehearsals is necessary in order to allow safe performances later in the week. Occasionally, when laryngeal inflammation is severe, and when difficult performance material cannot be modified, it may even be necessary to cancel an important concert, play, or speaking engagement. Although this form of voice rest always feels like a disaster at the moment, the professional voice user must remember that his or her responsibility is to preserve the instrument in optimal health for as many years as possible. Risking a severe vocal injury is rarely justified.

For professional singers, voice rest is more complicated than simply keeping quiet. Like singing and speaking, voice rest is a vocal skill that should be understood by both the physician and patient, mastered, and used judiciously. The most important time during periods of absolute voice rest and relative voice rest is when the patient begins using his or her voice again. Patients also must be forewarned that abusing or misusing the voice after vocal fold surgery, vocal fold hemorrhage, laryngitis, or any other precursor to a prescription of vocal rest is detrimental to proper healing.

We suggest that a certified speech-language pathologist work with the laryngologist to determine candidacy for voice surgery. If the patient has not yet mastered techniques taught in voice therapy prior to surgery, then he or she may be prone to voice abuse and misuse after surgery and not enjoy optimal results. Using a protective, tentative voicing after insult to the mucosa is also deleterious to vocal fold healing, because it produces excess tension in the laryngeal musculature and may increase the risk of vocal fold scarring.[6] In our practice, a speech-language pathologist is responsible for taking patients off voice rest, as well. To take the burden off the vocal folds and hasten the healing process, patients should be trained in resonant voice therapy. Use of properly supported "confidential voice" may be helpful in some patients. In our experience and in the opinions of other authors,[7,8] a preventive, vocal health education program by a team of voice professionals is essential for the professional voice user.

Hidden Consequences of Voice Rest

We noted earlier that injudicious prescription of voice rest may damage seriously a performer's career and reputation. This is especially true early in a professional career when cancellation of a concert may mean missing a career-making break. When deciding whether to cancel a performance, a careful risks-benefit analysis should be made. The consequences of cancellation for the performer may be apparent or subtle;

consequences for the physician may be even less obvious. When a physician is uncertain regarding proper treatment recommendations, a prescription of voice rest may seem to the laryngologist to be the most conservative course of action. Clearly, a physician's first responsibility is to the individual patient. Nevertheless, it must be remembered that the physician accepts enormous responsibility and liability when deciding to cancel a performance. For example, the author (RTS) cared for a premier rock singer on world tour. The performer's medical problems necessitated cancellation of two performances during 1 week of a 12-month world tour. As a consequence, the singer's insurance company paid $250,000.00 for each concert, and substantial additional economic repercussions occurred due to loss of fees associated with rental of the sports stadium where the concert was to take place, monies for concessionaires, city police, parking attendants, cable television recording commitments, and other factors. Fortuitously, we had strobovideolaryngoscopic and objective voice laboratory documentation to substantiate the necessity for the voice prescription. Otherwise, it could have been difficult to defend.

References

1. Hoover CA, Sataloff RT, Lyons KM, Hawkshaw M. Vocal fold mucosal tears: maintaining a high clinical index of suspicion. *J Voice*. 2001;15:451–455.
2. Cho SH, Kim HT, Lee IJ, et al. Influence of phonation on basement membrane zone recovery after phonomicrosurgery: a canine model. *Ann Otol Rhinol Laryngol*. 2000;109:658–666.
3. Wong DLH, Adams SG, Irish JC, et al. Effect of neuromuscular activity on the response to botulinum toxin injections in spasmodic dysphonia. *J Otolaryngol*. 1995;24(4):209–221.
4. Arnstein DP, Berke GS, Trapp TK, Natividad M. Regional blood flow to the canine vocal fold at rest and during phonation. *Ann Otol Rhinol Laryngol*. 1989;98:796–802.
5. Solomon NP, McCall GN, Trosset MW, Gray WC. Laryngeal configuration and constriction during two types of whispering. *J Speech Hear Res*. 1989;32:161–174.
6. Emerich KA, Spiegel JR, Sataloff RT. Phonomicrosurgery III: pre- and post-operative care. *Otolaryngol Clin North Am*. 2000;33:1071–1080.
7. Broaddus-Lawrence PL, Treole K, McCabe RB, et al. The effects of preventive vocal hygiene education on the vocal hygiene habits and perceptual vocal characteristics of training singers. *J Voice*. 2000;14:58–71.
8. Sataloff RT, Anticaglia J, Hawkshaw MJ. Patient history. In: Sataloff RT. *Clinical Assessment of Voice*. San Diego, Calif: Plural Publishing, Inc; 2005:1–16.
9. Murray T, Rosen CA. Vocal education for the professional voice user and singer. *Otolaryngol Clin North Am*. 2000;33:967–981.

6

Increasing Vocal Effectiveness

Bonnie N. Raphael and Robert Thayer Sataloff

Preparation for Oral Presentations

Physicians, speech-language pathologists, teachers, students, executives, and people in most walks of life are called on at some time or another to speak in public. Few people are naturally skilled, organized, comfortable public speakers. Most people are somewhat uncomfortable about speaking in public, some are terrified, and nearly all make less than optimal use of their vocal and dramatic skills without some instruction and preparation. Although this book is not intended as a text to teach singing, conversational speech, or public speaking, we have included it in this text, because speaking before a group of people is a common concern for most of our readers.

Modifications facilitating greater vocal effectiveness go far beyond vocal adjustments. For example, many vocal stresses can be lessened by eliminating psychological stress, by understanding room acoustics, by organizing material to be presented, and by acquiring other basic presentational techniques. This chapter describes our basic initial approach to training someone such as a physician to present a paper or lecture. Although it includes some basic vocal exercises, they are no substitute for formal training with a speech-language pathologist, a singing or speech teacher, or an acting coach. This chapter also includes descriptions of some physical and vocal warm-up exercises used by actors. Such exercises may be regarded as superfluous by the physician, but professional performers have found them extremely helpful in many different performance situations. Appropriate preparation helps to make a speaker appear more relaxed, effective, and well-focused. Such preparation is also invaluable for controlling performance anxiety. Most outstanding speakers do, in fact, work hard to acquire basic communication skills that make their presenta-

tions appear natural and unrehearsed. All too often, intelligent and well-intentioned speakers will spend considerable time in preparing the content of upcoming presentations but will spend virtually no time preparing themselves for the most effective spoken presentation of their research or position papers. Content that is interesting, valuable to the listeners, and important to the profession is too often lost or shortchanged because of ineffective presentation. Far too many speakers present what they have to say in a way that makes it either too difficult to grasp or too dull to have a favorable impact on a listening audience. This chapter outlines a methodical procedure through which oral presentations can be more effectively prepared. Furthermore, there are a number of useful texts available to supplement the material presented in this chapter.[1-4]

Preparation of Written Materials

Ideally, the research should be completed and all materials to be presented should be available to the speaker no later than 1 month before the date of the presentation. This allows the speaker sufficient time to get the presentation into a form best suited to communicate the chief features of the research. Approximately 1 month before presentation, the speaker should write out as many drafts of the presentation as are necessary, until it expresses orally what he or she wishes to say in the clearest and most effective manner possible. Rather than simply reading from the same text submitted for publication, the speaker would do better to substitute words that are easier on the tongue and to use grammatical structure that is easier on the listener's ear. Sentences should be shorter and more concise for listeners than they might be for readers. The speaker should check the effectiveness of the presentation by reading the speech aloud a number of times, making certain that it fits easily into the time allotment assigned and it is stylistically suited to the particular audience to be addressed. Effective speakers will prepare two drafts of a given presentation at this stage: one to meet the needs of the oral presentation and another that meets the needs of publication.

If the speaker is more experienced or more comfortable working in a somewhat but not totally structured manner, then he or she may decide to work from note cards or a simple outline of the presentation. Less experienced presenters or those dealing with a large amount of information that needs to be precisely stated may prefer to work from a written text of the speech. Even this written text, however, can be prepared in such a way that it does not intrude between the speaker and the audience.

One way in which the written presentation can be moved toward effective oral performance is via a structural rewriting of the speech. In a structural rewriting, the way in which the speech appears on the page to the reader's eye is the way he or she wishes to phrase it when reading it aloud. Use of a structurally rewritten text is particularly important to presenters for whom English is not their native language and to presenters inexperienced in formal speaking before large audiences. A structural version of a speech makes phrasing and pausing at appropriate intervals far easier for the speaker, because it replaces arbitrary margin settings with functional form. To better understand how this works, read aloud both versions of the Gettysburg Address shown in Figures 6–1 and 6–2. Most readers will find that, with virtually no preparation, the second rendering of the same written material (Fig 6–2) is far easier to deliver than the first; because, in the second version, the eyes see the text in the very phrases that the mouth will utter.

Just through this simple demonstration the reader should be able to see the benefits of creating and rehearsing with a structured rendition of the presentation. The Gettysburg Address was, in fact, written as a speech rather than an essay. Presenters who are both rewriting materials for oral presentation and restructuring their texts for more effective reading will find this technique of even greater value when dealing with materials that are more technical and less poetically phrased than this memorable address.

After creating the structural rendition of the presentation, the presenter can then spend the next week or so continuing the preparation process in one of two ways:

1. The speech can be read aloud twice a day from the structural script until the phrasing and pausing seem very natural and comfortable to the presenter; or
2. The presenter can tape-record the speech after just a few readings through of the structural script. This way, if rehearsal time is severely limited but commuting time to work or meetings is not, the tape can be played in a car, train, or airplane until it is virtually memorized as a result of the repeated listening.

If the presenter wishes to work from a written text of the speech but, because of excessive length, the structural version of it seems to involve too many pages, then it can be retyped into manuscript form, but with the following modifications:

1. The text should be double or triple spaced between lines.
2. The text should not extend lower than two inches from the bottom of any page, so that, if the podium has a "lip" to it, no lines are lost from view.
3. No sentence should begin on the bottom of one page and conclude on the top of the next page.
4. The speaker may choose to have the text of the speech photocopied in a way that the type is enlarged or darkened in the duplication process and, therefore, easier to read.
5. The text should be enclosed in some kind of cover or loose-leaf binder with the pages consecutively numbered, so that it is easier to handle and keep under control in the days preceding delivery of the paper and while traveling to the performance site. However, the pages should be loose rather than bound or stapled during the presentation. This allows the speaker to slide pages quietly during the talk.

If the speaker prefers to work from an outline or a series of note cards, then these can be prepared in a similar manner.

Audiovisual Materials

The decision as to whether to use audiovisual aids and the specific aids selected will depend on the speaker's style, on the size of the room in which the presentation will be made, and on the subject matter. An exhaustive review of audiovisual devices to assist presentations is beyond the scope of this chapter. However, a few principles and suggestions warrant inclusion. Visual aids are used much more commonly than audio aids. The two most common types of visual aids are handouts and slides.

The Gettysburg Address

by: Abraham Lincoln

Fourscore and seven years ago our fathers brought forth on this continent a new nation, conceived in Liberty and dedicated to the proposition that all men are created equal.

Now we are engaged in a great civil war, testing whether that nation, or any nation so conceived and so dedicated, can long endure. We are met on a great battlefield of that war. We have come to dedicate a portion of that field, as a final resting-place for those who here gave their lives that this nation might live. It is altogether fitting proper that we should do this.

But, in a large sense, we cannot dedicate—we cannot consecrate—we cannot hallow this ground. The brave men, living and dead, who struggled here, have consecrated it far above our poor power to add or detract. The world will little note nor long remember what we say here, but it can never forget what they did here. It is for us, the living, rather, to be dedicated here to the unfinished work which they who fought here have thus far so nobly advanced. It is rather for us to be here dedicated to the great task remaining before us—that from these honored dead we take increased devotion to that cause for which they gave the last full measure of devotion—that we here highly resolve that these dead shall not have died in vain—that this nation, under God, shall have a new birth of freedom—and that government of the people, by the people, for the people, shall not perish from the earth.

Fig 6–1. The Gettysburg Address presented in an unstructured format.

The Gettysburg Address

by: Abraham Lincoln

Fourscore and seven years ago

    our fathers brought forth on this continent

        a new <u>nation,</u> conceived in liberty,

            and dedicated to the proposition that <u>all men are created equal.</u>

Now we are engaged in a great civil war,

    testing whether that nation,

        or <u>any</u> nation so conceived and so dedicated,

            can long endure.

    We are met on a great battlefield of that war.

    We have come to dedicate a portion of that field, as a final resting-place

        for those who here gave their lives that this nation might live.

    It is altogether fitting proper that we should do this.

But, in a large sense, we cannot dedicate—we cannot <u>consecrate,</u>

    we cannot hallow this ground.

The brave men, living and dead, who struggled here,

    have consecrated it far above our poor power to add or detract.

The world will little note nor long remember what we <u>say</u> here,

    but it can never forget what they <u>did</u> here.

    It is for us, the living, rather,

        to be dedicated here to the unfinished work

            which they who fought here have thus far so nobly

            advanced.

    It is rather for us to be here dedicated to the great task remaining before us

        — that from these honored dead we take increased devotion

            to that cause for which they gave

                the last full measure of devotion—

that we here highly resolve

    that these dead shall not have died in vain—

that this nation, under God, shall have a new birth of freedom—

and that government of the people, by the people, for the people,

    shall not perish from the earth.

Fig 6–2. The Gettysburgh Address structurally rendered for speaking.

Handouts

Handouts vary from a brief outline of the material presented to a word-for-word transcription of the talk. They may include a bibliography of sources that amplify the material presented. All handouts should have a definite purpose. That purpose will determine the time of distribution, the length of the handout, and the size of the print. In general, if the speaker intends to refer to the handouts during the presentation, they should be prepared in large, bold type that can be read in dim light. Pages should be numbered, and each item should be marked for easy reference. Naturally, under these circumstances, handouts should be distributed prior to the presentation. It is often helpful to have figures in the handouts duplicated on slides for the speaker's use.

If the handouts will not be referred to, they will only distract the listener's attention away from the presentation. Under such circumstances, the handouts should be distributed after the presentation. This is also advisable when the handouts duplicate the speech. If handouts are distributed in advance by the host of a conference and a speaker wishes to prevent them from distracting his audience, then he or she should direct the room lights to be turned all the way down, so that the audience cannot see the handouts. This nullifies their potentially distracting effect and encourages the audience to focus its attention on the speaker. It is often helpful to supplement brief outlines with suggested readings. All handouts should include the speaker's name and address, so that listeners can write for additional advice, information, or to invite the speaker for future presentations.

Slides

Slide projectors are available in most lecture halls, and slides can be easily stored, transported, and seen when properly prepared. A well-organized slide lecture highlights important concepts for the audience, serves as an outline to the speaker, and projects figures important to the talk. Each slide projected should have a specific purpose. In general, a speaker can rarely use effectively more than approximately one slide per minute.

Slides should be prepared in bold type and are unusually unreadable if they exceed six lines. Limiting each slide to four or five lines is recommended. As a rule of thumb, it should be possible for the speaker to read each slide held toward a room light at arm's length. If this is not possible, the slide will generally not project well in a large hall. In addition to being easy to read, slides generally should be easy to look at. Diazos, the standard white-on-blue slides, can be made inexpensively and are much easier on the eye than is typed print on a white background. Computer-generated slides are also relatively easy and inexpensive if the speaker has access to the necessary hardware and software. Slides should always be numbered, so that, if a slide tray is spilled at the last moment, the lecture can be reorganized. It is also advisable for the speaker to put his or her name on each side, especially when the speaker does not use his or her own carousel. Whenever possible, the speaker should bring the slides already inserted in the carousel and checked in advance for order and position. In this case, the speaker's name should appear on the outside of the carousel. It is important to inquire in advance as to whether a standard carousel projector is available and whether front projection or rear projection will be used. In rear projection, the slides must be turned around from their usual position. When one is traveling, slides should always be carried with the speaker, not checked through airplane, ship, or train luggage. This is true for any important visual or auditory aid.

In some cases, dual projection (use of two projectors at the same time) may be desirable. When needed, both sets of slides should be numbered, so that the projectors can be easily coordinated (for example, slide 1A in one projector, and 1B in the second projector). If slides will be shown on only one projector during the middle of the talk, it is advisable to match them with blank slides in the second projector. Keeping the same number of slides in both projectors decreases the risk of losing synchronization between the two projectors.

Transparencies

In general, traditional transparencies are not as good as slides. They may work fairly well in a small classroom, but in large halls they are difficult to see and frequently look as if they have been made just moments before the lecture. If a speaker wishes to use transparencies to draw a figure and show the development of a concept or design, this can be done equally well (usually better) by a sequence of prepared slides. Traditional transparencies are not significantly easier to make or cheaper than well-prepared slides. If used, it is best to prepare transparencies in advance. Transparences can now be generated on a computer and printed onto a transparent template so that they are easy to read and look quite attractive; and they are an acceptable option especially if the lecture space is not too large.

Videotape

Videotape has become extremely popular and is a fine teaching tool. To be effective in a public presentation, it must be well-made, neatly edited, and self-sufficient. It is undesirable for the speaker to have to talk over the video in order for its message to be understood. In addition, there must be enough high-quality monitors in the auditorium to allow easy viewing by everyone in the audience. If the subject of the videotape is highly detailed, as may occur with microsurgery or histologic slides, numerous high-quality monitors often provide better resolution than projection video, and front projection usually provides better resolution than rear projection. It is important to be certain that the speaker's video format is compatible with the auditorium's equipment. This is a special concern if the speaker is presenting in a foreign country.

Film

With the advent of videotape, 16 mm sound movie projection has become less popular. However, this medium still provides excellent audio and video reproduction, and it may be preferable in some cases. Movie projection is especially useful if the speaker is required to use one central screen in a large room.

Computers

Computer-assisted presentations have become popular, for good reason. Using programs such as Power-Point (Microsoft-Redmond, Washington) it is possible to customize presentations, change the order and content of slides rapidly, integrate video seamlessly into a lecture, and utilize special effects (such as fade-in and fade-out slide changes). Many lecture sites do not have computers and projectors available; and sometimes those that do do not have all computer formats available. So, equipment availability must be checked in advance, and it is often best for the lecturer to bring his or her own computer. Even most venues that do have equipment provide only one computer and projector; so, dual projection (side-by-side) of computer presentations is not available readily, yet. Nevertheless, computer-assisted presentations can be elegant and convenient, as long as all the equipment necessary is available and functions well.

If computer presentations are utilized, the speaker should be certain to boot up the computer prior to starting the presentation. It is not good to waste the first 2 or 3 minutes of a 10-minute presentation trying to get the information to appear on the screen!

One other advantage of computer presentations is the presence of a laptop screen in front of the speaker. This allows the speaker to see the information that is being projected to the audience without having to turn to look at the screen in the front of the room. Howev-

er, this arrangement can also work against the speaker. Care must be taken not to spend too much time looking at the screen and keyboard, at the expense of eye contact with the audience. At present, computer presentations generally tie the speaker to the podium, because it is necessary to touch the computer keyboard to change slides. For speakers who prefer to move about the stage with a remote control slide changer, this can be problematic. It is likely that technological advances will solve this problem soon.

Pointers

Pointers are designed to direct the attention of the audience to specific items on the visual aids. If a mechanical pointer is being used, it is imperative to be sure it is long enough to reach the top of the projected images and that the microphone and slide controls are long enough to allow the speaker to get close enough to the screen to point. When using electrically lit pointers, the arrow should be focused in advance of the presentations; and the speaker should make sure that the pointer is bright enough to be seen from the back of the room. Laser pointers are now used most commonly. They, too, should be checked for visibility. In any case, pointers should be used only for their intended purpose. The speaker must avoid the tendency to tap mechanical pointers, or flash electric or laser pointers randomly. These gestures are distracting and diminish the effect of the pointers when they are used appropriately at other times during the lecture.

Audiotapes

Talks often are enhanced by the playing of audiotapes, bur effective audio reproduction requires as much thought, planning, and equipment as videotape or film. Generally, playing an audio sample from a pocket cassette recorder through a podium microphone is ineffective. Such demonstrations are usually difficult to hear and understand, the sound is distorted, and they appear improvised. If audio samples are important to a talk, arrangements should be made in advance for high-quality audio playback equipment. The tapes should be cued for the sound engineer, and short leaders of known time duration should be placed between audio samples. If it will be necessary to turn tapes on and off several times during the presentation, it is helpful to put an audio signal (such as beep) at the end of each sample, so that the sound engineer will know when to turn the tape off. The next sample should come approximately 10 seconds after the beep, allowing adequate time for the sound engineer to react and turn the tape recorder off, and for the tape recorder to be turned on and resume steady speed before the next example is heard. Either cassettes or reel-to-reel tapes may be used, but reel tapes can be repaired and played again more easily if they are damaged during the presentation. It is advisable to bring a backup copy and to bring both formats if equipment arrangements have not been confirmed.

Warm-up and Preparatory Exercises

Approximately 1 month before the presentation, effective presenters will begin an exercise regimen to get the voice primed for performance. A simple developmental warm-up done on a regular basis (every day for at least 3 weeks before performance) will get body alignment, breathing, and voice in condition to present research and opinion in the manner they deserve. Use of such a warm-up can make the difference between a bland, forgettable rendering of a presentation and a dynamic delivery of the materials in a way that will more than do them justice.

The following series of exercises is divided into four parts. It is important that they are done regularly. Doing them all with attention to the sensations experienced as they are done will produce the most noticeable results. These exercises are very helpful if done correctly, but they may be difficult to master from written descriptions alone. Speakers interested in perfecting these skills will benefit from a few sessions with a performance coach or from a public speaking workshop such as those offered by Executive Performance in Training Centers.[5] If pressed for time, the presenter should select and do at least one exercise in each of the four categories. As they are done, it is important to make them enjoyable rather than hard work.

I. General Relaxation and Energizing

The first category of exercises can serve to relax a speaker on days he or she is feeling tight or tense and to energize a speaker on days he or she is feeling weary or spent. If the speaker will take a moment to scan the body to ascertain physical and psychological state, then he or she will know best which exercises need to be emphasized and how much time to spend with each.

A. Full-body yawns, physically stretching out in all directions. Loosen belt and/or tie if necessary to give the stretches full excursion. Yawns should be genuine and not mere tokens.

B. Gentle shaking in many different areas of the body to loosen tension or to energize: hands, arms, shoulders, legs, small of the back, and so on. (Some individuals prefer energetic dancing to music, jumping rope, yoga, or stair climbing).

II. Breathing and Alignment

If there are any back problems that restrict flexibility or make certain movements uncomfortable, the exercises below can and should be modified accordingly.

A. Breathe out easily on a voiceless sigh and then simply soften the belly to initiate effortless inhalation without any shoulder involvement. Allow the air out again easily and completely but without postural collapse. This can be done on just breath or with full sound (haaaaaaaahhhhhhh). Repeat slowly and enjoyably a half-dozen times and notice the calming and energizing effect.

B. Place the palms of the hands on the rib cage (without tensing the shoulders in order to do so) to encourage rib flexibility during inhalation and exhalation. During inhalation, allow the ribs to move out in the direction of the palms of the hands. During exhalation, use the palms of the hands to encourage the ribs to move back in, but without any postural collapse in the spine. Repeat slowly four to five times, then drop the arms and shoulders heavily at the sides and enjoy the free movement of the rib cage when not inhibited by the pressure of the hands.

C. Slowly roll down through the spine, leading with the head and relaxing over with knees slightly bent, going only as far down as is comfortable. Slowly and comfortably, "rebuild" the spinal column, initiating the upward movement by pressing the soles of the feet into the floor and releasing the legs out of the hip joints, making sure that the head is the last thing to be added to the upright spinal column. Repeat three to four times until the body fully appreciates the connection between the feet and the head and moves as one connected and coordinated unit with no sharp division. Use full breaths to help maintain the sensation of internal space.

III. Top Quarter of the Body

A. Intertwine the fingers of both hands and place them on the back of the skull. Without tensing the shoulders or holding the breath, pull forward with the elbows and back with the head steadily for about 20 to 30 seconds. Release the isometric pull and enjoy the freedom that results in the cervical area of the spine.

B. With hands on shoulders, and while breathing freely, allow elbows to touch in front and to approach each other in back. Repeat until the muscles facilitating this activity fatigue just a bit. With hands on shoulders, "flap your wings" slowly until the muscles involved fatigue slightly. With hands on shoulders, allow elbows to make large, full circles first forward and then backward until muscles fatigue. Lift and drop shoulders easily in a shrug until muscles fatigue somewhat. Notice any changes that may occur in your ability to breathe freely as a result of this shoulder loosening.

C. Stand tall through the spine with shoulders relaxed and spread. Reach your right hand across the chest to your left shoulder and firmly massage the band of muscles that extends from the shoulder to the base of the neck. If any knots are present, gently knead them and coax the tension to melt away, helping with free and easy breathing throughout. Repeat this activity on the other side.

D. With your face continuing to remain forward instead of facing either shoulder, use a slow, even count of 16 to complete one full head roll to the right, enjoying an easy relaxing stretch in each direction through which the head passes as it makes a single rotation. Reverse, making a full, slow rotation to the left. This can be repeated a few times, keeping the rolls slow and easy and the breath moving throughout.

E. With the heels of the hands, use even, steady pressure right in front of the ears as you make big circles releasing and relaxing the jaw on both sides. If the urge to yawn occurs, so much the better. Allow the hands to slide down the jaw on both sides, toward the chin, easing the jaw down as they do so. Yawn again to feel the deep relaxation. Use the thumbs on either side of the face, in the vicinity of the molars, to locate and firmly press into the masseter muscles. Continue the pressure while breathing deeply for about 30 seconds before releasing the thumbs and enjoying the freedom and release in the jaw itself. (This exercise can be repeated anytime during the day when the jaw is feeling held and tight.)

F. Move the tongue around in the mouth to loosen up. Use it to count the teeth, or stick it out in the direction of the nose, then the right ear, then the chin, and then the left ear. With a loose, relaxed jaw, move just the tongue from top lip to bottom lip to top lip to bottom lip as you say or sing, la-la-la-la-la-la-lala-la-laaaahhhh.

G. Move the different parts of the face around slowly and quickly. Stand in front of a mirror, if necessary, to make sure that movement is actually taking place: eyebrows, eyes, bridge of nose, nostrils, cheeks, lips. See whether you can appear very surprised, very happy, very angry. Repeat these manipulations easily, without holding the breath, until the muscles being used are a bit fatigued.

IV. Voice and Speech

A. Drop the jaw, take a breath, and release a long sigh, which starts high and finishes low in the pitch range (haaaaaahhhh). Repeat three to four times, each time starting just a bit higher in pitch and finishing a bit lower without allowing the voice to either screech or growl. Explore the full extent of available range.

B. Use the fingers to rub and stimulate the face gently. Unfurrow the brow and relax the jaw. With the hands gently covering the cheeks and eyes and the lips touching, hum directly into the palms of the hands, feeling and enjoying the vibrations produced by the voice. Allow the pitches to move up and down while continuing to rub the face and hum. Then drop the hands and feel the vibrations in the bones of the face and skull instead of the palms of the hands as the humming continues.

C. With the jaw relaxed (mouth open) and the tip of the tongue gently tucked behind the bottom front teeth, raise and lower the back of the tongue in order to move easily from "ng" (as in sing) to "aaaahhhhh," keeping the focus of the sound forward. This combination can be either spoken or sung, but primary vibration of sound should ideally move from the nose to the mouth as the sounds alternate. Repeat enough times to make this comfortable.

D. Use full and steady breath from the midsection as you call out easily on full voice: "Hey, Joe! O.K.! Hello! How are you?"

E. Use a combination of different tongue twisters to help train the articulations to move more efficiently: red leather, yellow leather, blue leather, nuclear regulatory commission; blue-backed blackbird; delectable delicacy, and so on. (A number of bookstores carry collections of enjoyable tongue twisters. Some children's books [eg, the Dr. Seuss series] are quite useful in this regard as well.)

The more often these exercises are done attentively, the easier they become. They are representative of a far greater range of warm-up and developmental exercises available to the presenter who wishes to build the voice into an effective and expressive communication tool.

Final Rehearsal and Presentation

Approximately 2 weeks before performance, the opening sentence, the closing sentence, and any key ideas or quotations that would benefit from direct eye contact with the audience should be memorized.

The speech should be rehearsed at least once a day until the presenter is very familiar and comfortable with its contents, its structure, and any accompanying visual materials to be included.

If possible in the final week of presentation, the presentation should be rehearsed with a podium, at a microphone, and/or to a camera. The more the presenter can simulate the actual conditions under which the speech will be delivered, the fewer surprises will occur when the speech actually takes place. If someone can videotape a performance of the presentation, the presenter can use it to make any necessary corrections or adjustments in either content or style.

About 1 week before the presentation, the speaker should add two important exercises to the warm-up regimen:

1. *Visualization.* Sit or lie down, do some deep breathing to relax your muscles, and focus your concentration; then imagine you are watching yourself giving the presentation perfectly—without a hitch from beginning to end. Include details, colors, emotions throughout; take your time. Get into the habit of envisioning it perfectly done so that the actual performance is a simple, direct repetition of a task already mastered.

2. *Directing Energy.* People who suffer "stage fright" often describe a sensation of self-consciousness. All those eyes focused right on the speaker can be intimidating if the presenter does not know how to direct that energy. As the speaker continues to practice the presentation, he or she should imagine the audience as a large slice of pie, which can be divided into six different sections. No matter how large an audience may be, it may help the speaker to remember that each person seated in that audience is only one human being. Instead of speaking to an undefined mass of faces, the speaker can think of presenting to a series of individuals seated in different locations throughout the audience. Figures 6–3 and 6–4 indicate possible movement sequences for eye contact. If the speaker allows his or her gaze to linger with a specific individual for the length of a sentence or two and then to travel from section one to section two and so forth during transitions, then these individuals feel themselves an important part of the event rather than merely present. Any speaker who learns to make genuine rather than token eye contact with specific individuals in each section of the audience invites participation and interest in the presentation; he or she succeeds in making those present actual participants in the event. An act of communication demands not only a sender but an implied or actual recipient of the message.

Be sure to talk to rather than at your listener(s). Stage fright and self-consciousness can be dramatically lessened if and when the speaker shifts attention away from the self and to the members of the audience. If the speaker gives full attention to receivers (Are they paying attention? Are they understanding what I am saying? Do they need me to repeat that statement or to slow down a bit? Am I loud enough for

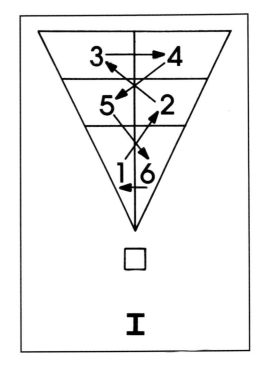

Fig 6–3. Practiced, planned patterns of eye contact help ensure that members of the audience will feel as if they are being spoken to personally. This figure contains one suggested eye-contact pattern that is particularly well-suited to relatively narrow and/or deep auditoriums.

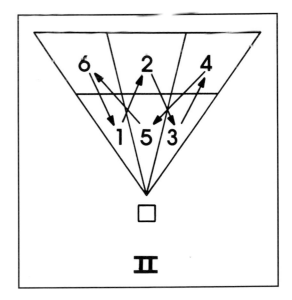

Fig 6–4. This alternate pattern of eye contact may be better suited in a shallow and/or wide auditorium than that illustrated in Fig 6–3.

the people in the back?), the focus of attention shifts from the self to them, and the task of communicating is that much more enjoyable.

During this final stage of rehearsal, a room of decent size should be used, in which should be placed three or four individual listeners, each sitting in a different section. After the presentation, the speaker can check with each listener to make sure he or she felt as though all present were being talked to rather than at. In the absence of cooperative helpers, the speaker can place specific objects in different locations in the room (a trash bin, a coffee mug on a seat, a sweater over another chair, etc) and make sure really to speak to each object in turn.

Reading the Room

It is extremely helpful for any speaker to assess the room or hall prior to speaking. While this may not be quite so critical for the physician presenting research results through a microphone as it is for a singer presenting an unamplified recital, the comfort gained from the mistakes avoided is comparable. Whenever possible, the speaker should inspect the room before presenting: during coffee break or lunch break or on a previous day. Any inconvenience is worth the effort. If this inspection is absolutely impossible, the speaker may gain some of the necessary information by observing and listening to the earlier presenters.

In assessing a room, the speaker should investigate acoustics (Can speakers be heard well from all portions of the room?), type of microphones available, room temperature, availability of water, lighting on the podium, availability of a pointer, placement of slide or film projector controls, number and position of stairs leading to the stage, location of the nearest bathroom for possible use shortly before presentation, presence and quality of projectors, type of projection (front versus rear screen), location and operation of lighting controls, and presence or absence of a stage manager and projectionist. Familiarizing oneself with these matters can prevent numerous embarrassing moments. If the presentation is long and there is no water available, the speaker can place a glass of water under the podium before the audience arrives. If a fixed microphone is used, the speaker must be prepared to maintain a reasonably constant mouth-to-microphone distance and direction. With fixed microphones (such as those attached to the podium), the microphone needs to be adjusted immediately prior to the speech. It should be approximately at chin level (no higher) and should be no more than 4 to 6 inches away from the speaker's face. Whenever possible, it should be tested prior to the arrival of the audience.

If a lavaliere microphone is used, the speaker must remember not to brush the microphone cord by putting his or her hands into pockets and not to brush papers across the microphone. If a wireless microphone is used, the speaker should be certain to turn it off at the end of the presentation. There are many stories, humorous to everyone except the speaker, of presenters who have left microphones on during bathroom breaks or exceedingly frank conversations about previous speakers or hosts of the event. Many high-quality wireless microphones work well even through the walls!

If a stage manager or projectionist is provided, the speaker should introduce him or herself ahead of time. These colleagues can greatly facilitate the smooth flow of the performance. They are used to being ignored by most speakers. However, they deserve and generally appreciate a little recognition. Taking a few moments prior to the presentation to discuss one's needs or at least shake hands is worthwhile.

Occasionally, disasters occur. Some of them can be anticipated. For example, the author (RTS) depends heavily on slides for many presentations. Consequently, he generally travels with a carousel replacement bulb and pointer; sometimes with a remote slide changer; and with a projector when speaking in a nonacademic building where audiovisual arrangements are questionable. However, any speaker should be prepared, in the event of major problems, to proceed with no amplification or visual aids at all.

Room temperature can also be a potent detriment to good delivery. If the air conditioning is turned up so high that the speaker is shivering, the audience will perceive this as nervousness. Identifying this problem in advance allows the speaker to dress appropriately and/or have the room temperature adjusted. At the opposite extreme, a room that is too hot or stuffy can make the audience uncomfortable enough to lessen the effectiveness of even the best speaker; adequate ventilation may make all the difference to his or her success.

Delivering the Speech

On the day of the performance, the speaker should make sure he or she is rested and physically comfortable. Shoes should be comfortable, breathing should not be restricted by either belt or collar, and even new clothing should have been tested in advance to ensure that the speaker will be comfortable performing whatever range of movement is called for during the presentation. Time should be allowed for a concentrated, uninterrupted warm-up and a visualization of the presentation perfectly performed. The speaker should make sure not to overeat before speaking and should drink enough water to maintain a good level of hydration without unduly taxing the bladder in the process.

If there are a series of speakers in one program and/or the introduction is lengthy, there are some "hidden" warm-up activities that can be done in the interim: easy, gentle head and neck movement; small sips of water; moving tongue easily around the mouth; releasing the jaw with lips closed; deep, easy breathing through the nose into the midsection of the body; finding supportive friends in the audience.

Finally, there is a "trick" that a number of successful speakers use to increase their degree of comfort during a presentation. They think of someone who loves their work, who thinks they can do no wrong; who is an ardent fan; and, in their imaginations, they bring this friend right into the audience they are about to address. It can be a young son, a grandmother who is no longer alive, or even a family dog. The speaker can just place this admirer in the audience and allow unqualified approval to inspire a confidence and ease that might otherwise be elusive.

During the presentation, the body should be fully erect but loose and easy rather than tight and held. Remembering to breathe easily and fully will be of great assistance in this regard. The speaker's feet should be slightly apart (one may be a few inches in front of the other), the weight should be forward over the metatarsal heads, the knees should be unlocked, and the speaker should be well balanced. This is an athletic "ready" stance, not far different from that seen in a shortshop or the other athlete prepared to perform. It is also approximately the same position used in recital by classical singers.

The lectern should not be used as a weight-bearing surface but rather as a script holder. A few gestures, all of which are directly related to the content of the material, are all that is needed. Constant shifting of weight from one leg to another and arbitrary waving one's arms needlessly in the air simply serve to communicate the speaker's general discomfort and lack of real communication skills to the audience members. If the speaker makes genuine eye contact with specific peo-

ple in different locations in the audience in the beginning of the speech, at key times during the speech, and again at the end, then there is a real sense of significant communication taking place.

Instead of simply twisting the head at the neck, if the speaker can face different sections of the audience at different times during the speech with the whole body (keeping the microphone between him- or herself and the audience at all times), then a sense of real commitment to what one is saying is effectively and easily transmitted; and the head and trunk of the body are both in a better position to produce free breathing and well-produced vocal sound. If the voice has been well prepared and exercised enough to respond easily and fully—in terms of pitch, loudness, rhythm, pause, quality—to the content of the speech, then what is being said by the speaker is wonderfully augmented by how the content is being transmitted. Finally, if the speaker can avoid any sense of collapse or visible relief when the speech is over—if, instead, he or she can make the final point, reestablish real eye contact with specific individuals, and then accept and acknowledge applause and reaction—then the delivery will be at least as remarkable as the content itself. Such techniques not only maximize a speaker's communicative impact but also help to minimize both the physical and the psychological stresses related to public speaking. Learning to present comfortably and effectively in person can make sharing one's research and opinions both effective and enjoyable.

References

1. Barton R, Rocco DV. *Voice: Onstage and Off.* Orlando, Fla: Harcourt Brace College Publishers; 1995. (An accompanying cassette tape is available as well.)
2. Eisenson J. *Voice and Diction: A Program for Improvement.* 7th ed. New York, NY: Macmillan; 1996.
3. Rodenburg P. *The Right to Speak.* New York, NY: Routledge; 1993.
4. Wilder L. *Professionally Speaking.* New York, NY: Simon & Schuster; 1986.
5. Executive Performance Intraining Center (EPIC). 1721 Pine Street, Philadelphia, Pa 19103. (215-735-3742).

7

The Singing Teacher in the Age of Voice Science

Richard Miller

What should a responsible voice teacher be teaching in a scientific age? Perhaps we should recall William Faulkner's opinion that the past is all that anyone living in whatever age actually has. What a responsible voice teacher does in this scientific age is not really different from what responsible voice teachers have been doing over several centuries, most of which have been replete with people who considered themselves enlightened and "scientific." Still, in light of recent expansion in knowledge and technology, it seems particularly important in the 1990s for singing teachers to be cognizant of developments in related fields and their potential to enhance teaching.

There is a prevalent opinion that, in past centuries, singers had little interest in science. That viewpoint is not supported by historical review. Consider, for example, the following description of respiration in singing:

The ribs raise outwardly, and . . . the diaphragm . . . descends and compresses the abdomen . . . . For good expiration . . . air must be made to leave with more or less force, with more or less volume, according to the character of the song.[1]

Those words were written not by Bouhuys in the 1970s, nor by Hixon in the 1980s, but by Jean-Baptiste Berard in 1775. Similarly, current interests in the study of vowel tracking were preceded by generations of interest in acoustic adjustments, as expressed by Mancini in 1774.[2]

If the harmony of . . . the mouth and "fauces" is perfect, then the voice will be clear and harmonious. But if these organs act discordantly, the voice will be defective, and consequently the singing spoiled.

Manuel García, inventor of the laryngeal mirror and a renowned singing teacher, clearly appreciated the practical importance of scientific knowledge about the voice. His comments of 1847 could easily have been written today[3]:

The capacity of the vocal cords to vibrate, the dimensions of the larynx, the thorax, the lungs, the pharyngeal, buccal and nasal cavities, the disposition of these cavities to resonate, constitute the absolute power of the voice of an individual . . . . The singer, in order to dominate the material difficulties of his art, must have a thorough knowledge of the mechanism of all these pieces to the point of isolating or combining their action according to the need.

A case could be made that teachers of singing have always wanted to know how the instrument functions. Certainly, both the great Lampertis made use of then-current scientific information. In the 20th century, such noted voice teachers as Marchesi, Shakespeare, Bachner, Herman Klein, Bartholomew, Mills, Curtis, Plunkett Greene, Witherspoon, Frank Miller, Clippinger, Martienssen-Lohman, Stanley, Westerman, Coffin, Appelman, and Vennard (the list could be greatly expanded) have called on factual information in support of pedagogical tenets. Rather than being new, interest in the available factual information characterizes the mainstream of historical vocal pedagogy.

We should not fool ourselves, however, into believing that what generally takes place today in vocal studios is based on intimate acquaintance with the current literature of science. Most teachers of singing give a nod of approval to the helpful scientist, and exhibit tolerance and indulgence toward those who want to play with machines, but, deep down in our hearts, we "know" that singing and teaching are matters of "instinct" and "artistry," and that there is no real possibility of improving on what Madame X handed down to Maestro Y, who in turn gave it unadulterated to my teacher.

Comparative vocal pedagogy reveals an immense stratified structure of both fact and nonsense. There exist systems of vocal technique built on assumptions without foundation in fact. Several brief illustrations will suffice: a world-renowned premier tenor recently explained during a master class that the vowel /i/ was the only vowel narrow enough to enter the frontal sinuses, while a rival tenor who occupies the very pinnacle of the heap informed his master class participants (while demonstrating slight laryngeal descent on inspiration) that, for the "open throat," the epiglottis must be held low at all times. A third noted artist advised "squeezing the uvula with the tonsils." Results from students trying to apply such advice were just short of disastrous.

What should today's voice teacher be doing in the studio? In any age, the main duties of a teacher of singing, with regard to technique, have always been chiefly to (a) analyze vocal problems and (b) design proper solutions for them. It is a pleasure to have students who exhibit few vocal problems, but teaching such pupils is not really teaching voice so much as it is sophisticated coaching and performance preparation. The teacher who helps the less natural singer establish a solid technical basis is a real voice teacher. The potential of the student must be discovered and technical means offered for rectifying problems impeding fine performance. How can this be done?

One choice is to try to pass on to the student what the teacher has learned about his or her own instrument. However, no teacher of singing has personally experienced all the possible forms of uncoordinated function that are exhibited daily in every active studio. In attempting to communicate impressions, instincts, and sensations through impressionistic, instinctive, and descriptive language, the teacher may not communicate the concrete information that the student requires.

Another choice is to teach by modeling—by imitation. If a teacher can demonstrate a beautifully free vocal sound, one may gain some insight into how it is produced. If the teacher has been a great singer, an astute student may glean certain subtle aspects of style and even a little technique. If the teacher is an over-the-hill opera diva, one may also pick up some tendencies it might be better not to have picked up. If a teacher has never mastered his or her own instrument sufficiently to be professionally useful, the student may be in real trouble when he or she models the master's voice!

It is important for the teacher to have a basic knowledge of bodily function and vocal acoustics and to be able to explain what students are doing wrong and why, in whatever language is necessary to reach any individual student. The *main* prerequisite for teaching singing today is none of the following: a fabulous ear, excellent musicianship, highly refined taste, a bubbling personality, goodwill, or a successful singing career, although *all* of these factors are helpful. The main prerequisite is to know what is malfunctioning in a singing voice and how to correct it. It is foolhardy to think one can reach a wise and consistently accurate assessment and resolution if one does not know something about how the vocal machine operates.

How much scientific information does the voice teacher need? As much as he or she can get. There is a growing, credible body of information to help the voice teacher understand what is really happening to a singer's voice, what various exercises can and should be done, and the real intent of the images used traditionally in voice teaching. In addition, learning such information increases the teacher's vocabulary, providing new language for those students in whom traditional constructs have not worked. There exists a fair battery of helpful scientific instrumentation that provides some exact information on singing. It includes a number of electronic devices. The spectrum analyzer tells us much about what singers describe as "resonance." The fiberscope and the electroglottograph also provide new possibilities.[4] (Studio uses of instrumentation are discussed in greater detail in chapter 10.)

Unfortunately, many of the physiological explanations put forth in the voice studio are still surprising to all but those of us who are singers, and most "acoustic" explanations are pure fantasy. Yet, as soon as a teacher of singing requests alteration in vocal sound, he or she is dealing in physiology and acoustics. However, unlike the car mechanic, the voice teacher is not dealing simply with a mechanically complex instrument. Knowing how the voice functions has never yet produced a great teacher of singing. A fine teacher combines mechanistic information with the psychological and the aesthetic.

Once having chosen to pursue such a complex profession and accept the enormous responsibility (and liability) for a student's vocal health and longevity, to rely entirely on imagery is to saddle oneself with a serious handicap. For example, when the relative amplitudes of overtones in the voice do not produce the particular goal the teacher has in mind, how much helpful information is conveyed by requesting, "Put more space around the tone"? Although a teacher has a distinct tonal concept in mind, the student putting "space around the tone" may make alterations to the acoustic tract, to the laryngeal position, and in airflow rate that have no relationship to a teacher's tonal aesthetic. Trying to "sing on the breath," "spin the tone," "place the tone in the forehead," "send it up and over," and so on, will, without doubt, have immediate influence on resulting timbre. By hit and miss, the teacher and student may finally get what the teacher wants. Persons using divining rods have also been known to locate underlying groundwater.

Today's singing teacher has access to a greater body of solid information and rational tools than ever before. We owe it to our students to be able to take advantage not only of everything that was known 200 years ago, but also of everything that is known today.

The advice of Bartholomew,[5] a pioneer in the study of the acoustics of the singing voice, still is appropriate:

Imagery should be used merely to suggest indirectly through its psychological effects a certain muscular setting which is awkward for the beginner. The teacher, though using it, should bear in mind at all times the true facts, because when imagery becomes so vivid that it is transferred into the physical field and used to explain physiologic and acoustic phenomenon, it becomes extremely dubious, unreliable, and even false. It is this misuse which is largely responsible for the bitter controversies over vocal methods, as well as for their often comical explanations. Furthermore, since imagery is largely individual and thus variable, when it is trusted as a physical explanation, the so-called "True Method" becomes as variable as the individual temperament, instead of as stable as Truth is usually expected to be.

It is the responsibility of the singing teacher in a scientific age to interpret and expand vocal traditions through the means of current analysis so that the viable aspects of tradition can be communicated in a systematic way. The advantage of teaching singing in the era of the voice scientist is that today's teacher has the means of sorting through what is offered, both historically and currently, at the vocal pedagogy smorgasbord, and of choosing rationally what is most nutritious, while discarding the garbage, of which there is plenty.

How can emerging information for use in the studio be expanded? Singers of stature should be willing to cooperate in noninvasive investigations of the singing voice. To make such information useful, various schools and techniques of singing should be identified in research reports. Participants should not all be indiscriminately lumped together as "professional singers," nor should students, even at graduate level, be designated professional opera singers in published reports. The subtle individual properties that set one voice apart from another should not be averaged out.

For scientific research to be valid and have practical value in the studio, teachers of singing must be involved, knowledgeable, and interested. Our input, in areas of expertise best understood by voice teachers, is essential.

Unless it is recognized that a number of separate techniques of singing exist, conclusions reached in studies about singers need to be read cautiously. There is little doubt, for example, that if five baritones studying with Dr. X have been taught to modify the vowel /ɑ/ to the vowel /o/ at the pitch B$_3$, spectral analysis will reveal changes in the region of vowel definition at that point. It cannot, therefore, be concluded that professional baritones modify /ɑ/ to /o/ at the pitch B$_3$, but only that baritones involved in the study who have been taught that particular method have learned their lesson well. Singing teachers must learn to read studies critically, so that the lessons they learn are the correct ones. They must also learn enough to know what kind of studies to seek out. For example, although perceptual studies are necessary, singing teachers really want to know more about how the vocal instrument produces the timbres singing voices are capable of making. They already hear those timbres. They need practical information on the mechanisms so it can be applied in the studio.

Much of what goes on in the vocal studio today is extraneous activity, or even counterproductive. This is true in the teaching of all athletic skills (of which singing is one). For example, in discussing sports biomechanics in 1984, Abraham[6] reported:

Analysis of high-speed films of elite performers has led to many interesting observations. Baseball pitchers, for instance, have been apparently wasting much time in the past strengthening their wrist flexor muscles to improve speed of their pitches. Research at the University of Arizona has revealed that the wrist "snap," which does contribute heavily to the speed of the pitched ball, is actually caused by the sudden deceleration of the forearm and occurs so fast that the wrist flexor muscles cannot even keep up, much less contribute to the motion.

Many exercises thought to strengthen or relax the musculature of singing may have no more relationship to actual function than do those for the major league pitcher mentioned above. Learning to "relax," or to "energize," or to "strengthen" certain muscles of the face, neck, and torso may have little to do with singing, yet some vocal instruction is largely directed to such activities.

A main goal of teaching in this and any age should be to do no harm. Every aspect of vocal technique must be in agreement with what is known about healthy vocal function. Any teacher assuming responsibility for a student's artistic and vocal health is obligated to educate him- or herself in the wisdom of a wide community of experts. There is no such thing as a unique vocal method or a unique teacher of singing. It is not necessary for each student and each teacher to rediscover the art of singing alone. There is a body of information that ought to be drawn on by anyone who claims to teach anything to anybody. No one can know it all, but we must be willing to modify what we do know as information expands. Demythologizing the language of vocal pedagogy is part of that process. Consultation with experts in related disciplines, through reading and offering our professional services to help discover new information, is another. Above all, as teachers of singing in a scientific age, we must ask ourselves how much we really know about the subject matter we deal with. Do we have facts, or do we rely on anecdotal opinions? Do we know the literature of our own field, as well as that of related fields?

Singing today is not a dying art. It is very much alive and growing. At this moment, it occupies an advantageous position where the traditions of the past and the information of the present can be combined in an exciting way. The responsibility, excitement, and reward of our profession lie in rising to the challenges of new opportunities to make the present and future of voice teaching even greater than the past.

References

1. Berard JB, Murray S, trans-ed. *L'Art du chant*. Milwaukee, Wisc: Pro Music Press; 1969.
2. Mancini G, Foreman R, trans. *Practical Reflections on Figured Singing*. Champaign, Ill: Pro Music Press, 1967.
3. Garcia M. *A Complete Treatise on the Art of Singing, Part One*. New York, NY: Da Capo Press; 1983.
4. Titze I. Instrumentation for voice research. *NATS Bull*. 1983;38(5):29.
5. Bartholomew WT. *The Role of Imagery in Voice Teaching*. Proceedings of the Music Teachers National Association, 1935.
6. Abraham L. Sports biomechanics: application of high tech to Olympic engineering. *Tex Prof Engineer*. 1984;July–August:16–19.

8

Historical Overview of Vocal Pedagogy

Richard Miller

The vocal instrument does not need to be constructed; it is available for immediate use. Lodged in a physical machine, it receives its impetus from mental and spiritual parameters of human personality. Its adaptability in channeling communication is the foundation on which human civilizations are built.

The capacity to communicate through vocal sound inevitably led to the voice of singing. Singing predates all other forms of music performance. In every primitive society, a few individuals were more attuned to the inherent emotive power of voicing than were others. They are the ancestors of the solo singer. As the potentials of the singing voice became increasingly evident, techniques for the realization of enhanced vocal skills were developed and passed on.

People of all ages and cultures have crafted indigenous styles of singing. Witness the Greek tragedian searching beyond the boundaries of normal speech for the best method by which to become audible in the amphitheater (however grateful its architectural acoustic); the citharoedus accompanying himself on the lyre or cithara in public Olympic competition; David singing and playing his harp privately before distressed King Saul; the cantor leading vigorously sung ancient liturgies—the synagogue *hazan*, the mosque *muezzin*; the ascetic monk intoning initial phrases of subdued Gregorian chant; the occult shaman inciting emotive responses in his listeners; the operatic soprano and tenor bringing down the house with ringing high Cs.

In early records of secular song, the late Medieval Goliards (students who protested the moral strictures of the universities), the early Renaissance trouvères and troubadours, the Minnesingers, and the Meis-

tersingers exemplify solo balladeering. Almost no evidence exists as to how these singers executed technical aspects of their art. References to breath management, laryngeal action, and resonation (the three components of the tripartite vocal instrument) are so minimal as to be of little use in determining how vocal color was achieved. Internal evidence from existing musical fragments suggests that vocal demands seldom exceeded those of speech.

Treatises written before the 19th century restrict themselves largely to matters of style. To the 16th century and the 17th century writer, codification of performance rules was of primary concern. Even in the 18th century, technical aspects of the singing voice were only tangentially treated. Indeed, there is peril in applying information from those centuries to vocal literature general performance, because much of what was written about performance practice could not pertain to the singing voice. Given the structure of the vocal instrument, it is clear that a singer was never expected to match the sounds of the mechanically constructed instruments with which he performed.

Current assessments of the character of pre-19th century vocalism are largely speculative, based on personal tonal preferences that enjoy minimal scholarly documentation. Beyond general aesthetic guidelines, both pedagogic and critical period literatures reveal little as to how vocal qualities were produced. Especially regarding late vocal Baroque literature, current "historically authentic performance" most probably remains wide of the mark.

A 15th century voice-pedagogy note comes from Franchinus Gaffurius in the *Practica musicae* of 1496[1]:

Singers should not produce musical tones with a voice gaping wide in a distorted fashion or with an absurdly powerful bellowing, especially when singing at the divine mysteries; moreover they should avoid tones having a wide and ringing vibrato, since these tones do not maintain a true pitch and because their continuous wobble cannot form a balanced concord with other voices.

Clearly, for Gaffurius a wide vibrato and a bellowing voice were as common and as undesirable in his day as are broad vocal oscillations and shouting in present-day singing. He did not suggest that the singing voice should avoid natural vibrancy but that an uncontrollable vibrato was not acceptable. Graffurius offered no instruction as to how these technical errors were to be avoided.

At Venice in 1592, in his *Prattica di musica utile et necessaria si al conpositore per comporre i canti suoi regolatamente, si anco al cantore*, Ludovico Zacconi recommended continuous use of vibrato, which he termed *tremoloy*[2]:

> This tremolo should be slight and pleasing; for if it is exaggerated and forced, it tires and annoys; its nature is such that, if used at all, *it should always be used*, [italics added] since use converts it into habit. . . . it facilitates the undertaking of passaggi [ornamentation]; this movement . . . should not be undertaken if it cannot be done with just rapidity, vigorously and vehemently.

Bénigne de Bacilly (c. 1625–1690) in *Remarques curieuses sur l'art de bien chanter* (Paris, 1668) made a distinction between *cadence* and *tremblement*. A.B. Caswell[3] translates Bacilly's *cadence* as "vibrato," a phenomenon not to be equated with the rapid oscillatory *tremblement*. Bacilly indicated that the singer's *cadence* is a "gift of nature" that sometimes becomes too slow or too fast. The *tremblement* may produce an undesirable *voix chevrotante* (bleating or wobbling). Slow and rapid oscillations are used only as ornaments. Clearly, there was no intention of outlawing natural vibrato. For Bacilly a pretty voice "is very pleasing to the ear because of its clearness and sweetness and above all because of the nice *cadence* [here, *vibrato*] which usually accompanies it. [11]

Other treatises from the late Renaissance make frequent reference to unwanted nasality and to the common fault of singing out of tune. They insist on beauty and consistency of timbre but remain mostly silent as to how desirable vocal quality can be managed. A chief reason for lack of attention in early treatises to the training of the singing voice is that extensive individual solo artistic expression did not emerge until the close of the 16th century. Prior to the "invention of opera" by the Florentine camerata in the last years of the 16th century and the early decades of the 17th century, although replete with complex technical and musicianly demands that required high-level performance, vocal literature had largely been directed to ensemble, not soloistic concerns. It is clear that early singers were highly trained and capable of executing pyrotechnical passages for individual voices, but singing was still adjunctive to social or religious functions, taking place in monastery, chapel, cathedral, salon, or parlor. In the 17th century the individual solo singer became a public performer in his own right, exhibiting remarkable ascendancy by mid-century.

Passing references to vocal technique prior to 1600 are of limited practical value to current performers of the vocal music from those eras. Further, aesthetic tastes are by no means stable from decade to decade, let alone century to century. To achieve "authenticity" by imitating each assumed aesthetic stratum of the past, the professional singer would need to develop technical maneuvers deleterious to vocal health. It is tempting to react to the layers of stylistic information available by nostalgically looking back to some period of lost vocal perfection. It is incumbent upon today's lyric artist to distinguish among vocal styles appropriate to diverse literatures, but Herbert Witherspoon's remark[4] may provide a needed counterbalance:

> There have always been few good singers and fewer great ones so a tirade about present-day conditions in comparison with the glorious past is of no use. . . . Perhaps if we heard the singers of a century or two ago we should not care for them. . . . Our task is with today, not yesterday.

However, to understand the several current strands of today's vocal pedagogy, a knowledge of their roots is essential.

Technical prowess is essential for all solo vocal performance that goes beyond speech or folksong idioms. In order to discover and disseminate technical principles for extended tasks, the discipline of vocal pedagogy arose. Vocal pedagogy of 17th century was mostly directed to the male voice, not to the castrato and female instruments as is sometimes falsely assumed. During the 18th century, a number of treatises concerned the castrati, whose techniques, as documented by such researchers as Duey,[5] Heriot,[6] and Pleasants,[7] were clearly of the highest order. However, it is easy to overlook the fact that public esteem for the female soprano at times rivaled that afforded the castrati. During the first half of the 18th century, the low female voice also gradually gained acceptance as a viable vocal instrument for the stage. Male and female larynges are affected differently by puberty. (The effects of puberty were largely avoided with the castrato.) But techniques of breath-management and articulation apply to every gender and category of singer. It is not the case that 17th- and 18th-century vocal instruction was intended only for the altered male larynx.

It is to 18th-century Italy that one must turn in tracing origins of an international vocal pedagogy capable of matching the tasks found within the vocal literature. Even today, much of the early Italian heritage remains dominant among competing national and regional schools. A brief survey of the pedagogic tenets of the historic Italian School follows.

Francesco Antonio Pistocchi (1659–1726) founded a Bolognese singing school around 1700. In pyrotechnical skill, it rivaled the proficiency of the string playing. He was the teacher of Antonio Bernacchi (c. 1690–1756), who in turn taught two of Handel's favorite castrati, Senesino and Carestini.

Another school of outstanding singers flourished under the tutelage of tenor/composer Nicola Porpora (1686–1768) at Naples, and quickly became international. The ability to sustain (*cantabile*) and to move (*cabaletta*) the voice were the pedagogic aims of the Neapolitan vocal school. (These skills became preeminent in the *cavatina/cabaletta* aria form of the following century.) Among Porpora's many successful pupils were two famous castrati, Caffarelli and Farinelli, and the highly regarded female sopranos Mingotti and Gabrielli.

Jean-Baptiste Bérard (also known as Jean-Antoine Bérard), discussing respiration for singing in his *L'art du chant* of 1755,[8] is in accord with the international Italianate School by advocating an outwardly raised ribcage, diaphragmatic descent, and controlled breath emission as technical essentials.

An early significant written source on solo vocal pedagogy[9] comes from the hand of the castrato Pier Francesco Tosi. His *Opinioni de' cantori antichi e moderni sieno osservazioni sopra il canto figurato* was first published in Bologna in 1723, when Tosi was more than 70 years old. It thereafter (1742) appeared in an English translation by a German emigrant to England, Johann Ernst Galliard, and has long been known in British and North American vocal pedagogy circles as *Observations on the Florid Song*. A German translation with commentary by J. H. Agricola, *Anleitung zur Singkunst*, was issued in 1757. Although largely concerned with the execution of embellishments such as the appoggiatura and the shake, and with the management of roulades and scales, Tosi makes general references to technical matters, but he mostly avoids specific advice. For example, with regard to breath management:

> . . . to manage his respiration . . . [the singer must] always be provided with more breath than is needful; and may avoid undertaking what, for want of it, he can not go through with.

Castrato Tosi designated the vocal registers as *voce di petto* (chest voice) and *voce di testa* (head voice) without precise advice as to how they were to be facilitated. He offered more specific information as to the effects of the articulators on the resonator tract. In keeping with the age-old Italian preference for front vowels over the back vowels in upper range, he maintained that the vowels /i/ and /e/ were less fatiguing than the vowel /ɑ/.

Although singing technique may not have adhered to uniform instructional ideals endorsed by all, common technical threads run throughout early treatises. Despite the commonality of pedagogic viewpoints on breathing and enunciation, one is struck by the frequent complaint from renowned teachers that the rest of the pedagogic world has lost the true art of singing (reminiscent of some of today's pedagogic and critical lamentation). Tosi was not happy with the existing status of the singing art:

> Gentlemen! Masters! Italy hears no more: [1723] such exquisite voices as in times past, *particularly among the women*) [italics added], and to to the shame of the guilty I'll tell the reason. The ignorance of the parents does not allow them to perceive the badness of the voices of their children, as their necessity makes them believe, that to sing and grow rich is the same thing, and to learn music, it is enough to have a pretty face. Can you make anything of her?

Tosi's comments on the role of the performing artist as teacher of singing are as sagacious for our era as for his:

> It may seem to many, that every perfect singer must also be a perfect instructor but it is not so; for his qualifications (though ever so great) are insufficient if he cannot communicate his sentiments with ease, and in a method adapted to the ability of the student.

Giambattista Mancini is another oft-cited 18th-century source on the art of singing,[10] yet his *Pensieri, e riflessioni pratiche sopra il canto figurato* of 1774 is, as its title implies, largely devoted to practical reflections on vocal ornamentation. Mancini (b. 1714, Ascoli; d. 1800, Vienna) had studied singing with Bernacchi and must have have had a good grasp of the accepted singing techniques of the period. Much of his pedagogic comment is directed to the resonator system, with particular attention to the maintenance of natural postures of the buccal cavity, and to the smiling posture as an adjustor of the vocal tract. Berton Coffin was struck by Mancini's awareness of the variation in physiologic structure among singers:[11]

> He acknowledged that all faces differ in structure, and some are better proportioned for singing than are others; nevertheless certain positions [of the mouth] were best for a smooth, pure quality of tone, and certain positions would bring out a suffocated and crude tone (too open) or a nasal tone (too closed). He thought the Italian vowels /(a, e, o, u/ could be sung on each note in the position of a smile with the /o/ and /u/ being slightly rounded. . . . Mancini felt the /i/ vowel was difficult and should be sung in the position of a "composed smile."

Another Mancini pedagogic tenet was that in order to be distinct and executed with the greatest possible velocity, all runs and agility passages should be supported by a robust chest, assisted by graduated breath energy, and with light "fauces" [the passage from the mouth into the pharynx].

W. Crutchfield[12,p293] remarks that Domenico Corri (1746–1825) is "probably the most valuable single theorist as far the provision of practical examples is concerned." Corri's extensive variations and cadenzas on Sarti's *Lungi dal caro bene*[12,p302] is cited as an example of vocal embellishment practices of the period. E. Harris[2] quotes Corri's 1810 comment on performance and style[13]:

> The vocal art affords various characters—the sacred, the serious, the comic, anacreontic, cavatina, bravura, etc., etc.—and though each style requires different gifts and cultivation, yet true intonation, the swelling and dying of the voice, with complete articulation of words, is essential to all.

Corri suggested that the voice should increase in volume as it rises and decrease in volume when descending. However, he does not offer significant advice to a reader searching for clues on how best to accomplish the technical complexities of the vocal literature considered.

Tenor Manuel del Popolo Vincent García Rodriguez (1775–1832) is known as García *père* to distinguish him from his son Manuel Patricio Rodriguez García (1805–1906). His vocal technique book *Exercises pour la voix*[14] was published in Paris between 1819 and 1822. It was fully within the pedagogical tradition of the 18th-century Italian school. (An English translation was published in London in 1824.) One of García's teachers was Giovanni Ansoni, a member of the Neapolitan singing school. Having already estab-

lished himself as a premier singer in his native country, García left Spain in 1808 to build an international opera career, performing in Paris, Turin, Rome, and Naples. The role of Count Almaviva (*Il barbiere di Siviglia,* by Rossini) was written for him: it is ample evidence of the capability of García *père* in executing the two major aspects of bel canto technique: sostenuto and velocity. In a brief introduction to the 340 vocalises of his technical system, García *père* presents explicit pedagogic advice:

> The position of the body must be erect, the shoulders thrown back, with the arms crossed behind; this will open the chest and bring out the voice with ease, clear and strong, without distorting the appearance of either face or body.
>
> . . . .[the singer ought] never to commence singing in a hurry, always to take breath slowly and without noise, which would otherwise be unpleasant to those who listen, and injurious to the singer.
>
> . . . .The throat, teeth and lips, must be sufficiently opened so that the voice may meet with no impediment, since the want of a strict attention to either of these three is sufficient to destroy the good quality of the voice and to produce the bad one, of the throat, nose, etc.; besides, proper attention to the mouth will give that perfect and clear pronunciation indispensable to singing, and which unfortunately, few possess.

Early 19th-century García *père* resides solidly in the tradition of the 18th-century Italian School. Among his pupils were his daughters (Viardot and Malibran, perhaps the most celebrated female vocal artists of the era), his son Manuel, and Adolphe Nourrit, the leading French tenor of the first half of the 19th century until the advent of Gilbert Duprez.

A thorough examination of the contribution of his son, Manuel García *fils* (1805-1906), becomes all the more intriguing because much subsequent critical comment implies that the younger García introduced technical directions that withdrew from previous tenets of the Italian School. When accounts of his entire teaching career are taken into consideration, it becomes doubtful that such a break with tradition took place. A case (admittedly controversial) could be made that García the younger used his new knowledge of laryngeal and vocal tract anatomy and physiology to verify and enhance what he had learned from his father.

Manuel García's appearance in New York at age 20 as Figaro in Rossini's *Il barbiere* (with his father as Almaviva, his sister as Rosina, and his mother as Berta) indicates that 10 years of vocal study with his father had produced a precocious baritone voice. (It also makes one question if performance standards were as high as current idealization of past vocal eras may imagine.) García's strenuous performing routine while still so young (sometimes even as substitute in tenor roles for his ill father) may well have contributed to his early vocal deterioration. In any event, he was unable to emulate the performance successes of his father and his siblings, and he turned to teaching. His *Traité complet de l'art du chant*[15] appeared in 1840.

In 1841, Manuel García's *Mémoire sur la voix humaine*[16] was presented to the French Academy. His growing curiosity about physical function was further sparked by anatomical observations made at military hospitals. In 1854 these interests led him to the invention of a primitive laryngoscope. (Note that it was a voice teacher, not a physician, who first saw the vocal folds in action during spoken and sung phonations.)

García devised register terminology with the designations Chest Voice, Falsetto Voice, and Head Voice, based on physiologic information and practical knowledge of then-current performance practice. These registration divisions are confusing to modern-day voice researchers. He discussed laryngeal positioning in detail as well as the *coup de glotte* (the stroke of the glottis). His descriptions later generated a variety of pedagogic assumptions, some of which, if one is to believe reports of his students, went far beyond principles he himself taught. In a summary of his method, undertaken in 1870 and published in 1872,[17] one finds distinct parallels with what his father had proposed, even to the inclusion of similar technical exercises. For example, he advised that the head and neck should remain erect on the torso, that the shoulders ought to be well back without stiffness, that the chest must remain in an expanded position, and that inspiration should occur silently and slowly without sudden diaphragmatic lowering. He recommended the use of a breath-management exercise that had come down by word of mouth from the previous century, Farinelli's Exercise, in which the breath cycle is accomplished through a slow tripartite maneuver consisting of an inspiratory gesture, a subsequent suspension of either inhalation or exhalation, and a concluding expiratory gesture, the three segments being of equal duration. He recommended use of *the attacco del suono* (onset) as a basic exercise for the development of breath-management skill. His "open" and "closed" vocal timbres are in line with the *voce aperta/voce chiusa* (open voice/closed voice) and the *copertura* (cover) terminology of the traditional Italian School. Laryngeal posture should be low and stable. His instruction on the relationship of vowel integrity to vowel modification in ascending pitch is a pillar of today's vocal art.

A thorough analysis of Manuel García's technical principles requires extensive consideration not possible here. Proof of the efficacy of his teaching lies in the large number of outstanding singers of many nationalities who were among his pupils. Further insight into García's pedagogy is to be found in *An Essay on Bel Canto* written by his pupil and close associate Herman Klein.[18] Never in the history of solo singing has one individual so influenced vocal pedagogy as did Manuel García. It is fair to suggest that current international mainstream vocalism and many of its divergent nationalist rivulets can be traced directly to interpretations of García's admonitions. His own assessment of the state of singing (when many thought it at its peak) was that singing had become as much a lost art as that of the manufacture of Mandarin china or the varnish used by the old string-instrument masters.

An interim figure, surfacing in the Italian school between the Garcías and the Lampertis, is the Neapolitan Luigi LaBlache (1794–1858), whose career as outstanding *basso* of the era took him to La Scala, Vienna, Paris, and London. Yet his *Méthode de chant*, published undated in Paris, as was the English edition,[19] came late in life. It offers little precise information as to how the art of singing ought to be taught. Evidence of his successful teaching lies in the number of his pupils who managed professional careers.

A Treatise on the Art of Singing[20] by Francesco Lamperti (1813–1892) is undated but is presumed to have appeared after 1860. F. Lamperti's chief contribution to the historic Italian School is his description of the *lutte vocale* (It. *lotta vocale*), the basis for the *appoggio* breath-management that is a fundamental precept of the 19th-century Italian School:

> To sustain a given note the air should be expelled slowly; to attain this end, the respiratory [inspiratory] muscles, by continuing their action, strive to retain the air in the lungs, and oppose their action to that of the expiratory muscles, which is called the *lutte vocale* or vocal struggle. On the retention of this equilibrium depends the just emission of the voice, and by means of it alone can true expression be given to the sound produced.

Although the term *appoggio* appears to have first come into use in the second half of the 19th century, the *lutte vocale* (which is analogous to the *appoggio* technique) already existed in the exercise that Farinelli is reputed to have learned a century earlier from Porpora (see above) in order to acquire his phenomenal breath management.

Francesco Lamperti held to the three-register designation of the 19th century Italian School (allowing for gender differences) and he was adamant that whether singing softly or loudly, timbre must be consistent. The *messa di voce* (sung on a single note or phrase beginning at *piano* or *pianissimo* dynamic level, crescendoing to *forte* or *fortissimo*, then returning to the original decibel level) was an important part of his pedagogy. He stressed the need for full, complete-toned production at all dynamic levels.

His son, Giovanni Battista (Giambattista) Lamperti (1839–1910), left an even more enduring mark on international vocal pedagogy: He taught singers who would become identified with the "second golden age" of vocalism, and these students carried on his system well into the first half of the 20th century. Lamperti's advice regarding general posture and events of the breath cycle[21] parallels that of his predecessors: "The shoulders [must] be slightly thrown back to allow the chest due freedom in front." For G.B. Lamperti, breath management was the prime factor in skillful singing. He recognized the unique relationshp of vocal registers to each vocal category and to the individual instrument. Breath renewal should be silently incorporated into the release of the tone at each phrase termination, with subsequent precise onset (attack). Singing *piano* was in all regards the same as singing *forte*, only softer. Above all, good singing necessitated command of the art of legato, which depended on efficient breath-management.[21] Lamperti's opposition to the "relaxed" posture then being advocated by the German school is eminently clear. In contrast to that school's lowered thoracic postures, the singer was to feel broad-shouldered and high-chested, straightened up like a soldier. Despite the reputation of many turn-of-the-century singing artists, Lamperti lamented the general deterioration of the art of singing and of voice teaching:

> There has never been so much enthusiasm for the singing art, nor have there been so many students and teachers as of late years. And it is precisely this period that reveals the deterioration of this divine art and the almost complete disappearance of genuine singers and worse, of good singing teachers.

Could Giambattista Lamperti have had in mind inroads the national schools were making into the historic international Italianate school?

A telling influence in 20th century North America vocal pedagogy is William Earl Brown's *Maxims of G. B. Lamperti*. The book first appeared in print in America in 1931,[22] but the maxims were collected in 1891–1893 when Brown was Lamperti's student and assistant in Dresden. He maintained that the quoted maxims were taken directly from studio notes he made during that period.

> At no time during the song or series of exercises must you relax while replenishing the breath or you [will] lose the feeling of suspension. Only when the song is over may you let go. . . . [Maintain] sustained intensity of initial vibration and continuous release of breath-energy. . . . Tone and breath "balance" solely when harmonic overtones appear in the voice, not by muscular effort and "voice placing."

He said legato was achievable only through the presence of constant vibrancy, a result of the *appoggio*. Lamperti held that loose breath escaping over the vocal folds and not turned into tone was destructive to good function, causing irregular vibration and disruption of breath energy.

> Until you feel the permanency of your vibration you cannot play on your resonances. . . . [E]nergy in regular vibration is constructive. The violence in irregular vibration is destructive.

The influence of the Lamperti maxims has never been surpassed by other pedagogic writing of the 20th century.

In the interest of chronology, the treatises of two other representatives of the Lamperti school, William Shakespeare and Herbert Witherspoon, are considered later. For additional commentary regarding the influence of this school's *appoggio* technique on modern vocal pedagogy, the reader is directed to C. Timberlake's astute remarks on historic pedagogy and performance styles.[23]

The historic Italian School dominated all European professional vocalism; its proponents taught in the major cities of Europe (García in London and Paris, G.B. Lamperti in Munich and Dresden, for example). In the latter half of the 19th century, with the emergence of European nationalism, the conscious development of indigenous regional cultures, and divergences stemming from application of new scientific findings to the art of singing, the reign of Italian vocalism became less encompassing. Whereas opera, the chief performance vehicle for professional singing, had been Italian-centered during the 17th, 18th, and early 19th centuries, in the latter half of the 19th century other performance literatures, such as the *Lied*, the *mélodie*, the orchestrated song, and the oratorio, began to flower, gaining increasing importance toward the close of the century. These literatures continued to burgeon as the 20th century dawned, garnering new impetus in subsequent decades. Even though the Italian model was still preeminent in the international world of professional vocalism, disparate, identifiable tonal aesthetics began to flourish in France, in Germany and Northern Europe, and in England, while

Italy persistently held firm to historic tradition through at least the first third of the 20th century. It is worthy of note that Manuel García is frequently cited in support of the many pedagogic strands that became alternatives to the original Italianate model. National digressions resulted from differing emphases in tonal ideals, from emerging vocal literatures, and above all, from an increasing interest in achieving synthesis of word and music, transcending the traditional Italian emphasis on vocalism as the chief aesthetic concern.

The unification of the German political states into a national body, the increasing importance of liturgical choral traditions such as the Germanic/Scandinavian Lutheran and the Anglican, the emergence of the public *Liederabend*, the rise of Romantic German opera, the impact of Wagner, and the shift from royal to public patronage altered the dominant role of the international Italian school, but did not obliterate its influence on national schools. (All pedagogic threads were woven into the North American vocal-pedagogy garment.)

The modern pedagogue may best understand the wide diversity among systems of vocal technique, most of which had their origins in the late 19th century, by gauging the extent to which they break away from the earlier international model and the extent to which they retain its premises. In a number of instances, divergent modern pedagogics continue the late 19th-century search for justification of techniques by applying modern scientific measurement. Some treatises of the latter half of the 19th century were written by teachers with one foot located south of the historic Italian pedagogic alp, the other foot planted north of it. "New" 20th-century pedagogic systems are seldom more than extensions of those diverse formulae.

Julius Stockhausen was born in Paris in July, 1826, and died in Frankfurt-am-Main in September, 1906. Beginning in 1845, Stockhausen undertook theoretic studies at the Paris Conservatoire, but privately studied voice with Manuel García, whom he followed to London in 1849. Despite Stockhausen's future impact on Germanic/Nordic and North American vocal pedagogy, he did not excel chiefly in opera. He was second baritone at the Mannheim theater from 1852–1853. Stockhausen's chief performance successes lay in oratorio and *Lieder* repertories. His public performance of *Die Schöne Müllerin* took place with great success in 1856 at Vienna. Brahms and Stockhausen first collaborated in recital in Hamburg in 1861, performing a program that included Schumann's *Dichterliebe*. Stockhausen's subsequent selection over Brahms as the director of the Hamburg Philharmonische Konzertgesellschaft and of the Singakademie did not interfere with their continued artistic coalition. Stockhausen premiered the baritone role of Brahms's *Ein Deutsches*

Requiem in 1868; the rangy, dramatic vocal writing was considered ungrateful to Stockhausen's instrument. The composer's remarkable Magelone cycle was written with Stockhausen in mind. It demands stamina and sensitivity, two facets that the singer seemed able to deliver equally well in the *Lieder* of Schubert, Schumann, and Brahms. After serving as a singing teacher at several institutions, Stockhausen founded his own school of singing in 1880. In 1884, *Gesangsmethode*,[24] translated as *Method of Singing*, appeared.

Stockhausen's publication is a significant step in the history of vocal pedagogy because of its continuing influence on the Germanic/Nordic vocal schools and on a sizable segment of North American pedagogy and because it raises questions as to the accuracy of Stockhausen's interpretation (and that of his disciples) of Manuel García's pedagogic orientation. One of Stockhausen's chief departures from the tenets of the 18th- and 19th-century Italian school lies in his advocacy of a constantly low laryngeal position while singing. Although it remains unclear as to how low Stockhausen's "low larynx " was, he advised a position lower than that of the normal speaking voice. In itself, this admonition is not in conflict with the historic Italian pedagogic tenet that requests the noble posture and silent breath renewal, in which limited laryngeal descent will occur and remain. But most of Stockhausen's followers interpret him as having taught retention of the yawn position, with depressed larynx, as being ideal for sung phonation. His avoidance of a pleasant facial expression, together with his promotion of the lowered jaw, diminished the supraglottic vocal tract flexibility so characteristic of the Italianate school. However, Stockhausen specifically outlawed both nasal and pharyngeal timbres. Inasmuch as it is difficult to envision how distended pharyngeal timbre can be avoided while one consciously induces throat-wall expansion, Stockhausen's comments may invite varying pedagogic interpretations.

Stockhausen requested that the lips be drawn backward on back and mixed vowels, and that for /e/ and /ɑ/ the lips be pursed in forward position. These are withdrawals from the *si canta come si parla* (one sings as one speaks) maxim of the traditinal Italian School. Yet, more in keeping with the Italian pedagogic heritage, Stockhausen recommended the use of closed vowels in ascending pitch patterns, and of open vowels in descending pitch patterns.

Although he did call for full rib expansion in the *respiro pieno* (full breath), another departure from the Italian School was Stockhausen's minimal attention to breath-management. His *passaggio* registration points are located similarly to those of García. He advocated the use of the *messa di voce* so dear to the Lampertis.

The modern pedagogue must conclude that Julius Stockhausen severely adapted traditional Italianate-schooled principles to the performance of the emerging Germanic repertoire in which he excelled and to national tonal preferences. Given his commitment to non-Italianate technical devices, one wonders how well Stockhausen may have managed vocalism and diction in the Italian and French operatic repertoires during his 3-year stint in the Paris Opéra Comique (1856–1859). Stockhausen's pedagogic orientation raises the question as to how far vocal technique can be altered for the performance of different literatures.

Not even a brief overview of historic vocal pedagogy can dispense with at least passing reference to Emma Seiler (c. 1875). Her own experiences as a singer, which she describes as having been in both Italian and German traditions, appear to have been frustrating. She finally associated herself with the eminent physicist/acoustician Hermann Helmholtz, who expressed indebtedness to her in his formulation of acoustic theories of voice production. Some of Seiler's assumptions regarding the function of the laryngeal mechanism are insupportable. In explaining her vocal registration hypotheses, she heavily relied on proprioceptive sensations of mouth, throat, stomach, and sternum. Her treatise[25] is largely important as a prototype of forthcoming Germanic pseudoscientific pedagogic literature that attempts in imaginative ways to apply physiology and acoustics to the singing-voice.

British vocal pedagogy was not immune to Germanic influences. Emil Behnke's *The Mechanism of the Human Voice* published in 1880,[26] and his *Voice, Song and Speech*,[27] in collaboration with Lennox Browne, were highly regarded in turn-of-the-century British pedagogy circles. Yet he was not a follower of Stockhausen, nor were his ideas in line with the Germanic techniques later developed by Armin. Behnke was particularly enamored of the male falsetto.

Enrico Delle Sedie (1822-1907) was a highly successful baritone in Italy, Paris, and London, singing the Verdian roles Di Luna (*Il trovatore*), Renato (*Un ballo in maschera*), and Germond (*La traviata*). Figaro (*Il barbiere di Siviglia*) and Malatesta (*Don Pasquale*) were in his repertoire. In 1876, he published *Arte e fisiologia del canto*, and in 1886, *L'estetico del canto e l'arte melodrammatica*. In 1894 *A Complete Method of Singing*,[28] which included material from his earlier publications, appeared in New York. Drawing on physiologic and acoustic information of the time, Delle Sedie exemplified those singers and teachers who increasingly began to turn to science as a means for verifying tenets of the historic Italian School. His method deals with the resonator tract as a filtering source for laryngeally generated sound. He unites the registration and timbre terminologies of the historic Italian School with emerging acoustic information, especially as regards vowel modification. As such, his writing has had considerable impact on American vocal pedagogy.

An American publication containing accurate drawings of the larynx and confirmable explanations of diaphragmatic function was E. B. Warman's *The Voice: How to Train It and Care for It* (1889). This treatise[29] is a successful effort to undergird the tenets of the Italianate school with scientific information.

A teacher of singing who left no written advice but whose outstanding pupils indicated his impact on vocal pedagogy, is the Neapolitan tenor Giovanni Sbriglia (1832-1916). Sbriglia made his debut at San Carlo in 1853 and his 1860 New York debut at the Academy of Music, where he appeared in *La sonnambula* with Adelina Patti. Both Edward de Reszke and his brother Jean (who underwent change from baritone to tenor), Pol Plançon (who also studied with Duprez), and Lillian Nordica were products of the Sbriglia studio.

Summaries of Sbriglia's teaching have been recorded by his pupils. Assuming these reports to be reliable, it appears that Sbriglia lies within the historic Italian School that extends from García *père* through the Lampertis and into the 20th century. Sbriglia opposed the *Bauchaussenstütze* (outward abdominal-wall thrusting) that became characteristic of the late 19th- and 20th-century Germanic school. According to Byers[30]:

> . . . he believed that all great singers breathed alike—"the same natural way." He did not like what he called 'the new pushing method of singing with the back of the neck sunk in the chest, and the muscularly pushed out diaphragm.
>
> . . . . The foundation of this teaching is perfect posture. Foremost is a high chest (what nature gives every great singer), held high without tension by developed abdominal and lower back muscles and a straight spine—this will give the uplift for perfect breathing. . . . Your chest literally must be held up by these abdominal and back muscles, supported from below, and your shoulder and neck will be free and loose.

It is easy to assume that Mathilde Marchesi was a proponent of the Italian School. However, Mathilde Marchesi (b. 1821, Frankfurt-am-Main; d. 1913, London) was a German mezzo-soprano who in 1852 married the singer Salvatore Marchesi. Her early training took place in Germany. In 1845, she went to Paris to study with Manuel García for a period of several years. Although she had some success as a public performer, her energies were largely devoted to teaching. Outstanding female singers were numbered among her pupils, among them Eames, Calvé, Garden, and Melba.

Theoretical and Practical Vocal Method[31] and *Ten Singing Lessons*[32] attest to Marchesi's organized approach to vocal pedagogy. Her description of the singing-voice as a three-part instrument consisting of motor, vibrator, and resonator system has a remarkably modern ring. In regards to posture for singing, she is directly in the lineage of García *père*, Manuel García, and both Lampertis, as evidenced by her suggestion that students should position the arms at the back in order to achieve proper chest elevation and to induce low breathing. She taught the *coup de glotte* (probably the balanced *attacco del suono*) which she described as producing firm, complete approximation of the glottis, and which she believed used minimal air to set the vocal folds in vibration. She adhered to the three-register concept of the Italian School. Marchesi modified the Italianate model by suggesting that the jaw drop into low position and remain nearly immobile during singing. Much of her success as a teacher appears to have been a result of her systematic approach, which was summarized in the maxim "First technique, afterwards aesthetics."

Lilli Lehmann's *Meine Gesangskunst* (1902), published in 1914[33] as *How to Sing* (later revisions appeared), has exerted lasting influence on aspiring North American, European, and Asian singers. It is not easy to classify Lehmann (1848–1929) by school because her language, both subjective and specific, borrows from several traditions and appears ultimately to be a search for justification of her personal vocal technique through physiologic and acoustic verification, much of it inaccurate. This combining of the subjective and the objective were expressed as follows:

> Technique is inseparable from art. Only by mastering the technique of his material is the artist in a condition to mold his mental work of art. . . . [M]uscles contract in activity, and in normal inactivity are relaxed. . . . [W]e must strengthen them by continued vocal gymnastics so that they may be able to sustain long-continued exertion; and must keep them elastic and use them so. It includes also the well-controlled activity of diaphragm, chest, neck, and face muscles. . . . Since these things all operate together, one without the others can accomplish nothing; if the least is lacking, singing is quite impossible, or is entirely bad.

One of the most influential pages in vocal pedagogy contains Lehmann's schema for subjective tone-placement sensations that move upward into the bony skull in response to ascending pitch. Lehmann's reputation as a gifted artist who could sing widely diverse roles, together with the longevity of her career, helped establish the importance of her opinions.

A major figure in 20th-century German-language vocal pedagogy literature is Franziska Martienssen-Lohmann, who precisely describes breath-management procedures, registration practices, and timbre designations within the Germanic/Nordic School.[34–36] By taking exception at times to typical Germanic practices of heavy Deckung (covering), excessive *Kopfstimme* (head voice) and the *Tiefstellung* (low positioning) of the larynx, Martienssen-Lohmann appears to move in the direction of the international Italianate school, as do many contemporary Germans.

The teaching of Georg Armin, beginning in the 1930s, left a lasting imprint on the "heroic" segment of the German School and on its North American derivative. His breath-damming *Staumethode*,[37] by which he believed the *Urkaft* (primal strength) of the vocal instrument could be rediscovered,[38] led to several techniques of induced low-trunk breath-management maneuvers, including anal-sphincteral occlusion and the cultivated grunt (extension of the vocal fold closure phase during phonatory cycles, with sudden release of glottal tension at phrase terminations).

Frederick Husler, with his collaborator Yvonne Rodd-Marling, made a 20th-century attempt to recover a presumed primitive vocal Atlantis. Through a series of exercises (including what he considered to be prespeech maneuvers), he meant to reestablish the vocal freedom he believed to have been lost through civilization's harnessing of the vocal instrument to the functions of speech.[39] A large group of teachers follow the Husler Method; they are found mostly in German, British, and Canadian conservatory enclaves.

The great Polish artist Jean de Reszke (1850–1925) stated that he did not wish to establish a method but only to express his personal ideas about the art of singing, yet his influence on the future of singing in France was monumental. Despite some study with Cotogni (a representative of the Lamperti school), Reszke did not advocate postural attitudes of the Italian school, preferring that the student discover "relaxed" breathing by sitting with collapsed and rounded shoulders and by dropping all muscles of the torso except the diaphragm. According to reports,[40] he advised, "Imagine yourself to be a great church bell, where all the sonority is round the rim." He aimed for local control of the diaphragm and recommended that "the body sit down on the diaphragm." He suggested the use of the sigh, together with hot-air expulsion to be felt on the hand, as means for "relaxing" the glottis, the throat, and the tongue. These admonitions are in line with a number of non-Italianate models that would take root in mid-20th-century North American soil. Reszke also advocated principles that remain characteristic of current (but by no means all) 20th-century French voice instruction: (1) Raised head posture (singing to the gallery). (2) Placement of the tone in the masque and at the bridge of the nose. (3) Producing "the singers grimace" (*la grimace de la chanteuse*) for high notes. One of his favorite exercises was based on a phrase containing a series of French nasals: *Pendant que l'enfant mange son pain, le chien tremble dans le buisson.*

For years, Paris was the international operatic center of the world. However, with a few notable exceptions, French singers have not enjoyed international careers in the later decades of the 20th century. Many observers, including French singing teachers, tend to view 20th-century French vocalism as being, at least in part, a Reszke heritage. A return to international pedagogic orientation is increasingly in progress in France.

At the close of the 19th century, the international Italianate pedagogy model was represented by non-Italian pupils of Giovanni Battista Lamperti. Englishman William Shakespeare's end-of-the-century treatises, made available in 1921 versions called *The Art of Singing*[41] and *Plain Words on Singing,* reiterate the *lutte vocale* of the Lamperti School: opposition between the muscles which draw in the breath. Noiseless and imperceptible breathing was the aim; a phrase was never to be terminated by allowing the torso to collapse. Although some aspects of traditional British vocal technique (such as spreading of the upper back) entered into Shakespeare's pedagogy, in general he was in line with the historic international school.

The same is true of Shakespeare's countryman H. Plunket Greene, who at the close of his 1912 book, *Interpretation in Song,*[42] appended two chapters, one devoted to breath management, the second to legato. Both could have been written by either of the Lampertis. Plunket Greene wanted an axial posture "with the chest as high as ever it will go." He detailed techniques for inducing the *appoggio* and delineated factors that contribute to legato singing.

Current British vocal technique seems to be of two minds, one filled with historic Italianate pedagogic ideals, the other aimed at "purity" of timbre based on influences from the treble-voice liturgical tradition—"cathedral tone." However, the one concept tumbles into the other, so that typical British tonal ideals often take on a recognizable insular flavor. (It is hardly possible to mistake British-trained operatic tenors, sopranos, or mezzo-sopranos for Italian-trained singers.)

At the beginning of the 20th century, the E. G. White Society proposed the theory of sinus tone production.[43] Despite a lack of scientific verification for its basic tenet, the society still claims more than 200 active members, most of them English and North American. It is closely allied with British notions of "tonal purity."

More recently, E. Herbert-Caesari attempted in several volumes[44–46] to fuse the mystical with the mechanical. His books remain influential in British vocal pedagogy.

In 1935 Herbert Witherspoon became director of the Metropolitan Opera Company, where he had already sung for eight seasons. He was a key figure in the performance world and in academia and was one of the founders of the oldest voice-teacher organizations in the world: the American Academy of Teachers of Singing and the Chicago Singing Teachers Guild. As mentioned earlier, Witherspoon is a direct descendant of the historic international Italian School. His 1925 *Singing*[4] remains a classic of modern vocal pedagogy. He studied with G.B. Lamperti and continued that tradition. Witherspoon's unique contribution originated in his conviction (1) that the singing voice primarily is a physical instrument that obeys the laws of efficient physical function, and (2) that the singing voice is an acoustic instrument that must be produced naturally in accordance with the laws of vocal acoustics. His dictum that we do not perform any physical act through relaxation, but with correct tension and action, places him in direct opposition to Germanic/Nordic techniques of the lowered, relaxed torso. His "lifts of the breath," meaning breath-energy increase at registration pivotal points, correspond to the passaggi registration demarcations of the Lamperti school. His treatment of vocal tract filtering is in complete accord with that school. A typical passage reads:

> . . . as pitch ascends . . . the tongue rises coördinately upwards and forwards, changing the shape of the throat and the mouth, the fauces point forward and narrow, or approximate; the uvula rises and finally disappears, the soft palate rises forward, never backward; while the epiglottis, rising up against the back of the lower tongue, seems to have a law of its own regarding quality, clear or veiled.

Not all of his observations precisely corresponded to what modern investigation verifies, yet Witherspoon masterfully combined past international vocalism with then-available scientific and acoustic information; tradition and modern pragmatism found a happy marriage. His pedagogy was based on the language of function, yet Witherspoon stressed that singing deals not simply with mechanics ("muscles and organs cannot be locally controlled") and that it is linguistic and musical interpretation that finally control technique.

In the period immediately before and following World War II, a plethora of writings on vocal technique emerged in Germany. In general, they tend to support low-abdominal breath-management techniques and fixated resonator tracts. Some American pedagogics were not far behind in building on those premises. Pedagogic cultivars of all the national schools flourish on the North American continent, yet the international Italian model is still the predominant exemplar for the professional singer.

The influence of Douglas Stanley, beginning with his 1929 *The Science of Voice*,[47] has been enduring on a small but devoted segment of American voice teaching circles. His viewpoints on register separation and unification have been further expanded by the skillful writing of Cornelius Reid.[48-50]

Among publications that have exerted influence on mid-20th-century vocalism, none has been more forceful than William Vennard's *Singing, the Mechanism and the Technic*.[51] This volume is a reliable source for the study of anatomy, physiology, and acoustics of the vocal instrument. As regards his use of the yawn/sigh device and his stances on "belly breathing," the *passaggi,* vocal registration, and postures of the vocal tract, Vennard indicates partial allegiance to the historic Germanic/Nordic camp. In other respects, he appears to be in tune with international vocalism.

Another important pedagogic strand in recent North American pedagogy comes from the prolific Berton Coffin,[52-54] whose premises unite his knowledge of the phonetic properties of the singing voice with scholarly interest in historic vocalism. Coffin's advocacy of elevated laryngeal and head postures described as "the sword-swallowing position," and his championing of male falsetto as a legitimate extension of the upper voice, ally him with segments of the modern French School, although in most other respects he retains allegiance to the international Italianate school.

A splendid singer himself, D. Ralph Appelman attempted to unite vocal pedagogy and scientific principles in his ground-breaking volume, *The Science of Vocal Pedagogy*,[55] which is filled with detailed information on physiology and acoustics. It has been difficult for Appelman's admirers to translate his highly systematized pedagogy into accessible lay language.

Even the briefest survey of vocal pedagogy must append a list (by no means definitive) of voice professionals, past and present, who have contributed significant articles or books on the relationships of function, artistic singing, and vocal pedagogy: L. Bachner; R.M. Baken; W. Bartholomew; M. Benninger; M.P. Bonnier; D. Brewer; M. Bunch; V.A. Christy; T. Cleveland; D. Clippinger; R. Colton; A. Cranmer; R. Edwin; J. Estill; V.A. Fields; T. Fillebrown; V. Fuchs; W.J. Gould; J.W. Gregg; T. Hixon; C.H. Holbrook; H. Hollien; R. Husson; J. Klein; J. Large; V. Lawrence; P. Lohmann; R. Luchsinger; M. Mackenzie; M.S. MacKinley; L. Manén; P.M. Marafiotti; W. McIver; B. McClosky; J. McKinney; C. Meano; D.C. Miller; D.G. Miller; F. Miller; R. Miller; G.P. Moore; R.C. Mori; M. Nadoleczny; G. Newton; D. Proctor; A. Rose; R. Rosewal; R. Sataloff; H.K. Schütte; N. Scotto di Carlo ; C. Seashore; R. Sherer; T. Shipp; D. Slater; A. Sonninen; A. Stampa; R.H. Stetson; J. Sundberg; J. Tarneaud; R. Taylor; J. Teachey; I. Titze ; J.B. van Deinse ; W. van den Berg; H. von Leden ; K. Westerman; H. W. Whitlock ; J. Wilcox; C. Wilder; P.S. Wormhoudt; and B.D. Wyke.

Recent contributors to the literature on vocal pedagogy apply fiberoptic stroboscopy, spectrography, fluoroscopy, and other forms of measurement to the events of voicing. Their intention has not been mostly to invent new ways to sing but to objectively compare traditional, international, national, regional, and idiosyncratic pedagogies in matters of their vocal efficiency and their relationship to vocal aesthetics and to vocal health.

Conclusion

The history of vocal pedagogy may be traced over a period of centuries. The earliest writings discussed in this chapter date from the 15th century. The Italianate School developed in the 18th century, and a subsequently diverse school of pedagogy emerged. A variety of influences have determined the progress of singing pedagogy and the techniques of singing and teaching utilized most widely today.

References

1. Jander O. Singing. In: Sadie S, ed. *The New Grove Dictionary of Music and Musicians*. New York, NY: Grove's Dictionaries of Music; 1980:17.
2. Harris E. The Baroque era voices. In: Brown HM, Sadie S, eds. *Performance Practice: Music After 1600*. New York, NY: WW Norton; 1989.
3. de Bacilly B; Caswell A, trans. 1968. (Originally published as *Remarques curieuses sur l'art de bien chanter*. Paris: 1668.)
4. Witherspoon H. *Singing*. New York, NY: G Schirmer; 1925.
5. Duey P. *Bel Canto in its Golden Age*. New York, NY: King's Crown Press; 1950.
6. Heriot A. *The Castrati in Opera*. New York, NY: Da Capo Press;1964.
7. Pleasants H. *The Great Singers*. New York, NY: Simon and Schuster; 1966.
8. Bérnard J-B (J-A). *L'ai-t due Chant*. Paris; 1755.
9. Tosi P-F; Galliard JE, trans. *Observations on the Florid Song*. London; 1742.

10. Mancini G; Buzzi P, trans. *Practical Reflections on the Art of Singing*. Boston, Mass: Oliver Ditson; 1907.

11. Coffin B. Vocal pedagogy classics: practical reflections on figured singing by Giambattista Mancini. In: Miller R, ed. *The NATS Bulletin*. 1981;37(4):47–49.

12. Crutchfield W. The 19th century: voices. In: Brown HM, Sadie S, eds. *Performance Practice: Music after 1600*. New York, NY: WW Norton; 1989.

13. Corri D. *The Singer's Preceptor*. London: 1810.

14. García M.P.V.R. *Exercices pour la voix*. Paris: A Parite; c.1820.

15. García M.P.R. *Trait complet de l'art du chant*. Paris: French Academy of Science, 1840.

16. García M.P.R. *Memoire sur la voix humaine*. Paris: E Suverger; 1841.

17. García, M.P.R. *Garcia's Complete School of Singing*. London: Cramer Beal and Chappell; 1872.

18. Klein H. *An Essay on Bel Canto*. London: Oxford University Press; 1923.

19. Lablache L. *Lablache's Complete Method of Singing: or, a Rational Analysis of the Principles According to Which the Studies Should be Directed for Developing the Voice and Rendering it Flexible*. Boston, Mass: Oliver Ditson.

20. Lamperti F; Griffith JC, trans. *A Treatise on the Art of Singing*. New York, NY: G Schirmer.

21. Lamperti G-B; Baker T, trans. *The Techniques of Bel Canto*. New York, NY: G. Schirmer; 1905.

22. Brown WE. *Vocal Wisdom: Maxims of Giovanni Battista Lamperti*. New York, NY: Crescendo Press; 1957.

23. Timberlake C. Apropos of appoggio, parts I and II. In: McKinney J, ed. *The NATS Journal*. 1995;52(3,4).

24. Stockhausen J. *Method of Singing*. London: Novello; 1884.

25. Seiler E. *The Voice in Singing*. Philadelphia, Pa: JB Lippincott; 1875.

26. Behne E. *The Mechanism of the Human Voice*. London: J Curwen & Sons; 1880.

27. Browne L, Behnke E. *Voice Song and Speech*. New York, NY: GP Putnam's Sons; 1897.

28. Delle Sedie E. *A Complete Method of Singing*. New York: private printing; 1894.

29. Warman EB. *The Voice: How to Train It and Care for It*. Boston, Mass: Lee and Shepard; 1889.

30. Byers MC. Sbriglia's Method of Singing. In: *The Etude*. May 1942.

31. Marchesi M. *Theoretical and Practical Vocal Method*. New York, NY: Dover; 1970.

32. Marcesi M. *Ten Singing Lessons*. New York, NY: Harper & Brothers; 1901.

33. Lehmann L. *How to Sing*. New York, NY: Macmillan; 1903.

34. Martienssen-Lohmann F. *Das bewusste Singen*. Leipzig: CF Kahnt; 1923.

35. Martienssen-Lohmann F. *Der Opernsänger*. Mainz: B Schott's Söhne; 1943.

36. Martienssen-Lohmann F. *Der wissende Sänger*. Zurich: Atlantis-Verlag; 1963.

37. Armin G. *Die Technik der Breitspannung: In: Beitrag über die horizontal-vertikalen Spannkräfte beim Aufbau der Stimme nach dem "Stauprinzip."* Berlin: Verlag der Gesellschaft fur Stimmkultur; 1932.

38. Armin G. *Von der Urkraft der Stimme*. Lippstadt: Kistner & Siegel; 1921.

39. Husler F. Rodd-Marling Y. Singing: *The Physical Nature of the Vocal Organ*. London: Faber and Faber; 1960.

40. Johnstone-Douglas W. The teaching of Jean de Reszke, In: *Music and Letters*; July, 1925.

41. Shakespeare W. *The Art of Singing*. Bryn Mawr, Pa: Oliver Ditson; 1921.

42. Greene HP. *Interpretation in Song*. London: Macmillan; 1912.

43. White EG. *Sinus Tone Production*. Boston, Mass: Crescendo; 1970.

44. Herbert-Caesari E. *The Alchemy of Voice*. London: Robert Hale; 1965.

45. Herbert-Caesari E. *The Science and Sensations of Tone*. Boston, Mass: Crescendo; 1968.

46. Herbert-Caesari E. *The Voice of the Mind*. London: Robert Hale; 1969.

47. Stanley D. *The Science of Voice*. New York, NY: Carl Fischer; 1929.

48. Reid C. *Bel Canto Principles and Practices*. New York, NY: Coleman-Ross; 1950.

49. Reid C. *Psyche and Soma*. New York, NY: J Pattelson Music House; 1975.

50. Reid C. *The Free Voice*. New York, NY: Coleman-Ross; 1965.

51. Vennard W. *The Mechanism and the Technic*. 5th ed. New York, NY: Carl Fischer; 1967.

52. Coffin B. *Historical Vocal Pedagogy*. Metuchen, NJ: Scarecrow Press; 1989.

53. Coffin B. *Overtones of Bel Canto*. Metuchen, NJ: Scarecrow Press; 1982.

54. Coffin B. *The Sounds of Singing: Vocal Technique with Vowel-Pitch Charts*. Metuchen, NJ: Scarecrow Press; 1977.

55. Appelman R. *The Science of Vocal Pedagogy*. Bloomington, Ind: Indiana University Press; 1967.

9

The Singing Voice Specialist

Robert Thayer Sataloff, Margaret M. Baroody,
Kate A. Emerich, and Linda M. Carroll

How many people have wished "If only I could sing..."? The fact is, virtually everyone can. Anyone who has pitch variation in his or her speaking voice and can tell whether two musical tones are the same or different can be taught to sing. That does not mean that he or she will be the next Luciano Pavarotti, but such a person can usually develop the muscle strength, ear–voice coordination, and confidence to enjoy singing and to be enjoyed by others. However, love of music is not the only reason for learning to sing. The muscles trained in coordination, ear training, and breath control during singing lessons can be extremely helpful in strengthening the speaking voice. A comprehensive voice team incorporates the benefits provided by a singing teacher with those of a speech-language pathologist and acting-voice trainer to optimize and expedite voice improvement.

Singing Lessons: An Overview

Pedagogy

To understand the special considerations for singing voice specialists (SVSs), teachers who specialize in working with injured voices, one must be familiar with singing training under normal circumstances. Within the academic world of voice teachers, the study of the workings of the voice and the techniques for training are known as *vocal pedagogy*. There are traditions and schools of thought in vocal pedagogy that date back centuries. They have been reviewed in numerous works by authors such as Richard Miller.[1] Over the years, many approaches have become popular enough to be known as "schools." There are German, French, Italian, and Russian schools, schools that follow the tenets of various famous teachers, and countless articles and books on teaching methodology. Many of the ideas and principles of one school of thought conflict with those of others.

Unfortunately, choral pedagogy is another matter. Choral singing has great influence on singers throughout the world, including young singers. Many choral conductors are trained as organists or instrumental conductors and have little or no formal training in singing or vocal pedagogy. Although specific methods for healthy choral singing have been promoted by various farsighted choir masters, there are few formal training or degree programs in choral pedagogy for the serious choral conductor who wishes to study the methods of producing optimal choral sound with optimal vocal health. Attention is just now being directed to this pervasive problem, as discussed in chapter 75.

Training of Singers

There are basically two types of traditional singing instructors: voice teachers and vocal coaches. The voice teacher works primarily on developing vocal technique through building coordination of musculature in the vocal mechanism. The vocal coach works primarily on repertoire (songs) and interpretation. The SVS is a voice teacher who works with injured voices, as discussed in the following sections. Many singers work with both a voice teacher and a vocal coach. Singers also need to be able to move on stage and feel comfortable with an audience, so some sort of body movement training can be necessary. Singers with a desire to sing opera or musical comedy may take some acting and stage combat training, as well. Aspiring classical singers also require language courses in at least Italian, German, and French. Study of Russian, Spanish, and other languages may also prove useful.

The beginning singer should, first and foremost, learn to omit any abusive vocal behaviors not only in singing, but also in speech. Although many singing teachers work with the speaking voice, most are not formally trained speakers or teachers of speech. Speech-language pathologists are trained and licensed to work with normal and pathological voices. Many, however, have little training or experience working with the refinements of technique required by the professional voice. Speech-language pathologists who have a particular interest in the professional voice attend symposia, obtain internships, and seek mentors. Fortunately, some speech-language pathologists have a great deal of experience and knowledge in voice, and it is ideal (but still unusual) for a singing teacher to affiliate with such a colleague. At present, it is illegal in most states for anyone but a licensed speech-language pathologist to treat a pathological speaking voice. Pathology, of course, is diagnosed only by a laryngologist. Voice trainers also exist, but there is no licensing or quality control for people who designate themselves in this category. They generally work with the voices of actors or public speakers and can be an invaluable asset to the voice team. There is no set of requirements that must be fulfilled in order for one to call him- or herself a singing teacher. Consequently, it is essential for other professionals to investigate the quality, training, experience, and reputation of singing teachers with whom they anticipate collaborating in patient care. Membership in the National Association of Teachers of Singers (NATS) is an encouraging sign, but the requirements for membership are certainly not rigorous enough to ensure that all members are high quality teachers.

Application of modern scientific insights to improve the training of teachers and singers has been prominent in the last few decades, and was popularized particularly by Vennard.[2] In recent years, increasing interest in interdisciplinary information disseminated through gatherings such as The Voice Foundation Symposia and NATS meetings has resulted in wide availability of undergraduate and graduate training programs in vocal pedagogy.

In this chapter, we make no effort to define good singing teaching or to promulgate any one technique as the *correct way*. In fact, there is great variation in responses from students in the studio, and good singing teachers have a large repertoire of techniques and exercises that allow them to individualize approaches to accomplish the goals of voice training.

In the next few pages, we present a few basic principles that can be used to understand singing teaching in general. Naturally, many details are omitted. However, for the reader who is not a voice teacher, this chapter should provide a basic idea of what a singing teacher does; and for the singing teacher, we have included information on documentation of voice lessons, correspondence with other professionals, and approaches to teaching people with injured voices. These topics frequently are not included in routine training for singing teachers.

In general, singing teaching begins with an assessment of the student. This leads to a determination of the singer's talent and problems, which guides the development of a lesson plan. Specific exercises are chosen to correct problems and improve vocal control and eventually artistry. Training occurs in all areas of the singer's anatomy. Abdominal exercises, pulmonary control, and correct alignment of posture cultivate the power sources of voice. Vocal exercises increase neuromuscular strength and coordination at the laryngeal level, improving not only range, quality, and vibratory symmetry, but also smooth control over changes in subglottal pressure, registers, and other variables. The supraglottic vocal tract is also trained, developing optimal vocal tract position and shape to create the desired harmonics without unnecessary muscle tension and with improved resonance. In general, principles of artistic economy apply. That is, if a good sound can be made without involving a specific muscle group (eg, those muscles that retract the tongue), then using extraneous muscles is generally wrong and deleterious to vocal health and performance. In most cases, voice lessons result in steady, gradual improvement in voice quality, range, efficiency, and endurance. Voice lessons should not end in hoarseness or physical discomfort in the neck or throat (although abdominal and back muscles are often fatigued and ache).

The principles of proper voice production are largely the same in speaking and singing. In fact, many people believe that the singing voice is simply a natural extension of a good speaking voice. In any case, training supplied by a singing teacher and a speech-language pathologist should be compatible and symbiotic. If a singer is receiving contradictory information from these two voice professionals (and is correctly interpreting their instructions), it could be indicative of incorrect training from one of them. Close scrutiny is warranted.

Singing Voice Specialist

As stated previously, singing voice teachers who work primarily with injured or abused voices of singers and nonsingers are known as "singing voice specialists" (SVS). The SVS is an experienced and specially trained voice teacher, usually with a degree in voice performance or pedagogy, who has professional voice performance experience, training in anatomy and physiology, training in the rehabilitation of injured voice users, and other special education. In addition to these basics, the SVS must acquire familiarity with objective voice measurement equipment and assessment; gain a basic understanding of the principles of laryngology and medications used commonly in this patient population and their potential effects, if any, on the voice; and have a fundamental knowledge of the principles and practices of speech-language pathologists. Being able to relate to performance demands based on personal experience is most helpful. It is critical that a singing voice specialist has an exceptional ability to hear minute changes in vocal quality and be an astutely demanding perfectionist. It is also desirable (but not essential) for the SVS to have reasonably good keyboard skills. He or she should be able to play scales for the patient, accompany simple songs, and make individualized practice tapes. It is not essential for the SVS to be a highly skilled pianist.

The SVS who works in an arts-medicine or voice care center may encounter differences from the routine studio work. The range of individual vocal potential is enormous. Some patients have great talent and potential for excellence, others may already be world-class professional singers and/or actors but require special instruction while recovering from vocal injury, and many are avocational singers. Also, there are other patients who have no interest in singing but can benefit from breath management, relaxation, resonance, and musical training in an effort to improve their speaking voices. Singing training for nonsingers should be pursued only in collaboration with traditional voice therapy provided by a certified speech-language pathologist.

The SVS must first be an excellent singing teacher, should have extensive training in the singing voice and, ideally, have personal experience as a professional singer. Being able to relate to performance demands on the basis of personal experience is most helpful. It is also desirable (but not essential) for the SVS to have reasonably good keyboard skills. He or she should be able to play scales with the patient, accompany simple songs, and make individualized practice tapes. It is not essential that the SVS be a highly skilled pianist. However, it is critical that he or she has an exceptional ability to hear minute changes in vocal quality and be an astutely demanding perfectionist.

At present, there are no formal training programs in the United States that teach singing teachers to work with injured voices. In fact, there are few good programs to train interested persons in "how to teach singing" in general. It is illegal in most states for a singing teacher to provide therapy for an injured or pathological voice unless he or she meets licensure requirements, most of which are equivalent to certification by the American Speech-Language-Hearing Association (ASHA). As stated earlier, however, speech-language pathologists generally do not receive training in the care of the professional voice. Very few speech-language pathology training programs provide instruction on care of the professional speaker, and most have no training in the singing voice at all. There is, however, a joint committee of ASHA and NATS that has compiled a list of professionals who have partially or fully met requirements for interdisciplinary training. Information on this joint committee may be obtained by contacting either ASHA or NATS. A few graduate programs have made great strides in combining the knowledge required from both fields, such as the vocology program at the University of Iowa. At present, if an independent voice teacher accepts a student for "voice rehabilitation" without having the student work concurrently with a licensed speech-language pathologist, that teacher may be subject to litigation, even if the student is referred by a laryngologist. A good interdisciplinary team working under one roof not only provides optimal patient care, but also obviates potential legal problems of this sort.

To acquire the necessary knowledge to become a SVS, it is helpful for the interested singing teacher to take advantage of available graduate level courses in speech science, neuroanatomy, neurophysiology, and speech-language pathology. There are also an increasing number of symposia dedicated to the professional voice. These offer additional training by practitioners skilled in the field. The Voice Foundation offers the most extensive annual symposium on care of the professional voice. Information may be obtained by writing to The Voice Foundation, 1721 Pine Street, Philadelphia, Pennsylvania 19103. Important information can also be gleaned from many of the publications listed as suggested readings near the end of this book. In addition, even for experienced voice teachers, a professional internship of some sort is almost imperative. The duration varies with the teacher's experience and need, and it may be broken up into short observation periods. However, a singing teacher interested in becoming active in caring for the injured voice needs to observe laryngologists in the office and operating room, speech-language pathologists specializing in professional voice care, SVSs working with injured voices, and voice laboratory technicians working with instrumentation. Access to such opportunities is limited, but it is available.

The trained SVS aids in the remediation of voice disorders utilizing singing voice exercises specific to the patient's vocal condition. The SVS works with a voice patient when recommended by the otolaryngologist, following strobovideolaryngoscopic examination and objective voice assessment (acoustic, aerodynamic, and other measures). A SVS should never work with a patient without a comprehensive medical examination and diagnosis from an otolaryngologist, because (among other reasons) voice work is contraindicated in some conditions such as recent vocal fold hemorrhage.

An SVS can be useful in the remediation of singers and nonsingers. However, it is *essential* that singers work with the SVS to ensure safe, healthy vocal production and to identify and eliminate potentially dangerous compensatory technical errors that often develop in response to vocal injury or dysfunction. The SVS is not a replacement for the patient's customary voice teacher. Rather, the SVS works with the patient's voice teacher to educate him or her about the patient's voice disorder, includes the voice teacher in the sessions (if approved by the patient), and instructs the patient and teacher regarding appropriate vocal exercises and goals in light of medical limitations established by the laryngologist.

For nonsingers, supplementing traditional voice therapy (by the speech-language pathologist) with singing voice training often facilitates and expedites therapy. There are many differences between singers and typical speakers. For example, the pitch range of conversational speech usually encompasses about a major sixth. Most singers possess at least a 2-octave range. Interestingly, physiological frequency range is about 3½ octaves in both singers and nonsingers, so most people have more potential than they realize. Pulmonary demands are also much greater during singing than speaking. In speech, we typically use 10% to 25% of vital capacity. The singer frequently uses closer to 65% of vital capacity. In many ways, singing is to speaking as running is to walking. In rehabilitating a patient who has difficulty walking, once a patient has learned to jog and run, walking becomes relatively trivial, since the patient is not working at his physiological limits during this activity. Likewise, once patients have acquired some of the athletic vocal skills employed routinely by singers (including increased frequency range, frequency and intensity variability, prolonged phrasing, breath management and support, etc), the demands of speech seem much less formidable. In many cases, even nonsingers utilize a more relaxed and anteriorly placed voice while performing sung or chantlike exercises. This helps facilitate a more resonant voice quality in the speaking voice, while eliminating pressed phonation.

Assessment

In evaluating a potential student, most singing teachers listen to a song or two, ask the singer to sing a few specific exercises, and discuss the singer's previous training. This process (history, diagnosis, treatment) is the same as that used by physicians and speech-language pathologists. More enlightened singing teachers also discuss matters of vocal health and hygiene in greater detail. Good singing teachers who hear any-

thing abnormal in a voice (hoarseness, breathiness, diplophonia, aphonia) routinely refer the prospective student for a laryngologic evaluation. Although rarely required by music schools, medical assessment and vocal fold visualization of all voice majors prior to matriculation would be beneficial.

The SVS's assessment protocol is more involved, not only because the singers have vocal problems, but also because it is necessary that the SVS have extensive knowledge of the experience, habits, and health of the patient. In an arts-medicine setting, the laryngologist has usually examined the patient before the SVS begins the evaluation. Regardless of these circumstances, we find value in a systematic, comprehensive assessment of each patient by the SVS. The SVS takes his or her own history from the patient, even though he or she may have been present when the laryngologist obtained a similar history. Repetition frequently yields additional information of importance to the voice team. Taking a history also allows the SVS the opportunity to more closely observe the speaking habits of the patient and to establish a comfortable rapport with the patient. The questions asked in the history are the same as those asked by the physician and are summarized in Appendix II. If a history form has not been completed for the laryngologist, the SVS asks the patient to complete a similar questionnaire. If a patient history form has already been completed for the physician, the SVS reviews this information and asks additional questions about previous teachers and training, specific techniques used, and other singing experience. The patient is asked to estimate the number of hours that he or she is speaking and singing throughout a typical day and high/low voice use days, if usage varies dramatically. Other questions regarding voice use are asked of the singer-patient, such as:

1. What kind of music do you perform most of often?
2. Do you sing in different voice ranges or classifications?
3. Are you playing any instruments while singing?
4. What is the environment like where you are performing?
5. Is there an amplification system? If so, are monitor speakers utilized?
6. Are special costumes and staging involved during singing?
7. How many years of formal singing training have you had?
8. How many teachers have you had?
9. What are your career goals?
10. What is your current career status?
11. Do you have recordings and/or videos of your voice at its best and at its worst?

The singer and nonsinger are asked about vocally abusive habits during speaking, such as:

1. Are you exposed to passive smoke?
2. Do you do any yelling (for or at pets, children, spouses)?
3. Do you do any coughing (in the morning, following meals)?
4. Do you find yourself talking loudly (on the telephone or over ambient noise)?
5. Do you clear your throat frequently?
6. Do you work out with weights? If so, do you breathe on exertion? Do you do aerobics?
7. Do you whisper?

If the patient is a singer, the next portion of the evaluation involves listening to the singer's usual warm-up exercises or warming-up the singer with scales, then listening to a song of the singer's choice. The entire evaluation is tape-recorded, and videotaped, if possible, as are subsequent lessons. Such tapes are good not only for documenting progress, but also for feedback for teaching purposes. In addition to the tape recorder and video camera, basic equipment for a voice studio includes a piano (or keyboard), full length mirror, hand-held mirror, and good lighting. The studio should have reasonably "live" acoustics, with a minimum of sound-treatment materials. It should also be properly heated and humidified, and drinking water should be readily available. The singing evaluation is usually done with the patient standing unless the patient routinely sings in a seated position. The patient is assessed for stance/posture, breath control, support, jaw and oral cavity position, general tension, range, and quality of sound. Range should be assessed with a series of scales, beginning comfortably in the patient's lower or middle range. The patient is asked to sing three-note or five-note ascending and descending scales on /ɑ/ or /ma/. The scales should proceed past the upper passaggio (including the falsetto in men) up to the highest musically acceptable note and descend to the lowest musically acceptable note. Voice breaks and other difficulties are noted. The voice should not be strained, and it is the SVS's responsibility to decide when the patient has reached his or her limit. The authors use a form for the SVS to record observations conveniently (Fig 9–1). Specific characteristics are assessed in each area, and a training program is designed to correct any errors observed.

Stance/Posture

The head, neck, and shoulders should be in neutral position. The shoulders should not be elevated, rolled forward, or held back, as these maneuvers introduce unnecessary tension. A singer should stand comfortably straight, but not in a stiffly erect, military fashion. Knees should be slightly bent and flexible, not locked, and weight should be centered over the metatarsal head (balls of the feet), not the heels. The feet should be apart, but not more apparent than the width of the shoulders. Many singers prefer to have one foot slightly forward. This athletic, well-balanced stance opti-

---

SUBJECTIVE EVALUATION: SINGING VOICE

TAPE # _____

☐ PROFESSIONAL VOICE USER
☐ NONPROFESSIONAL VOICE USER
☐ CLASSICAL SINGER
☐ NON-CLASSICAL SINGER
☐ NONSINGER

NAME: _____

DATE OF EVALUATION: _____

AGE: ____ DATE OF BIRTH: _____

SEX: ☐ MALE ☐ FEMALE

OTOLARYNGOLOGIST: _____

MEDICAL DIAGNOSIS: _____

SPEECH-LANGUAGE PATHOLOGIST: ____

OCCUPATION: _____

YEARS VOICE STUDY: _____

VOICE TEACHERS: _____

LONGEST TEACHER: _____

LAST VOICE LESSION: _____

Fig 9–1. Evaluation form used by singing voice specialists. +, minimal cues; ++, considerable tactile and visual cues required. *(continued)*

CHARACTERISTIC	CORRECTS TECHNIQUE		
	+ CUES	+ + CUES	UNABLE
STANCE/POSTURE:			
FEET POSITION			
WEIGHT FORWARD			
KNEES UNLOCKED			
UPPER TORSO/STERNUM			
SHOULDERS			
STRAP MUSCLES			
LARYNGEAL MOVEMENT			
FOREHEAD TENSION			
HEAD/NECK PROTRUSION			
HEAD/NECK ELEVATION			
BREATH:			
ABDOMINAL/DIAPHRAGMATIC			
THORACIC			
CLAVICULAR			
SHALLOW			
RAPID			
AUDIBLE			
EXCESSIVE ABDOMINAL MOVEMENT			
SUPPORT:			
EFFECTIVE			
DEFICIENT			
INEFFECTIVE			
LATE			
INVERSE PRESSURE			
ORAL CAVITY:			
REDUCED OPENING			
RISORIUS TENSION			
JAW JUTTING			
ANTERIOR JAW TENSION			
POSTERIOR JAW TENSION			
ANTERIOR TONGUE RETRACTION			
ANTERIOR TONGUE CURL			
POSTERIOR TONGUE ELEVATION			
POSTERIOR TONGUE DEPRESSION			

Fig 9–1. (continued)

```
RESONANCE: _____

FOCUS: _____

RANGE: _____SCALES: _____

QUALITY: _____

PLAN: _____
```

Fig 9–1. *(continued)*

mizes breathing and support. It behooves the SVS to acquire special knowledge of posture analysis and muscle conditioning. In many cases, it is advisable for the patient to include physical exercises to improve posture and strengthen support muscles. Basic principles of posture analysis and exercise programs can be found in the literature,[3] and consultation with a skilled physiatrist or physical therapist may be valuable in selected cases. The Alexander and Feldenkrais techniques, which are designed to deal with more efficient postural alignment, also may prove beneficial.

Breathing

The rib cage should be erect, so that the upper thorax appears slightly more full than during comfortable speech, but it should not rise excessively or cause muscle tension in the upper thorax, supraclavicular area, or neck. Most of the active breathing is abdominal, and distension should occur in the front, back, and sides. Breathing should be relatively relaxed, quiet, and nasal breathing is preferable when time between phrases permits. High thoracic breathing patterns, rapid intake, and noisy inspiration frequently indicate tension, which may be carried over into vocalization. Abdominal movement during inspiration and expiration should be efficient. Excessive abdominal activity may occur in singers consciously struggling to optimize breathing and support. Such excessive inflection, contraction, and distension of abdominal muscles undermine the adjustment process between breathing and initiating effective support.

Support

Support is a difficult concept for many singers to coordinate efficiently, and various constructs are used to teach it. The fundamental principle is to generate a vector of force under the airstream, supporting it upward between the vocal folds. Support should be continuous, not static. Some good abdominal and thoracic support may occur spontaneously in people while singing a rolled /r/, and singing scales on /v/. Good support may also be experienced during various spontaneous maneuvers such as laughing, coughing, or the act of blowing out a candle. Muscles in the lower abdomen, upper abdomen, and lower thorax and back are actively involved. Coordinated support should be initiated just before a tone is heard. In many cases, if a teacher advises a student to bring abdominal muscles in and up, the student will also raise his or her shoulder, chest, and neck muscles. Consequently, many teaching constructs have been created in which students are advised to think of their support as going "down and out" (the inverse pressure approach), rather than "inward and upward." This effort may also be an attempt to more precisely balance the flow of air needed for singing. Any teaching imagery can be effective, so long as the student and teacher understand the difference between the language of the imagery and the physical effect they are really trying to achieve. Good support should be present not only when singing high notes, but also in lower ranges. Singers frequently support well going up a scale but relax excessively during descending passages and have virtually no effective support in portions of their mid and lower ranges.

Support may be assessed visually and by palpation. It is often best to evaluate support while testing range, when the singer is not aware that support functions are being scrutinized. Good support is essential. When the power source is not working adequately, many voice users compensate with excess muscle tension in the neck, tongue, and jaw. Such muscular tension dysphonia is inefficient and potentially hazardous to the vocal folds.

Laryngeal Position

For most classical Western singing, the larynx is usually slightly below its neutral vertical position. The larynx should remain relatively stable and should not rise appreciably with ascending pitch or fall with descending pitch. These caveats are not necessarily true in other styles such as pop music, Asian music, and certain other cultural and ethnic styles. In general, note-by-note laryngeal articulation of pitch indicates improper singing technique.

Extrinsic Laryngeal Muscle Tension

All patients are visually evaluated for extrinsic laryngeal muscle tension during voice use. Protrusion of the strap muscles or any of the extrinsic laryngeal musculature may be indicative of muscle tension dysphonia, and such activity is considered indicative of hyperfunctional vocal behavior. Patients exhibiting this kind of behavior will often complain of throat pain lateral to the larynx with prolonged voice use and will present with "throaty" voice production. They commonly also have trouble singing softly, and they may develop a pitch wobble and voice fatigue.

Jaw Position

Jaw position may be assessed while singing /a/. The jaw should be allowed to open to its maximum, relaxed position, but it should not be forced open excessively. Appropriate jaw position is similar to that seen in most people just before the initiation of a yawn. It is generally close to a two-finger span, although no-one should be forced to meet this guideline if this degree of opening introduces jaw tension. The corners of the mouth should not be tensed, and the jaw should not quiver or alter position with changes in pitch. The posterior jaw should also be relaxed for all vowels. Decreased oral resonance due to limited mouth opening is often a tell-tale sign of jaw tension. Teeth clenching is characteristic of extreme jaw tension. However, mouth opening may change in relation to pitch.

Tongue Position

Tongue position may also be assessed on /a/. The tip of the tongue should rest in a relaxed posture against the mandibular central incisors or slightly behind. It should not retract, curl anteriorly, or rise posteriorly. The pharynx should generally be visible, not obscured by arching of the posterior aspect of the tongue. The tongue should be noted particularly at the moment when tone is initiated. Sudden tongue tension and retraction upon initiation of tone often indicate delayed or ineffective abdominal support. It is important to assess visually and by listening to the sound of the voice not only the anterior tongue position, but

also the posterior position of the tongue. Most well-trained singers know that the tongue is supposed to be relaxed and should not pull back from the teeth. However, it is possible (especially for the more advanced singer) to maintain the anterior tongue in good position and still introduce excessive posterior tongue tension. This excessive tension may result in voice fatigue and sometimes limitation of range. In addition to the criteria noted, tongue position should not change with alterations in pitch, and there should be no tongue activity apparent during routine five-note scales on /a/. The tongue and jaw should be able to function independently.

Face

While singing scales on /a/, virtually no facial muscle activity should be required. Excessive tension in the corners of the mouth, lips, corrugation of the chin, forehead tension, or other extraneous muscle use may indicate hyperfunction and may be associated with insufficient support. The facial expression should be pleasant, but no specific facial muscle gestures should be required to produce an /a/. Eliminating dependence on facial hyperfunction is important not only to optimize technique, but also because the singer and speaker need to be able to use facial muscles independently to show expression and emotion without affecting voice production.

Tone Placement

Singers and nonsingers often present with posterior tone placement in addition to tongue and jaw tension and extrinsic laryngeal muscle tension. A posterior tone will sound heavier and more mature, at least to the singer; and some singers will use this type of placement in an effort to sound older or to achieve a bigger sound. Unfortunately, posterior tone placement is usually indicative of excess muscle tension and improper singing technique. It also impairs the efficiency of the resonator (decreased singer's formant) thereby limiting projection and making the singer work harder to be heard.

Summary

At the completion of the assessment process, observations and findings are reviewed with the student. Fatigue, nervousness, and other variables must be taken into account during the first lesson, but an experienced SVS usually can draw accurate conclusions during the initial evaluation. Specific deficiencies are explained, and plans to remedy them are established.

Specific exercises are selected, and the SVS teaches them to the student or patient in the singing studio. A practice schedule is assigned, and arrangements for follow-up and further lessons are made.

To appreciate the special considerations involved in working with injured voices, it is helpful to understand the kind of exercises used routinely in training noninjured voices. Many of these are useful for patients with vocal injuries, as well; but modifications are often necessary. The following section reviews exercises commonly used to train singers.

Exercises for "Routine" Singing Lessons

Singing lessons involve selected exercises to build muscle strength, coordination, and efficiency. Throughout training, a combination of tactile (hands), verbal, visual, and auditory (live and recorded) feedback is used to correct errors and ensure that the singer can tell which techniques and sounds are correct and which are not. The exercises are designed to develop all parts of the vocal mechanism. Like other muscle-building exercises, it is often better to structure such exercises in short sessions to be repeated a few times throughout the day. In beginners, sessions should rarely be more than 20 minutes in length until muscle strength is developed and technique becomes consistent. Exercises to warm-up the voice first thing in the morning and to cool-down the voice following each practice session, rehearsal, performance, and in the evening are especially important. Although the efficacy of vocal warm-up has been understood, the benefits of a vocal cool-down have not been as widely appreciated and followed.

General Body Exercises

The singing teacher must make an assessment of the student's general physical condition. Good aerobic conditioning, abdominal muscle strength, and back muscle development are particularly important. In any student with health problems, or in older students, exercise programs should always be developed in conjunction with medical supervision. Vocal development should include some form of aerobic activity (eg, jogging, fast walking, swimming, aerobic dance, etc), abdominal muscle exercises (eg, sit-ups), and exercises that affect the back and lower abdomen (eg, leg lifts). Only exercises that the singer can perform without inappropriate strain should be chosen. Singers must be instructed to avoid forceful glottic closure and other forms of voice abuse while exercising. Groaning during sit-ups or weight lifting or counting numbers during aerobic dance can cause vocal injury (in fact, hoarseness and vocal nodules are seen commonly in aerobics instructors). Nevertheless, if a singer cannot run up a couple of flights of stairs without getting excessively winded, pulmonary function should be evaluated.

Breathing

There are many exercises that work well for teaching breath management for singers. In some cases, the teacher simply explains thoracic and abdominal breathing and the desired principles and helps the student experiment with correct and incorrect breathing techniques and postures by pointing out which techniques are correct. In most students, some sort of tactile feedback helps. Placing a student in unusual positions frequently helps him or her sense aspects of breathing technique that are harder to feel in normal positions. Such exercises may be done with the student lying on the floor with a small book under his or her head and with knees bent and feet flat on the floor. Another useful technique is to ask the student to bend from the waist and place his or her hands laterally on the waist, take a full breath and feel rib expansion. The breath is taken slowly, avoiding elevation of the shoulders and maximizing expansion of the lower portion of the rib cage. The student is instructed to exhale slowly and repeats the exercise several times. This exercise is then performed with the student standing one third to one half of the way up, maintaining proper balance. The exercise steps are repeated, trying to maintain the same abdominal and lower back sensations. They are then repeated while standing erect. It should be remembered that these exercises are intended as facilitators. Actually, these positions create modifications in respiratory function that are not appropriate for long-term voice development. These maneuvers are intended to help establish body awareness early in the training process, and students must be cautioned not to practice excessively or vocalize in these unusual postures. Many alternate exercise regimens are also effective. The student may stand with arms perpendicular to the floor, palms upward, elbows slightly bent, shoulders relaxed, and sense upper torso alignment, ease of breath, and efficiency of support. Students are also instructed to practice breathing and to combine relaxed breathing with flexion and relaxation of support musculature periodically during the day, not only during practice sessions, but also while speaking or simply walking from place to place.

Support Exercises

It is important for each student to realize that it is possible to vocalize without hyperfunctional muscle activity. Many students, especially those with previous singing experience, habitually engage superfluous muscle groups in preparation for each sung phrase. For such students, it is often best to start teaching support by eliminating as much extraneous muscle activity as possible, teaching the student simply to breathe in a relaxed fashion, and then adding support and sound. For other students with fairly good technique and no significant hyperfunctional abuse, it may be appropriate to proceed directly to discussions of im-proving support musculature strength and coordination. The latter group of students is easier to teach, and the exercises listed below are examples of the kind of approach used for the former group. Such students may be advised to:

1. Take slow, deep breaths in and out through the mouth, eliminating all muscle tension in the oral cavity, head, and neck. These exercises are done facing a mirror.
2. Take a slow, deep breath, and exhale slowly for as long as possible on "wh," being careful to maintain good posture and not allow the chest to collapse.
3. Take a slow, deep breath, exhale on /s/, /ɑ/, and /ʃ/, being careful to maintain good posture and slow exhalation.
4. Take a slow breath, and initiate a descending sigh on /u/, /o/, and /ɑ/. These vowels are then repeated but initiated with the consonants used in the previous exercise. In particular, /s/ has a tendency to help elicit support. The student is instructed to maintain the same abdominal and lower back sensations during the vowel as initiated during the consonant. The student should not be afraid if this exercise encompasses more than one register. Smooth transition between registers in the long descending sigh should be encouraged.
5. Take a slow breath, and exhale, permitting a gently voiced sigh during the exhalation. The exercise is then repeated, and the singer is asked to sustain the sigh on a descending scale.
6. Take a slow, deep breath, relax the jaw, engage the support musculature as previously explained, and sustain the vowel /ɑ/. Observe the tongue and neck closely. Abdominal support should not create any visible change in the oral cavity, head, or neck.
7. Take a deep breath, initiate support, and sing five-note ascending and descending scales beginning on the note identified during deep sigh exercises. The scales should be done on /ɑ/, and later on /o/ and other vowels (Fig 9–2). Initially, the notes should be connected (legato), and the student should take care to avoid laryngeal rise and fall while changing pitch. For some beginners, even

five notes is too great a range to sing when using improper techniques such as tongue retraction. However, for most students, five-note scales can be performed throughout low and high ranges. Later, when technique is more consistent, more advanced exercises are used.

8. Rolled /r/, /v/, /ʃu/ and lip trills (continuous "br") in descending passages are also good for developing breath management and increasing consciousness of correct skeletal posture (Fig 9–3). The student must be monitored carefully for laryngeal and throat tension. Students who cannot produce a rolled /r/ or lip trills without inappropriate muscle tension should avoid these exercises until later in training.

Technical Exercises

Technical exercises are used to develop agility, increase range, and improve pitch accuracy. Such exercises include (among others):

1. Rapid and slow five-note ascending/descending scales while humming and on various vowels (Fig 9–4). This exercise is good for virtually all students, but should be monitored closely for laryngeal tension as well as posterior tongue and jaw tension that often accompany humming efforts. It may be preceded by a descending five-note slide.
2. Slow sliding scales ascending and descending a major third on /ɑ/ and on /o/ → /ɑ/ (Fig 9–5).

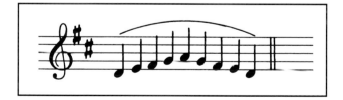

Fig 9–2. Five-note ascending/descending scale.

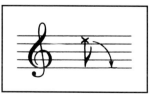

Fig 9–3. Five-note ascending/descending scale.

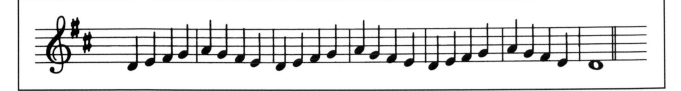

Fig 9–4. Repeated ascending/descending scales.

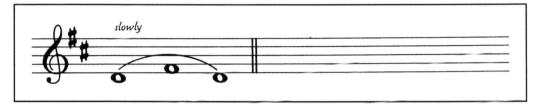

Fig 9–5. Slow ascending/descending slide of major third interval.

3. Arpeggio scales on /ɑ/ and /o/→/ɑ/, slowly, with careful legato connection from note to note (Fig 9–6). This exercise is good for the intermediate singer.

4. Slowly descending five-note scale, beginning on /u/ and changing to /ɑ/ on the last note, with a trill (Fig 9–7). This exercise should be used in the lower part of the voice to increase vocal control and effective use of support in the lower register. The trill should be a true half-step or whole-step trill, not simply excessive vibrato.

5. Lip vowel variation (/ɑ/ to /o/ to /u/ to /o/ to /ɑ/) exercises sung on a sustained tone (Fig 9–8). Tongue vowels may also be approached in this manner. This exercise may be done with tactile cues to keep the sound from "spreading." The vowel variation exercises are good for focusing the voice.

6. A great number of additional exercises are used during the training process. They involve connected and disconnected scales, patterns of scales involving various intervals rather than adjacent notes, exercises at different dynamics, exercises bridging different registers (eg, crescendo/diminuendo singing from falsetto to modal register and back), and many other patterns. Such vocalises may be found in numerous published collections and texts on vocal pedagogy.

Placement, Resonance, and Projection

Detailed discussion of tonal placement, sensations of resonance, and projection is bound to be controversial. For the purposes of this chapter, suffice it to say that, as respiratory control, muscle strength, and laryngeal coordination improve, various techniques are used to optimize the shape of the vocal tract. The tongue, soft palate, pharynx, jaw, and other regions of the supraglottic vocal tract are trained to generate with minimal effort the desired harmonic spectrum. In particular, the resonators enhance the desirable formant. Exercises to accomplish these goals include use of vowels, nasals, consonants, songs, chanting, ear training, and a considerable amount of trial and error with feedback from the teacher. Feedback from instrumentation such as spectrographs may also be helpful in selected cases.

Songs

Building repertoire may begin when the student has mastered several of the vocalises and has developed voice control over a large enough range to permit comfortable singing of the vocal literature. Singers who wish to sing classical repertoire do well to begin with an anthology of early Italian songs and arias and with simple English and American songs. Nonclassical singers should start with standard lyric-legato songs. Rock singers should also begin with balladlike rock songs rather than up-tempo pieces, and use songs that vary between modal and falsetto register, if possible. It is usually easier to begin with new repertoire, rather than trying to relearn old material in a technically correct fashion. Active performers should concentrate on incorporating the new technique into slower songs,

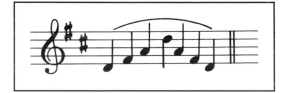

Fig 9–6. Arpeggio scales.

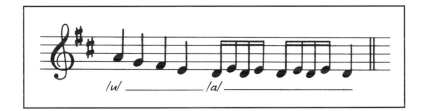

Fig 9–7. Descending scale with trill on last note.

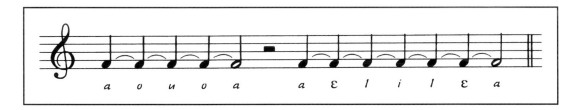

Fig 9–8. Vowel variation exercise.

gradually building the repertoire into an entire set or concert. If the student has been performing actively prior to studying with the teacher, it is especially important for the teacher to attend a performance of the singer. This allows a much deeper understanding of the singer's vocal needs, problems, and progress. Technical aspects of singing are the singer teacher's domain. Many singing teachers also provide training in interpretation, staging, and other artistic aspects of performance, although these matters can be relegated to voice coaches, acting teachers, and other professionals.

Training the Injured Voice

Special Considerations for the Singing Voice Specialist

In designing and individualizing training protocols, SVSs commonly work toward goals different from those familiar to most singing teachers. For example, in many instances, the SVS must be disciplined enough to ignore vocal quality, and to train the patient to practice appropriate techniques regardless of the sound. This is not a natural concept for singers, singing teachers, or even speakers. Ordinarily, a "good" sound is considered paramount, and singers will do whatever they can to sound attractive. This natural tendency may have gotten many of them into medical difficulty in the first place in the form of hyperfunctional muscle compensations. While rehabilitating the singer following disease, injury or surgery, it is essential to develop good technique, healthy muscle use, and to avoid muscle atrophy from prolonged voice rest or abstinence from singing. Neuromuscular rehabilitation can and should begin for many patients long before professional (or even attractive) vocal quality can be achieved. The timing of advancement in vocal training for such patients is determined by the SVS in collaboration with a laryngologist and speech-language pathologist. Early specially designed voice training (as soon as medically safe) is helpful in avoiding reinjury.

One of the most important aspects of training for an SVS is developing the ability to understand medical limitations, goals, prognosis, and expected duration of recovery (often months). Only with a clear understanding of these issues, and with full appreciation of the patient's activities and progress with the speech-language pathologist, can the SVS develop a singing protocol that is medically safe and appropriately helpful to the patient's voice rehabilitation. Training the singing voice with skillfully chosen exercises in the medical setting provides invaluable rehabilitation. Incorrect exercises can easily result in serious permanent vocal injury. Once the SVS has learned when the training process should be guided by tactile versus visual versus auditory feedback, and has mastered the other necessary skills and information, his or her contribution to the medical voice care team is invaluable not only for singers, but also for nonsingers.

Exercises

Singing voice sessions are designed to build muscle strength, coordination, flexibility, and efficiency. They are also designed to eliminate abusive vocal behaviors, promote easy and relaxed phonation, improve abdominal breathing and support, and promote frontal tone placement and resonant voice quality. This should lead to reduction, elimination, or prevention of vocal pathologies, optimal preparation for vocal fold surgery when necessary, and safe vocal production following surgery or injury.

There are no magic sets of vocal exercises. Each patient has his or her own specific needs depending on the pathology, extent of injury, age of injury, and vocal demands. It is important to understand the nature of the patient's vocal pathology, be able to identify probable causes of the pathology, identify compensatory technical behaviors, and understand the physiological and histological effects of the pathology in order to adequately work with an injured voice. Carefully chosen exercises are utilized, addressing each area of deficiency. In general, exercises are designed to develop all parts of the vocal mechanism. Like other muscle-building exercises, it is often better to structure such exercises in short sessions to be repeated a few times throughout the day. In beginners and patients with recent vocal injury, such sessions should rarely be more than 15–20 minutes in length (often less) until muscle strength is developed and technique becomes consistent.

When utilizing singing voice exercises, the patient should take frequent rest periods in order to reestablish appropriate muscle relaxation. Numerous man-euvers can facilitate this relaxation including gentle exhalatory gestures on a quiet, open-throated /hɑ/ or other vowel, stretching and gentle to vigorous movements of the body, massage, or even simply sitting or lying down. The duration of practice periods is strictly dictated by the laryngologist and the individual patient's ability to sing without any inappropriate strain or discomfort. Particularly in cases of resolving vocal fold hemorrhage, vocal fold tear or post-vocal fold surgery, 3–5 minutes of singing 2–4 times a day may prove sufficient. Duration and frequency of practice periods are increased according to the patient's comfort and skill level. It is absolutely critical that the patient be well-informed concerning general vocal hygiene and the need for appropriate stress management and sleep. The need for adequate hydration cannot be overemphasized. The exercises discussed below may be used for injured singers and nonsingers, according to the patient's abilities.

The previous instructions regarding general body exercises, breathing, and breath support exercises are applicable for the injured voice. When applying breath support to ascending/descending scales, however, it is often easiest to begin with limited note excursion. A sliding sung scale on a major second may eventually open more comfortably to a major third, then to a major fifth, and so on. Other ascending/descending patterns may also be used. Range in all exercises is strictly determined by the patient's ability to phonate the notes without inappropriate tension. Gentle sliding from note to note as opposed to strict delineation efforts on each note may be less traumatic to the vocal folds. Also, the easy stretching motion of the vocal folds on ascending/descending scales is believed to be effective in helping to regain vocal fold flexibility and in establishing appropriate compensation in the vocal mechanism. Lip and tongue trills may also prove useful on these scales and may be utilized on broader scales such as octaves, ninths, and elevenths, as the voice permits. Sliding sung scales and lip and tongue trills may be used in the rehabilitation of numerous vocal fold injuries including, but not exclusively, vocal fold scarring, vocal fold masses, superior laryngeal nerve paresis, and any resolving disruption of the vocal fold mucosa (I in Figure 9–9).

Legato, lightly sung three-note and five-note descending scales are recommended to help regain vocal fold agility. Ascending/descending scales sung in this fashion are also useful. Vowel choice is optional with open vowels such as /ɑ/ and /o/ usually providing the most exposed presentation of the voice. Again, scale excursion and overall range are determined by the patient's ability to maintain reasonable vocal technique (breath support, resonance space and placement) with minimal counterproductive compensatory muscle tension. This exercise is potentially useful in the remediation of most vocal fold injuries. Extreme caution is always recommended during the first sessions following disruption of the vocal fold mucosa (Fig 9–9II).

Exercises involving changes in volume appear to be useful in strengthening the vocal mechanism. They seem particularly effective in cases of superior laryngeal nerve pareses, when the ability of one or both vocal folds to stretch has been compromised. The concept of mezzo-piano to piano to mezzo-piano or piano to mezzo-piano to piano and later, mezzo-forte to piano to mezzo-forte and piano to mezzo-forte to piano may be applied to any number of scale patterns. The patient must be carefully monitored, particularly aurally and visually, to be sure that these alterations in loudness are not accomplished with inappropriate changes in the vocal tract, but rather through subtle breath support adjustments (Fig 9–9III). For patients with superior laryngeal nerve paresis, pitch-stretching exercises are also essential, such as sliding (glissando) passages. These may be combined with volume-variable exercises.

Most singing exercises may be performed on a hum, usually /ŋ/ or /m/. Humming is frequently performed incorrectly so care must be taken to monitor for inappropriate tensions. The /ŋ/ is best utilized with the mid or back portion of the tongue resting lightly against the roof of the mouth and the anterior tip of the tongue relaxed and in contact with the lower front teeth. The lips may be gently closed. The /m/ is most effective when the tongue is relaxed and forward in position but not touching the roof of the mouth, and the lips are resting gently against one another, not tightly pressed. With both hums, no amount of jaw, tongue or throat tension should be allowed. When done correctly, humming can be a particularly effective exercise for establishing better tonal placement and for stabilizing the delicate balance between the breath support system and the larynx. These exercises also help some patients improve kinesthetic recognition of muscle tension. Many patients get improved vocal function and tonal quality by first humming a scale pattern and then immediately repeating the pattern on a vowel sound (Fig 9–9IV).

When working with vocal fold paresis/paralysis patients, especially recurrent laryngeal nerve weakness where adduction and abduction are affected, the goal of more efficient glottic closure may be aided by the use of staccato exercises. Several patterns may prove useful. Vowel choice is optional, but several vowels should be used in the design of any patient's exercise program. Using /p/ or /b/ as an initial consonant can help facilitate the sensation of increased forward tonal placement. /H/ may also be used, but careful monitoring of laryngeal position and tension should be maintained (Fig 9–9V).

When working with the nonsinger, the SVS can offer significant contributions to the speaking voice. First, singing voice exercises may be effective in hastening the patient's adaptation of efficient vocal technique which is needed for correct speech production. Second, singing exercises can also strengthen specific areas of weakness within the vocal system and help establish appropriate compensations for permanent vocal fold injury. When working with the nonsinger, the SVS must choose exercises that allow for smooth carryover of vocal production from singing to speaking.

1. One useful concept is to establish technically well-sung phrases in the general frequency range of the speaking voice and then alternate between singing the phrase and speaking the phrase. Chantlike speaking may be utilized as a bridge between singing and the more normal inflection of the speaking voice. The consonant-vowel construction of the words can provide a useful tool in identifying and maintaining appropriate breath flow and placement of tonal resonance (Fig 9–9VI) during singing and connected speech. Also, note patterns may vary to more closely represent the pitch movement patterns of melodic speech (Fig 9–9VII).

2. Some patients are unable to sing technically well in or near their speaking registers but can produce a better singing voice in their middle or upper singing registers. Obviously, the goal would be to extend the more appropriate method of voice production into the speaking range. A descending scale, starting at the point of optimum vocal production, can be moved stepwise or gliding downward, finally resting on a note at the upper end of the speaking range. That final note is sustained and gradually moves from singing to speaking voice. This should be done all on one breath, if possible. Each successive scale pattern is one half step lower until the speaking range has been covered. Maintaining steady breath support and the more "open" resonance sensations of the singing voice as the patient moves into speech is the optimum goal. A descending scale on a vowel with the bottom note blended into spoken counting is also helpful (Fig 9–9VIII).

3. The relationship between recitative and speech can be very useful for singers with good speaking voices. Singing teachers frequently teach recitative

by having the student speak the words in rhythm and then add notes in a natural fashion. The connection can be bridged in the opposite direction, as well. Opera and oratorio singers skilled in recitative can start a familiar recitative passage with notes and gradually eliminate specific pitches, slipping into speaking voice. This concept of moving from singing voice smoothly into speaking voice can be utilized with various text passages and may prove useful for nonsingers as well as singers. Such exercises often expedite traditional voice rehabilitation. However, any SVS working with the speaking voice should do so only in conjunction with therapy provided by a speech-language pathologist.

4. Rap music can also work well for nonclassical singers and nonsingers with speaking voice problems. Rap music provides bridging material similar to recitative. When using rap music, the rhythm tract may be gradually faded out during the rap. It is surprising how many singers can sing and rap with appropriate technique, but speak poorly and have trouble grasping traditional speech therapy approaches. Like recitative, rap exercises should be combined with instruction from a speech-language pathologist to facilitate rehabilitation.

We have suggested only a few of the many possible singing voice exercises useful in the treatment of the injured voice. These exercises must not be considered prescriptive. Rather, individual programs must be contoured to the special strengths and weaknesses of each patient. Often, the patient has more than one problem, for instance: reflux, plus bilateral masses; superior laryngeal nerve paresis; reflux and a unilateral cyst; and so forth. The vast majority of patients present with some degree of hyperfunctional voice use. Even the most technically sophisticated classical singer can succumb to the use of counterproductive compensatory muscle tension. Furthermore, no attempt has been made in this chapter to address the extraordinarily complex psychological issues that often accompany voice problems. This infinite combination of variables presents the SVS with many unique challenges. It is important to remember that a singing voice exercise is a means to an end, not an end in itself. The SVS must call upon a refined and educated listening ability, broad practical experience with numerous vocal technical approaches, and a working knowledge of pertinent human anatomy, physiology, and voice disorders to efficiently and effectively impact this important patient population.

Singing Styles

It should be recognized that there are many styles other than classical Western operatic singing. It is essential for laryngologists, singing voice specialists, and all other members of the health care team to avoid biases common to those of us steeped in Western classical tradition. Although the singing techniques and behaviors discussed throughout this book, and in this chapter particularly, represent a healthy, established approach, other singing styles can also be healthy despite significant technical differences. For example, rock, pop, and country western singers may perform two to four 45-minute sets each night, six nights each week for years without vocal problems. These artists do not always use a laryngeal position slightly below neutral, as advocated for operatic singing. Some sing with a raised larynx, others with a neutral or low larynx, and still others vary laryngeal position throughout their pitch ranges. Many use much less respiratory volume than classical singers. However, they also use amplifiers and do not try to project their voices into large halls over orchestras and choirs. Singers in other cultures such as Persian, Turkish, Chinese, African and Tibetan singers use a variety of techniques that initially strike us as abusive. Yodeling, which involves leaps from chest voice to falsetto, also seems potentially hazardous, although it often is accompanied by more breath support than "regular" singing in the same performer. Countertenor singing is a style that utilizes the male falsetto. Incorrect falsetto singing can be extremely abusive; but technically skilled yodelers and countertenors can produce beautiful sounds for decades without vocal problems. Any of these styles may be vocally abusive if performed incorrectly. This is also true of classical operatic singing. However, we must recognize that it is technically possible to perform music in almost any style in a manner that is not only idiomatic, but also vocally safe. The voice team, and especially the laryngologist and singing voice specialist, must be familiar with the special techniques, demands, and problems of the singing style of each individual patient. It is neither helpful nor scientifically justified to dismiss any particular genre (including hard rock) as medically unacceptable. With sufficient understanding, patience, voice team skill and patient compliance, a vocally "right way" can be found to do almost anything.

Frequency of Lessons

Singing lessons should be given every week when possible, and every 10 to 14 days, at least, if weekly

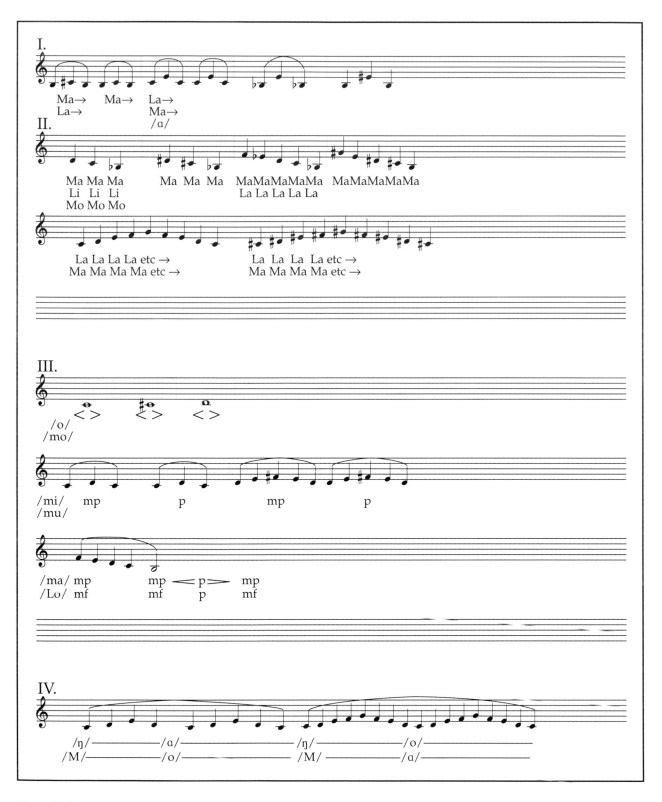

Fig 9–9. Carryover exercise from singing voice to speaking voice.

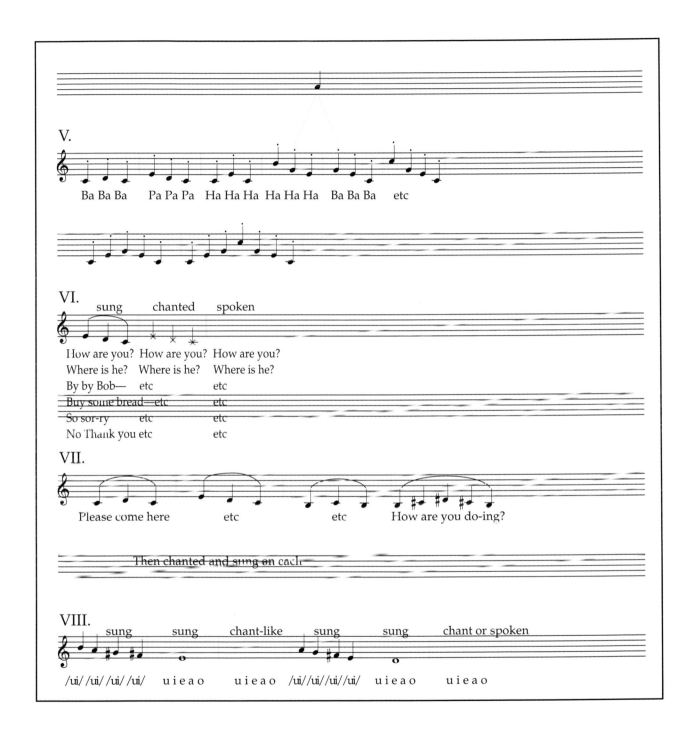

Fig 9–9. *(continued)*

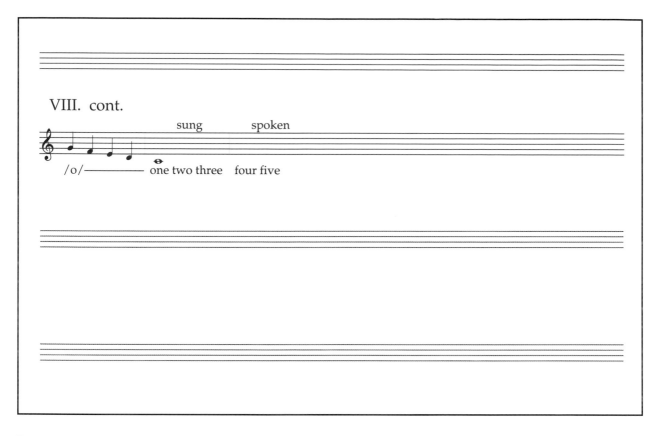

Fig 9–9. *(continued)*

sessions are not possible. Frequent lessons are especially important early in training to be certain that techniques are being implemented correctly in practice sessions between lessons. Often, short lessons, two or three times a week may be most productive at this time. If the patient is working with an SVS and speech-language pathologist, it is particularly helpful if he or she can see both of them on the same day. Ideally, they should be in the same location. The combined team approach is highly effective for singers and speakers, and it is often helpful for the SVS and speech-language pathologist to work together with the patient part of the time. This provides an opportunity to be certain that singing lessons and voice therapy are coordinated and that any potential misconceptions in the patient's mind are resolved.

Reports and Documentation

It is necessary for the SVS to communicate in writing with the laryngologist and speech-language pathologist. An initial report should be sent to the referring professional and should include the behaviors exhibited, exercises used, effectiveness of therapeutic intervention, and treatment plan. If the singer-patient is

from a distant area, this report (along with the reports of the laryngologists, speech-language pathologist, and voice laboratory) will serve as a guideline for the voice teacher in the patient's locality. If the patient intends to continue studying with the SVS, each session is documented on audio (and often video) tape and with progress notes similar to those used by physicians and speech-language pathologists. In our office, these progress notes are kept in the medical chart, along with notes by the other team members. Periodically, summary progress reports are prepared as well. Record keeping is not traditionally a requirement of the singing teacher. However, professional standards have been established in a medical milieu, and SVSs must observe them like any other medical professional. Such documentation may be useful for students without health problems in private studios, as well. A sample initial report is provided in Appendix IV.

Conclusion

Working with injured voices is a complex and challenging process. Nonsingers can benefit from working with an SVS by learning abdominal breathing/support, improved resonance and placement, and an overall relaxed and easy manner of production during singing, and by learning how to carry these techniques over into the speaking voice. Singers benefit from work with an SVS by learning specific exercises to improve vocal function, eliminate abusive vocal behaviors, reduce or eliminate vocal pathologies, maintain muscle tone and coordination during periods when singing is restricted, and, in general, receiving reinforcement in the rules of safe and efficient singing. Singing teachers who acquire special skills in training patients with vocal injuries provide invaluable help in the medical setting. Hopefully, the current demand, along with increasing interest among singing teachers, will result in high quality, interdisciplinary training programs to make it easier for voice teachers to enter this exciting new field.

References

1. Miller R. *English, French, German and Italian Techniques of Singing: A Study in National Tonal Preferences and How They Relate to Functional Efficiency*. Metuchen, NJ: The Scarecrow Press Inc; 1977.
2. Vennard W. *Singing: The Mechanism and Technic*. New York,NY: Carl Fischer Inc; 1949 (1st ed); 1968 (5th ed).
3. Kendall FP, McCreary EK. *Muscles: Testing and Function*. Baltimore, Md: Williams and Wilkins; 1983:269–320.

10

Use of Instrumentation in the Singing Studio

Robert Thayer Sataloff

Voice Training Applications of Medical Technology

For generations, both medical care and voice teaching have been hampered by the need to rely on subjective assessment of the voice. On those fortunate occasions when the doctor or teacher has a skilled, unbiased ear and excellent auditory memory, subjective assessment may work fairly well. However, the health and safety of patients and students in general are better served by more objective methods of voice assessment. For voice teachers, dependence on the ear alone gives rise to special problems. For example, there is sometimes disagreement as to which vocal productions are good and which are bad; whether a voice is the same, better, or worse after a year or two of training; what exactly is meant by "good" or "bad"; and so on. Consequently, it would be valuable for a singing teacher or music department to be able to assess accurately the vocal performance and progress of each student through objective measures of voice function repeated over time. Such technology is no substitute for traditional, excellent voice training. Rather, it provides an extra set of tools for the voice teacher to help identify specific problem areas and to assure steady progress. Physicians have been faced with the same needs in diagnosing voice abnormalities and assessing the results of treatment. Consequently, instrumentation has been developed for medical voice assessment, and much of this instrumentation has potential application in the studio.

Although instrumentation to perform all the tests utilized in a clinical voice laboratory is not widely available, much of it can be found in large cities with medical schools, especially if there is a laryngologist specializing in voice in the area. All the relevant tests are painless, and occasionally they have the added advantage of detecting an unsuspected and treatable medical problem that may affect vocal training and performance. Even the singing teacher who is not in a position to utilize such technology regularly should be familiar with it, because such analysis may prove extremely revealing and helpful in selected students with special problems that do not respond to a teacher's usual approach.

Without restating information discussed in *Clinical Assesment of Voice*[1] on each of the six components of objective voice assessment, a few additional comments are worthwhile to shed light on potential teaching applications of medical instrumentation.

Vocal Fold Vibration

For the purposes of vocal training, we include in the category Vocal Fold Vibration not only true measures of vocal fold vibration, but also visual evaluation of laryngeal posture. The flexible fiberoptic laryngoscope has revolutionized our ability to visualize the larynx. It is small (usually about 3.5 mm in diameter) and passes painlessly through one nostril. Occasionally, a gentle topical anesthetic is placed in the nose, but most people do not find the tube uncomfortable in the nose, even with no anesthetic at all. When connected to a video camera, the flexible fiberoptic laryngoscope allows the student, teacher, and physician to watch the position of the palate, pharynx, tongue base, epiglottis, false and true vocal folds, and other vocal tract structures during speech and singing. At some institutions, such as the Academy of Vocal Arts in Philadelphia, recordings of this sort have been made routinely for many years, prior to each student's matriculation as a freshman. Laryngeal posture, degree of tongue retraction, signs of strain, and other factors can then be compared with future recordings over the course of training. Such recordings are not only instructive for the student and teacher, but they may also provide invaluable feedback in selected cases. For example, occasionally, teachers are faced with a student with extremely "throaty" production, marked tongue retraction, and markedly excessive tension during singing. Most such students can have their techniques improved through traditional exercises, but an occasional student finds it very difficult to change technique to a more relaxed posture. Some such students do extremely well when the usual constructs and abstractions of the studio are supplemented by visual feedback. The student can watch his or her vocal folds and tongue base during singing and eliminate the hyperfunction and tongue retraction. While such situations do not occur often, it is useful for the voice teacher to know that such assistance is available for special cases. In a great many more cases, students and teachers find visual inspection of the larynx and pharynx during singing interesting and useful, although not essential.

Vocal fold vibration can be asssessed by several means. The most common and best is strobovideolaryngoscopy. It allows detection of scars, small masses, subtle neurologic weaknesses, and other problems that may be heard in the voice as hoarseness, breathiness, or weakness. It is invaluable for a singing teacher to have such information so that the teacher and student know whether the vocal problems they are hearing are merely training deficits or are the result of a physical problem that requires special training methods.

Phonatory Ability

Objective measures of phonatory ability are easily and readily available. Maximum phonation time is measured using a stopwatch along with physiological frequency range and musical frequency range, which can be measured at the piano. These and other tests of phonatory ability should theoretically improve during vocal training, except for physiologic frequency range (which probably remains about the same). The student or patient is instructed to sustain the vowel [ɑ] for as long as possible on deep inspiration, vocalizing at a comfortable frequency and intensity (loudness). Ideally, the frequency (pitch) and intensity are monitored using inexpensive equipment that can be purchased at a local radio electronics store. Physiological

frequency range of phonation disregards quality and measures the lowest and highest notes that can be produced. Musical frequency range of phonation measures the lowest and highest musically acceptable notes. Such tests can be performed into a high quality tape recorder and sent to a laboratory for formal analysis, including spectrographic analysis. Frequency limits of vocal registers may also be measured, as well as several other parameters. Combinations of tests of phonatory ability allow measures of glottal efficiency that may be valuable and should theoretically improve during vocal training.

Aerodynamic Measures

Aerodynamic tests may be especially valuable to the professional voice user and teacher. In some singers and actors, lung capacity may be substantially less than expected. It is important to identify such vocalists and optimize their pulmonary function through aerobic exercise and other means. In other singers and actors, initially good lung function gets progressively worse during singing or other exercise. Such singers may have unrecognized asthma induced by the exercise of performance. It is essential to identify such singers and treat them, or usually they will develop the same kinds of hyperfunctional voice abuse problems seen in people with poor support technique, even if they are trained well.

In addition to measures of lung function, airflow can be measured across the vocal folds. This provides a good measure of glottal efficiency and an objective way to identify voices that are excessively breathy, pressed, or well adjusted. These parameters should also improve during training, and this should be especially noticeable with many beginning students.

Acoustic Analysis

The best acoustic analyzers are still the human ear and brain. Unfortunately, they are still not very good at quantifying the information they perceive, and we cannot communicate it accurately. Acoustic analysis equipment used to be expensive for use during routine voice teaching. However, since most of the tests can be performed from a good quality tape recording, they are always at a singing teacher's disposal. Moreover, fairly sophisticated systems can now be accessed free over the Internet, as discussed below. It is sometimes useful to document progress in vocal stability, vibrato regularity, pitch accuracy, or development of desirable harmonics (the singer's formant). In non-voice majors required to study singing, visual feedback instruments are available to assist students in learning to match pitches.

Teachers interested in using more elegant technology to analyze and document voice performance, as well as for feedback during singing lessons, can now do so without investing in expensive equipment. Technological, computer-based resources and their integration into traditional voice teaching have been summarized nicely by Nair in his book and its coordinated CD-ROM.[2]

Laryngeal Electromyography and Psychoacoustic Evaluation

Laryngeal electromyography and formal psychoacoustic evaluation have relatively little applicability in routine voice teaching. However, the principles of psychoacoustics may provide useful guidance for school faculty juries judging singers, actors, and other speakers. Traditionally, such juries are composed of people with differences in opinion, taste, and sometimes personality; and the biases inevitably introduced in such situations are very difficult to identify and negate. Most music and acting schools handle this problem simply by trying to have enough people on each jury to have such problems "even out." However, study of formal techniques of psychoacoustic evaluation would probably lead to improvements in the jury system.

Discussion of Studio Applications

Currently available techniques for looking at, analyzing, and documenting voice function have been used successfully by physicians and a few farsighted voice teachers. They are not substitutes for good studio teaching technique but rather are extra tools in the teacher's armamentarium. As such, it behooves the modern voice teacher to become familiar with available technology that may enhance teaching efficiency and consistency.

There are also other reasons why singing and acting teachers should be familiar with and concerned about objective voice assessment. Political and legal developments over the past several years have made it clear that voice teachers are eventually (and probably soon) going to have to introduce the same kind of peer review and quality control practiced in other professions such as medicine and speech-language pathology. At present, most teachers and music schools rely on very little beyond personal opinion to define good singing, healthy singing, successful training progress, or even a "good voice." In modern times, such subjective vagaries may be insufficient for the individual voice teacher and especially for the music school trying to assess voice teachers and select an optimal voice faculty. Objective voice analysis may help. Not only can it define parameters and progress for individual students, but it can also help teachers in self-assessment and improvement and music schools in faculty assessment. Any good teacher is eager to identify his or her strengths and weaknesses, so the introduction of objective assessment should be viewed as a blessing by most high-quality people in the profession. For example, consider a school with four voice faculty members each of whom is assigned 15 freshmen. Each freshman can be recorded on high-quality audio- and videotape singing standardized scales and an audition aria and can undergo comprehensive objective voice analysis. Such recordings can be repeated at the end of the first and second semesters, and annually (or more often) thereafter. Assume further that in each studio there are four new students with the same technical problems: tongue retraction, ineffective support, poor soft singing, and slight tremolo. Then assume that these problems disappear within the first year in students of three of the teachers, but the problems shown by students of the fourth teacher get worse, and two or three students of that teacher who initially did not have those problems develop them. Objective voice assessments detect such patterns early, document them in a clear, scientific fashion that eliminates the perceived personal persecution with which such information is often greeted, and allows the teacher, students, and administration to make appropriate adjustments before significant (and possibly compensable) harm is done to the students.

Clearly, objective voice assessment has been a boon to laryngologists and can be a valuable adjunct to the individual singing and acting teacher. Moreover, it may provide our first real means to define good, healthy singing, acting, and teaching and to help promulgate high standards of practice among those who choose to call themselves "voice teachers."

References

1. Heuer R, Hawkshaw MJ, Sataloff RT. The clinical voice laboratory. In: Sataloff RT. *Clinical Assessment of Voice.* San Diego, Calif: Plural Publishing Inc; 2005:33–81.
2. Nair G. Voice: *Traditional and Technology: A State-of-the-Art Studio.* San Diego, Calif: Singular Publishing Group; 1999.

11

Choral Pedagogy and Vocal Health

Brenda J. Smith and Robert Thayer Sataloff

Amateur and professional singers of all ages participate in choral music in schools, churches or synagogues, community choruses, or other civic venues. Choral pedagogy, the newest academic field in performing arts medicine,[1] addresses the need for choral conductors to be better informed about vocal health. Most choral conductors are instrumentalists or keyboard players, not singers. For decades, choral conducting was taught as an adjunct activity to orchestral conducting. More recently, several authors have addressed the special issues of choral conducting that can strengthen voices rather than injure them and of vocal health in singers, both choral and solo. In an article entitled "The Development of a Choral Instrument," Howard Swan, conductor of the Occidental Glee Clubs and founder of the Choral Conductor's Guild, wrote:

Choral conductors, even more so than teachers of singing, are divided in their opinions concerning vocal technique. Some refuse to employ any means to build voices. Either they consider such procedures to be unimportant, or they are afraid to use an exercise, which is related to the singing process. Sometimes the choral director cloaks his own ignorance of the singing mechanism by dealing directly with the interpretive elements in a score and thus avoids any approach to the vocal problems of the individuals in his chorus. [2(p5)]

Therefore, when evaluating the health and well-being of a singer engaged in choral activities, a health care professional or singing teacher should pose a number of questions, such as:

- Is the choral conductor primarily a singer? An instrumentalist?
- Does the choral rehearsal begin with a period of warm-up and end with a cooldown? If so, what is the nature of the warm-up? The cooldown?
- Is there a policy regarding choral posture for sitting and for standing?

- Does the singer sight sing music easily?
- Is music taught in the rehearsal using the piano or the voice?
- Are the text and music taught simultaneously?
- What is the level of discipline within the choral group?
- Does the conductor offer the choir a breath gesture?
- Are singers often asked to sing in extreme vocal ranges?
- Is there a seating chart for the choir? Is the seating arrangement determined by vocal qualities? By height?
- How frequently does the choir perform? What level of difficulty is the repertoire? Is it sung with piano? Orchestra? Organ? A cappella (without accompaniment)?
- Is there a break during the rehearsal? Is food served? Are caffeinated beverages consumed?

Warm-up and Cooldown Procedures

If the choral conductor is a singer, the rehearsal is likely to begin with a warm-up period. The purposes of any warm-up period are to:

- adjust the voice from speaking to singing,
- align the body and free the breathing mechanism for the act of singing,
- create a physical awareness of the vocal mechanism being used correctly,
- stretch gently and exercise the skeletal muscles used in phonation following the principles of muscle physiology that highlight the importance of muscle warm-up prior to any athletic activity.

In a choral rehearsal, these adjustments are best made when a well-trained singer or qualified conductor sings patterns and gives verbal instruction regarding their execution. In the introduction to the book *Voice Building for Choirs*, the authors write:

A choral conductor who feels incapable of presenting choral voice building exercises to a choir may wish to call upon a professional voice teacher or a trained choir member to fulfill the assignment. In any case, one must resist the temptation to employ the organ or the piano as a mechanism for voice building because of the percussive nature of both instruments. The conductor who is involved with performing as an accompanist for the choir is not capable of hearing critically.[3(pxi)]

If the choral conductor is an instrumentalist who has chosen to assume the role of leadership with a choir, it is probable that the preparation for singing will be a series of tuning exercises or a set of patterns played on the piano. If tuning exercises begin the choral rehearsal, singers may attempt to sustain the speaking voice to achieve proper pitch levels. The mechanism of the piano is a percussive action in which internal hammers hit metal strings. Singers instinctively imitate its sound by pressing on the back of the tongue while producing tone. Constriction and tension then follow in the pharyngeal and laryngeal areas. Generated by pressed phonation, this initial choral sound may continue for the entire rehearsal. This is not only tiring, but also potentially injurious because of excessively increased forces of vocal fold contact. Choral singing should be refreshing to the voice, not fatiguing. This is not to say that the piano can never be used during warm-ups. Many good choral conductors and singing teachers use the piano without adverse effect, but only if they are aware of the pitfalls and expert at obtaining good vocal technique despite the piano. The choral rehearsal should be a forum for developing singing voice techniques that are healthy with or without piano accompaniment; but the instrument must be built on proper posture, breath, and resonance techniques, under expert guidance.

Only recently have vocal pedagogues realized the importance of a cooldown at the conclusion of a period of singing. Just as the voice adjusts during a warm-up from speech to song, a cooldown returns the voice from the extremes of the singing range to a comfortable speaking condition. Physiologically, cooldown vocal exercises are analogous to stretching exercises advised after running or weight lifting. In general, choral rehearsals last from 90 minutes to as long as 3 hours. After an extended period of vocal activity, it is helpful to assist the vocal mechanism in identifying the speaking range of the voice and to reinforce or restore appropriate muscle relaxation, tone, and flexibility.

The cool-down period can be brief but must not be forgotten. A steady, extended sigh from the highest to the lowest ranges of the voice, a gentle shrug of the shoulders, or a simple recitation of poetry on a supported tone will prepare the singers for conversational speech, and will help relax muscles just as cool-down exercises do after sporting events.[4(p162)]

Choral ensembles have adopted various strategies regarding warm-up and cooldown procedures. Church musicians, for whom the pipe organ is the primary performing medium, frequently ask church choir members to rehearse the hymns for the coming worship service as an act of warm-up or cooldown. This may be an efficient use of time, but it can be detrimental to the singers. Many choral singers cannot read text and music simultaneously with ease. A good warm-up separates vowel shapes from consonants, allowing the voice to flow on the breath before introducing the complexities of forming consonants. When text and music are required simultaneously under pressure in rehearsal circumstances, inexperienced singers may tighten jaw and neck muscles and sing without proper support for several verses of music, thus tiring the voice unnecessarily, and risking vocal injury.

In some choral settings, singers are asked to arrive at the rehearsal prepared to sing. Because most choral ensembles convene in the evening after a full day's work or in the midst of an academic schedule, few singers can be expected to have either the time or the discipline to complete a useful warm-up prior to arrival at the rehearsal. If a student of singing complains of hoarseness or vocal fatigue after choral singing, the teacher's first inquiry should investigate the opening moments of the rehearsal. The seeds of tension are often planted there. Should warm-ups be unproductive or cooldowns absent, the teacher of singing must provide the choral singer with a short regimen of exercises to insure adequate preparation for the tasks of choral singing. Ideally, if the teacher can delicately communicate these suggestions to the conductor as well, they may benefit the whole choir, not just one student.

Posture

Choral conductors must be responsible for the posture of the choir in seated or standing positions. Posture is important because of its effect on the efficiency of support musculature, and therefore on the degree of tension or efficiency with which laryngeal muscles are used during singing. This affects vocal fold contact forces and injury potential, as well. Fearing the appearance of tyranny or nagging, many choral conductors refrain from admonishing their choral singers regarding poor posture. Others may assume that singers, like instrumentalists, have learned their singing techniques through years of private instruction. Such a presumption can be very harmful to the vocal health of choral singers, most of whom are untrained. In the eyes of the choral singer, the choral conductor is an authority in the area of vocal music. If the conductor allows poor posture habits among the singers, this failing can produce not only bad singing technique in untrained choral singers, but also a wide gap between studio teaching and choral training.

It is important for choral conductors, vocal coaches, and teachers of singing to discuss the maintenance of good posture at all times. To date, few chairs are designed to encourage proper support of the spine for singing. Students of singing must be taught to stand, sit, and walk with erect, balanced posture even if the matter is ignored by the choral conductor.

Teaching of Choral Repertoire Music

A healthy singing tone evolves from a process of neurological signals that are expressed through the vocal tract. Therefore, a clear mental image of the pitch and the vowel must be created before a clear, ringing tone can emerge. The act of *audiation,* the term used in music education for hearing the vocal sound mentally before phonation, requires training, practice, and timing. In the corporate setting of a choral rehearsal, participating singers present with various levels of musical skill. Some may sing music readily at sight; but the majority might rely heavily on the power of imitation to learn notes, rhythms, and words. Thus, choral singers who read music readily tend to lead those with less skill. This practice causes the weaker singer to avoid the opportunity to train the ear and create a mental image of the desired pitch/vowel combination, and it may also stress the more skilled singer who may sing too loudly in order to lead the section. These singers should be advised to lead by example, singing as if they were giving a demonstration lesson to the one person on each side of them rather than trying to sing louder than the whole section.

It is very difficult for any choral conductor to accommodate the strengths and weaknesses of each singer. If the singers in the choir are for the most part inexperienced, the conductor may use the piano as a leveling tool, playing the notes on the keyboard to assist those who read notes and rhythms slowly. Some conductors record the choral parts on cassette tapes for their singers to hear outside the rehearsal. Rehearsal techniques that depend heavily on the piano as a means of teaching the notes may foster inaccurate, nonlegato singing among the choir members unless these issues are addressed specifically in other aspects of the rehearsal technique. Singers who learn their music by any form of passive listening are stifling their own musical growth. If a choral singer complains of vocal fatigue or hoarseness after rehearsals, the physician, speech-language pathologist, or voice teacher must consider the singer's ability to sight sing and the methods for music teaching practiced by the choral conductor.

Just as solo singers sing the music into their voices, choral singers must teach the individual contours of melody and rhythm into their voices. The singing instrument runs by mental impulses that must be trained carefully. Time and patience are required if the voice is to learn to produce the pitch and the vowel accurately on each rhythmic pattern. Ordinarily, well-designed rehearsals do not result in tired, hoarse voices.

Text

The goal in healthy singing is the achievement of a flowing, legato line. Singing on the breath is the cornerstone of bel canto, or beautiful singing. In the papal choirs of the 16th and 17th centuries, the high art of bel canto singing was taught to young boys using exercises on vowel sounds only. Documents of the time indicate that the young singers were asked to demonstrate the steadiness of their legato singing techniques by singing a series of vowel sounds over a lighted candle. Each vowel sound was sung and a steady crescendo to decrescendo or *messa di voce* (literally, a measuring of the voice) was performed. A voice capable of making measured dynamic changes without disruption of the tone shows evidence of firm breath control and vowel purity. If the flame did not flicker, the voice was considered competent to execute consonant sounds and to endure the rigors of regular performance at worship.

Most voice teachers agree that the teaching of vowels should precede the teaching of consonants, establishing first the flow of tone before interrupting it with the articulation of consonants. Vocalises (exercises) are built from vowel patterns to which consonants are added gradually. The teaching of solo repertoire begins often by singing the musical lines on vowels to establish tone and manage breath support. Developed over centuries, these pedagogical methods have proven their worth in the achievement of healthy vocal technique.

Lack of vocal techniques and the press of time often preclude choral conductors from using the vocal wisdom of the ages in the teaching of repertoire to choirs. In all too many choral rehearsals, the text is used as a tool for the eye of inexperienced singers. Choral singers, having based their membership on a strong ability to imitate sound and memorize melody by ear, are generally novices in the area of rhythm. The rhythm of choral music is founded on the rhythmic patterns of the text. In an effort to save rehearsal time, choral conductors often invite the choir to sing unfamiliar repertoire directly on the text. Singers with less rhythmic skill can follow the words and avoid frustration. Oddly enough, some choral conductors will use this method even with repertoire written in foreign languages loaded with uncommon sounds and symbols. This common choral method invites vocal harm through its seek-and-find philosophy. Singers cannot sing healthfully unless the mind understands the vowel shapes on proper pitches in the right rhythmic patterns. Slow, careful learning produces healthy, confident singing. Several hours of frenzied singing in a choral rehearsal can compromise overall vocal technique and health. If students of singing experience mental and vocal fatigue after choral rehearsals, the voice teacher should inquire about the method of teaching of repertoire.

Like learning a foreign language, sight singing improves with use. Incorporating some sight singing into every rehearsal will yield benefits.[4(p165)] There are many published and reliable methods for teaching sight singing to choirs, some of which have been cited already in this chapter.[2,3,5]

Discipline

Choirs are drawn together by the charisma of the choral conductor. The conductor determines the nature of the organization, its goals, and its methods. A choir is not a democratic society, but a group of people governed by its leader. In some choirs, the discipline is very strict. In others, singers are allowed to whisper or talk at will. The level of discipline within the ensemble is of significance to the health and well-being of the individual choral singers. If the discipline of the choir is held firmly enough to produce effective results but flexibly enough to allow moments of relaxation, healthy singing will evolve. Where discipline is lax, choral singers may abuse their voices. If the choral conductor has a tyrannical nature, a spirit of fear may pervade the rehearsal, creating unwanted tensions of potentially serious consequence to the voices.

Breath Gesture

For decades, American choral conductors were taught orchestral conducting techniques. Adjustments to the choral setting were made on an as needed basis. Orchestral conductors assume rightly that each member of the orchestra has had private instruction on the instrument. Orchestras are organized by section with

leaders who provide hints about the execution of difficult passages to others in the section. The orchestral conductor indicates the tempo and the character of the music with a single flick of the baton. Instrumentalists have trained themselves to respond to the signal and produce tone on demand.

The singing instrument requires considerably more time and a great deal more coordination to prepare than most orchestral ones. Singers must hear the pitch, imagine the vowel shape, and prepare the breathing mechanism. The coordination of this set of activities in choral music is organized by the choral conductor's breath gesture. Unfortunately, not every choral conductor has been taught this basic skill; because it is not always part of instrumental conducting technique (although it provides substantial benefit for instrumentalists, as well). Many conductors use orchestral conducting techniques, giving a downbeat and hoping for a choral sound. Unprepared, the singers grab for breath and produce tone. This method of creating choral music can be very harmful to the singer through excessive tension and forceful, poorly supported attacks.

Range and Tessitura

The selection of choral repertoire is a complicated process. Public choral concerts are expensive. The repertoire must appeal to the potential audience. In religious settings, the text must be appropriate to the event. Frequently, neither the disposition and skill of the singers nor the range and tessitura of the music are considered adequately. Choral conductors may attempt to balance the choral sound by asking certain singers to depart from their normal singing ranges and join the ranks of other sections. Baritones may be asked to sing in falsetto for extended periods to strengthen the tenor section. Sopranos who read music easily are often added to the alto section to insure a harmonic balance. Altos may be asked to sing tenor parts. An occasional, gentle venture out of one's range is not necessarily harmful to a skilled singer. A long departure (such as a season) from the normal classification, however, can be very detrimental to the choral singer.

The range and tessitura of the repertoire have a significant impact on the comfort level of each singer in the choir. The range, the highness and lowness of the notes of a given vocal part, may be reasonable. However, the tessitura, the range of notes in which the majority of the melodic material lies, may be at the extreme end of the range. When choral singers are asked to produce voice in extreme tessituras for long periods of time, vocal fatigue or injury may result. Some choral conductors question the stamina of their singers, believing in prolonged full-voice repetition as a means of strengthening the ability of the choir to sing at extreme tessitura. This practice is unwise and dangerous. It is more likely to cause injury than to build stamina.

Seating

In the best of circumstances, the experience of singing together can fortify the body, mind, and spirit of the choral singer. In less favorable settings, choral experiences have the adverse effect of inhibiting vocal growth and confidence. Group dynamics affect choral singing strongly. The abilities of singers vary widely. Personality traits, musicianship skills, and size and timbre of vocal gifts foster competitive attitudes. If a choral conductor considers the personal, musical, and vocal capacities of singers when organizing the sections of the choir, choral singing can promote positive human and artistic growth. Singing instruments respond best in a relaxed and receptive atmosphere.

Unfortunately, many choral conductors take little note of individual characteristics, positioning choir members within a section by height or by seniority. Other choral conductors allow singers to arrange themselves. Usually, leaving group dynamics to chance creates conflict between weaker and stronger personalities, untrained and trained singers. Singers with less vocal gift or training may refrain from singing, sensing competition with singers of more ability or experience. These inhibitions cause physical tensions that could compromise vocal health. Choral singers should be seated based on the qualities of their sound and skill, with weaker singers nestled artfully among stronger ones. This practice fosters a blended choral sound without intimidating the singers. Choral singing is teamwork. Every member of the choir must feel as if he or she is an important element of the musical organization. The choral conductor should encourage this attitude with a welcoming spirit and supportive tolerance.

Performance Schedule

Choral concerts are peak experiences. In preparation for performances, choral groups rehearse extra hours. Generally, choirs stand on risers, creating an uncomfortable elevation in somewhat claustrophobic circumstances. It is important to recognize the hazards for students of singing who participate in long rehearsals in cramped postures. Choral folders may contain several pounds of music. Singers on the back row may extend their chins to see the conductor who is placed many feet away. Conductors can (but often do not) mitigate these problems through a few extra minutes of adjusting position and posture of singers on the

risers. If the choral performance experience is to be a healthy one, singers must also be taught to conserve their vocal and physical energy during the week leading up to performance.

The repertoire and type of accompaniment must be appropriate to the size and ability of the choir if healthy singing is to occur. Choral conductors and singers are ambitious musicians. Often the love of a particular work may override reason, setting up vocal or intellectual demands that pose perils for the singers. For instance, smaller choirs may aspire to sing *Ein deutsches Requiem* by Johannes Brahms with an orchestra but might be better served presenting the work with its duo-piano accompaniment. It is important to advise students and choral conductors about the negative effects on individual voices when confronted with overwhelming instrumental accompaniments. A cappella singing tends to be spontaneously the healthiest form of choral music-making, based firmly in the bel canto traditions; but healthy choral singing is possible with any ensemble provided the conductor and choir are trained properly.

Rehearsal Traditions

Until recently, singers were unaware of the detrimental effect of certain foods and beverages on the singing voice. Most choirs have associated singing with social life, designing rehearsal routines around a coffee break or fellowship period. If the refreshments consumed during the break contain chocolate, refined sugars, caffeine, or citrus, the voices of many of the singers will be at risk for gastroesophogeal reflux (GERD) in the subsequent rehearsal period. When students of singing complain of hoarseness in the latter portion of choral rehearsals, reflux could be one source of the distress.

Benefits of Choral Singing

A choral rehearsal can be an ideal forum for strengthening musicianship skills, vocal technique, and self-esteem. The singer has the opportunity to relax within the choral tone, participating in arching phrases of greater length than any single voice can manage. The student of singing can develop an historical context for the solo repertoire being studied in private lessons. Because smaller voices perform equally with larger ones, choral singing teaches acceptance and offers a sense of accomplishment. The goals of choral singing are different from those of solo singing. Cooperation in choral singing demands that singers contribute to the choral sound but never dominate it. Choral singers respond to the artistic demands set by the conductor.

In solo singing, the individual vocal and interpretive traits of the singers are paramount. The teacher of singing is wise to train the student of singing to make appropriate adjustments in either context with comparable skill. The ability to do so (sing well in solo and ensemble settings) is a sign of technical and artistic vocal facility that is usually associated with healthy singing. There is nothing intrinsically unhealthy about singing in choirs, as long as solo singers who do so are trained properly.

The Role of the Voice Teacher in the Choral Context

Ideally, every singing teacher would be affiliated with a choral organization, acting as a consultant on vocal matters whenever possible. In order to advise students wisely, singing teachers should be acquainted personally with the choral conductors within their immediate area. Solo singing and choral singing are compatible but different vocal activities. Teachers of singing and choral conductors must work together to ensure the vocal health of students of singing.

The Role of the Laryngologist and Speech-Language Pathologist in the Choral Context

Laryngologists and speech-language pathologists who care for singers have important roles in the choral context. First, many medical professionals are enthusiastic singers themselves. Some are even trained in singing. Whether or not a laryngologist or speech-language pathologist is a skilled, trained singer, it is helpful for medical professionals to participate personally in choral singing. If the medical professional is not a trained singer,

the choral experience provides invaluable insights that are helpful in the evaluation and treatment of patients. In addition, the physician and speech-language pathologist should act as consultants for the choral conductor and choir members on matters of vocal health. The active participation of health professionals in a musical community fosters the kind of interdisiplinary collaboration among physicians, speech-language pathologists, singing teachers, choral conductors, and performers that is most likely to lead to effective voice building and healthy vocal performance. Good, secure choral conductors ordinarily not only welcome such collaboration but moreover seek it out.

References

1. Sataloff R. *Performing Arts Medicine*. 2nd ed. San Diego, Calif: Singular Publishing Group; 1999.
2. Swan H. *Choral Conducting: A Symposium*. Englewood Cliffs, NJ: Prentice-Hall, Inc; 1973.
3. Ehmann W, Haasemann F. Voice *Building for Choirs*. Smith B, trans. Chapel Hill NC: Hinshaw Music, Inc; 1980.
4. Smith B, Sataloff R, *Choral Pedagogy*. San Diego, Calif: Singular Publishing Group; 2000.
5. Sinclair C. *The Effect of Daily Sightsinging Exercises on the Sightsinging Ability of Middle School Choir Students*, St. Paul, Minn: University of St. Thomas; 1996.

Selected Bibliography

Finn W. *The Art of the Choral Conductor*. Boston, Mass: CC Birchard and Co; 1939.
Sataloff R. *Professional Voice: The Science and Art of Clinical Care*. 2nd ed. San Diego, Calif: Singular Publishing Group; 1998.
Sataloff R. *Vocal Health and Pedagogy*. San Diego, Calif: Singular Publishing Group; 1997.
Smith B, Sataloff R, *Choral Pedagogy*. San Diego, Calif: Singular Publishing Group; 2000.

12

The Role of the Acting-Voice Trainer in Medical Care of Professional Voice Users

Sharon L. Freed, Bonnie N. Raphael,
and Robert Thayer Sataloff

Acting-voice trainers are also called voice coaches, drama voice teachers, and vocal consultants. Traditionally, these professionals are closely associated with the theatre. Their skills may be useful on the medical voice team not only to restore a voice recovering from injury, but also to strengthen and develop the voice in ways that help prevent future injury.

This chapter is written to acquaint physicians, speech-language pathologists, singing voice specialists, and others with the profession of voice and speech training (acting-voice trainers) and to acquaint acting-voice trainers with many of the special issues that must be considered when they join a medical voice team.

An Overview of Acting-Voice Training for Noninjured Speakers

It is important for all members of the medical voice team to understand the teachings of acting-voice trainers and the various approaches they may use in the training process. This chapter is not intended as a comprehensive review of the profession, but rather as an overview to help the other team members understand the training and background of acting-voice trainers. Raphael has presented a similar overview in previous literature.[1] Such understanding is helpful in clarifying the value of their participation on the medical voice team.

Because voice training involves behavior modification, acting-voice trainers have developed a variety of approaches that may be used for the education of any individual. In addition to having particular vocal agen-

das, different people find themselves more receptive to one mode of learning than another and to one style of presentation than another. Certain speakers, for example, do best when information is auditory. Systems based on listening to a model and then making the necessary adjustments in their own sound are helpful to auditory learners. Other speakers succeed when they can obtain information visually, by observing a particular facial posture or shoulder relaxation technique and then duplicating it as well as they can while observing themselves in a mirror. Still other speakers respond most quickly when the information they receive is kinesthetic, when they can learn by being either physically touched or told what they might experience in their own breathing or postural or facial muscles and then seeing whether they can voluntarily produce the desired kinesthetic sensations.

Obviously, there is no such thing as a learning mode that is purely auditory or visual or kinesthetic; virtually all behavioral modification techniques involve stimulation and information provided in all three modes, but one or another might be more prominent and therefore more useful to a particular individual or more compatible with the style of a particular teacher. Similarly, certain voice patients or students might be more comfortable working with a teacher or coach on an individual basis while others are more comfortable as a member of a workshop or a small class. Some speakers do best with a speech-language pathologist specializing in voice rehabilitation. If the voice is free of medical problems (eg, vocal nodules or polyps, contact ulcers, vocal trauma or paralysis, chronic laryngitis), most voice patients or students can be helped by one of the four basic types of training common among acting-voice trainers, as described in this chapter: Traditional, Skinner, Linklater, or Lessac.

Traditional Approaches and Education of Acting-Voice Trainers

It is important for physicians and other health-care professionals to understand approaches to acting-voice training, the contributions of the trainer on the medical voice team, and the possible training biases and approaches of actors who seek our care as patients. Individual acting-voice trainers have various educational, training, and practical experiences that influence their techniques. Those traditionally trained, for example, may have completed undergraduate and graduate-level coursework in communication and speech education, public speaking, or oral interpretation, and perhaps in the anatomy and physiology of speech and phonetics. Typically, their training has included education in basic anatomy and function of the voice mechanism, techniques fostering the elimination of stage fright, the development of a warm-up routine, the acquisition of techniques for better breathing and development of individual vocal dynamics (ie, pitch, rate, loudness, and quality), and the elimination of subclinical problems common to many speakers, such as hypernasality, insufficient loudness, mumbling, monotony, poor phrasing, excessive speed, and insufficient consonant articulation. Their training also frequently includes some performance experience.

Some traditional acting-voice trainers may encourage selected patients or students to pursue the same kinds of didactic introductory education the trainers received themselves. Some voice patients and students do well with this approach, preferring introductory courses in colleges or conservatories for acquiring enough basic information and skills both to speak and perform more effectively. Advocates of traditional approaches enjoy the straightforward, easily understandable presentation of basic information and skills and feel that, by the end of a good introductory course, they know how to continue to build vocal technique by working on their own. However, the more demanding a professional voice user's vocal challenges, the more likely it is that he or she will need additional supervised training and development. This can be provided by acting-voice trainers who offer individual instruction in the skills discussed above. Critics of some traditional approaches find them too academic or cerebral, and deficient in getting knowledge and skills beyond the "brain" and down to the "gut" where they are needed to express and control the emotional content of speech.

The Work of Edith Skinner

Edith Skinner, one of the most famous students of the noted Australian phonetician William Tilly, came to the United States to teach his work in the early part of this century. After learning the International Phonetic Alphabet and techniques of sound transcription, Skinner applied them to the speech training of actors, teaching for a great many years at Carnegie-Mellon University and then at Juilliard, training a considerable number of actors and teachers to use what she called good American speech. In her work, a carefully defined and prescribed series of rules for pronunciation is applied to speaking, reading, and acting by students who have been taught the International Phonetic Alphabet and phonetic transcription. After intensive articulation drill practice, these pronunciation standards are then applied to a wide variety of materials in performance until they become habitual.

Proponents of Skinner's work observe that many judgments are made about people on the basis of how they speak and that acquiring "good American speech" will help those who wish to sound more cultured or better educated. Several sounds acquired through this training also carry more easily in large performance spaces and are more easily understood by listeners from different parts of the United States or those for whom English is a second language. The resulting speech patterns have proven extremely useful for performances of the works of Shakespeare, other classical plays, and plays in translation, as well. For example, when producing classical plays, directors often choose to identify royalty or upper class characters by having them use a pronunciation pattern similar to standard British, and then take servants or others toward something like Cockney—a bit ludicrous when you recall that *Romeo and Juliet* is set in Italy and *Hamlet* in Denmark. Subtle but effective class distinctions might be achieved in a manner that is far less obtrusive or foreign to American audiences by the juxtaposition of "good American speech" with general American speech instead. In addition, acquisition of a fairly standard sound provides the actor with an effective base for stage dialects with results that are consistent across all members of a given cast. Finally, advocates say that, by teaching consistent and optimal placement of individual speech sounds, Skinner's approach improves resonation, projection, and healthy vocal production in general. Skinner's approach can be reviewed in her manual *Speak with Distinction*.[2]

Critics note that what is identified as good American speech is not a neutral American accent but rather a somewhat affected sound, based on a Southern British model rather than on native American speech, and also based on Skinner's race and cultural standard. They feel it eradicates or undervalues the great diversity of speech patterns characteristic of different areas and cultures present in this country and is more relevant to an older generation of American stage and film actors. Nonetheless, Skinner's work produces speakers with beautifully precise speech and excellent "ears."

The Linklater Method

Kristin Linklater was trained as an actress at the London Academy of Music and Dramatic Art in England. She received her voice and speech training under the eminent master teacher Iris Warren, whom she later assisted. In 1963, she introduced Iris Warren's work to this country by training a select number of US and Canadian teachers and coaches for an extended period of time. She continues teaching and coaching actors throughout the world.

Linklater's work is based on the premise that each of us has a beautifully functioning, natural voice with which many of us interfere (because of insidious tension and habitual inhibition) as we attempt to communicate our thoughts and feelings. Her approach, as best described in her book, *Freeing the Natural Voice*,[3] involves a process of freeing the vocal channel from habitual physical and psychological impediments that may prevent the voice from emerging in its most expressive, unadulterated form.

Linklater's method begins with and never abandons a connection with breath and impulse to speak from deep within the body. Exercises deal with allowing the free passage of this breath, especially when dealing with emotionally charged material; freeing up the vocal channel via loosening the shoulders, neck, jaw, tongue, and lips; with developing greater vocal range through contact with and exploration of a series of resonators; and immersing oneself in the intricacies, subtleties, implications, and layers of the language itself, of the text being spoken. Physical, psychological, and cultural blocks to full connection with text are confronted and worked through in both individual and group coaching sessions.

Linklater has trained a great number of teachers, directors, actors, and public speakers through a month-long intensive workshop which she taught for several years at Shakespeare & Company, the courses she now teaches to undergraduates at Emerson College in Boston, and the private workshops she continues to offer in the Boston area and elsewhere. She has written two excellent texts that are widely used and available.[3,4] In addition to training a number of people who base their own teachings on her work, she has intensively trained and certified a select number of teachers whom she feels are most qualified to pass on the essence of her technique and philosophy. A voice patient seeking to undertake Linklater's work should inquire of any potential teacher about the exact nature and extent of his or her training and qualifications.

Critics of Linklater's work describe it as a long and too psychologically oriented warm-up process that shortchanges both attention to clear articulation and development of the actor's ability to characterize vocally; they say those trained solely in Linklater work may be capable of very fine and compelling acting, but only in their own personae.

The Lessac System

Arthur Lessac began his own training as a singer at the Eastman School of Music in Rochester, New York. As his interest in the workings of the human voice developed, he supplemented his musical training with formal study in the anatomy and physiology of the voice and then, later on, in the workings of the human body in general. He began to develop his system of behavior modification in a search for something organically American rather than derived or adapted from late 19th and early 20th century British acting schools. He has been investigating, experimenting, and evolving a detailed system for the use and training of the human voice for at least 40 years. During the past 20 years or so, he has expanded his consideration of the actor's body, as well.

Lessac's system is based on the proposition that the speaker must eliminate all anesthetic-deadening habits in his or her communicative behavior and replace them with an ongoing state of habitual awareness. *Awareness*, according to Lessac, is a matter of being present and conscious on a moment-to-moment basis as one breathes, produces voice, and speaks. Instead of seeking to imitate or duplicate any other models, each speaker uses kinesthetic awareness to rediscover and enjoy his or her own sounds that are both aesthetically pleasing and based on natural behavior.

Lessac approaches voice through the acquisition of three complementary vocal actions. In using structural action, the speaker rediscovers the ability of the natural forward structure of the face and oral cavity to produce vowels that are rich, full, and free of restricting habitual tensions. In tonal action, the speaker becomes aware of and learns to produce buzzing and ringing vibrations on the hard palate and up into the top front quarter of the skull to focus the tone so that it will project effortlessly and protect the speaker from any vocal injury or discomfort, even when speaking in inhospitable vocal environments or when using the voice in potentially harmful ways (eg, screaming). In using consonant action, the speaker treats each of the consonants as a musical instrument, learning to taste its particular identifying vibrations, explore its range, communicate emotional feelings and connections through it, and then incorporates these new found awarenesses into spoken language.

By leading with one vocal action or another, the actor learns to utilize different vocal and dramatic colors, interpretations, or readings of dramatic material and to adapt effortlessly to different playing spaces. By learning to explore while performing memorized materials, the actor learns to be in the present moment and to allow the performance to be a discovery rather than a reproduction of what has been rehearsed in a particular way or habituated through repeated performance.

Advocates of Lessac's system cite its ability to heal and strengthen voices that have suffered from hyperfunction and strain and its ability to produce speech sounds that are clear, communicative, and beautiful in actors who do not respond well to traditional articulation exercises and drill sheets. Some critics are put off by Lessac's untraditional terminology. Others observe that, until students fully understand and internalize their training, they may look and sound forced or uncomfortable as they speak and that, when taught incompletely or incorrectly, the system might produce a way of speaking that is self-conscious or even pretentious. They feel, contrary to Lessac's best intentions for his work, that a little learning can be a dangerous thing when it comes to the acquisition of the vocal actions. Nonetheless, actors who have mastered its basics have a system for vocal developments that can serve their needs for the rest of their lives. Lessac's system and philosophy are described in detail in his two books, *The Use and Training of the Human Voice*[5] and *Body Wisdom: The Use and Training of the Human Body*.[6]

Other Options

There are several other excellent approaches to training that actors may encounter in their training. Several excellent voice and speech teachers base their work on the writings and teachings of three highly reputed coaches in England: Cicely Berry,[7,8] Clifford Turner,[9] and Patsy Rodenburg.[10,11] Other actors and speakers

who feel that limitations or restrictions in their voices are physically based have benefitted greatly from work with an Alexander teacher,[*] a Feldenkrais practitioner,[†] or a physical therapist.

Physicians should also be aware of other areas of expertise that are common among voice trainers. Some speech-language pathologists and many acting-voice trainers also specialize in accent reduction or elimination. Through a process of auditory training and articulation practice, foreign or regional accents can be reduced significantly in many cases. However, speakers of English as a second language and even those with heavy American regional accents must be willing to make a long-term commitment if significant and permanent accent reduction or elimination is to be achieved. These issues may be of considerable importance to some professional voice users. Moreover, untrained attempts at accent reduction can be vocally taxing in some people, as can speaking a foreign language. In such situations, the right acting-voice trainer or speech-language pathologist can improve vocal technique and safety while simultaneously reducing accent.

Some voice patients and clients either really enjoy singing or have always wanted to learn to sing and discover a very strong connection between singing training and significant development of many facets of the speaking voice, including breath control, projection, resonation, range, and phrasing. Those techniques were discussed in preceding chapters.

Considerable additional information about voice and speech training techniques has been published by the Voice and Speech Trainers Association (VASTA). VASTA has also prepared an extensively annotated bibliography of books and articles on voice production and speech training, text analysis, dialect, body awareness training, speech science, and singing.[‡]

Acting-Voice Training for Injured Voices

As important as a wide repertoire of training techniques is for those who teach speakers who fall into the "normal" category, mastery of many approaches is even more critical for acting-voice trainers who work either in a medical setting or as a consultant to a

---

[*]Certified Alexander Teachers can be located through the North American Society of Teachers of Alexander Technique (NASTAT), 8710 Delgany Ave #2, Playa del Rey, CA 90293; telephone (310)827-8106.

[†]Qualified Feldenkrais practitioners can be located through the Feldenkrais Guild, 706 Ellsworth St, PO Box 489, Albany, OR 97321-0143; telephone (503)926-0981 or (800)775-2118.

[‡]For membership information, contact Barry Kur, Past President, Voice and Speech Trainers Association (VASTA), Dept of Theatre, 103 Arts Bldg, Pennsylvania State University, University Park, PA 16802; telephone (814)865-7586. For an extensive annotated bibliography of books and articles on voice production and speech training, text analysis, dialect, body awareness training, speech science, and singing, contact VASTA Bibliography, University of Utah, Theatre Department, 206 PAB, Salt Lake City, UT 84112.

medical team. The acting-voice trainer might be called on to deal with patients who are under the simultaneous care of the laryngologist, speech-language pathologist, and/or singing voice specialist. Some patients will have relatively mild vocal problems such as muscular tension dysphonia, while others may be recovering from nodules, hemorrhages, vocal fold surgery, cancer, or other organic conditions. In this setting, the acting-voice trainer must understand the disease process, the medical implications of a diagnosis, the team's overall therapeutic plan and goals, and the patient's limitations and potential. The acting-voice trainer must individualize the training plan, taking all of these factors into account. Approaching such complex problems requires an acquaintance with all of the techniques mentioned earlier in this chapter, as well as with methods used by speech-language pathologists and singing voice specialists, plus the ability to integrate these otherwise diverse approaches into a unified sequence.

Education for the Acting-Voice Trainer in a Medical Setting

First, the acting-voice trainer working in a medical office must be an expertly trained, experienced voice trainer. Ideally, he or she should also have performance experience. However, this training and experience must be supplemented with additional knowledge.

Many of the special educational requirements for acting-voice trainers who work in medical settings are the same as those discussed in chapter 9, The Singing Voice Specialist. Unfortunately, there are no organized academic programs to prepare acting-voice trainers to work with injured voices. Consequently, unless the voice trainer is willing to complete a master's program and certification in speech-language pathology (an ideal, but long route), it will be necessary to acquire training through selected courses, observation, and apprenticeships with well-established voice teams. Similarly, all of the recommendations for singing voice specialists who wish to work with injured voices apply. The acting-voice trainer needs indepth knowledge of anatomy, physiology, neurogenic voice disorders, phonetics, voice science, and laboratory instrumentation and its interpretation. He or she must spend time with an otolaryngologist, becoming familiar with the style and substance of medical practice. This process includes observation of office-based patient care, strobovideolaryngoscopy and its interpretation, surgery, and medical report writing. The acting-voice trainer also needs to observe and study the new techniques of voice therapy employed by speech-language pathologists (see

chapter 4, Voice Therapy). In addition, singing lessons are helpful and should be supplemented by observation of a singing voice specialist in a medical setting. The knowledge acquired in these approaches is invaluable in allowing the acting-voice trainer to clearly understand the function of everyone on the medical voice team and to integrate his or her training plan into the team's overall vision for each individual patient.

Assessment

As a member of the medical voice team, the acting-voice trainer must learn to perform and report a systematic assessment. Each member of the team provides a written summary of the initial encounter with a patient. Although writing such reports is routine for physicians and speech-language pathologists, it is not customary among acting-voice trainers or singing voice specialists. Chapter 9, The Singing Voice Specialist, details the assessment process and report format developed for high performance singing voice analysis. It has been used as a model in developing practices for the acting-voice trainer. A sample report can be found in Appendix IV. In general, the initial evaluation approach proceeds as follows.

History

The acting-voice training session in the medical setting begins with a thorough case history of the patient. This history partially duplicates the one taken by the physician and is summarized in Appendix Ib. The acting-voice trainer also obtains additional history to pinpoint the activities, habits, and behaviors in the daily life of the professional voice user that may cause or aggravate voice problems. Special attention is paid to the number of hours in a day of professional voice use, the type of performance space used by the patient (auditorium, classroom, indoor, outdoor), audience size, use of amplification, environmental factors (background noise, dust, smoke), and other issues, as discussed in *Clinical Assessment of Voice*.[12] Special attention must be paid to simultaneous employment (the "day job") that actors frequently maintain for economic stability. Many such second occupations (such as waiting tables) are vocally abusive. The acting-voice trainer is also interested in the patient's level of stress and tension, both overall and occupation-specific. Additionally, information is obtained about how the patient prepares for a professional speaking engagement or performance.

The acting-voice trainer further questions the patient about any prior voice or speech training. Surprisingly, many highly successful professional voice users (even actors) have had no voice training at all. If a patient has had some training, this can be useful in designing an effective training program. For example, if a patient has had some positive experience with Linklater training, exercises can be given during the session using the principles of this approach as a foundation for further training.

The acting-voice trainer also inquires about the patient's goals. In some cases, patients are committed to training their voices to become more efficient and powerful, whereas others are satisfied with their present voices and only want techniques to ease their discomfort.

During this portion of the evaluation, the acting-voice trainer is not only getting valuable information about the patient's vocal use; he or she is also listening to how the professional voice user is using his or her voice during conversational speech. This helps the acting-voice trainer evaluate and assess the strengths and weaknesses of the patient's vocal function.

Evaluation

The next section of the assessment consists of evaluating technical proficiency in the patient's conversational and performance voice. The patient is asked to read a passage of a dramatic monologue or present a portion of a lecture or speech that he or she frequently gives. The presentation is audio- or videotape recorded both for documenting later progress and as a teaching tool. During this time, the patient is evaluated for alignment, body tension, breath support, relaxation and isolation of the articulators, forward placement, and overall presentation style.

Alignment. The acting-voice trainer pays close attention to the alignment of the patient's body during the initial session. The head should be balanced on a lengthened and released neck and spine. The shoulders should be relaxed, open, and wide. The hips are balanced over the knees, the knees are easily released forward over the toes. Special focus is given to the patient's head, neck, and torso relationship. Poor alignment in these areas can create tension and inefficiency, which can contribute to voice problems.

Body Tension. The patient is closely observed to see whether tension in the body is adversely affecting the voice. The acting-voice trainer looks for specific areas of body tension such as facial tension, clenched jaw, retracted tongue, lifted shoulders, locked knees, contracted buttocks, contracted abdomen, extrinsic neck muscle tension, arms held at sides, or clenched fists. It is also noted if body tension is getting in the way of the performer's overall communication.

Breath Support. As in initial singing and speech sessions, the acting-voice trainer looks for relaxed abdominal breathing. Although many patients are highly trained professionals, even the most well-trained professional voice user can lose efficient breath support when struggling with a voice injury.

Relaxation and Isolation of Articulators. It is essential for the professional voice user to be able to both relax and separate the function of the individual articulators. The more one articulator can function in isolation; the more relaxed the overall articulation can be. The acting-voice trainer must assess whether the patient is using only what is necessary to create the sound and allowing everything else to stay relaxed. Specifically, the trainer looks for tension in the jaw, tongue, and lips, and the ability of the tongue and lips to function separately from the jaw.

Forward Placement. When the voice is well placed, it is easy to project in large spaces without strain. The voice is taking advantage of its own amplifier. Professional voice users with vocal injuries, because of poor technique or counterproductive muscle compensation, usually attempt to project by pushing from the throat instead of connecting the breath through to the resonating chambers.

Evaluation, Summary, and Treatment Plan

After the initial evaluation is completed, the acting-voice trainer discusses his or her analysis with the laryngologist, and then with the patient. Technical deficiencies are explained and recommendations to improve them are made. Goals are specifically defined. The patient is informed of the need for outside practice in order for sessions to be effective. Exercises are then taught to the patient, and the patient is given his or her first limited opportunity to address vocal problems using these techniques. Ideally, selected exercises will help the patient feel and/or sound better, thus encouraging compliance. Sessions are tape-recorded for ease of home practice, and a practice schedule is assigned. Arrangements for follow-up sessions are made. In addition, if the patient is an actor, the acting-voice trainer is usually the best person on the team to maintain contact with the actor's coaches, teachers, and directors if the patient plans to continue working with the team during or after treatment. Coordinated arrangements must involve not only diverse aspects of medical intervention, but also all other aspects of the patient's vocal life.

Treatment

After the assessment and establishment of a treatment plan, the plan is communicated to the other members of the medical voice team. When all team activities have been coordinated and all components of the plan are compatible and symbiotic, the acting-voice trainer proceeds with "treatment" or training, under medical supervision. This portion of the habilitation or rehabilitation process may begin immediately or be delayed until the patient has worked with the speech-language pathologist and/or singing voice specialist. In people who have had significant vocal injuries or recent surgery, acting-voice training may be delayed, but it often continues after therapy with the speech-language pathologist has been completed.

We have already noted the importance of individualizing approaches and having access to and knowledge of all available techniques from various disciplines. However, we wish to emphasize a few important differences from the work with which most voice trainers are familiar. First, the rate of progress is often different. In the theater, voice coaches are routinely under pressure to prepare performers almost instantaneously for imminent stage obligations. In theater schools, voice trainers may have 2 to 4 years during which to accomplish vocal goals with their students. In the medical setting, the rate of progress is determined by the condition of the weakest part of the system (such as the edge of a recently injured vocal fold). In patients who have sustained a vocal injury, the healing and overall rehabilitation process, as determined by the laryngologist, establish the speed at which vocal advances can be made safely. It is essential for the acting-voice trainer to understand the vocal fold and vocal tract condition of each individual. If inappropriate exercises are used, or if appropriate exercises are used too vigorously in an effort to speed progress, vocal injury may result. Such occurrences are potentially disastrous and must be avoided through proper training, communication, and pacing of training. At the same time, however, many patients are impatient. So progress must be made as quickly and safely as voice use allows. Making judgments about which approaches and exercises to use when, how vigorously, and for how long at each practice session can be difficult. That is one of the principal reasons why acting-voice trainers need extra education and close team collaboration in the medical setting.

Second, the acting-voice trainer must be acutely aware and suspicious of any voice deterioration, however subtle. People who have had vocal fold injuries frequently have fragile vocal folds. As much as voice trainers try to protect the voices of experienced actors,

the acting profession challenges and taxes voices, as discussed in chapter 11; and acting-voice trainers are accustomed to helping actors rise to the challenge and overcome their vocal limitations. Although this goal applies to patients as well, it must be pursued with much greater caution. When acting-voice trainers hear a healthy actor develop a bit of voice fatigue or slight hoarseness, they commonly teach him or her how to relax and work through it. With a patient, especially early in the training process, this is generally not appropriate. Instead, we need to stop, allow the voice several minutes to return to baseline, and request medical examination (looking at the vocal folds) if it does not.

Third, the acting-voice trainer must be prepared to work toward goals that may be different from those acting-voice trainers are accustomed to in theatrical professionals. Many patients developed their vocal injuries by straining to achieve a preconceived sound. Such straining leads to muscular tension dysphonia, which can be associated with vocal nodules, cysts, hemorrhages, and other problems. If the vocal folds have been injured, auditory memory and feedback may not be the best guides for the recovering patient or his or her acting-voice trainer. Rather, like other members of the medical voice team, the acting-voice trainer must be prepared to work toward comfortable, technically correct, and safe vocal production, in some cases ignoring breathiness, hoarseness, and other vocal qualities that no one considers desirable. However, hyperfunctional efforts to eliminate them are even less desirable! The acting-voice trainer must help the patient to work with the sound achieved when technique is correct, and enhance that voice through the use of interpretation, expression, pitch, and rhythm variability, and the many other components of speech that are so important in training actors. Providing non-stage speakers with these skills allows them to fulfill their communication needs using components of speech that do not tax the vocal folds, and it gives them specific tools and skills under their conscious control which they may call upon when they need to express themselves in routine or extraordinary circumstances. Mastering these aspects of the craft of dramatic speaking gives them controlled alternatives to the brute force usually invoked by untrained patients with vocal injuries who do whatever they can to try to sound better, frequently to their own vocal detriment.

Exercises

Numerous exercises may be used in voice training. Those listed below are intended as examples of techniques found useful for many patients. The list is not intended to be complete, nor does it imply that these exercises are suitable in all cases. They are presented to provide the reader with better insights into some of the approaches commonly used by acting-voice trainers.

The Warm-up

Initial sessions with a professional voice user usually begin with some type of body warm-up. These exercises help the patient develop a sensory awareness of his or her body in space, as well as an awareness of the muscles used in voice and speech production. This kind of awareness is useful in retraining muscles to work more efficiently. The warm-up also helps to strengthen and condition these muscles. The exercises should become a part of the professional voice user's daily routine and preperformance preparation. This not only helps the voice to function more efficiently, but can allow the speaker to appear more relaxed and focused in performance.

The specific warm-up exercises recommended vary depending on the individual patient's needs, but usually include exercises for general relaxation and energizing, breathing and alignment, stretching and releasing the upper body, energizing the articulators, and voice placement. Some specific examples of these exercises can be found in chapter 6.

Relaxation

When patients have excessive tension that contributes to voice difficulties, actor relaxation techniques may help them cope with life and occupational stressors, or stress related to the voice injury. Some of these techniques include progressive relaxation and imaging, modified yoga positions for stretching and releasing larger muscle groups, range of motion exercises to stretch and release specific areas of tension such as the jaw and tongue, and gentle shaking either to release tension or energize different areas of the body. Additionally, relaxation work as part of a team session can be useful in speeding the recovery process. During a singing session, for example, the acting-voice trainer can work physically with the patient by releasing specific areas of tension while the patient is doing vocal exercises with the singing voice specialist. Something as simple as placing a hand on the patient's shoulders as a reminder to keep the shoulders relaxed while inhaling or gently manipulating the head and neck to keep the extrinsic muscles released while singing often is enough to help patients kinesthetically understand the process of making sound with less effort.

The Articulation Warm-up

For patients with extreme jaw and tongue tension, a series of exercises to warm up the articulators is often useful. These exercises train patients to release tension in the jaw and tongue and develop strength and dexterity in the tongue and lips so that the voice is produced with much less effort. The following exercises are based on work condensed from and adapted by Ralph Zito from Edith Skinner's *Speak with Distinction*.[2] Ralph Zito heads the voice faculty of the Drama Division at the Juilliard School in New York City.

The Preparation

1. The exercises always begin with gentle stretching. The patient is asked to sit forward on the edge of a chair and let his or her spine lengthen up toward the ceiling. Keeping this length, the chin drops toward the chest to give the back of the neck a gentle stretch. With each outgoing breath, the weight of the head releases the back of the neck a little more. The patient then uses the hands to gently lift the head back into an upright position. This trains the neck muscles to use minimal effort while in motion.

2. The head is then released over the right side with the right ear directly over the right shoulder. The patient is encouraged to do this exercise without collapsing the spine so that the torso remains upright and aligned. The patient is then asked to breathe easily in and out, and imagine that with each exhalation the muscles along the side of the neck are softening, and the space between the left ear and shoulder is increasing. The head then rolls across the chest to the left side and the exercise is repeated on the opposite side. The head is again lifted back in place with the hands.

3. Next, the patient is asked to wiggle the muscles of the face, brow, and head for a minute or so as if mosquitos were landing on the face and he or she had no hands to brush them away. The patient is then asked to squeeze the face into a tiny ball and then stretch it wide open while the jaw drops and the tongue stretches out of the mouth. This is repeated a few times and then the patient is asked to blow out across the lips (like a horse) a few times. The patient is asked to observe how the face feels after the exercise to encourage developing a keener kinesthetic awareness of the muscles of articulation.

4. While maintaining the upward energy of the spine, the heels of the hands are brought up to the sides of the head, and in one easy motion the jaw is gently massaged open. The jaw is allowed to hang open

for a few moments while the patient checks the position of the tongue (ideally, resting at the bottom of the mouth with the tongue tip placed behind the lower front teeth), and breathes. A mirror is used to facilitate the patient's awareness of any jaw or tongue tension that may cause the jaw to close or the tongue to retract. The patient is then asked to tilt the head forward and slide the tip of the tongue forward over the lower lip and continue to breathe. With each outgoing breath, the patient uses gravity to increase the ability of the tongue to stretch up and out of the throat. The head then lifts by uncurling from the back of the neck, and the tongue slowly slides back into the mouth with the tip of the tongue remaining behind the lower front teeth.

The Lips

The next series of exercises is designed to help the patient learn to relax and energize the lips. They also train the patient to isolate the lips from the jaw so the lips can spread without having to close the jaw, and the jaw can open without losing the rounding of the lips.

1. First, with the jaw closed gently, the lips are pursed as far forward as possible and then spread into a smile as wide as possible, keeping the lips together. The goal is to do the exercise as slowly and smoothly as possible. This is repeated 10 times.
2. The exercise is now done with the jaw slightly open and the lips slightly parted throughout the exercise. The patient imagines sipping soda through a straw. The patient is reminded that it is important not to close the jaw as he or she smiles. A mirror is used to monitor this.
3. The sequence is repeated once again with the lips and jaw even more open and the lips moving forward into a wide oval. The patient is given the image of the face of a choir boy to use as a model. The lips are then spread into an open grin while the jaw remains still. It is helpful to have the patient place a finger on his or her chin to monitor any movement of the jaw.
4. Another exercise that is helpful for isolating and relaxing the lips and jaw is repeating *wee-wee-wee-wee-wee-wee*. The patient is trained to make these sounds lightly and easily and with minimal tension and lateralization. The patient then repeats *waw-waw-waw-waw-waw-waw*. The patient is made aware of the necessity to keep the lips rounded over the open jaw so that the sound does not become "wah." Finally the two sounds are spoken alternately (*wee-waw-wee-waw*) keeping the jaw still for the first sound and the lips rounded for the second.

The Tongue

The goals of these exercises are to increase the overall relaxation and dexterity of the tongue, to isolate the tongue from the lips and the jaw, to develop control of the tip of the tongue, and to isolate the parts of the tongue from each other.

1. With the jaw slightly open, the patient is asked to stick the tip of the tongue straight out. It is then moved slowly left and right as slowly and smoothly as possible without moving the jaw. This is repeated several times. The patient continues to use a mirror to monitor the movement. Next the tongue tip moves from the upper lip down to the lower lip, again working as slowly and smoothly as possible. These movements are then combined so that the tongue moves left, right, up, and down.
2. The patient then makes a big circle clockwise with the tip of the tongue as if the tongue is a paint brush and the patient is an artist painting a circle on the air in front of him. Reverse directions so that the movement is counterclockwise. The patient is asked to observe which parts of the movement are difficult and which parts are easy.
3. With the jaw quite open, the tongue tip moves from gum ridge down to the lower front teeth several times, as if the patient were silently saying *lu-lu-la*. The tongue should move straight up and down as smoothly and steadily as possible. The mirror is used to make sure the jaw remains still. The patient then releases the tongue and blows out across the lips.
4. With the jaw remaining open, the back of the tongue moves up to the soft palate and down for the sound *gah-gah-gah*. The jaw stays relaxed, and the tip of the tongue remains resting behind the lower front teeth.

It is important to do this work in short increments of time, as tension can be created by working so specifically on individual articulators. In between each of these exercises, it is helpful to do some of the stretching and shaking exercises mentioned previously.

Efficacy of the Acting-Voice Trainer in a Medical Office

We believe that the acting-voice trainer is an extremely valuable part of the medical voice team. In addition to individual sessions, many voice training sessions have been held jointly with a singing voice specialist, speech-language pathologist, or both, working simultaneously with the acting-voice trainer. The concurrent use of more traditional medical approaches and acting-voice training (both voice and body techniques) has facilitated compliance and carryover and expedited recovery. In addition, the acting-voice trainer has been invaluable for advanced training in patients whom we formerly would have discharged from therapy. Although speech-language pathologists and singing voice specialists do address high-performance speaking voice needs, the added dimension of the professional acting-voice trainer has contributed enormously to our ability to carry our patients further toward reaching optimal speaking performance. In future years, we anticipate the addition of acting-voice trainers to other medical teams and the development of educational programs to make it easier for acting-voice trainers to provide more knowledgeable intervention in patients with vocal injuries.

References

1. Raphael BN. A consumer's guide to voice and speech training. *N Engl Theatre J*. 1994;5:101–114.
2. Skinner E, Mansell L, ed. *Speak with Distinction*. New York, NY: Applause Theatre Book Publishers; 1990.
3. Linklater K. *Freeing the Natural Voice*. New York, NY: Drama Book Specialists; 1976.
4. Linklater K. *Freeing Shakespeare's Voice*. New York, NY: Theatre Communications Group; 1992.
5. Lessac A. *The Use and Training of the Human Voice*. 2nd ed. Mountain View, Calif: Mayfield; 1967.
6. Lessac A. *Body Wisdom: The Use and Training of the Human Body*. Claremont, Calif: Arthur Lessac; 1978.
7. Berry C. *Voice and the Actor*. London: Harrap; 1973.
8. Berry C. *The Actor and His Text*. London: Harrap; 1987.
9. Turner JC: *Voice and Speech in the Theatre*. 3rd ed. London: Pitman; 1977.
10. Rodenburg P. *The Right to Speak*. London: Methuen Drama; 1992.
11. Rodenburg P. *The Need for Words*. London: Methuen Drama; 1993.
12. Sataloff RT, Anticaglia J, Hawkshaw MJ. Patient history. In: Sataloff RT. *Clinical Assessment of Voice*. San Diego, Calif: Plural Publishing Inc; 2005:1–16.

13

Laryngeal Manipulation

Jacob Lieberman, John S. Rubin,
Thomas M. Harris, and Adrian J. Fourcin

This chapter, written by an osteopath, two laryngologists, and a speech scientist, is on manipulation of the larynx and the perilaryngeal structures. This is a young science, perhaps still more of an art than a science, but which takes as its predecessors, principles from anatomy, physiology, osteopathy, and physical therapy. We present a synopsis of the role that laryngeal manipulation plays in our clinical practice. Concepts presented in this chapter are fresh and still undergoing change. Many come out of an ongoing collaboration with the Sidcup Voice Unit.

Certain aspects of manipulation, for example, side-to-side movement of the larynx, have been used by physicians as a part of the routine clinical examination for well over a century and by performers for centuries. One or two quick side-to-side movements of the larynx to help relax the larynx are part of many performers' routine preparations.

Recently, manipulation of the larynx has been reported on by practitioners as one form of treatment in patients presenting with functional voice disorders,[1-7] and more generally in patients with muscular tension dysphonia (Murray Morrison, Instructional Course, Annual Meeting of the American Academy of Otolaryngology Head and Neck Surgery, September 1999; Murray Morrison, Laryngology Research meeting, AAOHNS annual meeting, San Antonio, 1998; John Rubin, Laryngology Research meeting, AAOHNS annual meeting, San Antonio, 1998).

Currently, the core team of the voice clinic at Sidcup consists of laryngologist(s), speech and language pathologist(s), an osteopath, and a singing teacher. The osteopath is also a certified child, family, and adolescent psychodynamic psychotherapist; similarly, the speech and language pathologist has taken extra training in counseling. There is also immediate access to a psychiatrist, other singing teachers, and coaches.

The role of the osteopath is to examine the relationship of posture, breathing mechanics, and the function of the larynx to voice production. In the Sidcup clinic the osteopath is frequently called on to assist in the diagnosis, as well as to assist at an early stage in the rehabilitative management (Table 13–1).

In this chapter we discuss laryngeal manipulation from an osteopathic perspective. Anatomy and physiology, indications for manipulation, the osteopathic examination, tenets of basic manipulation and advanced manipulation, treatment outcomes, and our current hypotheses for the underlying mechanisms involved are presented.

Biomechanics of the Larynx

The larynx is a complex structure consisting of cartilages, muscles, ligaments, joints, and mucous membranes, all interacting in highly precise and timed functions, that is, synergetically. Given the sphincteric nature of laryngeal closure, it is our view that it is overly simplistic to argue that any given phonatory behavior occurs on the basis of a single muscular activity. The relative pull of each muscle is balanced by the activities of other muscles. The overall vectors of pull and joint axes determine the actual position of the arytenoids and, hence, of the vocal folds.[8] This is particularly apt when discussing the various muscles (interarytenoid, lateral cricoarytenoid, and so forth), that have direct attachment to the muscular process of the arytenoid cartilages and are involved in medial positioning of the vocal fold.

Table 13–1. Lieberman's Protocol (Revised)(Reproduced with permission from Lieberman J. Principles and techniques of manual therapy. In: Harris T, Harris S, Rubin JS, Howard DM, eds. *The Voice Clinic Handbook.* Whurr Medical Publishers, London, 1998, appendices 6.1 and 6.2: 132–137.)

Assessment of Posture and Laryngeal Apparatus (Joints and Muscles) in Hyperfunctional Dysphonia

This protocol is a nonexhaustive reference for the assessment of posture and the laryngeal apparatus. It is designed to accompany the instructional course on the detailed anatomy of the larynx, its palpatory assessment, and the assessment of posture-related aspects of voice dysfunction. It can be used in multidisciplinary voice clinics as part of the overall assessment of voice patients to provide a framework for practitioner agreement and research.

1. POSTURE and LARYNGEAL ACTIVITY

1.1 OBSERVATIONS:

Sitting: (while patient is providing history): (tick as appropriate)

Anterior neck compartment:

Signs of increased muscular activity:	Smooth		Conspicuous Rt	Conspicuous Lt	
Static (patient is silent)					
Dynamic (talking)					
Level and position of thyroid lamina		Normal	High	Low	Deviated
Bulging omohoid muscle activity in speech			Absent	Present Rt	Present Lt
Skin crease asymmetry			Absent	Present Rt	Present Lt
Head position in the sagittal plane — Tilt			Absent	Present Rt	Present Lt
Head gestures (head nodding in speech/swallowing)			Absent	Present Rt	Present Lt
Jaw movement (vertical and lateral plane)* — Asymmetric			Absent	Present Rt	Present Lt

1.1.2 **Standing:** (lateral view): (tick as appropriate)

Weight bearing (sagittal plane, observed from the side):	Normal	Anterior sway	Posterior sway
Spinal curve (exaggerated: hyperhypolordosis):			
Lumbar	Normal lordosis	Decreased lordosis	Increased lordosis
Thoracic	Normal kyphosis	Decreased kyphosis	Increased kyphosis
Cervical	Normal lordosis	Decreased lordosis	Increased lordosis
Rib cage:			
Flexibility	Normal	Decreased	
Function	Normal	Raised	Held
Breathing patterns:			
Diaphragmatic	Normal	Decreased	Paradoxical
Upper chest	Absent	Present	Increased
Clavicular	Absent	Present	Increased
Head position (cervical translation):			
Anterior	Absent	Present	
Cervical thoracic hump	Absent	Present	Cervical level

1.1.3 Spinal Curves

Standing: (anterior/posterior view):

Lumbar-thoracic (including scoliosis)	Normal	Asymmetry Rt	Asymmetry Lt
Scapular level	Normal	Raised Rt	Raised Lt
Head level	Normal	Tilt Rt	Tilt Lt

1.1.4 Spinal Curves

Standing: (vertical axis):

NOTE: the normal larynx moves with the torso

Torso rotation	Normal	Clockwise	Counterclockwise
Pelvis rotation	Normal	Clockwise	Counterclockwise
Head rotation	Normal	Clockwise	Counterclockwise

2.1 PALPATION:

(tick as appropriate)

Cervical spinous processes: Palpable	No	Yes	Cervical level
Suboccipital musculature (above C2): Tonus	Normal	Increased Rt	Increased Lt
Symmetry	Normal	Increased Rt	Increased Lt
Tenderness	No	Increased Rt	Increased Lt
Cervical musculature (other): Tonus	Normal	Increased Rt	Increased Lt
Symmetry	Normal	Increased Rt	Increased Lt
Tenderness	No	Increased Rt	Increased Lt
TMJ: Movement	Normal	Asymmetry Rt	Asymmetry Lt
Opening	Normal	Asymmetry Rt	Asymmetry Lt
Tenderness	No	Increased Rt	Increased Lt
Sternocleidomastoid muscle: Tonus	Normal	Increased Rt	Increased Lt
Symmetry	Normal	Increased Rt	Increased Lt
Tenderness	No	Increased Rt	Increased Lt

3.1 The LARYNGEAL APPARATUS:

OBSERVATION:

(tick as appropriate)

Superior suspensory muscles: Tone	Normal	Low	High
Laryngeal range of movement (in speech and swallowing):	Normal	Increased	Decreased
Inferior suspensory muscles: Tone	Normal	Asymmetric Rt	Asymmetric Lt

(continues)

Table 13–1. *(continued)*

4.1	The LARYNGEAL APPARATUS: PALPATION	(tick as appropriate)

Palpate for position, tone, symmetry, tenderness both in static (passive) and dynamic (swallowing, speech singing):

Item	Parameter	Options
Hyoid		Normal | High | Low
Geniohyoid: static	Tone:	Normal | Asymmetric
	Tenderness:	None | Present
Geniohyoid: dynamic		Normal | Asymmetric
Superior suspensory muscles: static	Tone:	Normal | Asymmetric Rt | Asymmetric Lt
	Tenderness:	None | Rt | Lt
Superior suspensory muscles: dynamic		Normal | Asymmetric Rt | Asymmetric Lt
Inferior suspensory muscles: static	Tone:	Normal | Asymmetric Rt | Asymmetric Lt
	Tenderness:	None | Rt | Lt
Inferior suspensory muscles: dynamic		Normal | Asymmetric Rt | Asymmetric Lt
Thyrohyoid apparatus: static	Coronal: attitude hyoid to thyroid:	Parallel | Tilt Lt | Tilt Rt
	Size of gap:	None | Diminished Rt | Diminished Lt
	Tenderness:	None | Rt | Lt
	Symmetry:	Normal | Asymmetric Rt | Asymmetric Lt
Thyrohyoid apparatus: dynamic (movement)		Normal | Rotation Rt | Rotation Lt
Cricothyroid muscles: static	Tone:	Normal | Asymmetric Rt | Asymmetric Lt
	Tenderness:	None | Rt | Lt
Cricothyroid visor (joint)(head neutral): static	Resting state:	Closed | Mid position open | Open
	Anterior arch:	None | Present
Cricothyroid joint: dynamic	Changes with siren:	No change | Closes
	Changes with yawn:	No change | Opens
	Posterior glide of arch with pitch rise:	No change | Diminishes
Constrictor muscles: (perform lateral shift test):	Mobility:	Absent | Present Rt | Present Lt
	Tenderness:	None | Asymmetric Rt | Asymmetric Lt
Internal laryngeal structures (for experienced therapists only):	Accessible:	No | Rt | Lt
	Tenderness:	None | Rt | Lt
	Movement:	None | Rt | Lt

Furthermore, the larynx is suspended from the basicranium, not by direct bony attachment, but by a series of muscular and ligamentous attachments.

The larynx can be considered to be an "intrusion" into the pharynx. Its major role is that of airway protection, and this is critical to life itself. The larynx protects the lower airway biomechanically both by creating a diversion for the food particles around the endolarynx and by closing sphincterically and moving in an upward and forward fashion with each swallow.

Another critical role is pressure-valving. Pressure-valving prevents ingress or egress of air and allows sudden increases in intrathoracic and intra-abdominal pressures to occur. This permits activities such as coughing, defecation, and weight-lifting.[9]

Phonation has been considered as a more recent activity and has been related to the lowering of the larynx from the basicranium.[10] Scherer has noted that phonation only occurs in a narrow range of overall vocal fold movement, approximately 10 to 15%, that brings the vocal folds nearest to one another.[11]

Hast published his study on the physiology of the cricothyroid muscle over 30 years ago,[12] yet the biomechanics of the larynx remain poorly understood. That said, investigators have correlated laryngeal injury with inefficient or abnormal laryngeal function or have identified vocal improvement through reduction in mechanical strain via voice therapy or other techniques.[12-15]

More specific techniques involving manual circumlaryngeal therapy have been espoused for such conditions as functional dysphonia[1-4] and more generally for hyperfunctional conditions (Murray Morrison, Instructional Course, Annual Meeting of the American Academy of Otolaryngology Head and Neck Surgery, September, 1999; Murray Morrison, Laryngology Research meeting, AAOHNS annual meeting, San Antonio, 1998; John Rubin, Laryngology Research meeting, AAOHNS annual meeting, San Antonio, 1998).

Much further investigation is needed, emphasizing the development of methods to recognize and quantify biomechanical dysfunction and restoration.[15] For the physical therapist who is attempting to improve muscular or joint efficiency or position and thereby improve the voice, the entire vocal tract needs to be considered. This should include the deep and superficial postural muscles as well as the muscles, joints, and ligaments directly related to the sound source. In that regard, the importance of posture has been identified by individuals such as Alexander, Pilates, Feldenkrais, Rolf, and others.[16-19] While physical therapy has

become integrated into rehabilitation of sports injuries, it is only recently that these fields have been applied to voice research or rehabilitation.

Laryngeal Joints

There are two pairs of joints of particular importance to the position and configuration of the vocal folds, the cricothyroid and the cricoarytenoid.

The Cricothyroid Joint

The cricothyroid joint is a synovial joint that consists of a circular facet on the medial aspect of the inferior horn of the thyroid cartilage, articulating with an articular facet on the side of the lamina of the cricoid. This articular facet lies at the junction of the arch and the body of the cricoid, and faces in a dorsolateral and superior manner. Of note, the two cricoid facets are often asymmetric.[20] The joint is stabilized by its capsule as well as by a posterior and a lateral ligament. The posterior ligament is said to control movement of the inferior horn of the thyroid, while the lateral ligament limits posterior displacement of the thyroid, with respect to the cricoid.[21]

The cricothyroid joint is considered by Lieberman to be a key element in the tensioning mechanism of the vocal ligament.[14,22] The radiating fibers that moor the lower horn of the thyroid to the cricoid permit rotation about a (predominantly) transverse axis, and allow it to "rotate up and down like the visor of a helmet."[21(p699)] This in turn leads, indirectly, to stretching and tightening of the vocal ligament with a corresponding increase in fundamental frequency of the voice. In a study of fresh cadavers, this was found to correspond to a stretch of 25% in the length of the vocal ligament.[20,23]

Lieberman and Harris[8] (Jacob Lieberman, unpublished data, 2000) have also identified, through palpation, some movement of the cricoid in an anterior-posterior (A-P) direction in relation to the thyroid during phonation. This movement has also been identified by Boileau Grant.[21] By pulling the thyroid cartilage anteriorly with respect to the cricoid cartilage, such movement increases tension in the vocal ligament. It lacks the mechanical advantage that the lever mechanism provides through rotation about the cricothyroid joint, however (Tom Harris, personal observation, 2002).

A-P movement in the cricothyroid joint is observed in many young female singers who perform in musical theater. It is worth noting that the dorsolateral orientation of the facets is designed to stop such a movement. It is therefore quite possible that the flexibility of the inferior horns of the thyroid cartilage, as well as stretched ligament, allow such a movement to take place. Although such A-P movement seems to increase the vocal range, for instance in belting, it may also render the joint to be less stable.

The Cricoarytenoid Joint

The cricoarytenoid is a synovial joint of the saddle type. Each arytenoid has a deeply grooved base with a facet that articulates with an elliptical joint facet in the posterior aspect of the upper cricoid. Each cricoid facet is a raised structure, convexly curved and measuring approximately 6 mm along its major, longitudinal axis. This axis runs as (very nearly) an arc with its center based at the anterior commissure along the posterior, lateral, and superior margin of the cricoid cartilage. As this axis exceeds the transverse diameter of the corresponding arytenoid articular surface, a degree (only a few millimeters) of sliding along the axis is made possible.[9,15,21,23,24] It may be utilized during forceful laryngeal closure.

The primary motion, however, is forward and backward gliding along the minor axis of the cricoid facet[23,24] (or looked at from a different perspective, revolving about the long axis [Tom Harris, personal observation, 2002]). This bidirectional movement results in changes not only anterior and posterior, but also vertical, because of the oblique setting of the long axis. It resembles the movement of a rocking chair, thus "rocking" is a common description. "Rotation" is also described but by and large ignores the vertical displacement, which is significant. Letson notes that, for each "unit" of vertical displacement, there are two units of medial-lateral displacement.[24]

To summarize, arytenoid motion occurs in three directions. Anterior and posterior movements and vertical movements are caused by "revolving" or "pitchlike" motion along the minor axis of the cricoid. The medial and lateral motion is determined by the orientation of the cricoarytenoid facet. During adduction, the outward angulation of the vocal process away from the body of the arytenoid permits the length of the vocal process to approximate at the proper vertical height.[24-26]

Ligaments of the Cricoarytenoid Joint

A fibrous articular capsule and two ligaments stabilize and limit movement of the cricoarytenoid joint. The posterior cricoarytenoid ligament attaches to the superior rim of the cricoid lamina between the two cricoarytenoid facets and extends anteriorly to the medial surface of the arytenoid cartilage.[20,23] Together with the articular capsule, its primary function is, most likely, prevention of lateral dislocation of the arytenoid on forced abduction of the vocal folds.[20,23]

The anterior ligament of the cricoarytenoid joint is the vocal ligament.[23] It extends from the vocal process of the arytenoid and then condenses to form Broyle's ligament and inserts into the thyroid cartilage just inferior to the thyroepiglottic ligament. It stabilizes the arytenoid and maintains the positional integrity of the true vocal fold, thereby allowing the vocal fold to be acted upon by the intrinsic laryngeal muscles.

The vocal ligament forms the upper border of the triangular membrane (also known as the cricothyroid ligament and the conus elasticus). This membrane attaches below to the whole length of the upper border of the arch of the cricoid; in front it blends into the median cricothyroid ligament. After curving medial to the lower border of the thyroid cartilage it ends above in the free upper border, the vocal ligament.[9,21,23]

The quadrangular membrane is a fibroelastic sheath, more delicate than the cricothyroid ligament. It extends bilaterally from either side of the epiglottis and curves backward to the lateral border of the arytenoid cartilage. Its free upper edge condenses slightly to form the aryepiglottic ligament. Its free lower border condenses to form the vestibular ligament, the basis of the false vocal fold.

Intrinsic and Extrinsic Laryngeal Muscles

From the standpoint of manipulation of the larynx, it is helpful to think in terms of groups of muscles, phonatory function, and overall activity. The laryngeal muscles are definable in this manner. Useful groupings include:

1. "Special muscles" of phonation: the thyroarytenoid and cricothyroid;
2. Intrinsic muscles that insert into the epiglottis and/or quadrangular membrane;
3. Intrinsic muscles that insert into the muscular process of the arytenoids;
4. Extrinsic muscles that elevate the larynx: the suprahyoid suspensory group;
5. Extrinsic muscles that depress the larynx: the infrahyoid suspensory group;
6. The constrictor muscles which elevate and pull the larynx backward against the deep cervical fascia and the cervical spine.

Special Phonatory Muscles

The *vocalis muscle* is the medial body of the thyroarytenoid muscle. It travels in an anterior-posterior (A-P) fashion with the vocal ligament forming the substance of the true vocal fold. Contraction of the vocalis causes bulking and shortening of the free edge of the vocal fold and stiffening of the muscle. It acts to help control pitch production, thereby causing lowering of the fundamental frequency, at least during soft phonation.[9,27-31] While it is not possible to access this muscle digitally, it can be manipulated through the articulation of the cricothyroid joint.

The *cricothyroid muscle* is readily accessible to manipulation. Although often considered to be an intrinsic laryngeal muscle because of its impact upon pitch, the cricothyroid is really an extrinsic laryngeal muscle. Unlike the other intrinsic laryngeal muscles (innervated by the recurrent laryngeal nerve), its innervation is from the external branch of the superior laryngeal nerve. The cricothyroid originates on the anterior surface of the arch of the cricoid. It divides into two parts, the pars recta (anterior or oblique part) that passes upwards to the ala of the thyroid, and the pars oblique (posterior or horizontal part) that passes more outward to the inferior cornu of the thyroid. Contraction, particularly of its vertical belly, causes increased tension and stretch on the vocal ligament, thereby affecting pitch.[32-34] The oblique part of the cricothyroid muscle is probably responsible for the A-P movement described above.

Harris and Lieberman have named the opening and closing action of the cricothyroid joint on the anterior thyroid and cricoid cartilages the "cricothyroid visor."[8,14] The resting state, and contraction, of the cricothyroid muscle have a marked impact on the "cricothyroid visor," and is believed by them to be significant in voice production. Furthermore, they postulate that abnormal patterns of muscular activity can occur in the cricothyroid muscle and in the "visor" mechanism leading to voice problems, and that manipulation of this muscle and joint can markedly improve these problems.[8,14]

Intrinsic Muscles That Insert into the Epiglottis and/or Quadrangular Membrane

Intrinsic muscles that insert into the quadrangular membrane are recognizable by having the name "epiglottis" as part of their title: for example, aryepiglotticus. Such muscles have as one of their actions the drawing down of the epiglottic cartilage over the larynx. They work as part of the swallowing mechanism, helping to protect the endolarynx from food particles.

They act in synchrony, one with another, in a vegetative fashion under reflexogenic control.[35,36]

It is unclear if these muscles participate significantly in patterns of voicing or voice disorders. Estill has postulated that one vocal quality, "twang," may be associated with constriction of the epiglottis in association with aryepiglottic contraction.[37] More research is required to confirm these suggestions. While these muscles are difficult to access via basic laryngeal manipulation, it appears that they relax subsequent to general relaxation of the laryngeal musculature.

Intrinsic Muscles That Insert into the Muscular Process of the Arytenoids

Muscles that insert into the muscular process of the arytenoid cartilage (and thereby have "arytenoid" as part of their name) are invariably linked to movement and/or tensioning of the true vocal fold. All these muscles are true intrinsic laryngeal muscles and are innervated by the recurrent laryngeal nerve.

During swallowing the true vocal folds are brought and held tightly together by several of these muscles acting in synchrony. The posterior cricoarytenoid has been generally posited to be the one intrinsic laryngeal muscle that causes the vocal folds to abduct. That said, it is clear that the laryngeal intrinsic muscles do not act in a vacuum. There are patterns of muscular movements that bring the vocal folds to the desired position or level of stretch or tension (and we postulate that the vector for maximum abduction involves the lateral cricoarytenoid as well as the posterior cricoarytenoid[8]).

These muscles are accessible to the experienced practitioner in laryngeal manipulation. However, it is rarely appropriate to manipulate them directly as they are so intricately linked to fundamental reflexogenic activities. Attempts at such manipulation, unless the patient is adequately prepared, are likely to lead to throat discomfort, and are not recommended for the beginner.

Extrinsic Muscles That Elevate the Larynx: the Suprahyoid Suspensory Group

The suprahyoid suspensory muscle group are powerful muscles that play an important role in the act of swallowing. These muscles extend upward from the hyoid bone into the base of the tongue, and skull base. It is not at all uncommon for patients to present to the voice clinic with a "raised" larynx, and "held" suprahyoid musculature. There are many potential reasons for this to occur.

From a physiologic perspective, one understandable cause is as follows: muscular imbalances between the deep flexors and the deep extensors of the neck are commonplace, with the almost inevitable outcome being the deep extensors "triumphing." The end result of this (and associated muscular imbalances) is recognizable to all of us: "slumped" posture, rounded shoulders, head held forward, and chin tilted up. Chin tilt can be exacerbated by the necessity of performing on a raked stage. As the head translates farther forward, there is a tendency for adaptive "shortening" of the stylohyoid muscle, one of the suprahyoid suspensory muscles (E. Blake, personal observation, 2001).

Other causes might typically include performing with laryngeal edema or with nodules on the vocal folds, and, in an attempt to obtain vocal fold closure, recruiting extrinsic laryngeal muscles and thereby raising the larynx.

Lieberman has also found an association between a tight and foreshortened thyrohyoid muscle (with the clinical correlate of a foreshortened and "held" thyrohyoid membrane) and unresolved emotional issues.[22]

This group of muscles is readily accessible to laryngeal manipulation.

Extrinsic Muscles That Depress the Larynx: the Infrahyoid Suspensory Group

The sternothyroid, sternohyoid, and omohyoid muscles are a part of the muscles known as "strap" muscles or "ribbon" muscles. They are involved in the swallowing mechanism to lower the larynx and assist in "resetting" the mechanism.[35,38] These muscles are readily accessible to the beginner in laryngeal manipulation.

Although not strictly relevant to this section, note that the geniohyoid and strap muscles working synchronously tend to pull the larynx in an anterior direction, and thereby act in an antagonistic fashion to the constrictors.[8,39,40]

The Constrictor Muscles

The constrictor muscles form a muscular sling that defines the posterior and lateral parts of the pharynx. There are three constrictors, superior, middle, and inferior, one overlapping the other, extending from the basicranium to the cervical esophagus. Each is fan-shaped, attaching to its counterpart via a tough raphe of fibrous tissue just anterior to the prevertebral fascia. The middle constrictor is the only muscle of the constrictor group that "anchors" the hyoid bone; the inferior constrictor "anchors" the thyroid cartilage, with attachments from the upper border of the thyroid cartilage to the lower border of the cricoid cartilage.[21]

In our view, the constrictors are involved in many presentations of hyperfunctional voice disorders. The

patient's ability or failure to relax these muscles, with or without manipulation, is a useful indicator of prognosis for treatment outcome (J. Lieberman, personal observation, 2002).

Deep Muscles of the Neck

The deep muscles of the neck can be divided into the posterior extensors, the suboccipital muscle group, the deep anterior neck flexors, and the superficial anterior neck flexors. We shall not spend much time on these important groups of muscles as they are outside the scope of the chapter, but discuss them briefly as problems therein can lead to foreshortening of muscles involved with voicing (as described above).

The Posterior Extensors

The key group of muscles here are the erector spinae muscles. They span the vertebrae, give support, establish, and maintain appropriate extension of the vertebral column. The muscles attached to the skull produce extension, lateral flexion, and rotation of the head.

The erector spinae includes, superficially, the iliocostalis, longissimus, and the spinalis. Deeper muscles include the semispinalis, the deep short muscles, the multifidis, and cervicis.[41]

Suboccipital Muscle Group

These muscles extend the skull at the atlanto-occipital joint and rotate it at the atlanto-axial joint. They are important for stereoscopic vision. Muscles include the rectus capitis posterior major and minor, and the obliquus capitis superior and inferior.

Deep Anterior Neck Flexors

These include the three scalene muscles and the prevertebral muscles (the longus colli, longus capitis, rectus capitis anterior and lateralis). Their actions include: scalenes—weak neck flexion, and lifting and stabilizing the upper two ribs; prevertebral muscles—twisting the head on the neck and flexing the neck.

Superficial Anterior Neck Muscles

These include the sternocleidomastoid, levator scapulae, trapezius, and splenius. The sternocleidomastoid turns the head obliquely to the other side. When working with its opposite member it pulls the head downward and forward. The levator scapulae raises and helps rotate the scapula. The trapezius holds the shoulder back and up, steadies and raises the scapula, draws the head backward and to one side. The splenius supports the spine.[41]

These muscles are readily accessible to osteopathic manipulation and often held in a contracted state in patients with voice disorders (also in individuals with musculoskeletal related headache). As previously noted the deep extensors frequently are found to be held in a contracted state. Another common finding is for various fibers of the trapezius to be contracted and tender in patients with voice disorders (E. Blake, personal observation, 2002).

It is facile to believe that any one muscle works in isolation in the larynx or elsewhere, but this is generally not the case. Several muscles work together both synergistically and antagonistically in the same reflex arc. For example, the tensor fascia lata is an extensor of the hip when the knee is flexed less than 20 degrees, and acts as a flexor of the hip when the knee is flexed beyond 20 degrees (J. Lieberman, personal observation, 1999). In the larynx, as elsewhere, muscles work together, the net pull leading to movement or to stability.[8]

Indications for Laryngeal Manipulation in Voice Patients

As we have worked together over time as a team, we have identified more indications for referral to an individual specially trained in laryngeal manipulation. There are two basic indications for such a referral. The first is when the otolaryngologist has identified abnormal musculoskeletal patterns in a patient presenting with a voice problem. This indication is predominantly for treatment from the therapist. The second general indication is for assessment when the laryngologist is uncertain as to the cause of the dysphonia, for example, in the absence of obvious vocal fold mucosal pathology. Let us review these instances.

1. The otolaryngologist is reasonably certain that a musculoskeletal problem exists and is affecting voice production. Typical instances for referral might include:
   a. The patient with the high-held larynx and tightly held base of tongue musculature, with or without mucosal pathology of the true vocal folds. This type of referral is likely to lead to rapid improvement over one or two sessions. This pattern also responds quickly to Roy's or Mathieson's circumhyoid manipulation.[1-3]
   b. The patient with a forward-held (hyperlordotic) neck with a palpable "shelf" on palpation of the posterior spinous processes at, typically, C4/C5

or C5/C6, and a forward-held cricoid in relationship to the anterior thyroid. This, with or without mucosal pathology of the true vocal folds, is likely to represent a long-standing postural pattern. It is likely to respond to laryngeal manipulation but to take several sessions and possibly to require intermittent follow-up (J. Rubin, personal observation, 2002).
   c. The patient with reduced range of motion of the cricothyroid visor, with a voice that tires easily. This pattern, with or without mucosal pathology at the level of the vocal folds, is likely to be an end result of "guarding" the larynx, but responds rapidly to laryngeal manipulation.
   d. The patient with the low-held larynx, in association with tightly held sternocleidomastoid muscles; the phoniatric correlate being a gravelly voice with a marked amount of "creak" in the voice quality. This is likely to respond well to laryngeal manipulation, or to Mathieson's combination of manipulation and speech therapy.[2]
   e. The patient with the exquisitely tender and tightly held thyrohyoid membrane, usually unilaterally. This is likely to respond to manipulation; however, gentle investigation into possible unresolved emotional issues would not be amiss. Lieberman finds the combination of manipulation and application of psychodynamic models extremely beneficial in the management of such cases whose symptoms are considered as a physical manifestation of emotional state of mind (J. Lieberman, personal observation, 2002).
2. The otolaryngologist is uncertain as to the cause of the dysphonia. In this circumstance, the osteopathic assessment is likely to be of benefit in demonstrating whether or not there is any underlying muscular or joint pathology.

There are certain caveats. (1) A traditional course of therapy with a speech-language pathologist (SLP) may well successfully treat some or all of the patients treated by the physical therapist. Management is not exclusive; we frequently obtain opinions and/or management protocols from both SLP and osteopath. (2) In the patients with secondary hyperfunction, caused by, for example, a partial palsy, a sulcus, chronic pharyngolaryngeal reflux, and so forth, the underlying cause needs to be identified and treated appropriately. (3) Much as with speech therapy, any new pattern of musculoskeletal positioning needs to be internalized by the patient if it is to be long-lasting. This may require several sessions (see research section in this chapter).

Case histories follow, demonstrating some of the authors' indications for manipulation.

Case History 1: Acute Management

One of the authors was contacted only hours prior to performance by a performer suffering from increasing vocal difficulties.

He saw the performer and concluded that the performer was suffering from mild laryngeal edema, which could be managed medically with a single dose of prednisone. However, significant musculoskeletal issues were also identified; thus, an osteopath was contacted and came backstage to see the performer.

After explaining the process, the osteopath proceeded to perform a 10-minute period of general relaxation manipulation to the performer's neck, followed by a 5-to -10-minute period of manipulation directed specifically at the tender, held region. Ten to fifteen minutes post-therapy, the performer found that the laryngeal discomfort had eased markedly. The performer was then able to perform credibly in the role.

Case History 2: Subacute Management

A performer presented to one of the otolaryngologists following the acute onset of hoarseness brought on by an episode of violent coughing and retching. One vocal fold was noted to be discolored, consistent with a vocal fold hemorrhage. Judicious voice rest led to improvement to baseline from the standpoint of laryngeal appearance and stroboscopic function, but the performer continued to suffer from vocal fatigue. It was postulated that the performer had developed new musculoskeletal "habits" involving the perilaryngeal musculature because of (unconscious) protection of the larynx. Osteopathic consultation was requested together with consultation with the performer's singing voice teacher. Following two or three sessions of basic manipulation procedures of the perilaryngeal musculature and neck, as well as work with the singing voice teacher over a few weeks, the performer felt to be back at baseline.

Osteopathic Evaluation

The history and assessment of the patient by the osteopath should result in a functional diagnosis as well as a treatment plan. Much as with the otolaryngologist, history taking begins the moment the patient presents to the office. Body movements, both voluntary and involuntary, and general body positioning while the patient is absorbed in presenting his history,

frequently give subtle or obvious clues to the underlying musculoskeletal pathology. A conventional medical history is taken, with emphasis on problems affecting the gastrointestinal tract, respiratory system, central nervous system, or psyche. Sleep patterns, gynecologic issues, and the musculoskeletal system are all reviewed. For greater detail on the history see the chapters by Sataloff in *Clinical Assessment of Voice*.[42]

Osteopathic Assessment

The osteopathic assessment (see Table 13–1) begins with visual observation and then proceeds to palpation. Palpation is performed to assess the resting muscle tone, contracted muscle tone, resting joint position, range of motion, and ease of mobility.

If failure to relax a muscle following activity leads to hyperfunctional muscular behavior, and voice and swallow require repetitive, complex muscular activity, then it is hardly surprising that both the laryngeal and perilaryngeal musculature are at risk for hyperfunctional patterns. These patterns are identifiable by tight, tender, and contracted muscles. This results in loss of full joint range of movement and loss of movement pattern. It is experienced as stiffness.[43]

It should be recalled that, although the patient presents with a hoarse voice, the osteopath is interested in far more than the larynx; he or she needs to evaluate the entire vocal tract. Specifically, he or she will need to assess (1) general posture; (2) head position; (3) integrity of the deep and more superficial muscles of the neck; (4) integrity of the muscles, joints, and ligaments supporting breathing; (5) integrity of the muscles, joints, and ligaments of the pharynx and larynx; (6) position of the laryngeal cartilages and hyoid bone.

General Posture

The general posture of an individual plays a significant role in the development or perpetuation of voice problems. As noted above, there is a steady state between the extensors and the flexors of the body. In our society this balance is frequently abrogated. There is often peer pressure leading children to assume a "slumped" position. Adults spend much of their working day and evening seated in front of computer screens or televisions, often in unhealthy postural positions. Unfortunately, the media has paid much attention to bulging abdominal muscles (the "six pack" appearance) in individuals with flat stomachs. This has led to an emphasis in adults' sports time, on exercises designed to pull the lower rib cage down toward the pelvis. Thus, even during exercise, some adults tend to develop muscles that promote abnormal postural patterns.

These postural patterns lead to a cascade of compensatory postural changes with a resultant hyperlordotic neck. This in turn places the suprahyoid suspensory muscles at significant risk for the development of chronic spasm, and can lead to inefficient muscular patterns of voicing.

There are many other causes of general postural problems relating to spinal curvatures and asymmetries, injuries, or congenital problems affecting the pelvis, hips, legs, and feet, all of which can ultimately affect voice production.

Head Position

Head position has a direct effect on voice production. The adult head weighs 14 to 16 pounds. Position of the head can affect the resting length of the suspensory muscles. Hyperlordosis has already been discussed above. Head tilt or anterior-posterior displacement can affect voice. Examples of individuals with head tilt might include: teachers who work from a piano, with their students always singing from the same side of the piano; many instrumentalists (for example, some woodwind players, guitarists, violinists), and so forth.

Integrity of the Deep Muscles of the Neck

These muscles have been reviewed above briefly. All are involved in head, neck, or upper spine positioning or stability. Abnormalities in any of these muscles ultimately can lead to voice problems.

Integrity of the Muscles, Joints, and Ligaments Supporting Breathing

The mechanisms inherent to the "bellows" are crucial to voice production.[44] Limitation of motion, caused by injury, inflammation, infection, aging, and so forth, can decrease efficiency of these mechanisms. Examples might include: limitation of rib cage movement, for example, as caused by ankylosing spondylitis; reduction of efficiency of the muscles and ligaments supporting expiration, for example, stretching of the rectus abdominis muscles during pregnancy. Of note, at times the emotional state of the patient may also influence abdominal support or pattern of breathing.

Integrity of the Muscles, Joints, and Ligaments of the Pharynx and Larynx

These have been reviewed in some depth above. Palpation of these structures gives the osteopath insights into the voicing mechanism at the level of the sound source. Examples might include: (1) increased tension, tenderness, or guarding in the suspensory musculature; (2) a held cricothyroid visor with decreased range of motion of the cricothyroid joint, both changes often being found in prolonged voice misuse patterns.[22]

Much emphasis recently has been placed on the Morrison muscular tension dysphonia patterns, type 1 through 4[45,46]; however, they primarily have been identified by the patterns of visualized vocal fold closure. Harris has attempted to go one step further and characterize the specific muscular misuse patterns that have led to the observed vocal fold closure patterns.[47]

The relative size of the thyrohyoid space (and the thyrohyoid muscles) should be assessed. Lieberman notes that in individuals with hyperfunctional voicing disorders, the space is much reduced in surface area.[22]

Position and Mobility of the Laryngeal Cartilages and Hyoid Bone

1. Thyroid cartilage position. This can be observed readily as well as palpated. Deviation of the thyroid cartilage from center is frequently accompanied by major underlying postural changes. Examples might include rotation of the torso to one side, scoliosis, abnormal unilateral hypertrophy of the superficial muscles of the neck (for example, unilateral torticollis), surgery (for example, following a unilateral radical neck dissection), unilateral hyperostosis of the cervical spine, and so forth.

2. Limitation of movement of the thyroid cartilage on side-to-side movement (rotation). This finding may be associated with aging, hyperostosis of the cervical spine, or a tumor of the larynx or neck. In young, otherwise healthy performers, the most common cause of this limitation of movement, however, is increased resting muscular tone in the "strap" muscles. This is generally indicative of a musculoskeletal pattern associated with increased "holding" or "guarding" of these muscles. It is often associated with voice changes, including lowering of the fundamental frequency of the speaking voice and a gravelly quality to the voice. This muscular pattern is readily amenable to laryngeal manipulation.

3. Hyoid position. The hyoid bone is the principal structure below which the remainder of the larynx is suspended. It should lie in a horizontal plane, and be located just below the mandible. Typically it lies approximately 1/2 inch caudal to the body of the mandible. Angulation of either side toward the mandible suggests unilateral tight posterior hyoglossus or stylohyoid muscles or anterior thyrohyoid ligaments.[22] Such angulation may also be asso-

ciated with inflammatory lymphadenopathy in zone two (the jugulo-digastric region) of the neck (J. Rubin, personal observation, 2002). Lateral tilting of the hyoid bone may be associated with unilateral tightness of the superior suspensory muscles or to the unilateral pull of a tight thyrohyoid muscle. When the hyoid bone appears to be pulled forward anteriorly, a tight geniohyoid muscle should be suspected.[22] The reverse may occur should the middle constrictor muscle be hypertonic (J. Lieberman, personal observation, 2002).

In patients with a "held" larynx, or a posteriorly backed larynx, consideration should be given to the possibility of unresolved emotional issues. Aronson has noted that one common denominator of psychogenic voice disorders is a hypercontractile state of the intrinsic and extrinsic laryngeal musculature.[6] These considerations are very important to successful long-term intervention, but are outside the scope of this chapter (see Psychological Aspects of Voice Disorders in *Clinical Assessment of Voice*[48] for further insights).

The superior suspensory muscles consist of the stylohyoid, geniohyoid, hyoglossus, mylohyoid, and anterior and posterior bellies of the digastric muscles. As noted, excessively tight suprahyoid musculature in association with a high-held larynx signifies marked muscular hyperactivity often in association with unresolved emotional issues.[22] One example of such a clinical scenario is that not uncommonly found in mutational dysphonias.

The inferior suspensory muscles should be palpated. These include the sternothyroid, sternohyoid, and omohyoid muscles. These muscles are long, with thin bellies and are thus difficult to assess by direct palpation. Their quality can be inferred by assessing the resting level of the larynx and by stretching it upward and laterally (see below). An extremely low-held, or "anchored" larynx should be checked for. Koufman has classified one type of speaking-voice abuse pattern as the "Bogart-Bacall" syndrome, in which the patient speaks with a very low-pitched fundamental frequency. This is associated with a low-held larynx.[49,50]

Endolaryngeal Examination

Prior to laryngeal manipulation by an osteopath, the larynx should be examined by an otolaryngologist with a flexible or rigid endoscope, preferably with an attached stroboscope, and the results relayed to the osteopath. Particular attention should be paid to the characteristic appearance of any known patterns of dysphonia. Typically these include muscular tension dysphonia, as described by authors such as Morrison,

Koufman, or Harris,[44-46,48] or bowing. There may also be evidence of asymmetry of vocal fold movement or of arytenoid position (see below).

The otolaryngologic examination should include evaluation for evidence of extraesophageal reflux (posterior interarytenoid "heaping," piriform pooling, posterior laryngeal edema or redness, and so forth), and for subtle laryngeal mucosal pathology that may be the source of the abnormal muscular behavior. The stroboscope will be of critical importance here, as subtle asynchrony of the mucosal wave, areas of adynamism, and so forth may lead the examiner to infer the possibility of such pathologies as a partially resolved vocal fold palsy, a small cyst, sulcus, or scar, all of which could be the source of the muscular dyskinesia.

The arytenoid cartilages and the cricoarytenoid joints are accessible to palpation by the osteopathic practitioner with adequate experience, particularly in long, thin-necked individuals. Similarly, the posterior cricoarytenoid muscles and interarytenoid muscles can be palpated and compared for tenderness and hypertonicity. These maneuvers require considerable skill and can be very uncomfortable to the patient, however. Thus, they should be considered to be outside the scope of this chapter. It is worth noting that the patient's response to such an examination can assist in the diagnosis, one example being the irritable larynx (Murray Morrison, Instructional Course, Annual Meeting of the American Academy of Otolaryngology Head and Neck Surgery, September 1999).

Basic Laryngeal Manipulation

Generally speaking, common sense needs to be used when considering performance of laryngeal manipulation. For example, laryngeal manipulation is not advisable in patients with laryngeal or thyroid malignancies, or in instances of Graves' disease. In the presence of other anterior neck pathologies, the techniques should be modified appropriately to avoid unnecessary discomfort. Prior to manipulation, a thorough explanation of the proposed procedure, its risks and benefits, should be given to the patient, and his or her permission sought.

Particular care must be exercised when working in the area overlying the carotid artery and especially around the carotid body and sinus.

Prior to any manipulation, the osteopath gently palpates for any deviation from "normal" anatomic structures, for example, an unusually enlarged or prominent carotid sinus in relation to the hyoid bone and its attachments. Imaging has not been found to be necessary, as direct hands-on palpation is very sensitive to such abnormalities. While laryngeal manipulation proves to be a highly safe treatment in experienced hands, we teach that energetic or inadvertent manipulation should not be performed near the carotid; it can lead to rapid changes in blood pressure and/or pulse rate; it can also lead to loosening of atheromatous plaques in elderly patients.

Similarly, care should be exercised in instances of previous laryngeal trauma, surgery, or radiation where normal anatomy may be altered.

General

In cases of soft tissue damage caused by repetitive strain injury, similar to certain orthopedic problems, the muscles will be chronically shortened, fibrotic or scarred, and tender to touch. By working on the muscles, the osteopath is able to stretch scar contractures, lengthen the muscle belly, increase blood flow, and improve lymphatic drainage. The osteopath probably also affects the neuromuscular pattern of outflow locally and centrally, although this requires further clarification through research.[22]

Limitation of joint movement can also be addressed by direct joint manipulation, as well as by soft tissue techniques to surrounding musculature. In addition to reducing muscle spasm, the practitioner also attempts to alter head position, reduce hyperlordotic spinal curve, and improve mobility in the thoracic spine.

Treatment aims include restoration of joint mobility and muscle function. Perhaps as important is bringing to the conscious level the unconscious and habitual abnormal postural patterns that need to be corrected.[42]

General concepts of manipulation to attain these goals include those of:

1. Identification of the indicated muscle or structure to work on.
2. Stabilization of indicated muscle against a known, more fixed structure (for example, the cricoid cartilage).
3. Passive stretch where two structures (for example, hyoid bone and mandible) are held apart under gentle stretch for a period of time.
4. Dynamic stretch (the patient activates a muscle that the osteopath wishes to manipulate, and the osteopath works with or against the patient's own force).
5. Muscle kneading.
6. Working beyond guarding (the osteopath maintains stretch beyond the point at which the patient holds back).

Basic Manipulation: General Technique

Much of basic manipulation involves general soft tissue work on the posterior neck, shoulders, and upper back. The patient is treated while lying supine on a firm table or gurney with a movable head support.

First the cervical and upper thoracic spinous processes are carefully assessed for evidence of abnormal alignment, tenderness, and integrity or laxity of interspinous ligaments. The cervical and upper thoracic spine is gently investigated for range of motion. This will give the osteopath information as to what can be safely accomplished.

The posterior extensor muscles are then palpated and gently placed under stretch, during which time the osteopath checks for focal or point tenderness or guarding. Focal areas of spasm are identified and stretched to relax the hypertonic muscle, increase blood flow, and break the spasm.[22]

Not uncommonly the superficial neck muscles are addressed next. The levator scapulae and splenius are frequent sources of neck pain and often require specific work. The trapezius is another muscle frequently found to be tight or in spasm. Often certain fibers of the trapezius may be found to be contracted and others stretched, given the size of this muscle and its broad insertions.

Frequently the anterior neck, larynx, and laryngeal and pharyngeal muscles are next addressed. Areas particularly relevant to voice problems include: suprahyoid suspensory muscles, cricothyroid visor, scalenes, sternocleidomastoids, and lower strap muscles.

Suprahyoid Suspensory Muscles

As previously noted these muscles are at particular risk for chronic shortening, thereby causing the laryngeal complex to be elevated and effecting a change in resonatory pattern.

These are large powerful muscles and can be addressed individually. When using soft tissue techniques it is best to stabilize the hand against the mandible or the hyoid bone and work from this solid base.

The patient can actively assist by attempting to initiate a swallow (but not a full swallow) while the osteopath gently presses down against the hyoid. This type of combined patient/practitioner activity is termed "dynamic stretch."

Cricothyroid Visor

This "keystone" area has been anatomically characterized above. The osteopath can relax both cricothyroid muscles individually, applying soft tissue stretch techniques, working against the cricoid cartilage as his solid base. He can also work directly on each cricothyroid joint. Dynamic stretch, in this instance would involve the patient "sirening" the pitch up from low to high, thereby actively placing the cricothyroid muscle into contraction, while the osteopath stretches this muscle.

Scalenes, Sternocleidomastoids, and Lower Strap Muscles

The larynx frequently is found to be held in an abnormally low position, a typical correlate being tightly held and tender lower bellies of the SCM, scalenes, and lower strap muscles.

This is a common problem noted in 26% of Koufman's patients with "functional" voice problems,[50] but must be differentiated from a chronically high-held rib cage (as seen in some patients with severe emphysema).

These muscles can be stretched against the solid base of the upper sternum and medial clavicles, and are readily accessible to manipulation.

Successful Outcome After Larngeal Manipulation

In our clinical experience, albeit anecdotal, the following are comments frequently made by patients immediately following laryngeal manipulation: immediate change in pitch, audible to patient and practitioner; increased resonance; increased ease of swallowing associated with a sense of "openness"; decreased hoarseness; decreased "wobble"; decreased pain and discomfort.

In the longer term, it is not uncommon for there to be reported an increase in stamina, vocal flexibility, and range, better negotiation of the passaggio, and shorter duration of recovery time following laryngeal exertions. Research to confirm these anecdotal impressions is needed, as discussed below.

There is often resolution of the laryngeal "click" (that is caused by anterior movement of the hyoid bone over the thyroid cartilage and is frequently associated with chronically shortened and tightly held thyrohyoid muscles) and a decreased need to clear the throat. Finally, JL finds in many of his patients acknowledgment of underlying emotional issues related to the laryngeal pathology (Jacob Lieberman, unpublished data, 1999).

Because of the relaxed laryngeal musculature and the small alteration in laryngeal position, professional voice users occasionally experience what they call a "wild voice," momentarily. Warming-up type exercises are required to allow the performer to get used to the changes.

In the pilot study assessing the efficiency of manipulation versus conventional speech therapy, the two modalities were found to be dissimilar but complementary.[7] Manipulation was found to excel at rapidly reducing tension in muscles that were tightly held in the "unaware" patient. With manipulation, early vocal fatigue was found to be reduced as was laryngeal discomfort. While conventional speech therapy was found to address these problems as well, the progress was slower. Speech therapy, however, was found to be better at substituting more efficient voicing patterns over the pretreatment dysphonic patterns.

Advanced Manipulation

Advanced manipulation is designed for instances in which the laryngeal intrinsic muscles require direct address. This might include times when the laryngeal "set" needs to be altered. For example, Lieberman has directly manipulated the intrinsic muscles of certain patients with granulomas who have failed traditional therapy, the aim being to reduce the hard prephonatory gesture and resultant impact of the arytenoid cartilages. In Lieberman's practice, advanced manipulation is not uncommonly combined with elements of psychotherapy that focus on unresolved emotional issues.

It must be remembered that manipulation of the intrinsic muscles of the larynx involves working on the posterior aspect of the larynx on muscles that are designed for mainly reflexogenic activities. Such manipulation requires considerable palpatory skill, as well as great sensitivity in working with patients.

Ongoing Research

Laryngeal manipulation has been developed, and practiced in Queen Mary's Hospital Sidcup, Kent, for the last 14 years. Initially the team looked at the relationship of head position, shoulder girdle, and hyperfunctional voice disorders.[7]

The clinic has developed a research protocol with Professor A. Fourcin using the laryngograph to record vocal parameters prior to and immediately following manipulation, in an attempt to validate the anecdotal findings described above. Preliminary laryngographic data have often confirmed clinical findings, including: immediate change in fundamental frequency of the speaking voice, better control, and wider vocal range. As an example, a patient with spasmodic dysphonia treated with manipulation is presented (Fig 13–1). The project is ongoing.

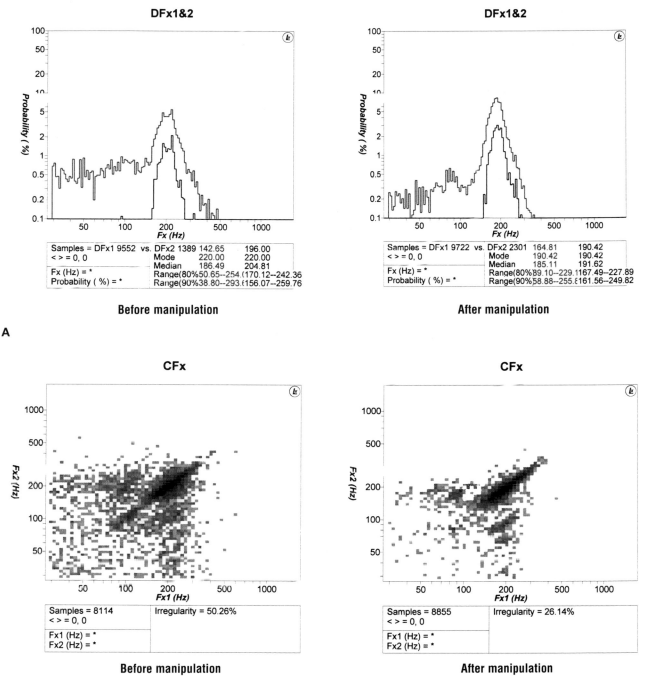

Fig 13–1. A. Laryngographic data taken from a patient with spasmodic dysphonia before and after one treatment with laryngeal manipulation. (Courtesy of Professor Adrian Fourcin) Plots shows range, before and after one manipulation. Range as defined herein refers to the range of frequencies contained within the speaking voice, while reading from a standard text. Note the reduction in spread of the first order distribution *(in red)*, and the slight improvement in range definition shown by the second order distribution *(in black)*, both following manipulation. **B.** Plots shows regularity, before and after one manipulation. Regularity as defined herein refers to the extent to which successive vocal fold periods are comparable, while reading from a standard text. Note the reduction in irregularity in the post-manipulation distribution. *(Continued)*

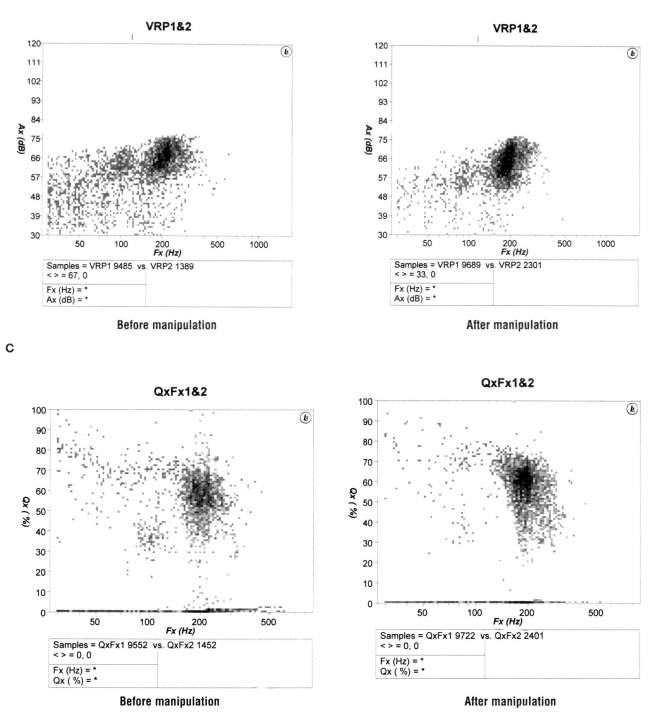

Figure 13–1. C. Plots show a phonetogram before and after one manipulation. The phonetogram as defined herein refers to the distribution of loudness against pitch, while reading from a standard text. Note that the post-manipulation plot demonstrates a more compact control of loudness (less dispersion) **D.** Plots show "quality" before and after one manipulation. "Quality" as defined herein refers to the extent to which the closed phase percentage of the total period is well defined in the speaking voice, while reading from a standard text. Note that there is a (somewhat) better definition of the closed phase in the post-manipulation plot.

Other research projects in planning involve assessing cricothyroid joint activity, diaphragmatic breathing, and the function of the thyrohyoid mechanism.

Conclusion

We have presented a synopsis of the role that laryngeal manipulation plays in our practice. Certainly in our voice clinics, the more we have considered the possibility of musculoskeletal issues in patients with voice disorders, the more reasons we have found for referring such patients for diagnostic investigation and treatment by a physical therapist, osteopath, or by practitioners with similar skills. The critical issue is for the therapist to participate actively in the voice clinic so that he or she will develop sensitivity to the needs of the patient.

That said, muscles do not work in isolation. The musculoskeletal system is driven by thoughts and affects. The effects of physical therapy, passive and active manipulation in particular, are immediate and frequently effective in (at least temporarily) breaking through unconscious neuromuscular pathways (habits). To be long-lasting, the "new" musculoskeletal behavior must be internalized by the patient. Many or most of our patients require refresher sessions to reinforce the beneficial behavior patterns.

Manipulation is a potent treatment modality, but it does not resolve underlying emotional conflicts. Hence, a small proportion of our patients will benefit from a short course of supportive counseling, or from more formal psychotherapy.

References

1. Mathieson L. Vocal tract discomfort in hyperfunctional dysphonia. *Voice.* 1993;2:40–48.
2. Mathieson L. *Greene and Mathieson's The Voice and Its Disorders.* 6th ed. London, England: Whurr Publishers Limited; 2001.
3. Roy N, Leeper HA. Effects of the manual laryngeal musculoskeletal tension reduction technique as a treatment for functional voice disorders: perceptual and acoustic measures. *J Voice.* 1993;7:242–249.
4. Roy N, Bless DM, Heisey D, Ford CN. Manual circumlaryngeal therapy for functional dysphonia: an evaluation of short- and long-term treatment outcomes. *J Voice.* 1997;11:321–331.
5. Aronson AE. *Clinical Voice Disorders: An Interdisciplinary Approach.* 2nd ed. New York, NY: Georg Thieme Verlag; 1985.
6. Aronson A. *Clinical Voice Disorders.* 3rd ed. New York, NY: Thieme Medical Publishers; 1991:117–145.
7. Harris S, Harris T, Lieberman J, Harris D. The multidisciplinary voice clinic. In: Freeman M, Fawcus M, eds. *Voice Disorders and Their Management.* London, England: Whurr Publishers; 2000:313–332.
8. Harris T, Laryngeal mechanisms in normal function and dysfunction. In: Harris T, Harris S, Rubin JS, Howard DM, eds. *The Voice Clinic Handbook.* London, England: Whurr Publishers; 1998:64–90.
9. Rubin JS. The structural anatomy of the larynx and supraglottic vocal tract: a review. In: Harris T, Harris S, Rubin JS, Howard DM, eds. *The Voice Clinic Handbook.* London, England: Whurr Publishers; 1998:15–33.
10. Laitman JT, Noden DM, Van de Water TR. Formation of the larynx: from homeobox genes to critical periods. In: Rubin JS, Sataloff RT, Korovin GS, Gould WJ, eds. *Diagnosis and Treatment of Voice Disorders.* New York, NY: Igaku-Shoin Medical Publishers; 1995:9–23.
11. Scherer RC. Laryngeal function during phonation. In: Rubin JS, Sataloff RT, Korovin G, Gould WJ, eds. *Diagnosis and Treatment of Voice Disorders.* New York, NY: Igaku-Shoin Publishers; 1995:86–104.
12. Hast MH. Mechanical properties of the cricothyroid muscle. *Laryngoscope.* 1966;76:537–548.
13. Cooper DS, Partridge LD, Alipour-Haghighi F. Muscle energetics, vocal efficiency, and laryngeal biomechanics. In: Titze IR, ed. *Vocal Fold Physiology: Frontiers in Basic Science.* San Diego, Calif: Singular Publishing Group; 1993:37–92.
14. Harris T, Lieberman J. The cricothyroid mechanism, its relationship to vocal fatigue and vocal dysfunction. *Voice.* 1993;2:89–96.
15. Rubin JS, Sataloff RT. Voice: new horizons. In: Sataloff RT, ed. *Professional Voice: The Science and Art of Clinical Care.* 2nd ed. San Diego, Calif: Singular Publishing Group; 1997.
16. Fisher K. Early experience of a multidisciplinary pain management programme. *Hol Med.* 1988;3:47–56.
17. Robinson L, Fisher H, Knox J, Thomson G. *The Official Body Control Pilates Manual.* London, England: Macmillan Publishers; 2000.
18. Feldenkrais M. *Awareness Through Movement.* New York, NY: Harper & Row; 1972.
19. Rolf IP. *Rolfing: Reestablishing the Natural Alignment and Structural Integration of the Human Body for Vitality and Well-Being.* Rochester, Vt: Healing Arts Press; 1989.
20. Dickson D, Dickson W. Functional anatomy of the human larynx. *Proc Penn Acad Ophthalmol.* 1971;29.
21. Boileau Grant JC. *Grant's Atlas of Anatomy.* 6th ed. Baltimore, Md: Williams & Wilkins; 1972.
22. Lieberman J. Principles and techniques of manual therapy: application in the management of dysphonia. In: Harris T, Harris S, Rubin JS, Howard DM, eds. *The Voice Clinical Handbook.* London, England: Whurr Publishers; 1998:91–138.
23. Dickson DR, Maue-Dickson W. *Anatomical and Physiological Basis of Speech.* Boston, Mass: Little, Brown & Co; 1982.
24. Letson JA Jr, Tatchell R. Arytenoid movement. In: Sataloff RT, ed. *Professional Voice: The Science and Art of Clinical Care.* San Diego, Calif: Singular Publishing Group; 1997:131–145.

25. Baken RJ, Isshiki N. Arytenoid displacement by simulated intrinsic muscle contraction. *Folia Phoniatr.* 1977; 29:206–216.

26. von Leden H. The mechanics of the cricoarytenoid joint. *Arch Otolaryngol.* 1961;73:63–72.

27. Arnold GE. Physiology and pathology of the cricothyroid muscle. *Laryngoscope.* 1961;71:687–753.

28. Choi HS, Berke GS, Ye M, Kreiman J. Function of the thyroarytenoid muscle in a canine laryngeal model. *Ann Otol Rhinol Laryngol.* 1993;102:769–776.

29. Fujimura O. Body-cover theory of the vocal fold and its phonetic implications. In: Stevens KN, Hirano M, eds. *Vocal Fold Physiology.* Tokyo, Japan: University of Tokyo Press; 1981:271–288.

30. Titze IR, Jiang J, Drucker DG. Preliminaries to the body-cover theory of pitch control. *J Voice.* 1988;1(4):314–319.

31. Vilkman E, Alku P, Laukkanen A. Vocal-fold collision mass as a differentiator between registers in the low-pitch range. *J Voice.* 1995;9:66–73.

32. Alipour-Haghighi F, Perlman Al, Titze IR. Tetanic response of the cricothyroid muscle. *Ann Otol Rhinol Laryngol.* 1991;100:626–631.

33. Alipour-Haghighi F, Titze IR, Perlman AL. Tetanic contraction in vocal fold muscle. *J Speech Hear Res.* 1989;32: 226–231.

34. Titze IR, Durham PL. Passive mechanisms influencing fundamental frequency control. In: Baer T, Sasaki C, Harris KS, eds. *Laryngeal Function in Phonation and Respiration.* San Diego, Calif: College-Hill Press; 1987:304–319.

35. Broniatowski M, Sonies BC, Rubin JS, et al. Current evaluation and treatment of patients with swallowing disorders. *Otolaryngol Head Neck Surg.* 1999;120:464–473.

36. Hellemans J, Agg HO, Pelemans W, et al. Pharyngoesophageal swallowing disorders and the pharyngoesophageal sphincter. *Med Clin North Am.* 1981;65:1149–1171.

37. Estill J. *Voicecraft: A User's Guide to Voice Quality. Vol 2, Some Basic Voice Qualities.* Santa Rosa, Calif: Estill Voice Training Systems; 1995.

38. Rubin JS. The physiologic anatomy of swallowing. In: Rubin JS, Broniatowski M, Kelly J, eds. *The Swallowing Handbook.* San Diego, Calif: Singular Publishing Group; 2000:1–20.

39. Sonninen A. The role of the external laryngeal muscles in the length-adjustment of the vocal cords in singing. *Acta Otolaryngol.* 1956;118:218–231.

40. Vilkman E, Sonninen A, Hurme P, Korkko P. External laryngeal frame function in voice production revisited: a review. *J Voice.* 1996;10:78–92.

41. Lumley JSP, Craven JL, Aitken JT. *Essential Anatomy.* Edinburgh, Scotland: Churchill Livingstone; 1973.

42. Sataloff RT. *Clinical Assessment of Voice.* San Diego, Calif: Plural Publishing, Inc; 2005:21–72.

43. Rubin JS, Lieberman J, Harris TM. Laryngeal manipulation. *Otolaryngol Clin North Am.* 2000;33:1017–1034.

44. Rubin JS. Mechanisms of respiration (the bellows). In: Harris T, Harris S, Rubin JS, Howard DM, eds. *The Voice Clinic Handbook.* London, England: Whurr Publishers; 1998:49–63.

45. Morrison MD, Rammage LA, Gilles M, et al. Muscular tension dysphonia. *J Otolaryngol.* 1983;12:302–306.

46. Morrison M, Rammage L, Nichol H, et al. *The Management of Voice Disorders.* San Diego, Calif: Singular Publishing Group; 1994.

47. Harris S. Speech therapy for dysphonia. In: Harris T, Harris S, Rubin JS, Howard DM, eds. *The Voice Clinic Handbook.* London, England: Whurr Publishers; 1998: 186–195.

48. Rosen, D, Heuer RJ, Levy SH, Sataloff RT. Psychological aspects of voice disorders. In: Sataloff RT. *Clinical Assessment of Voice.* San Diego, Calif: Plural Publishing, Inc; 2005:173–200.

49. Gould WJ, Rubin JS. Special considerations for the professional voice user. In: Rubin JS, Sataloff RT, Korovin G, Gould WJ, eds. *Diagnosis and Treatment of Voice Disorders.* New York, NY: Igako-Shoin Press; 1995:424–435.

50. Koufman J, Blalock O. Functional voice disorders. *Otolaryngol Clin North Am.* 1991;24:1059–1073.

14

The Effects of Posture on Voice

John S. Rubin , Ed Blake,
and Lesley Mathieson

This chapter looks at the potential adverse effects of abnormal posture on the vocal tract. Although it has been known for centuries that poor posture can have an adverse effect on voicing, there has been relatively little research into the subject. Recently, however, the importance of posture to well being has become popularized through the works of authors such as Alexander,[1] Pilates,[2] Feldenkrais,[3] and others. Physiotherapy and osteopathy have become integral to the field of Sports Medicine and to rehabilitation of musculoskeletal injuries. Only very recently has consideration of these sciences been applied to voice research and rehabilitation.

Posture could, in one sense, be considered to be a constant battleground between the deep extensor and flexor groups of muscles. The long bones and pelvis, the skull, and the spine are the obvious targets and (in many cases) the origins and/or insertions of these muscle groups.

The larynx is suspended from the basicranium, not by direct bony attachment, but by a series of muscles and ligaments. It could be viewed as a victim in this struggle, in part due to its location in the anterior neck, in part to its dense muscular attachments to the prevertebral fascia, and in part due to its attachments to the basicranium above and the trachea below.

Rolf has described the ideal state of posture (what she calls "equipoise") in which the individual stands upright.[4] The head is held vertically over the perpendicularly oriented shoulder girdle, vertically over the hip joints and the pelvis, and vertically over the forward-facing feet. A plumb line through the coronal plane formed by the ears would pass directly over the plane of the shoulders and hip joints. The eye plane is horizontal, the rib cage is neutral. The spine "rests in the pelvis much as a person sits in a rocking chair."[4(p175)] It

has four curves. The sacral and thoracic are concave ventrally, the lumbar and cervical are convex.

Posterior Extensors

In a free erect spine, the extensor system of the back (the "erector spinae" muscles) supply support and span the vertebrae. The erector spinae consist of three groups of superficial vertical fibers, which interweave, and numerous deeper oblique fibers.[5] The action of the erector spinae is to establish and maintain appropriate extension of the vertebral column. It contains three superficial muscles, the iliocostalis, longissimus, and spinalis. The iliocostalis is placed laterally. It extends from the iliac crest and angles of the ribs and inserts into the transverse processes of the cervical vertebrae. It has a lumbar, thoracic, and cervical portion.

The longissimus is intermediate in position, attached inferiorly to the transverse processes of the thoracic and cervical vertebrae. Its uppermost fibers, the longissimus capitis, reach the lateral surface of the mastoid bone. The medially placed spinalis passes alongside and is attached to the vertical spines.

Deeper muscles include the semispinalis and the deep short muscles (the levator costae, multifidis, rotatores, interspinus, and intertransversus muscles). Of the several parts of the semispinalis that run from the lower (tenth) thoracic vertebrae, upwards and medially to the occiput, the massive semispinalis capitis, supporting the head, is almost vertical. It is attached to the occiput between the superior and the inferior nuchal lines.

The multifidis, arising from the dorsal sacrum, runs from the transverse processes and inserts into the lower border of the third cervical vertebra. It also has some role in neck extension.

The splenius capitis and cervicis also support the spine. The splenius will be discussed again later as a superficial anterior muscle, because of its lateral location and action. The splenius capitis attaches inferiorly to the ligamentum nuchae and spinous processes of the upper three or four thoracic vertebrae and the seventh cervical vertebra. Superiorly, it attaches to the mastoid process and lateral part of the superior nuchal line deep to the sternocleidomastoid. The splenius cervicis has a similar inferior attachment but passes to the transverse processes of the upper cervical vertebrae.

The major action of the erector spinae is to maintain the upright position of the body. When standing at rest, the center of gravity lies just in front of the second sacral vertebrae. Body movement, however, frequently carries the center of gravity forward. This mass of muscle is then required to restore the upright position.

The muscles attached to the skull produce extension, lateral flexion, and rotation of the head.[5]

Suboccipital Muscle Group

The suboccipital muscles are important because they permit accurate head positioning and thus stereoscopic vision. They extend the skull at the atlanto-occipital joints and rotate it at the atlanto-axial joints. Muscles in this group include the rectus capitis posterior (RCP) major and minor and the obliquus capitis (OC) superior and inferior. The RCP major arises from the spine of the axis and inserts into the occiput below the inferior nuchal line. The RCP minor is anteromedial to the RCP major and passes from the posterior tubercle of the atlas to insert into the occiput behind the foramen magnum. The OC superior arises at the tip of the transverse process of the atlas and inserts into the occiput between the superior and inferior nuchal lines, lateral to the semispinalis. The OC inferior originates at the tip of the transverse process of the atlas and inserts into the spine of the axis.[5]

Deep Anterior Neck Flexors

The three scalenes together with the prevertebral muscles make up the deep muscles of the anterior neck. They attach to the anterior tubercle of the transverse processes of cervical vertebrae and are, by definition, the deep flexors of the neck.

Scalene Muscle Group

The scalenus anterior arises from the anterior tubercles of the third to sixth cervical vertebrae and inserts into the scalene tubercle of the first rib. The scalenus medius arises superior to the posterior tubercles of the second to seventh cervical vertebrae and inserts into the upper surface of the first rib, posterior to the scalene tubercle. The scalenus posterior is part of the medius but inserts into the second rib.

The action of the scalene muscle group is that of weak flexion of the head and neck. It also acts to lift and stabilize the upper two ribs.[5,6]

Prevertebral Muscles

The prevertebral muscles include the longus colli (cervicis), longus capitus, and rectus capitis anterior and lateralis. They lie in front of the cervical and upper thoracic vertebrae, and are covered anteriorly by the prevertebral fascia.

The longus capitis arises from the third through sixth anterior tubercles (the same as the scalenus anterior). It runs cephalad, ascending to the basi-occiput where it inserts behind the plane of the laryngeal tubercle. In so doing, it fills the hollow space between the bodies and the transverse processes.

The longus colli (cervicis) has vertical and oblique portions. The vertical portion arises from the body of the third thoracic vertebra to the fifth cervical vertebra. It inserts into the bodies of the second to fourth cervical vertebrae. The upper oblique portion arises from the anterior tubercle of the transverse processes of the third to fifth cervical vertebrae and inserts into the anterior tubercle of the atlas. The lower oblique portion arises from the bodies of the first through third thoracic vertebrae and inserts into the anterior tubercle of the transverse processes of the fifth and sixth cervical vertebrae. [6-8]

The rectus capitis anterior covers the atlanto-occipital joint, extending from the front of the lateral mass of the atlas to the basi-occiput. The lateralis extends from the transverse process of the atlas to the jugular process of the occipital bone. The action of these prevertebral muscles is to twist the head on the neck and to flex the neck (bend it forward).

Superficial Anterior Neck Muscles

In addition, four significant superficial muscles bind the neck to the shoulder girdle. These are the sternocleidomastoid, levator scapulae, trapezius, and the splenius. At times when neck function is compromised, these superficial muscles can become the major initiators and executors of neck movement.

Sternocleidomastoid

The sternocleidomastoid is a large anterior neck muscle that is of great functional importance to the neck. It extends posteriorly and superiorly up the entire front of the neck from its origins on the manubrium and medial aspect of the clavicle to its broad insertion into the mastoid process and outer half of the superior nuchal line of the occiput. Its action, alone, is to turn the head obliquely to the opposite side. More often, it works in concordance with its opposing member, at which time the two muscles pull the head downwards and forwards. Torticollis is a chronic condition that occurs when one of the sternocleidomastoid muscles goes into permanent contraction.

Levator Scapulae

The levator scapulae arises from the posterior tubercles of the transverse processes of the four upper cervical vertebrae. It runs downwards and backwards to reach the medial border of the supraspinous portion of the scapula. It raises the scapula. It also helps to rotate it, and thereby pulls the glenoid cavity downwards.

Trapezius

The trapezius is a large, triangular muscle of the posterior neck. Together, the two trapezius muscles form a trapeze, or table, across the upper back and neck. The origin of the trapezius is very broad, extending from the skull all the way down to the spinous process of the last thoracic vertebra. In its upper part, its origins are the medial third of the superior nuchal line of the occiput and all of the spines of the cervical vertebrae, through the medium of the ligamentum nuchae. Its insertion needs to be looked at in thirds, its upper, middle, and inferior fibers. Fibers of the upper third insert into the lateral third of the clavicle. Fibers of the middle and lower thirds insert into aspects of the scapula.

In health, the function of the trapezius is to hold the shoulders back and up, as in a "military carriage."[8] It raises, steadies, and rotates the scapula. When the trapezius is weak, the shoulder appears to droop or be bottlenecked. From the standpoint of head movement, the trapezius also draws the head to one side or backward.

Splenius

The splenius has already been described above.

Clavicle/First Rib Relationship

In "equipoise" the anterior attachment of the first rib to the clavicle is very nearly horizontal with its posterior attachment to the vertebrae. The more closely this approximates the horizontal, the more snugly the yoke of the shoulder girdle will fit and the more clearly the body will display a generally vertical-horizontal alignment.[4] Rolf believes that the postural fate of the neck depends on the pectoral girdle and its efficiency.

The clavicle is joined to the first rib by interclavicular ligaments. In conditions of poor posture, it is not uncommon for it to rest directly on the first rib, immobilized by a deterioration of the subclavius muscle. Generally, this process starts after the ventral rib cage becomes lax as a result of chronic shortening of the rectus abdominis (see below).[4]

Abdominal Wall Musculature, Psoas, and Lower Erector Spinae Axis

Rectus Abdominis

The rectus abdominis is felt by Rolf to be the primary anterior flexor of the mid body.[4] In general, as the rectus flexes, shortens, and thickens, there is compensatory lengthening and stretching of some of the lower fibers of the erector spinae.[4]

Ease and efficiency of movement require the psoas, rather than the erector spinae, to be the primary antagonist to the rectus abdominis. This psoas/rectus balance is thought by Rolf to be basic to the mechanism of walking and standing still.[4] Nonetheless, all three muscles, the rectus abdominis, psoas, and the lower fibers of the erector spinae, work together.

The rectus abdominis inserts into the anterior pelvis and arises from the rib cage. It exerts pull as high as the fifth rib and acts to pull the rib cage downward and the pelvic rim upward.

The psoas originates from the upper anterior lumbar spine in close proximity to the crura of the diaphragm. It inserts into the lesser trochanter of the femur via a tendon shared with the iliacus. It lengthens with every movement of flexion and helps prevent the lumbar vertebrae from slipping into compression and misalignment. Rolf states that it determines the structural position of the skeletal system[4]

Robinson et al, although not commenting specifically on this fulcrum, agree that the deep stabilizing muscles are critical to movement. They identify the transversus abdominis (which lies just deep to the rectus abdominis), muscles of the pelvic floor, and the multifidis as a group of muscles that stabilize the lumbar spine and act as a "girdle of strength."[2]

From the standpoint of this chapter we shall not discuss the lower body, although it clearly impacts both balance and posture and, when out of balance, may affect the functioning of the vocal tract. This correlates well with the concept that practically the entire body can impact upon vocal functioning.[9]

Posture and Muscular Balance

In our society, there are several factors that, taken together, may lead to a muscular imbalance between the deep flexors and extensors. For example, most of us spend much of our working and leisure time in a seated position in nonergonomically designed seats in front of various consoles or screens. We tend to sit in a slouched position with our pelvis tilted, our abdomen compressed, our abdominal flexors contracted, and our lower back extensors stretched. It is hardly surprising that so many of us suffer with chronic lower back pain.

Robinson et al,[2] in their Pilates manual, identified the following problems associated with prolonged sitting: weak transversus abdominis; tight upper rectus abdominis; tight dominant hip flexors; rounded thoracic spine; tight pectorals; medially rotated scapulae; tight levator scapulae (elevating the scapulae); head forward, leading to weak deep neck flexors and tight neck extensors; tight adductors and medial rotators of the hip; weak gluteals; a rotated, twisted spine. One can identify several effects on the neck immediately.

Rolf adds that chronic shortening and flexion of the rectus abdominis strains the entire body. The "neck and cervical spine are inevitably included in the compensation. The myofascial structures of the cervical spine become anteriorly shortened and therefore the head comes forward."[4(p105)] This problem may then be compounded by the exercise that we choose to do in our free time in an effort to "keep fit." Many of these activities have as their goal the strengthening of the abdominal musculature, which we may perceive to be poor, in part due to the protrusion of our abdomens from underlying abnormal posture. Our concerns regarding our abdominal appearance are heightened by the stereotype of tight rippling muscles fostered by many magazines and by Hollywood. Thus our exercises tend to include weight lifting, sit-ups, abdominal crunches, and so on. When incorporated into a well-defined exercise program, these exercises are beneficial. However, if performed incorrectly, the consequences of these activities can be even more serious than the structural implications of a sagging rib cage caused by abnormal posture when seated. A further muscular imbalance is created, with further advantage given to the flexors.

When further abdominal compression occurs, so does compression and strain of the three or four uppermost ribs. This may impact deleteriously on the function of the upper intercostals, which is important in singing, although perhaps not as important in conversational speech. In turn, continued ventral sag of the first and second ribs displaces and raises the first dorsal vertebra in the back. Anterior displacement of the entire group of lumbar vertebrae is a frequent spinal aberration.

Also in our necks, which are already being held forward, the muscle masses of the semispinalis and multifidis can often be felt through palpation to be amorphous, solid, unyielding."[4(p242)] Their inelasticity can crowd the cervical vertebrae into a shortened arc. Some of the segments may be forced into spaces anterior or posterior to the position of good function. A physiological consequence is what Lieberman calls a cervical dorsal shelf.[10]

Posture and Personality Traits

When discussing the vocal tract and muscular causes of dysphonia, personality traits and emotional issues also need to be taken into consideration. There are postural variations that may relate to self-image and psychosocial issues. For example, in pompous or insecure individuals, it is not uncommon to find a forcibly lowered chin and head retraction. In self-effacing individuals, rounded shoulders and a dropped head are observed commonly (L Mathieson, personal observation, 2001). Many "driven" persons who present with voice disorders are found to have a tightly bound, lowered larynx,[11] Lieberman has found an association between certain individuals presenting with high degrees of anxiety and a high-held larynx with tender suprahyoid musculature.[12] It has been well documented by Aronson and others that the intrinsic and extrinsic musculature of the larynx can be affected by the emotions.[13]

Stabilty Versus Mobility

Let us now examine the above-mentioned postural issues from a slightly different perspective, that of the musculature of the cervical spine. Muscular involvement of the cervical spine can be categorized into "stability" and "mobility" activities. At times, stabilizing muscles can act as mobility muscles. Stability muscles control the head and neck in a neutral position, thereby minimizing the loads placed on the stability mechanisms provided by annular fibers and facet approximation. The longus colli (cervicis) is the primary anterior muscular stability mechanism of the cervical spine.

Mobility muscles are the prime movers of the head, neck, and shoulder girdle. They also may serve to provide a stability mechanism in the event of reduced muscular support from the longus colli (cervicis). Examples of mobility muscles include the sternocleidomastoid, trapezius, and levator scapulae.

Stage direction that involves singing to the dress circle (upper level), often on a raked (canted) stage, frequently will position the upper and midcervical spine in a substantial degree of extension. Less specifically, but more commonly, shorter individuals have a tendency to tilt their heads upwards in the presence of taller individuals; taller individuals have a tendency to stoop, with one postural element including a forward head and neck.

The potential loss of anterior muscular stability in this position of forward head position can result in increased shearing forces through the intervertebral joints and facet joint compression. Reduced anterior muscular stability can be attributed to changes in the resting length of the longus colli (cervicis) muscle. The longus colli (cervicis) is placed at a mechanical disadvantage in cervical extension when compared to its antagonists, because cross bridge overlap is lessened in this lengthened position. Production of force from the main anterior stabilizer of the cervical spine is reduced substantially.

A situation of prolonged cervical extension will result in anatomical shortening of the antagonists to the longus colli (cervicis). The resultant increased cross bridge overlap and consequent improved force production levels from the sternocleidomastoid, levator scapulae, and upper fibers of the trapezius serve to pull the upper cervical spine into further extension. This positional dominance results in continued overactivity and eventual adaptive shortening (chronic contraction) of portions of these muscles. This, in turn, maintains the cervical spine in some degree of extension (hyperlordosis) at rest. The sternocleidomastoid is the most likely of these muscles to undergo such adaptive shortening as a result of its more mobile proximal attachments that allow even greater positional change with increased muscle activity than the sternum or clavicular articulations (E. Blake, personal observation, 2004).

The consequence of this, from a muscular perspective, is an imbalance between the activity and force production of the designed stability mechanism and that of the prime movers of the neck and shoulder girdle, which are now unopposed in pulling the spine in the direction of their anatomical pull. The severity of the imbalance is linked directly to the amount of extension in which the cervical spine is held. These loads are often too great to be tolerated by the more delicate structures of the cervical spine, and they are a common cause of facet and annular injury.

Muscular Imbalance and Voice

Upper and middle cervical extension results in a positional change of the styloid process of the mastoid, moving it anteriorly. This, we believe (E Blake, personal observation, 2003), allows for adaptive shortening of the stylohyoid muscle, as its origin and insertion have moved closer together as a consequence of head position. The stylohyoid muscle functions with improved force output in this position. It therefore elevates the larynx into a position that changes the shape of the vocal tract, altering resonance and pitch.

A muscular imbalance similar to that described earlier can now occur between the stylohyoid and sternohyoid muscles. The adaptive shortening that will occur in the stylohyoid will resist the forward translation of the hyoid bone and thyroid cartilage during singing. In turn, this may alter vocal fold length and tension (E Blake, personal observation, 2001). Consequently, there is potential loss of the singer's top range, in addition to the presence of breathy phonation. This is still postulation but fits with the clinical patterns seen in many of our patients.

Lieberman et al believe further that shortening (chronic contraction) of the cricothyroid muscle may occur.[10] This could be postulated to occur in response to the above-described laryngeal elevation or even to the forward translation of the larynx in relation to the hyperlordotic cervical spine. In this clinical scenario, the anterior cricoid ring often is positioned in a plane anterior to the inferior thyroid cartilage (J Rubin, personal observation, 2001).

As a correlate, Lieberman et al often note the resting anatomical relationship of the anterior cricoid ring / inferior rim of thyroid cartilage complex (which they designate the "cricothyroid visor") to be narrowed with little discernable space.[10] In this clinical scenario, they often identify a decreased range of motion of the cricothyroid visor as the individual changes vocal pitch from vocal fry to falsetto,[10] presumably in association with diminished cricothyroid muscle activity or efficiency. We have noted that some affected individuals recruit external muscles, particularly the suprahyoid muscles but also the strap muscles, and even at times other muscles of first and second branchial arch origin, to assist in pitch elevation. The physical consequence is an elevated larynx and tightened suprahyoid and perilaryngeal muscles.[12]

The issue of pain or discomfort in relation to muscular imbalance is relevant to this discussion, as well. A sense of discomfort commonly arises when muscles are not used appropriately. Further discomfort may occur as phonation is attempted while the anatomically related muscles are unduly tense. This can result in a cycle of muscle tension and pain, which further reinforces the behavioral muscular 'holding' pattern.[14]

Treatment

Various physical techniques have been developed to help alleviate the problems described above. Many are outside the purview of this chapter and can be found in texts on Alexander technique, in Pilates manuals, and so on. In essence, if we limit ourselves to the neck, physical techniques of use to our patients might include those that deal with:

1. release of tension/contraction of the suprahyoid musculature. Such techniques have been championed by workers such as Lesley Mathieson[14] and Nelson Roy[15];
2. release/stretch of the cricothyroid mechanism and release of tight strap muscles. Such techniques have been championed by Jacob Lieberman[10];
3. repositioning of the forward (hyperlordotic) cervical spine, including release of restriction of the cervical facet joints, release of contractions of the sternocleidomastoid and trapezius, stretch of the upper fibers of the erector spinae. These techniques are commonly used in physiotherapy, osteopathy, and to a lesser degree in massage. For voice patients, they have been championed by Ed Blake (E Blake, personal communication, 2001).

Lieberman et al[10] have described techniques for working directly on the cricothyroid joint and muscle and on the ligamentous and muscular attachments of the hyoid in such scenarios. They have identified rapid improvement of voicing in certain individuals. We have noted this as well but should note that laryngeal manipulation therapy may become possible only when other fundamental issues of posture have been addressed.

In her extensive work combining speech therapy with laryngeal manipulation, Mathieson has often found vocal improvement to occur immediately upon working on the muscular and tendinous attachments to the hyoid bone.[14] Roy has had similar experience.[15] Mathieson suggests that vocal improvement may occur when a muscle status is achieved that allows the larynx to respond easily to lateral digital pressure. This passive lateral laryngeal movement may well be an indicator that excessive tension has been eliminated or substantially reduced. As a result, vocal strategies can then be introduced in therapy, whereas previously they would have been counterproductive (L Mathieson, personal observation, 2001). Teachers and performers, through the ages, have reported that lateral movement of the laryngeal cartilages is associated with a sense of freedom of the voice.[9]

Case Report

A case report (fictitious but based on our clinical experience) will help elucidate our current management approach. A 45-year-old professional female singer and dancer presented to the author (JR) on the day of an evening performance with a 2- to 3-week history of throat pain and increasing difficulty with the top register of the voice. Some months earlier she had suffered from a back injury for which she received intermittent physical therapy. On laryngeal examination, there was a satisfactory mucosal wave on stroboscopy with no definitive mucosal pathology; but the neck was found to be held in extension, and the anterior neck musculature was tight and tender to palpation.

An urgent referral was made to a physiotherapist (EB) who identified several musculoskeletal abnormalities, including resting extension of the upper cervical spine, deficits in force production of the deep neck flexor stability mechanism, and stiffness in the upper and midthoracic spine. Palpation of the second and third cervical vertebral facet joints demonstrated restriction of movement and duplicated the discomfort noted by the patient. There were also trigger points in the upper trapezius and levator scapulae and spasm of the sternocleidomastoid; and the lower trapezius was found to be inefficient, with difficulty initiating contraction.

Initial therapy focused on altering the resting position the larynx. Specific technical aspects are outside the scope of this chapter, but it was accomplished through direct manipulation and mobilization of the upper cervical and thoracic vertebrae and through soft tissue work on the affected muscles. The performer was able to perform that evening.

Intermediate therapy was designed to continue releasing the restricted muscular and arthrogenic structures. An exercise plan was also developed to strengthen the deep neck flexors and lower fibers of the trapezius. Following three or four additional sessions, the performer felt that she was back to normal voicing.

Further Thoughts on Posture and Voicing

In discussing aspects of therapeutic intervention, one key issue is that changes in the resting position of the larynx often appear to be secondary to changes in the resting position of the cervical spine. These, in turn, may well be secondary to fundamental postural changes elsewhere in the body. Such postural issues require attention if local treatment of laryngeal position is to provide more than temporary relief of vocal symptoms.

Because this is a chapter on the effects of posture on voice, a final note should perhaps be referenced to posture with regard to breathing for speaking and or singing. Inappropriate posture frequently affects lung volume and subglottal air pressure; and inappropriate breathing patterns (eg, upper chest breathing) can affect posture, which in turn affects laryngeal position and phonation. Perhaps there will be a further chapter on this aspect of voicing in the fourth edition of this book as further clinical experience and research are accumulated.

Conclusions

Many types of musculoskeletal programs, including Alexander, Pilates, Feldenkrais, Rolf, and others, have emphasized the overall importance of posture to body "wellness." We believe that a clinical correlate to this is a balance of the deep flexor and extensor muscular systems of the body. An imbalance therein, even in the lower extremities or pelvis, can have far-reaching postural effects that ultimately affect the voice. We must emphasize that these are still, for us, early days in our interpretation and management of such complex musculoskeletal problems and the laryngeal manifestations thereof; but we believe these issues are important in the management of voice disorders and that further study is warranted.

References

1. Fisher K. Early experience of a multidisciplinary pain management programme. *Holistic Med.* 1988;3:7–56.

2. Robinson L, Fisher H, Knox J, Thomson. *The Official Body Control Pilates Manual.* London, England: Macmillan Publishers Ltd; 2000.

3. Feldenkrais M. *Awareness Through Movement.* New York, NY: Harper and Row; 1972.

4. Rolf IP. *Rolfing: Reestablishing the Natural Alignment and Structural Integration of the Human Body for Vitality and Well-being.* Rochester, Vt: Healing Arts Press; 1989.

5. Lumley JSP, Craven JL, Aitken JT. *Essential Anatomy.* Edinburgh, Scotland: Churchill Livingstone; 1973.

6. Ger R, Abrahams P, Olson TR. *Essentials of Clinical Anatomy.* 2nd ed. New York, NY: Parthenon Publishing Group; 1996.

7. *Stedman's Medical Dictionary.* 22nd ed. Baltimore, Md: Williams and Wilkins; 1972.

8. Boileu Grant JC, Basmajian JV. *Grant's Method of Anatomy.* 7th ed. Baltimore, Md: Williams and Wilkins; 1965.

9 Rubin JS, Korovin G, Epstein R. Care for the professional voice. In: Rubin JS, Sataloff RT, Korovin G., eds. *Diagnosis and Treatment of Voice Disorders.* 2nd ed. Clifton Park, NY: Thomson Delmar Learning; 2003.

10. Lieberman J. Principles and techniques of manual therapy. In: Harris T, Harris S, Rubin JS, Howard D, eds. *The Voice Clinic Handbook.* London, England: Whurr Publishers; 1998:91–138.

11. Koufman J, Blalock O. Functional voice disorders. *Otolaryngol Clin North Am.* 1991;24:1059–1073.

12. Rubin JS, Lieberman J, Harris TM. Laryngeal manipulation. *Otolaryngol Clin North Am.* 2000;33(5):1017–1034.

13. Aronson A. *Clinical Voice Disorders.* 3rd ed. New York, NY: Thieme Medical Publishers; 1991:117–145.

14. Mathieson L. *Greene and Mathieson's The Voice and Its Disorders.* 6th ed. London, England: Whurr Publishers Ltd; 2001.

15. Roy N, Leeper HA. Effects of the manual laryngeal musculoskeletal tension reduction technique as a treatment for functional voice disorders: perceptual and acoustic measures. *J Voice.* 1993;7:242–249.

15

Exercise Physiology: Perspective for Vocal Training

Carole M. Schneider, Keith G. Saxon, and Carolyn A. Dennehy

Aristotle wrote that "the animal that moves makes its change of position by pressing against that which is beneath it."[1(p489)] The study of movement in animals, as Aristotle pointed out, is characterized by two distinct concepts: the physical interaction that exists between the organism and the environment, and the skillful way organisms organize and carry out the physical interaction (pressing). Therefore, if we accept that movement is the result of the interaction between biological systems and the environment, we can study these concepts to learn how to improve human performance.

The study of human body functions, commonly referred to as *physiology*, emphasizes the cause and effect associated with specific mechanisms. Based on numerous scientific investigations, a large body of specialized information is gradually accumulated and generalized explanations for the results are formulated. Over time these explanations are tested and eventually distilled into principles that can be applied with consistent results.

Physiological principles associated with human activity have been extensively studied. These principles have been integrated into the science of exercise physiology and summated into training principles that can be applied across a spectrum of individuals from patients requiring rehabilitative services to elite athletes preparing for Olympic-caliber competition. It is, therefore, reasonable to assume that these basic tenets for physical training and conditioning could be applied to any type of activity involving movement, including vocal performance. Presently, there has been little research conducted that reports the benefits of exercise training on non-sport-related activities. However, a book published by Saxon and Schneider[2]

has introduced the principles of exercise physiology and applied these concepts to vocal training.

The enhancement of any physical performance is directly related to the level of fitness and conditioning of the performer. Improvement in physical performance can range from drastic alterations in the untrained to acute refinement of highly developed skills in the trained individual. Overall physical conditioning of the heart, lungs, and skeletal muscles during regular prescriptive exercise can have a profound effect on the performance levels of anyone along this continuum and can serve to protect individuals against injury and disease. Vocal performers can expect to benefit from general and specific physical conditioning in this regard.

Any activity that involves working muscles can be enhanced by regularly and consistently applying the principles of muscle training and conditioning. Vocal performance is no exception. Sound is the result of complex and dynamic interactions between various muscles and the physical environment. The better the muscles are conditioned to work as independent structures and in synergistic fashion, the better they will perform. The resulting effects of muscle activity, for example, sound production, will be enhanced. When vocal performers apply a technique to improve sound quality, they may not be utilizing the best physiological principles to train the musculature involved in producing sound. However, specific and individualized muscle training may result in better overall sound quality, greater range, and sustainable phrases, as well as improve the general fitness level of the performer and increase his or her resistance to injury and disease.[2]

Beyond exercises for more global cardiovascular conditioning comes muscle training for the vocal mechanism. It is difficult to isolate muscles of the pharynx, larynx, or respiratory system as one might to train the biceps or quadriceps femoris. However, it is possible to perform exercises that work groups of muscles in a coordinated fashion.

Improvement in physical fitness or condition leads to increased performance capacity, particularly as it pertains to the cardiorespiratory and skeletal muscle systems. Exercise physiology is based on a relatively simple premise that suggests that the more efficient these systems are, the higher the level of physical fitness and work capacity. Increasing heart and lung capacity to deliver more oxygen to working muscles and requiring less energy to perform the task allows physical activity to be extended for longer periods of time. Since these systems are essential contributors to voice production, performance quality, and endurance, training and maintaining them are important for vocalists. Furthermore, continuous refinement and maintenance of a desired level of conditioning implies that training and conditioning is a dynamic and specific process.

General Principles of Training

Training for an athletic competition involves the application of four basic principles to elicit a training effect: overload, specificity, individuality, and reversibility. Training for a vocal performance should incorporate the same training principles to produce a training effect in the musculature and energy systems utilized in vocal production.

Overload Principle

The *overload principle* states that physiological adaptations will occur in the working muscles with the appropriate stimuli. Appropriate stimuli include workloads that are greater than workloads encountered in daily life. Christensen[3] found that regular training at a constant workload gradually lowered the heart rate and produced a training effect such as an improvement of the oxygen-carrying capacity of the cardiovascular system. Additional training at the same workload did not change the heart rate response. When training involved a heavier workload, the heart rate response was even lower than the original heart rate. Adaptation occurs at a given workload. To develop further physical fitness, the training must incorporate an additional overload. Overload can be varied by manipulating the components of training as specified by the American College of Sports Medicine.[4]

These training components are frequency of exercise, duration of exercise, intensity of exercise, type (mode) of exercise, and exercise progression.

Overload in singing means requiring more of all or part of the entire vocal apparatus than it is used to doing. The obvious solution of producing greater sound pressure levels or increased airway pressure are among the least adaptive and most risky. Overload also can be produced by singing longer at more moderate volume, singing more frequently, and even without singing or making a sound while working on air flow control and varying airway resistance.

The application of training overload must be gradual. Intense training should be interspersed with easy workouts (decreasing exercise intensity and/or duration). There are limited data on the laryngeal musculature regarding loading and unloading specific muscles. A correlation has been found with high pitch and high intensity and high load on the cricothyroid and thyroid arytenoid muscles.[2,5] Additionally, sufficient rest should be given to the sport athlete or vocal performer to allow for adequate recovery.[6] Sport athletes overload by using periodization cycles, which helps prevent overtraining. Periodization has several cycles throughout the year. The *load cycle* is the building of the training program during the off-season or non-competitive season. The *recovery cycle* is active rest (low intensity, short duration) and separates the load cycle and the competitive season. Recovery periods are essential to allow for physiological adaptations to occur. The *peak cycle* develops maximum muscular conditioning and skill enhancement. The *conditioning cycle* is active rest for a few months following the strenuous competitive season.

Manipulation of these factors during vocal training will enhance vocal performance and may reduce the incidence of injury. Skilled teachers are applying some of these concepts in the studio when interspersing vocal exercises with rest. Varying rehearsal to multiple short sessions or extended long sessions also illustrates the application of the overload principle.

Specificity Principle

The training program must be appropriate for the activity or performance. There are two basic types of specificity: *metabolic specificity* and *skill specificity*. Metabolic specificity requires that the training program overload the energy (metabolic) system that supports the activity. The energy system rate and capacity must meet the demands of the activity or performance. McArdle[7] found that the cardiovascular and respiratory training responses were most pronounced when training stressed the specific muscle groups involved in the chosen activity. For example, if a superbly trained cyclist is compared to a superbly trained runner, the cyclist is going to lose when the task chosen for comparison is the treadmill. Despite equivalent cardiovascular conditioning, the runner had the advantage of having trained his or her muscles for exactly the task at hand. Such local skeletal muscle metabolic adaptation contributes to the improvement of fitness and performance.

Skill specificity means training the muscle groups and movement patterns (neuromuscular) involved in the activity of interest. In other words, training programs should contain activities closely related to the actual performance skills. To develop the vocal skill of attaining and sustaining a pitch at high volume, the muscles should be strengthened using intense contractions of short duration while increasing the frequency of practice sessions. To develop the voice for prolonged singing, the muscles should be strengthened using low intensity contractions for long durations.[2] It is axiomatic that the optimal training material to prepare a given repertoire is to use that specific repertoire.

Individuality Principle

The physiological responses to training vary between individuals. Similar training routines will not produce exactly the same physiological benefits to all athletes. The skilled voice teacher does not recommend the same training program to all students in the studio. Training is optimized when individual needs and capacities are addressed. The resulting effects are enhancement of performance for all skill levels.

Application of the individuality principle implies a level of sensitivity, assessment and creativity on the part of the trainer. Only through understanding an individual's skill set, level of training, innate talent, and even optimal method of learning will the most productive training occur.

Reversibility Principle

The majority of physiological benefits from training are lost within a short period of time when training is discontinued. The length of time is variable depending on the physiological parameter in question. The loss of the benefits of training can vary from several weeks to several months.[8] Saltin and Rowell[9] found that inactivity decreased physiological function 1% per day. Most physiological benefits of training are probably completely lost after 4 to 8 weeks of inactivity. These studies demonstrated that pulmonary ventilation and oxygen uptake were greatly affected by detraining. Since these are essential physiological components utilized during vocal performance, the

reversibility principle may indicate that absolute voice rest is not recommended except in specific cases, such as after injury or surgery. This is the prime muscle-based argument for continuing some kind of exercise even in the face of mucosa injury. There is some suggestion (Katherine Verdolini, PhD, personal communication, 2001) that continued exercise may hasten recovery by manipulating wound healing factors such as tissue anoxia.

The Exercise Prescription

The American College of Sports Medicine[4] has established components that must be included in the exercise prescription (training program) that will produce a training effect. The components include frequency of exercise, duration of exercise, intensity of exercise, type (mode) of exercise, and exercise progression. The same components can be used in the studio or voice therapist's office to elicit desired changes in vocal quality. The exercise prescription for a voice must include knowledge of the level of training, the skills possessed, the time available before the next performance, and the interval since the last performance. Underlying disease states, prescription and over-the-counter medications, and herbal preparations are also factors. Diet and sleep remain factors that require not only exploration but also modification to achieve optimal training effect.

Frequency of Exercise

Exercising three times per week has been established as the optimal frequency to produce a training effect. However, this time course is dependent on the intensity of the activity being performed. Research comparing the results of sport-specific training of comparable workloads 2 days per week, 3 days per week, and 5 days per week showed that training effects occurred with programs of 3 or more days per week.[10,11] Frequency of training, however, is dependent on the individual's initial fitness level. The lower the initial fitness level, the greater the conditioning effect even with a 2-day per week program. Training six or seven times per week provides minimal fitness improvement and increases the risk of overuse injury.[12] Exercise with short duration and low intensity requires more frequent training to produce beneficial physiological effects.

Duration of Exercise

The duration of training is directly related to the improvement of physical fitness.[13,14] The American College of Sports Medicine[4] has recommended that each exercise session be at least 20 minutes in duration with continuous exercise if the exercise intensity is low (50 to 75% of maximal heart rate reserve). If the exercise intensity is high (above 75% of maximal heart rate reserve: maximal heart rate minus resting heart rate times exercise intensity plus resting heart rate), the exercise duration is decreased. Training the energy and muscular systems required for specific vocal effects at comparable durations should enhance singing performance.

Intensity of Exercise

The maintenance of vocal efficiency may depend on the intensity of the training sessions, in addition to the frequency and duration of the training sessions. An important component of physical training is exercise intensity. Physiological changes from training occur primarily from intensity overload. Subjective evaluation from the performer can help determine if the training workload is too easy or too hard, but it cannot identify an optimal training intensity. Heart rate has a linear relationship with exercise intensity. For example, as the exercise intensity increases, heart rate increases. Because of this relationship and the ease of assessing heart rate, the most common method developed to determine the appropriate exercise intensity is heart rate. The exercise intensity should be strenuous enough to get the heart rate between 60% and 90% of the performer's heart rate reserve. The heart rate can be determined immediately after the activity by counting the pulse.

The determination of blood lactic acid (lactate) is another objective measure of exercise intensity. Lactate levels can be measured using a small drop of blood from the finger. Multiple blood samples can be collected to determine the blood lactate profile of the performer during the exercise or activity. These values are then plotted and a blood lactate profile curve is produced. The point at which there is a sudden rise in blood lactate is called the onset of blood lactic acid (OBLA). The goal of the training sessions is to have OBLA occur later and later during the exercise training workout. The occurrence of OBLA at a higher exercise intensity means that the performer is able to work longer before lactic acid accumulates in the blood, thus increasing the body's utilization and tolerance of blood lactic acid and delaying muscle fatigue.[15] The application of intensity of training may be useful during singing, especially in the laboratory setting where heart rate and blood lactic acid can be easily collected. Additionally, heart rate and lactic acid could be monitored during performance to judge the intensity of work while singing.[16]

Exercise intensity can also be determined using the measurement of oxygen consumption. The capacity of the cardiorespiratory system is limited. The maximal amount of oxygen that can be utilized by the working muscles is called *maximal oxygen consumption*. The maximal amount of oxygen the muscles can consume is dependent on an increased respiration and increased cardiac output (heart rate times stroke volume). The maximal amount of oxygen an individual can utilize in this manner can be measured in a laboratory setting. Oxygen consumption is linearly related to exercise intensity and heart rate. The greater the exercise intensity, the higher the amount of oxygen utilized. The greater the capacity of oxygen consumption, the more physically fit the individual. A more fit person can perform work with less energy demand, and therefore less oxygen demand. Thus, training a singer to become more physically fit would enhance the singer's ability to perform at a lower energy demand and, thus, perform longer or with less stress on the physiological systems involved.

The final determinant of exercise intensity, and one of the most important to singers, is ratings of perceived exertion (RPE).[17] The scale is a numeric qualifier for individuals to rate their own perception of the physical work demands. This scale ranges from 6 to 20. The RPE scale was developed to correspond to heart rate by adding a zero to the RPE value (eg, an RPE of 12 equals 120 bpm).[18] With practice an individual can learn to associate a heart rate response to an RPE value. Once this occurs, a performer can use the RPE value instead of monitoring the heart rate to determine the appropriate exercise intensity for a conditioning effect.

Type (Mode) of Exercise

The type of training modality should be specific to the activity. Training to acquire a particular skill should be consistent and directly designed to influence a particular effect. In addition to the practice of singing, exercises specific to the energy systems and muscles used during singing need to be incorporated.

Exercise Progression

The greatest physiological improvements in fitness are seen within the first 6 to 8 weeks of the training program. Further improvements require that the cardiorespiratory system and the muscular system continue to be overloaded by adjusting the duration and intensity of the exercise program to meet the new level of physical fitness. Exercise progression should be slow and gradual to avoid the incidence of injury. In regard to vocal performers, the present level of vocal conditioning would determine the stages of vocal training. The components (ie, intensity, duration) of the exercise training program do not change but the degree of progression is specific to the conditioning level of the vocal performer.

Phases of the Exercise Routine

The exercise workout for athletic performance or vocal performance should consist of a *warm-up*, a *conditioning phase*, and a *cool-down*. The function of the warm-up is to increase blood flow to the working muscles and increase the muscle temperature. This decreases the chance of muscle injury.[6] The warm-up activity should gradually intensify to prepare the muscles for the more demanding conditioning phase. The length of the warm-up should be 10 to 15 minutes.[19]

The conditioning phase should include activity at a predetermined exercise prescription, varying the frequency, duration, and intensity of the work. The conditioning phase should be specifically designed to produce the desired effects and should be adjusted as adaptations occur.

The cool-down incorporates the same activity used in the conditioning phase but at a much lower intensity. The reduced intensity facilitates venous blood flow back to the heart and avoids blood pooling in the arms and legs. Continuous movement during the cool-down prevents dizziness and the possibility of fainting.[20]

Application to Vocal Performance

Singing involves the whole body, the vocal and facial areas, the abdomen, chest, and the legs. Therefore, the muscles and energy systems utilized during performance need to be trained. The principles used for the development of a training effect in the systems involved in sport training can be applied to training the physiological systems involved with vocal performance.[2]

One example, to illustrate the point, is the requirement of proper posture for sound production. The development of proper body alignment involves correct body posture. Correct body posture involves an appropriate balance between the agonist and antagonist muscles involved with maintaining appropriate positioning of the upper thorax. Henderson[21] recommends pulling the shoulders straight back until the shoulder blades feel as if they are touching. Repeating this frequently will assist in establishing the correct postural position for the head and shoulders.

Performers have come to rely on methods such as the Alexander technique and Feldenkrais therapy to address this issue and others.

A better procedure for establishing correct posture would be to do an analysis of the muscles involved in maintaining desired posture and then develop an exercise prescription (type, frequency, duration, intensity, and progression) that involves training the muscles used to maintain the appropriate balance for enhanced posture, which would result in more effective use of the energy needed to perform.

Saxon and Schneider[2] have published a reference textbook for vocal performers. The text includes an analysis of the muscles and energy systems involved during vocal performance. The goal is to enhance vocal performance incorporating the established training principles from the area of exercise physiology.

References

1. Artistotle, Forster ES, trans. *Progression of Animals.* Cambridge, Mass: Harvard University Press; 1968:489
2. Saxon KG, Schneider CM. *Vocal Exercise Physiology.* San Diego, Calif: Singular Publishing Group, Inc; 1995.
3. Christensen EA, as cited in Astrand I, Astrand PO, Christensen EA, Hedman R. Intermittent muscular work. *Acta Physiol Scand.* 1960;48:448–453.
4. American College of Sports Medicine. Position statement on the recommended quantity and quality of exercise for developing and maintaining fitness in healthy adults. *Med Sci Sports.* 1978;10:vii–x
5. Shipp T, McGlone RE. Laryngeal dynamics associated with voice frequency change. *J Speech Hearing Res.* 1971;14:761–768.
6. Brooks GA, Fahey TD. *Exercise Physiology: Human Bioenergetics and Its Applications.* New York, NY: Macmillan Publishing Company; 1985.
7. McArdle WD. Specificity of run training on VO_2 max and heart rate changes during running and swimming. *Med Sci Sports.* 1978;10:16.
8. Cureton TK, Phillips EE. Physical fitness changes in middle-aged men attributable to equal eight-week periods of training, non-training and retraining. *J Sports Med Phys Fitness.* 1964;4:1–7.
9. Saltin B, Rowell LB. Functional adaptations to physical activity and inactivity. *Fed Proc.* 1980;39:1506.
10. Pollock ML, Cureton TK, Greninger L. Effects of frequency of training on working capacity, cardiovascular function, and body composition of adult men. *Med Sci Sports.* 1969;1:70–74.
11. Pollock ML, Tiffany J, Gettman L, Janeway R, Lofland H. Effect of frequency of training on serum lipids, cardiovascular function, and body composition. In: Franks BD, ed. *Exercise and Fitness.* Chicago, Ill: Athletic Institute; 1969;161–178.
12. Pollock ML, Wilmore JH. *Exercise in Health and Disease.* 2nd ed. Philadelphia, Pa: WB Saunders Company; 1990.
13. Milesis CA, Pollock ML, Bah MD, Ayres JJ, Ward A, Linnerud AC. Effects of different durations of training on cardiorespiratory function, body composition and serum lipids. *Res Q.* 1976;47:716–725.

14. Sharkey BJ. Intensity and duration of training and the development of cardiorespiratory endurance. *Med Sci Sports.* 1970; 2:197–202.

15. Brooks GA, Fahey TD. *Fundamentals of Human Performance.* New York, NY: Macmillan Publishing Company; 1987.

16. Saxon KG, Michel JF, Schneider CM. The singer as athlete: lessons from applied and exercise physiology. *Care of the Professional Voice, The Voice Foundation's 20th Symposium*; June, 1991; Philadelphia, Pa.

17. Birk TJ, Birk CA. Use of ratings of perceived exertion for exercise prescription. *Sports Med.* 1987;4:1–8.

18. Borg GV, Linderholm H. Perceived exertion and pulse rate during graded exercise in various age groups. *Acta Med Scand.* 1967;472 (suppl):194–206.

19. Heyward VH. *Advanced Fitness Assessment and Exercise Prescription.* Champaign, Ill: Human Kinetics; 1991.

20. Bowers RW, Fox EL. *Sports Physiology.* Dubuque, Iowa: Wm C Brown Publishers; 1992.

21. Henderson LB. *How to Train Singers.* New York, NY: Parker Publishing; 1979.

16

Medications and the Voice

Robert Thayer Sataloff, Mary J. Hawkshaw, and Joseph Anticaglia

Medications are used to treat many problems encountered commonly in professional voice users. Some are used to treat illnesses affecting the head and neck, others involve other organs and systems in the body and can potentially affect the larynx and voice production. Many medications that potentially affect the voice are discussed in the first two editions of this book and in other literature.[1,2] In many cases, the effects are minor and not clinically significant. However, physicians, nurses, and others caring for professional voice users should be familiar with drug-induced phenomena that may affect the voice.

In addition to the recognized effects and side effects of medications, when trying to predict or recognize the potential vocal consequences of pharmacologic agents, it is important also to consider biological variability in individuals An individual's response to medications is influenced also by gender, age, body size, metabolic status, and concurrent use of other medications or recreational drugs. "Recommended doses" are the amount of a drug generally required to achieve the desired balance between an effect or side effect. However, they are merely guidelines based on average responses in test populations. Optimizing the relationship between desired effects and undesirable side effects requires individualization, especially in professional voice users for whom even "minor" side effects may be vocally disabling.

Antihistamines

Antihistamines are used commonly to treat allergies. However, virtually all antihistamines can have a drying effect on upper respiratory tract secretions, al-though severity varies widely with different drugs and from person to person. In addition, antihistamines are often combined with sympathomimetic or parasympatholytic agents, which further reduce and thicken mucosal secretions and may reduce lubrication to the point of producing a dry cough. This may be more harmful to phonation than the allergic condition itself. Normal mucosal secretions are extremely important for free movement of the vibratory margin of the vocal folds. If vocal tract lubrication is suboptimal as a result of dehydration, or by shifting the normal balance of serous and mucinous secretions, alterations in phonation occur. Laryngologists frequently discover that a patient has self-medicated with an over-the-counter (OTC) antihistamine preparation, thus making it imperative to seek this information when taking a patient's medical history. When professional voice users develop thick, viscous vocal fold secretions during performance, results can be disastrous.

The majority of antihistamine agents are acetylcholine antagonists that have parasympatholytic activity, which probably accounts for the increased viscosity of secretions by directly affecting the salivary glands and mucus-secreting membranes of the respiratory tract. They may also have a sedative effect that can impair sensorium and disturb performance. Milder, newer antihistamines such as fexofenadine (Allegra, Hoechst, Marion, Roussel) and loratadine (Claritin, Schering) produce less drowsiness and often less dryness; but in many people, they are often less effective in treating symptoms than drugs with more disturbing side effects. Mild antihistamines in small doses may be helpful for performers with intermittent allergic symptoms, but the medications should be tried between or before performances, not immediately prior to professional engagements. When medication is needed to treat an acute allergic response shortly before performance, oral or injected corticosteroids rather than antihistamines usually accomplish the desired result without causing significant side effects. Antihistamines used to treat allergies are different from the antihistamines (H2 blockers) used to treat other conditions such as reflux. H2 blockers (ranitidine, Zantac, Glaxo Wellcome) are used to block the stimulant effects of histamine on gastric acid secretions.

The antihistamines most commonly used are those belonging to the alkylamine or chlorpheniramine family. Because they have been deregulated by the FDA and are now available over-the-counter (OTC), these agents are being used with increasing frequency. Diphenhydramine (Benadryl, Warner-Lambert) and scopolamine (Transderm, Novartis Consumer), which have a significant drying effect, are present in some OTC sleep aids, presumably for their sedative effect. Promethazine (Phenergan, Wyeth-Ayerst) is contained in several antitussive mixtures and can dry laryngeal secretions. Meclizine (Antivert, Pfizer), another OTC antihistamine used to treat dizziness and motion sickness, is also encountered commonly. All antihistamines provide some degree of relief from motion sickness; and to a greater or lesser degree, all cause drying of the mucous membranes, especially of the nose and oropharynx.

Mucolytic Agents

The lubricant viscosity of respiratory tract and vocal fold surface tension are essential to normal phonation. Dehydration and/or thickening of secretions may be caused by medications such as antihistamines, as discussed above, anticholinergics, generalized dehydration, and/or other factors. Dehydration may occur as the result of exercising, performing athletic or recreational activities, or from exposure to environmental factors such as the dry air on airplanes and the low humidity at high altitudes. Dehydration can also occur with febrile illness and/or prolonged vomiting or diarrhea. It must be remembered that the viscosity of respiratory secretions is directly related to available body water, assuming the absence of metabolic or pharmacologic interference. No medications, including mucolytic agents, are substitutes for adequate hydration. However, mucolytics may be helpful in counteracting the effects of antihistamines and in ameliorating the mucosal consequences of dehydration quickly. Guaifenesin is a useful wetting agent, expectorant, and vasoconstrictor that increases and thins mucosal

secretions. Guaifenesin (Humibid, Adams) is currently among the most convenient preparations available. Mucolytics are relatively harmless and may be helpful in singers who complain of thick secretions, frequent throat clearing, or postnasal drip, which is often caused by secretions that are too thick rather than too plentiful.

Corticosteroids

Corticosteroids are potent anti-inflammatory agents that can be helpful in managing an acute allergy attack and acute laryngitis. Many laryngologists recommend using steroids in low doses, such as methylprednisolone 10 mg. However, the author (RTS) has found higher doses for short periods of time to be more effective. Depending on the indication, the steroid dosage may be methyl prednisolone 60 mg (Medrol, Upjohn) orally or dexamethasone 6 mg (Decadron, Merck) intramuscularly followed by a short course of a high dose oral steroid tapered over 3 to 6 days. Regimens of oral steroid therapy, such as a dexamethasone (Decadron, Merck) or methylprednisolone (Depo-Medrol, Medrol, or Medrol Dosepak, Upjohn) may also be used. Physicians should be familiar with the dose relationship among steroids (Table 16–1).

Adrenocorticotropic hormone (ACTH) may also be used to increase endogenous cortisone output, thus decreasing inflammation and mobilizing water from an edematous larynx,[3] although the author (RTS) has found traditional steroid therapy entirely satisfactory. Care must be taken not to prescribe steroids excessively, and they should not be used habitually (or in females for monthly dysphonia premenstrualis). They should be used only when there is a pressing professional commitment that is being hampered by vocal fold inflammation. If there is any question that the inflammation may be of infectious origin, antibiotic coverage is recommended. Steroids, whether administered short-term or long-term, must be used with extreme caution in diabetics. Steroids elevate serum glucose; and in the diabetic patient, they can cause blood sugars to become uncontrolled. Laryngologists should have their patients consult their endocrinologist before starting steroids so that a schedule for monitoring blood glucose can be established while a patient is on steroid therapy.

Corticosteroids may have additional significant adverse effects; although they are not generally seen following short-term steroid use, they may occur in any patient. The side effects encountered most frequently include gastric irritation with possible ulceration and

Table 16–1. Steroid Equivalency.

Adrenocorticosteroids	Common Trade Name	Glucocorticoid (Anti-inflammatory Potency) Equivalent Dose (mg)	Mineralocorticoid (Sodium Retention) Relative Potency
Betamethasone	Celestone (Schering)	0.06	0
Cortisone	Cortone (M-S-D)	25	0.8
Dexamethasone	Decadron (M-S-D) Deronil (Schering) Dexameth (Major) Gammacorten (CIBA) Hexadrol (Organon)	0.75	0
Fludrocortisone	Florinef (Squibb)	0.1	100
Fluprednisolone	Alphadrol (Upjohn)	2	0
Hydrocortisone	Cort-Dome (Dome) Cortef (Upjohn) Cortenema (Rowell) Cortril (Pfizer) Hydrocortone (M-S-D)	20	1
Methylprednisolone	Depo-Medrol (Upjohn) Medrol (Upjohn) Solu-Medrol (Upjohn)	4	4
Paramethasone	Haldrone (Lilly) Stemex (Syntex)	2	0
Prednisolone	Delta-Cortef (Upjohn) Hydeltra T.B.A. (M-S-D) Hydeltrasol (M-S-D) Meticortelone (Schering) Nisolone (Ascher) Sterane (Pfizer)	5	0.8
Prednisone	Delta Dome (Dome) Deltasone (Upjohn) Deltra (M-S-D) Meticorton (Schering) Paracort (Parke-Davis) Servisone (Lederle)	5	0.8
Triamcinolone	Aristocort (Lederle) Aristospan (Lederle) Kenacort (Squibb) Kenalog (Squibb)	4	0

Note: M—S—D, Merck, Sharp & Dohme.

hemorrhage, increased appetite, increased energy, insomnia, mild mucosal drying, blurred vision, mood change (euphoria, occasionally psychosis), irritability, and fluid retention. These side effects can range from mild to severe depending on the dosage given and the patient's metabolism and response to the medication.

The author (RTS) routinely prescribes ranitidine (Zantac, Glaxo Wellcome) when treating patients with steroids, as prophylaxis against gastric irritation. Patients that are already taking H2 blockers and/or proton pump inhibitors (PPIs) might require increased dosages of their medication while on steroids. Long-term effects such as muscle wasting and fat redistribution are generally not encountered with appropriate short-term use of steroids.

Another potential problem peculiar to professional voice users is steroid abuse. Because the side effects of steroids generally are uncommon and because steroids work extremely well, there is a tendency (especially among singers) to overuse or abuse them and to share their medication with other performers. This practice must be avoided.

Diuretics and Other Medications for Edema

Diuretics are potent medications that help the body eliminate excess fluid and should be taken only with a physician's prescription and supervision. Like steroids, they should be taken only by the individual for whom they were prescribed. Diuretics are indicated and used to treat certain illnesses, such as heart or kidney failure, when the body is unable to excrete fluids at a rate needed to maintain its fluid and electrolyte balance. Diuretics also are used in conjunction with antihypertensive agents for the treatment of high blood pressure.

The premenstrual period is a temporary physiological condition in which women retain fluid as a result of decreased estrogen and progesterone levels associated with altered pituitary activity. An increase in circulating antidiuretic hormone results in fluid retention in Reinke's space as well as in other tissues. The fluid retained in the vocal fold during inflammation and hormonal fluid shifts is protein-bound, not free water.[4] Diuretics do not remobilize this fluid effectively and can dehydrate the performer, resulting in decreased lubrication and thickened secretions and persistently edematous vocal folds, and thus should not be used for vocal fold symptoms related to these conditions. If diuretics must be used for other medical purposes, the voice should be monitored closely.

Topical and systemic decongestants such as oxymetazoline hydrochloride (Afrin, Schering-Plough) and pseudoephedrine (Sudafed, Warner-Lambert) have also been used to treat edema/congestion in the upper respiratory tract. Oxymetazoline hydrochloride (Afrin) applied by a large particle mist to the larynx is particularly helpful in treating severe edema immediately prior to performance, but it should be used only under emergent and extreme circumstances. Afrin is more commonly used as a nasal spray to treat nasal congestion. Its primary action involves reduction in the diameter and volume of vascular structures in the submucosal area; however, it may also produce "rebound" phenomena and thus requires use with caution.

Sprays, Mists, and Inhalants

Diphenhydramine hydrochloride 0.5% (Benadryl, Warner Lambert) in distilled water, delivered to the larynx as a mist may be helpful for its vasoconstrictive properties, but it is also dangerous because of its topical anesthetic effect and is not recommended by the author (RTS). However, Punt advocated this mixture and several modifications of it.[5]

Five percent propylene glycol in a physiologically balanced salt solution may be delivered by large particle mist and can provide lubrication, particularly helpful in cases of laryngitis sicca after air travel or as associated with dry climates. Such treatment is harmless and may also provide a beneficial placebo effect. Water, saline, or other physiologically balanced solutions delivered via a vaporizer or steam generator are frequently effective and sufficient. This therapy should be augmented by oral hydration, which is the mainstay of treatment for dehydration.

Nasal steroid sprays such as beclomethasone (Beconase, Glaxo Wellcome), beclomethasone dipropionate (Vancenase, Schering), budesonide (Rhinocort, Astra), triamcinolone acetonide (Nasacort, Rhone-Poulenc Rorer), and mometasone furoate (Nasonex, Rhone-Poulenc Rorer) do not appear to harm the voice. The steroid in the nasal spray works topically on the nasal mucosa and is not absorbed systemically. However, certain propellants in these nasal sprays may cause mucosal drying. For this reason, the author (RTS) generally prescribes steroid nasal sprays that have an aqueous medium, such as budesonide (Rhinocort AQ, AstraZeneca LP).

Most oral steroid inhalers, such as triamcinolone acetonide (Azmacort, Rhone-Poulenc Rorer) used to treat asthma are not recommended for use in professional voice users.[6,7] Dysphonia caused by contact inflammation from oral steroid inhalers occurs in up to 50% of patients and is related to the aerosolized steroid itself and not to the Freon propellant. Steroid inhalers used for prolonged periods may result in *Candida* laryngitis; and as is common in asthmatics, prolonged use of steroid inhalers can cause atrophy of the vocalis muscle.[7,8]

Antibiotics

When antibiotics are used in professional voice users, high doses are recommended to achieve therapeutic blood levels rapidly, especially if important performances are imminent. When there is little time between initial treatment and performance, starting treatment with an intramuscular injection may be helpful. Selecting oral antibiotics that are absorbed rapidly and achieve optimal blood levels faster may also be helpful.

When patients have no pressing engagements, antibiotic use should be based on cultures whenever appropriate (eg, throat culture for streptococcus infection). However, in the common situation in which a performance must proceed and when there is clinical evidence of bacterial infection, antibiotics should be instituted after cultures are taken, without waiting for the results. The potential damage of delayed treatment in an active performer is greater than the potential harm of antibiotic use for an unproven organism.

Antiviral Agents

A limited number of antiviral agents are available commercially. Acyclovir (Zovirax, Glaxo Wellcome) is used specifically for treating the herpes simplex virus (HSV) types I and II and may be appropriate in patients with recurrent herpetic superior laryngeal nerve paresis or paralysis. Oseltamivir (Tamiflu, Roche) is a relatively new antiviral drug that can be effective in the treatment of acute influenza and for prophylaxis of influenza in adults and children, 13 years and older. It is not a substitute for a flu vaccination. Voice problems have not been reported with Tamiflu; however, rash and swelling of the face and tongue have been reported which could have a negative impact on vocal performance. Zanamivir (Relenza, Glaxo Wellcome) is another antiviral medication administered by oral inhalation, which delivers the medication directly to the respiratory tract. Relenza is indicated for treatment of influenza A and B in patients who have been symptomatic for no more than 2 days, and in adults and children 7 years or older. However, it is generally not recommended for patients with underlying airway disease; bronchospasm and decreased lung function have been reported with use of this drug. Recently, a new medication to reduce the length and degree of symptoms of the common cold has been introduced and should be available in less than one year pending FDA approval. Plecondril (Picovir, ViroPharma) specifically attacks the rhinovirus, which is the most common cause of the common cold. Pending FDA approval of this medication, it will be available by prescription only and its brand name will be Picovir.

Vistide (cidofovir, Gilead Sciences) is now being used as an intralesional injection in treating human papilloma virus (HPV) involving the larynx. Patients with human immunodeficiency virus (HIV) are also treated with antivirals such as zidovudine (Retrovir, Glaxo Wellcome), which was previously called azidothymidine (AZT). This drug has the potential to cause very severe side effects; however, it is often difficult to determine what is a side effect of a medication, because many of the side effects can be manifestations of the HIV disease process itself. Zidovudine can cause hoarseness, cough, pharyngitis, nervousness, muscle spasm, tremor, and many other systemic side effects, all of which can have a negative impact on vocal performance.

Amantadine (Symmetrel, Endo Labs) used in the treatment of Parkinson's disease, also has been found to be effective against influenza[9-12] and other viruses. If a performer must work in an area in which there is a flu epidemic, it may be reasonable to use this drug. However, agitation, tachycardia, and extreme xerostomia and xerophonia may occur. When these side effects occur, they are generally severe enough to require cancellation of a performance.

Antitussive Medications

Cough suppressants (antitussives) often contain an antihistamine and codeine, a narcotic, that can have a secondary drying effect on vocal tract secretions.[13,14] Benzonatate (Tessalon, Forest) is a non-narcotic antitussive that acts peripherally by anesthetizing stretch receptors in the upper respiratory tract, thereby suppressing the cough reflex. However, severe hypersensitivity reactions including laryngospasm and bronchospasm have been reported. Dextromethorphan is a non-narcotic, antitussive agent found in most cough syrups and has pharmacologic actions similar to those of codeine. Generally, the over-the-counter preparations that contain dextromethorphan and guaifenesin (Robitussin DM, Robins) work well for voice professionals. All patients, including singers, should be instructed to read the labels on all OTC medications. If there is any question regarding safety or ingredients of a product, it should be discussed with their primary physician and/or laryngologist.

Antihypertensive Agents

Almost all of the antihypertensive agents used currently have a parasympathomimetic action of varying degrees and thus dry mucous membranes of the respiratory tract. Often, they are used in combination with a diuretic that promotes dehydration. The authors have frequently noted dryness with reserpines and agents of the methyldopa group, and occasionally a dry cough with some of the newer medications used to treat hypertension. When mucosal drying and a dry, nonproductive cough are thought to be a side effect of an antihypertensive medication, the laryngologist may recommend that the patient's internist prescribe another antihypertensive agent. Beta-blockers such as propanolol (Inderal, Wyeth Ayerst) are also used in the treatment of hypertension but are not recommended treatment for preperformance anxiety.[15]

Gastroenterologic Medications

Medical management of gastroesophageal reflux disease (GERD) generally includes neutralization of gastric acid with antacids; suppression of acid secretion with histamine receptor antagonists (H2 blockers), such as ranitidine (Zantac, Glaxo Wellcome); blocking of the gastric proton pump enzyme (H+/K+ATPase) with antagonists such as omeprazole (Prilosec, Astra Merck); and modifications in lifestyle and diet. In the laryngologist's (RTS) practice, the authors frequently encounter patients who misunderstand their medical treatment for laryngopharyngeal reflux despite receiving oral and written explanations and instructions by the authors and being reinforced by other members of our voice team involved in a patient's care. The most common misconception is that H2 blockers and/or proton pump inhibitors (PPIs) eliminate the need for antacids and other lifestyle modifications. It is especially important for singers and all patients to understand the correct rationale for use of their medications; because inadequately treated reflux laryngitis can have deleterious effects on the voice over time

including cancer of the larynx or esophagus. A more in-depth discussion of reflux management can be found elsewhere. Laryngeal cancer and its treatment can be found in chapter 23.

Antacids can cause constipation, diarrhea, or bloating in some people, which may affect performance by impairing the support mechanism vital to singers and other musicians. Occasionally, they also have a drying effect. However, it is usually possible to find an antacid that can be tolerated by any individual. It is also possible to select antacids that do not contain chemicals (eg, aluminum) that some people wish to avoid (Tables 16–2 and 16–3).

H2 receptor antagonists have revolutionized the treatment of gastroesophageal reflux disease and proved beneficial for the treatment of reflux laryngitis (RL) and are now used widely by most laryngologists that treat a large number of professional voice users.

H2 receptor antagonists inhibit the stimulation of gastric acid secretion and are generally effective in reducing acid output from gastric parietal cells, although they have little affect on the basal rate of acid production. The H2 blockers most commonly used in-

Table 16–2. Contents of Liquid Antacids (in mg/tsp).

	Aluminum Hydroxide	Magnesium Hydroxide	Calcium Carbonate	Magnesium Carbonate	Magaldrate	Simethicone	Sodium
Alternagel	600						<2.5
Aludrox	307	103					
Amphojel	320						
Camalox	225	200	250				
Delcid	600	665					<15
Di-Gel	200	200				20	
Gaviscon (mg/tbsp)	95			412			
Gelusil	200	200				25	
Gelusil II	400	400				30	
Kolantyl	150	150					
Maalox	225	200					
Maalox Plus	225	200					
Mag-Ox		400				25	
Mylanta	200	200				20	
Mylanta II	400	400				40	
Riopan					540		0.1
Riopan Plus					540	20	0.1
Riopan Plus E-S					1,080	30	0.3
Uro-Mag		140					

Table 16–3. Contents of Antacids: Tablets-Chewables-Gums (in mg).

	Aluminum Hydroxide	Magnesium Hydroxide	Calcium Carbonate	Simethicone	Dihydroxy-Aluminum Na+ Carbonate	Magnesium Carbonate
Alka-Mints			850			
Algicon	360					320
Alu-cap			194			
Alu-tab			585			
Bisodol		178				
Calcitrel		120	585			
Chooz		500				
Remegel	Mg carbonate codried gel 476.4					
Rolaids (cherry)			550		334	
Rolaids (plain)		64	317			
Tempo	133	81	414	20		
Titralac			420			
Tums			500			
Tums E-X			750			

clude ranitidine (Zantac, Glaxo Wellcome), famotidine (Pepcid, Merck), cimetidine (Tagamet, SmithKline Beechman), nizatidine (Axid, Lilly) have been deregulated by the FDA and are now available OTC, but in much lower doses than prescription doses. Patients should be made aware of this. Although drying of the laryngeal mucosa (from its antihistamine action) is not a major side effect of the H2 blockers, it does occur and must be considered. Occasionally, the drying effects of H2 blockers can be severe enough to cause not only dry mouth, but also dry and irritated eyes. This condition makes it difficult to read scores and causes excessive blinking, especially under spotlights, which can be misinterpreted by an audience as nervousness.

Gastric proton pump (H+/K+ATPase) inhibitors (PPIs) suppress gastric acid production and are generally highly effective in the management of GERD and RL. Medications such as omeprazole (Prilosec, Astra Merck), lansoprazole (Prevacid, TAP), rabeprazole (Aciphex, Janssen), pantoprazole (Protonix, Wyeth-Ayerst), and esomeprazole (Nexium, Astra Zeneca) inhibit the H+/K+ATPase system, which is virtually unique to the gastric parietal cell. H+/K+ATPase competitive inhibitors cause inactivation of the H+/K+ATPase enzyme, suppressing both basal and stimulated gastric acid secretion for prolonged periods of time. In most patients, once or twice daily dosing usually provides excellent control of acid production. Proton pump inhibitors do not adversely affect the lower esophageal sphincter or esophageal motility, but they do slow the linear emptying rate of solids from the stomach.[16] Although the incidence of side effects of PPIs is low, they can cause diarrhea, abdominal pain, and nausea and elevation of liver enzymes (this is also true of most H2 blockers). Dry mouth, esophageal candidiasis, muscle cramps, depression, tremors, dizziness, fatigue, and headaches have also been reported. Resistance to omeprazole has also been reported.[17]

Hyperkinetic agents improve motility and help prevent reflux by increasing the rate of gastric emptying. For several years, metoclopramide (Reglan, Robins) was the only such agent available. Because of troublesome side effects, particularly neurological abnormalities in approximately 10% of patients, the drug was never used extensively in professional singers; and it has now been largely replaced by newer agents. At present, the most commonly prescribed medication in this drug class is cisapride (Propulsid, Janssen). Cisapride increases lower esophageal sphincter pressure and lower esophageal peristalsis, which significantly accelerates gastric emptying of liquids and solids. The most common side effects are headache, abdominal pain, nausea, diarrhea, constipation, dizziness, pharyngitis, depression, dehydration, and rhinitis. Dry mouth, tremor, and somnolence have been reported in less than 1% of patients; and numerous other adverse reactions are seen uncommonly.

Other medications used to treat disorders of the gastrointestinal tract include phenobarbital, prochlorperazine, isopropamide, and propantheline bromide. Members of the belladonna alkaloid group, including scopolamine and atropine, are widely used and prescribed for their antispasmodic effects. All of these agents have a significant drying effect on secretions in the vocal tract.

Not infrequently the laryngologist may encounter a patient who consumes large amounts of vitamin C (ascorbic acid) in an effort to maintain health or to prevent the common cold. However, large amounts of ascorbic acid can irritate the stomach lining and consequently aggravate gastroesophageal reflux laryngitis. In some patients, a drying effect may occur when vitamin C is taken in large doses, probably due to a mild diuretic effect.[18] Additionally, in patients with impaired renal function, high doses of vitamin C may produce acidic urine and possibly renal calculi.

Sleeping Pills

Sleeping pills generally should not be necessary for healthy people. Occasionally, the stresses of a tour and the aggravations of travel, along with frequent changes in time zones, can disturb sleep patterns. For this reason it is appropriate to take a small supply of a mild sleeping medication when traveling and to use it with great caution. These should be prescribed with instructions regarding rebound insomnia and the risk of habituation and physical dependence. Performers should avoid using diphenhydramine (Benadryl, Warner-Lambert), an antihistamine that is a common ingredient in many OTC sleep aids. It is a safe drug and works well, but it produces excessive drying of mucosal membranes.

Analgesics

Aspirin and other analgesics such as ibuprofen are prescribed frequently for relief of minor to moderate pain. The platelet dysfunction caused by aspirin predisposes an individual to bleeding and even hemorrhage, especially in vocal folds traumatized by excessive voice use in the face of vocal dysfunction. A vocal fold hemorrhage can be devastating to a professional voice user; and for this reason, the laryngologist (RTS) prohibits aspirin use and recommends minimal use of

NSAIDs in his singers and all voice patients. However, the author (RTS) has one exception to the aspirin rule for singers and other professional voice users. A low daily dose of aspirin, generally one children's aspirin (81 mg), is used commonly in the treatment of patients with known coronary artery disease and for the prevention of heart disease in others. Because this dosage of aspirin is so small, its potential for jeopardizing the voice is low; and treatment of heart disease always takes precedence over maintenance of a healthy voice. Acetaminophen (Tylenol, McNeil) is the recommended analgesic for mild to moderate pain. The nonsteroidal anti-inflammatory drugs (NSAIDs) such as ibuprofen (Motrin) and ketoprofen (Oruvail, similar to ibuprofen, but taken only once daily) may interfere with the clotting mechanism, and their use is also discouraged in professional voice users.

A new class of analgesics, selective COX-2 inhibitors, is now being used to treat acute and chronic pain. These medications do not interfere with the COX-1 pathway and do not cause bleeding dyscrasias or gastrointestinal side effects as seen with traditional NSAIDs.

Caruso used a spray of ether and iodoform on his vocal folds when he had to sing with laryngitis. However, such use of analgesics is extremely dangerous and should be avoided. Pain has an important protective physiologic function. Masking it risks incurring significant vocal damage that may not be recognized until after the analgesic wears off. If a singer requires analgesics taken orally or topical anesthetics to alleviate laryngeal discomfort, the laryngitis is severe enough to warrant canceling a performance. If the analgesic is used for headache or some other discomfort not directly associated with voice production, symptomatic treatment should be discouraged until singing commitments have been completed or cancelled.

Narcotic analgesics should not be used for any reason shortly before performance, especially if the medications are being used for laryngeal discomfort. Even when the pain is outside the head and neck, narcotics may cause sufficient change in sensorium to impair performance and risk vocal fold injury through unconscious technical voice abuse. As Damsté reported, sedatives and narcotics, in addition to impairing intellectual function, may cause an uninhabited drive to speak and symptoms of dysarthria.[19] Occasional exceptions can be made. For example, if a low dose of codeine early on a performance day is sufficient to control moderate menstrual cramping, its use is certainly not unreasonable. However, if menstrual cramps are so severe that high doses of codeine (in the

60 mg range) are required within a few hours of performance, cancellation may be more appropriate.

Hormones

The most significant group of drugs that can adversely affect the voice are hormones such as androgens and anabolic steroids.[20-25] These drugs cause changes in voice quality by alterations in fluid content and structural changes. Structural alterations in laryngeal architecture seldom occur as the result of pharmacologic influences, but androgens are an exception. They may produce irreversible lowering of fundamental frequencies and coarsening of the voice, especially in females.[22 30] Androgenic agents such as Danocrine (danazol, Sanofi) are used in the treatment of endometriosis, as part of chemotherapy regimens for some breast cancers, and to treat postmenopausal sexual dysfunction and other problems.[31-40] Birth control pills with relatively high progesterone content are most likely to produce androgenlike changes in the voice.[41-48] Most oral contraceptives marketed in the United States now have an appropriate estrogen-progesterone ratio, and voice changes are seen in only about 5% of women who use birth control pills (C. Carroll, MD, and H. von Leden, MD personal communication, September, 1992). These changes generally are temporary, abating when oral contraceptive use is discontinued.

Estrogen replacement is helpful in forestalling the typical voice changes that follow menopause. The conjugated estrogen preparation used most frequently in the United States is Premarin (Prempro). Until recently, the conjugated estrogens were thought to be preferable to estradiol; however, it now appears that there is no real difference with regard to the effect on the voice (J. Abitbol, personal communication, 2001). The progesterone, Provera is often prescribed in combination with Premarin (Prempro). In low doses, natural progesterones usually do not cause significant voice problems. However, some of the synthetic progesterone substitutes have androgenic effects and the potential for permanent virilization of the voice. Unless medical contraindications are present, professional voice users should be offered hormone replacement under appropriate medical supervision at the time of menopause.

Other hormone replacement medications may also affect the voice, often beneficially. Thyroid replacement may restore vocal efficiency and "ring" lost with even a mild degree of hypothyroidism. Agents used to treat maladies in any part of the diencephalic pituitary axis should be presumed to have laryngeal effects and warrant close monitoring of voice function.

Bronchoactive Medications

Phonation depends on the availability of a powerfully supported airstream passing between the vocal folds. Impairment of pulmonary function can cause severe problems for professional voice users. Pulmonary function is affected deleteriously by bronchoconstriction, which occurs in allergic reactions and asthma. These conditions may hamper or prevent vocal performance unless recognized and treated promptly. Bronchodilators can be used to counteract the bronchoconstrictive effects of such environmental factors as house dust, pollen, other inhalant allergens, and common air pollutants produced by our increasingly industrialized society. Bronchodilators often are used to treat patients with reactive airway disease, although inhaled bronchodilators may produce chronic laryngitis, as discussed previously. Clinically, inhaled cromolyn sodium appears to cause fewer problems than most of the other inhalant bronchodilators commonly used in the treatment of asthma. The bronchodilator used most often is epinephrine and its related compounds, including xanthines (aminophylline is an example). In professional voice users, the author (RTS) favors asthma management primarily with oral medications and minimal inhaler use.

Cystic fibrosis is an autosomal recessive disorder in which systemic dysfunction of the exocrine glands causes excessive mucus production in the airways and reduced pulmonary function. Dornase alfa (Pulmozyme, Genectech), an enzyme used in the treatment of cystic fibrosis, has been reported to cause sore throat, hoarseness and other voice alterations, laryngitis, and chest pain.[49] However, these side effects are not severe and generally will subside without adjustment of dosage.

Beta-Blockers

Propanolol (Inderal, Wyeth-Ayerst) and other beta-blockers have been used successfully in the treatment of hypertension, cardiac tachyarrhythmias, and migraine headaches. Beta-blockers also have been used to treat stage fright. British investigators[50] found that instrumental musicians given propanolol did, in fact, exhibit less anxiety during performance; however, a significant response was not seen in voice professionals or musicians.

A subsequent study reported that propranolol, given for preperformance anxiety, lessened anxiety and also produced an increase in salivation.[51] This investigation was conducted by measuring the weight increase in saliva-saturated dental rolls of cotton placed in the mouth during performance. This indicated that the problem of upper respiratory tract secretion dryness had been avoided and that some of the parasympathomimetic effects of performance anxiety had been negated.

Today, laryngologists generally agree that these drugs should not be used by singers or other voice professionals. Beta-blockers are potentially dangerous because they can slow the heart rate, decrease blood pressure, and cause bronchospasm that can trigger asthma attacks in susceptible patients. In addition, when given in doses sufficient to ameliorate stage fright, they produce a lackluster performance.[15] Any professional voice user who requires an ingested substance to perform the daily activities of his or her chosen profession is manifesting a more significant psychological problem and should be referred for appropriate counseling and treatment and not merely medicated.

Neurologic Medications

Professional voice users may be diagnosed with a neurologic disease during evaluation of their voice complaint or have a coexisting illness. A number of highly potent medications are used in the medical management of neurologic disorders. The side effects of some of these medications and/or the course of the illness itself may ultimately force the end of a performance career or, at the very least, require significant modifications. Some of the most common neurologic diseases and the medications used to treat them are discussed.

Parkinson's disease is treated with medications having anticholinergic properties such as L-dopa (and L-dopa in combination with other agents), dopamine receptor agonists, and monamine oxidase inhibitors (MAOIs.) Parkinsonian syndrome, not secondary to Parkinson's disease, may also be a focus of treatment with these drugs.

The MAOIs are also used in the treatment of depression. However, many other drugs used in the treatment of depression also have anticholinergic properties and have been associated with speech disorders, hoarseness, and aphonia.[52,53] Side effects are related to a drug's mechanism of action on the central nervous system and peripheral target organs.[54] Anticholinergic side effects include blurred vision, dryness, impaired urination, constipation, nervousness,

dizziness, and drowsiness, as well as confusion, memory loss, headache, hallucinations, and delusions[55] Side effects most commonly associated with L-dopa are gastrointestinal disturbance, orthostatic hypotension, syncope, oral dryness, blurred vision, and cardiac arrhythmia. Dyskinesias, nightmares, confusion, agitation, psychosis, depression, increased libido, and end-of-dose akinesia have been reported.[55] L-dopa in combination with other agents is used to decrease peripheral and systemic side effects. Amantadine (Symmetrel, Endo Labs) used in the treatment of Parkinson's disease is also used as an antiviral drug to treat influenza.

Dopamine receptor agonists can cause gastrointestinal (GI) disturbance, postural hypotension, and fatigue as well as skin rash, headache, involuntary movements, depression, and sometimes confusion or hallucinations.[49]

Myasthenia gravis is an autoimmune disease in which serum antibodies impair synaptic transmission at the neuromuscular junction by disturbance of the neurotransmitter acetylcholine.[56] Pyridostigmine bromide (Mestinon, ICN) is used to treat myasthenia. Mestinon enhances the action of acetylcholine by inhibiting the enzyme acetylcholinesterase. Excessive salivation and gastrointestinal disturbances are common side effects of acetylcholinesterase inhibitors. Skin rash, nervousness, confusion, or weakness is also reported. Attention deficit disorder (ADD) is a commonly diagnosed medical problem that affects children and adults. Once the diagnosis is confirmed and symptoms persist, medication is indicated. The medication prescribed most often is methylphenidate hydrochloride (Ritalin, Novartis). Most of the time, Ritalin, in appropriate doses, does not cause significant voice problems even in singers. However, it may produce a slight tremor that could, theoretically, be audible in singing.

Multiple sclerosis (MS) involves the progressive loss of myelin in white matter adjacent to the ventricles of the brain, optic nerves, brainstem, cerebellum, and spinal cord.[56] Drug therapy aims at reducing the frequency of exacerbations and/or reducing the degree of myelin loss during an attack. Medications are also used to treat associated symptoms such as spasticity, cerebellar dysfunction, and depression.[55] These medications include immunosuppressants such as corticosteroids, adrenocorticotrophic hormone, azothioprine, and cyclophosphamide. Corticosteroid side effects have been previously discussed. Other immunosuppressants may also be used in patients with an inability to tolerate corticosteroids, but these side effects are potentially extremely serious. Beta-interferon (Avonex, Schering) is a potent immunosuppressant given by injection; its side effects include local inflammation, flulike syndrome, fever, chills, muscle aches, and asthenia. The incidence of these side effects will diminish with continued treatment. The side effects of medications used to treat MS, along with symptoms of the disease, can affect performance but are reported to rarely cause speech disturbance.

Herbs and Supplements

Over the past decade or so, more and more individuals, including singers, are seeking alternatives to medications in the form of herbs and dietary supplements. Many common herbs have potential side effects for voice users; additionally, some herbs should never be taken by anyone because of potentially severe consequences. Some are highlighted in Table 16–4, and selected substances are summarized in greater detail in Table 16–5. In addition, it is helpful to be familiar with some of the most common dietary supplements and their intended usage (Table 16–6).

These dietary supplements are not to be considered prevention, treatment, or cure for any medical problem. Some supplements are dangerous. For example, glucosamine, which is extracted from shellfish, should not be taken by individuals with shellfish allergy. The ingredients of all supplements must be studied carefully, and patients should be encouraged to discuss the use of dietary supplements with their physician before using them. Nevertheless, their use is ubiquitous.

Table 16–4. Herbal Medications and Their Common Risks.

Herbal Medications	Risks Associated with Use
Chaparral, Coltsfoot, Comfrey	Potential for hepatotoxicity
Cowslip	Anticoagulation activity (salicylates)
Dong quai	Anticoagulation activity (coumadin), and alteration in hormonal activity
Dandelion	Diuretic, dehydration
Echinacea	Can be immunosuppressive if used > 8 weeks continuously. Also may induce allergic response.
Elder	Diuretic activity, dehydration
Ephedra (Ma Huang)	Stimulant, potential for seizures, HTN (hypertension), death;
Fennel	Anticoagulation activity (coumadin)
Feverfew	Anticoagulation activity, diuretic activity
Garlic, Ginger, and Ginkgo	Anticoagulation activity (inhibition of platelet aggregation)
Goldenseal	May elevate blood pressure, and cause allergic responses
Jack-in-the-pulpit	Anticoagulation activity
Licorice root	Hormonal activity (estrogen/progesterone); also a steroid and antidiuretic, capable of inducing a cushingoid syndrome/hypertension
Melatonin	Used by many as a sleep aid; it has hormonal activity and can also cause immune dysregulation
Nettles	Diuretic activity
Primrose	Anticoagulation activity (salicylates), hormonal activity
Red Root	Anticoagulation activity
Vitamin E	Taken in megadoses (4000 IU or greater), it has anticoagulation activity (anti-platelet)
Willow bark	Anticoagulation activity (salicylates)
Yam	Hormonal activity (potent progesterone)
Yohimbe	Hormonal activity (androgen/testosterone)

Table 16–5. Herbal Products.

Common Name	Scientific Name	Uses	Adverse Reactions	Comments
Ginkgo, Maidenhair tree	*Ginkgo, Ginkgo biloba*	Memory, and concentration, intermittent claudication, Alzheimer's, altitude sickness	Bleeding, GI upset, headache, palpations, restlessness, nausea, vomiting	Avoid using it with blood thinning medication (eg, coumadin, aspirin), insulin, thiazide diuretics, antidepressants, antipsychotics.
Echinacea, Purple coneflower, Black Sampson	*Echinacea purpura, E. pallida, E. angustifolia*	Common cold, upper respiratory infections (flu)	Liver damage; initially, it stimulates the immune system; after 8 weeks may be immunosuppressive	Avoid using it with liver toxic drugs (methotrexate), calcium channel blockers, (verapamil), anti-anxiety drugs (valium), steroids (prednisone), patients with autoimmune disease (eg, HIV/AIDS); Cross-allergenicity (eg, daisies, ragweed, marigolds).
St John's Wort, SJW, Amber, Goatweed, Klamath weed	*Hypericum perforatum*	Antidepressant, seasonal affective disorder (SAD), anxiety	Insomnia, anxiety, GI upset, vivid dreams, fatigue, photosensitivity, intermenstrual bleeding	Avoid using SJW with herbal or prescription products until you are aware of the adverse reactions and interactions of these medications. Refer to text.
Ephedra, Ma Huang	*Ephedra sinica*	Reduce weight, enhance physical performance	Heart attacks, strokes, seizures, hypertension, death	Avoid its use. Ephedra may be fatal.
Valerian, Phu, Garden heliotrope	*Valeriana officinalis*	Sedative-hypnotic, anxiolytic[81]	Morning drowsiness[82]	Can cause additive effects with alcohol, and other medications that have sedative properties.
Ginseng, Korean and American ginseng.	*Panax ginseng* (Korean); *Panax quinque-folium* (American)	Improves cognitive function;[83] lowers fasting blood glucose[84]	Agitation, insomnia nervousness; Estrogenic effects may cause vaginal bleeding	Avoid using with caffeine, blood thinning, and antidiabetic medications.
Saw Palmetto, Dwarf palm tree	*Serenoa repens,*	Benign prostatic hypertrophy, (BPH)	Infrequently, GI upset, an instance of intraoperative hemorrhage	Improves urinary symptoms of BPH with fewer side effects[85] compared to the drug finasteride (Proscar). Use cautiously if at all with blood thinning medication.

(continues)

Table 16–5. *(continued)*

Common Name	Scientific Name	Uses	Adverse Reactions	Comments
Horse Chestnut (seed)	*Aesculus hippocastanum*	Chronic venous insufficiency (CVI), varicose veins	GI upset, kidney toxicity[86]	Useful for CVI[87]; avoid use with blood thinning medication; monitor glucose levels in diabetic patients.
Pycnogenol, Pine bark extract	*Pinus maritime, P. pinaster*	CVI, varicose veins,[88] diabetic and other retinopathies	None reported	Reduces edema by decreasing capillary permeability
Milk Thistle	*Silybum marianum*	Cirrhosis of the liver, hepatitis, jaundice, liver poisoning (eg, mushroom poisoning)	Occasional laxative effects	A member of the daisy family, the German E Commission (comparable to FDA in USA) has approved its use for liver disorders as noted here under "use"
Garlic	*Allium sativum*	Lowers LDH (low density lipoprotein) & cholesterol[89]	Halitosis, GI upset	Can increase the risk of bleeding; The therapeutic effect is modest compared to other cholesterol-lowering drugs.
Kava, Kava-Kava	*Piper methysticum*	Stress, anxiety disorders[90]	Liver toxicity, gastrointestinal (GI) upset, headache, dizziness.	Avoid using it. Several European governments have banned its use. Especially harmful in combination with liver toxic drugs, sedatives, sleeping pills, alcohol, levadopa (Parkinson's disease).

Complementary, Alternative, and Integrated Medicine

Millions of Americans spend billions of dollars annually on complementary alternative medicine (CAM), and many of these are herbal products. Some CAM herbal preparations are useful, others have no proven efficacy. Some are safe, others are potentially harmful. The quality of the product may vary from one manufacturing company to another. Occasionally, the ingredients listed on the label do not correspond to the product in the bottle. The recommended dosage is not uniformly agreed-on, and the manufacturers of herbal products are not regulated sufficiently at this time. Some singers and other voice patients use CAM indiscriminately; and it behooves them, their teachers, and their health care providers to become familiar with the potential benefits and risks of taking complementary and alternative remedies.

Complementary medicine uses therapies "along with" conventional medicine (eg, the use of massage for low back pain "along with" muscle relaxants). *Alternative* medicine uses therapies "in place" of conventional medicine (eg, homeopathy to treat rheuma-

Table 16–6. Other Natural Products.

Other Natural Products	What They Are Used For

Supplements
    Glucosamine
    Chondroitin
    Calcium
    Vitamin D
    Sam-e
    Ipriflavone
	Bones and joints

Herbals
    Ginkgo biloba
    Ginseng
    Niacin
    Folic acid
    Riboflavin
    Zinc
    Copper
    Vitamin B6 and B12
	Memory and mental acuity

Stanol Esters
    Garlic
    Vitamin B complex
    Folic acid, E, D, and K
    Calcium
	Control cholesterol and healthy heart

Isoflavones Black cohosh (Botanical)	Supplements menopause symptoms

For Men: Herbals
    Jujube dates, Ginseng, Ginkgo biloba;
    Amino Acids—Arginine Alanine, Lysine,
    Glutamic acid, Vitamins, B-Vitamins
	Sex drive and function

For Women: Herbals
    Wild Yam, Chaste Berry,
    Avena Sativa, Vitamin E
	Sex drive and function

toid arthritis or the unsuccessful attempt to treat cancer with laetrile). *Integrative* medicine incorporates proven effective outcomes of CAM with conventional medicine.

CAM is not limited to herbal products. Homeopathy uses principles of similars and dilutions. Similars work on the concept that if a specific substance causes symptoms in a healthy person similar to that of an ill patient, that substance can be used to cure the sick individual ("like cures like"). Dilutions use the principle that small doses "stimulate" a beneficial immune response or "vital force" in the body.

Traditional Chinese medicine incorporates acupuncture and herbal remedies. Chiropractors and osteopaths use manipulation techniques. Some CAM practitioners utilize massage, hypnosis, biofeedback, or meditation; others use prayer and spirituality, energy, or naturopathy as well as a host of other modalities.

The field of alternative and complementary medicine is vast. As of February 2003, the on-line research resource Pub-Med of the National Library of Medicine cites more than 220,000 publications, abstracts or full articles. The challenge is to weed out the useful from the useless and the safe from the dangerous.

Herbal products come from plants that have been investigated for their biochemical composition and potential use as medication. The distinction between herbal products and conventional drugs is gradually being obliterated. All biochemical products are potential poisons. The side effects of medications, although usually minor, may at times be disabling, devastating, or even fatal, whether it is an herbal product or conventional drug. When one introduces a foreign substance into the body, there is the potential for an adverse reaction. Singers take herbal products for a variety of reasons, and many erroneously equate "natural" with safe and effective.

Quality Control and Product Regulation

Pharmaceutical companies must go through several phases before their drugs can be sold to the public. The safety, effectiveness, and side effects of the product must meet premarket standards of the Federal Drug Administration (FDA).

In contrast, when Congress passed the 1994 Dietary Supplement Health and Education Act (DSHEA), CAM manufacturers were allowed to put their products on the market without quality control standards. This "free ride" is now being challenged by the FDA, which proposed regulations regarding the purity, quality, and strength of the products (recommended daily doses).[57]

The FDA has documented cases of supplements that have been contaminated with lead, instances in which the declared amount of an ingredient (isoflavone) was lacking by 50%, probiotics, lacking by 99%, and an instance in which the strength of a product (niacin) had been increased by a factor of 10, resulting in nausea, vomiting, heart attack, and liver damage before the manufacturer recalled the product.[57] Contamination of herbal products has occurred with microorganisms (eg, *Staphylococcus aureus*), heavy metals (ie, lead, mercury, arsenic), radioactive agents (I-131), pesticides (DDT), microbial toxins (bacterial endotoxins), other plants (digitalis, belladonna), and fumigation agents (ethylene oxide) and adulterated with analgesics, diuretics, nonsteroidal anti-inflammatory medication, and steroids.[58]

Until better labeling and manufacturing controls are put in place, one must be especially diligent about purchasing supplements and herbal products from reputable companies with standardized formulations. The FDA has proposed rules regarding the labeling and manufacturing of supplements and herbal products; but it has not addressed the question of safety and efficacy of these preparations, yet.

Herbal Products

Hundreds of herbal products (alone or in combination) are marketed in the United States. CAM manufacturers are not allowed legally to claim their product cures or prevents disease; but they can and have claimed that products boost the immune system, burn fat, enhance stamina and energy, stimulate mental function, fight fatigue, improve memory, elevate mood, fight osteoporosis, and many other assertions. Below (and in Table 16–6) are selective considerations of herbal products.

Kava

Kava, also known as Kava-Kava, is derived from the plant *Piper methysticum,* and is a member of the piper family, a plant native to the South Pacific islands. People use kava to treat restlessness, and to reduce stress and anxiety. Studies support the effectiveness of kava for short-term use (1–8 weeks) for anxiety disorders.[59,60] Kava's ingredients, known as kava-lactones, have an anxiolytic (calming) and sedative effect.

One of the problems with kava is that it can cause unpredictable, severe liver damage, which has required liver transplants in several patients.[61,62] Hepatitis, cirrhosis, and liver failure have been reported, as well as adverse effects including jaundice (yellowing of the skin), gastrointestinal upset, and impaired motor reflexes. Of paramount concern, the use of kava has been implicated in deaths due to liver toxicity.

Some countries have limited its distribution or banned its use (Switzerland, Germany, Canada). If one cannot ascertain a set dosage for kava or the mechanism by which it is broken down in the body, the consumption of products containing kava poses an unacceptable health risk, and it should be avoided. Certainly, the health risk is heightened in patients with liver problems or those who use drugs, herbs, or products with effects or side effects similar to kava. For example, antihistamines, sedatives, alcohol, sleeping pills, St. John's wort, ginseng, and chamomile are among the substances that can heighten drowsiness, as well as place one more at risk for liver damage.

Ginkgo Biloba

The ginkgo tree, which comes from China, Korea, and Japan, has been around for more than two hundred million years, can live more than one thousand years, and is considered by some to be one of the wonders of the world, a "living fossil."[63] Extracts of the gingko leaves contain active ingredients such as flavonoids, terpenoids that have antioxidant and anticoagulant (blood thinning) properties. The majority of studies indicate that gingko is likely to be effective in helping concentration and memory and can help circulation for "intermittent claudication" (pain in the lower legs after walking due to vascular insufficiency).

The usual dose of ginkgo can cause palpations, gastrointestinal episodes, headache, and other side effects. Large doses can cause nausea, vomiting, and restlessness. One of the most worrisome, potential side effects of gingko is excessive spontaneous bleeding. There have been reports of spontaneous brain hemorrhage, and excessive post-operative bleeding associated with gingko use.[64-66] These are rare occurrences, but potentially devastating.

It is conceivable that inappropriate use of ginkgo in singers could be a contributing factor in vocal fold hemorrhage, particularly in combination with anticlotting products such as aspirin, nonsteroidal anti-inflammatory drugs (NSAIDs), coumadin, or other herbs such as garlic, ginger, or ginseng. Ginkgo extract can alter blood glucose levels. Therefore, in diabetic patients using insulin, glucose monitoring should be done more frequently.[67] Ginkgo may reduce the effectiveness of seizure medications and should be used cautiously or avoided totally in patients prone to seizures disorders.[68] Ginkgo might interfere with fertility and generally should not be used by couples who are trying to conceive.[69] People taking thiazide, a diuretic, should avoid using gingko leaves because it can increase blood pressure.[70]

Echinacea

Echinacea is a perennial herb that is native to the United States. *Echinacea purpura* is the plant most frequently used for research and herbal treatment. People use this American purple coneflower to treat upper respiratory infections, influenza, and the common cold, as well as a myriad of other conditions.[71] Echinacea seems to be most effective in reducing the duration and severity of certain symptoms of the common cold or influenza if it is taken when symptoms first appear and continued for 7 to 10 days. Certain allergic patients should avoid taking echinacea, particularly if they are allergic to ragweed, marigolds, daisies, chrysanthemums, or chamomile.

Echinacea, in the short term, can have a stimulating effect on the immune system. However, if it is used for more than 8 weeks, it may suppress the immune system and may cause liver damage.[72] Because echinacea might stimulate the autoimmune system, it should be avoided in individuals with autoimmune disorders such as multiple sclerosis, rheumatoid arthritis, and perhaps patients with HIV/AIDS.[73] If a patient has liver problems or is taking medications that potentially can cause liver toxicity such as methotrexate (a chemotherapeutic agent that is sometimes used for rheumatoid arthritis and autoimmune ear disease), he or she should avoid taking echinacea.

St John's Wort

St. John's wort is an herb with yellow flowers derived from *Hypericum perforatum*, which is cultivated in the United States, Africa, Asia, and Europe. In the Middle Ages, people used St. John's wort to cast out evil spirits for afflictions such as mental illness. Wort, not to be confused with "wart," comes from the old English *wyrt*, meaning plant. One explanation for the plant's common name is that its flowers typically blossom around June 24th, the birthday of St. John the Baptist. However, there are other folklore explanations for its name.

St. John's wort is as effective as traditional antidepressant medication with fewer side effects for mild to moderate depression[74] and for seasonal affective disorder (SAD), a depression peaking in the fall/winter and declining during the spring/summer when there is more sunlight.

The side effects of St. John's wort, although uncommon, include insomnia, dry mouth, upset stomach, fatigue, dizziness, photosensitivity (hypersensitivity to light), and headache. This herb should be used cautiously with other antidepressants such as nefazodone (Serzone, Bristol-Myers-Squib), sertraline (Zoloft, Pfizer), or paroxetine (Paxil, Glaxo-Smith-Kline), because it might cause serotonin syndrome, a serious complication resulting in an increase in serotonin levels that may result in hypertension, extreme anxiety, tachycardia (increase in heart rate), confusion, and coma.[75] The herb may reduce the therapeutic effect of digitalis, decrease the concentration of oral contraceptives causing break-through bleeding and possibly pregnancy, and decrease the concentration of protease inhibitors and medications used for HIV/AIDS patients. It should be avoided with tetracycline, sulfa, and quinolones (eg, Cipro); because in combination with these drugs, it can contribute to an increased sensitivity to sunlight with resultant dermatitis, inflamed mucous membranes, and oral blistering. The interaction of St. John's wort with certain amino acids, for example, tyramine-containing foods (red wine, chocolate, cheese, eggs) and tryptophan (cottage cheese, beef liver, fish, peanuts), might cause a hypertensive crisis.[76] People with hypertension should be especially alert to these interactions of St. John's wort.

Ephedra, Ma Huang

Ephedra comes principally from *Ephedra sinica*, a shrublike plant that is native to China. It should be distinguished from the alkaloid-free American ephedra or Mormon tea, which does not have either the toxicity or therapeutic effects of ephedra.

For thousands of years, the Chinese have used ephedra in pill or tea form for asthma, cough, and the common cold. Today, ephedra is used most commonly to lose weight and to improve physical performance. It is clinically related to amphetamine (speed) and is found in a variety of products. Aspiring singers may use it to lose weight. A milder form of ephedra, pseudoephedrine, is found in many decongestants, cold, and cough medicines.

Side effects from ephedra are not infrequent and can be life-threatening. It has been linked to heart attacks, hypertension, stroke, and seizures; and some such incidents have occurred in young professional athletes. Ephedra can constrict blood vessels, increase heart rate, and cause thermogenesis (elevation of the body temperature) and heat stroke. It has been associated with personality changes and dependency after long-term use.[77,78]

The interaction of ephedra with caffeinated drinks can increase the side effects of nervousness, insomnia, and dizziness. It can make some steroids less effective, elevate blood glucose, and should be avoided in patients with conditions such as angina, anxiety, heart disease, hypothyroidism, hypertension, and urinary retention (eg, patients with enlarged prostates).

The Federal Drug Administration has received hundreds of reports linking ephedra or ephedrine use to serious side effects including deaths. Until better guidelines are formulated, it is best to avoid ephedra products.

Surgery and Herbal Products

One should avoid herbal medications for at least 14 days prior to surgery according to the American Society of Anesthesiologists.[79] Ginkgo, ginger, ginseng, and garlic can contribute to excessive bleeding. Valerian and kava can potentiate (increase) the sedative effects of anesthetics. Ephedra can provoke hypertension, cardiac irregularities, and temperature elevation. Ginseng can lower blood sugar.[80] Kava and echinacea can cause liver damage, particularly in conjunction with certain anesthetic agents that may also be toxic to the liver. Preoperatively, patients should let their surgeon and anesthesiologist know about "all" of the medications they are taking including all herbal and other CAM products.

Conclusion

It is essential for laryngologists, nurses, speech-language pathologists, singing voice teachers, vocal coaches, and others involved in caring for professional voice users to be familiar with the potential vocal effects of all ingested substances, including medications. This chapter reviewed only a small number of the pharmacological agents that may affect voice adversely. It is also incumbent on health care providers to educate voice professionals about the action of medications and the potential consequences of drugs (prescription and nonprescription) on the voice, thus enabling individuals to make an informed consent for recommended treatment.

In general, herbal therapies and conventional drugs are safe. Legally, herbs are foods that do not treat or cure disease. However, in the medical world, they are drugs that can help or hurt one's well-being.

Even if the FDA imposes premarket safety and efficacy standards, singers and other voice professionals should take herbal products for the right reasons, at the right time, and from reputable manufacturers who have standardized the formulations of their products. They should let responsible people know what medications they are taking and recognize that at certain times they will be at greater risks compared to others because of the use of these substances.

The side effects, interactions, lack of quality control and proven effectiveness of some herbal preparations have serious ramifications for professional voice users and the risks may seriously outweigh the benefits. What is on the label may neither work nor be in the bottle. Until more randomized control trials are done to substantiate the safety and usefulness of herbal products, one should use caution in buying supplements.

Singing and acting teachers and laryngologists are in a unique position to influence the behavior of their clients. The examples given above highlight several of the great many herbal products available, and they emphasize the need for all of us who interact with voice performers to be aware of the strengths and limitations of CAM and to educate the singers and other voice professionals under our care.

References

1. Sataloff RT, Lawrence VL, Hawkshaw M, Rosen DC. Medications and their effects on the voice. In: Benninger, MS, Jacobson BH, Johnson AF, eds. *Vocal Arts Medicine: The Care and Prevention of Professional Voice Disorders.* New York, NY: Thieme Medical Publishers; 1994:216–225.

2. Lawrence VL. Common medications with laryngeal effects. *Ear Nose Throat J.* 1987;66(8):318–322.

3. Schiff M. Medical management of acute laryngitis. In: Lawrence VL, ed. *Transcripts of the Sixth Symposium: Care of the Professional Voice.* New York, NY: The Voice Foundation; 1977:99–102.

4. Schiff M. Comment at the Seventh Symposium: Care of the Professional Voice. The Juilliard School;1978; New York, NY.

5. Punt NA. Vocal disabilities of singers. Applied laryngology—singers and actors. *Proc R Soc Med.* 1968;61:1152–1156.

6. Williams AJ, Baghat MS, Stableforth DE, et al. Dysphonia caused by inhaled steroids: recognition of a characteristic laryngeal abnormality. *Thorax.* 1983;38:813–821.

7. Watkin KL, Ewanowski SJ. Effects of aerosol corticosteroids on the voice: triamcinolone acetonide and beclomethasone dipropionate. *J Speech Hear Res.* 1985;28:301–304.

8. Toogood JH, Jennings B, Greenway RW, Chuang L. Candidiasis and dysphonia complicating beclomethasone treatment of asthma. *J Allergy Clin Immunol.* 1980; 65(2):145–153.

9. Davies WL, Grunert RR, Haff RF, et al. Antiviral activity of 1-amantanamine (amantadine). *Science.* 1964;144: 862–863.

10. McGahen JW, Hoffman CE. Influenza infections of mice. I. Curative activity of amantadine HCl. *Proc Soc Exp Biol Med.* 1968;129:678–681.

11. Wingfield WL, Pollack D, Grunert RR. Therapeutic efficacy of amantadine-HCl and rumantidine-HCl in naturally occurring influenza A2 respiratory illness in man. *N Engl J Med.* 1969;281:579–584.

12. Council on Drugs. The amantadine controversy. *JAMA.* 1967;201:372–373.

13. Martin FG. Drugs and vocal function. *J Voice.* 1988;2(4): 338–344.

14. *Nursing '89 Drug Handbook.* Springhouse, Pa: Springhouse Corporation; 1989:236.

15. Gates GA, Saegert J, Wilson N, et al. Effect of beta-blockade on singing performance. *Ann Otol Rhinol Laryngol.* 1985;94:570–574.

16. Rasmussen L, Oster-Jorgensen E, Qvist N, et al. Short report: a double-blind placebo-controlled trial of omeprazole on characteristics of gastric emptying in healthy subjects. *Aliment Pharmacol Ther.* 1991;5:85–89.

17. Bough ID Jr, Sataloff RT, Castell DO, et al. Gastroesophageal reflux laryngitis resistant to omeprazole therapy. *J Voice.* 1995;9(2):205–211.

18. Lawrence VL. Medical care for professional voice. {[Panel.] In: Lawrence VL, ed. *Transcripts from the Annual Symposium: Care of the Professional Voice.* New York, NY: The Voice Foundation; 1978:3:17–18.

19. Damsté PH. Changes in the voice caused by drugs. In: Meyer L, Pach HM, eds. *Drug Induced Diseases.* Amsterdam, The Netherlands: Excerpta Medica; 1978:543–548.

20. Damsté PH. [Virilization of the voice due to anabolic steroids.] *Ned Tijdschr Geneeskd.* 1963;107:891–892.

21. Damsté PH. Voice change in adult women caused by virilizing agents. *J Speech Hear Disord.* 1967;32:126–132.

22. Derman RJ. Effects of sex steroids on women's health: implication for practitioners. *Am J Med.* 1995;98(1A):137S–143S.

23. Pinsky L, Kaufman M, Killinger DW. Impaired spermatogenesis is not an obligate expression of receptor defective androgen resistance. *Am J Med Genet.* 1989;32(1): 100–104.

24. Rolf C, Nieschlag E. Potential adverse effects on long-term testosterone therapy. *Baillieres Clin Endocrinol Metab.* 1998;12(3):521–534.

25. Pedersen MF, Moller S, Krabbe S, et al. Fundamental voice frequency in female puberty measured with electroglottography during continuous speech as a secondary sex characteristic. A comparison between voice, pubertal stages, oestrogens and androgens. *Int J Pediatr Otorhinolaryngol.* 1990;20(1):17–24.

26. Saez S, Francoise S. Recepteurs dandrogenes: mise en evidence dans la fraction cytosolique de muqueuse normale et d'epitheliomas pharyngolarynges humains. *CR Acad Sci (Paris).* 1975;280:935–938.

27. Vuorenkoski V, Lenko HL, Tjernlund P, et al. Fundamental voice frequency during normal and abnormal growth, and after androgen treatment. *Arch Dis Child.* 1978;53:201–209.

28. Arndt HJ. Stimmstörungen nach Behandlung mit androgenen und anabolen hormonen. *Munch Med Wochenschr.* 1974;116:1715–1720.

29. Bourdial J. Les troubles de la voix provoques par la therapeutique hormonale androgene. *Ann Otolaryngol Chir Cervicofac.* 1970;87:725–734.

30. Joura EA, Zeisler H, Brancher-Todesca D, et al. Short-term effects of topical testosterone in vulvar lichen sclerosus. *Obstet Gynecol.* 1997;89(2):297–299.

31. Hansen J, Eckert L, Mlytz H. Sex hormones and carcinoma of the larynx in women. *Arch Klin Exp Ohren Nasen Kehlkopfheilkd.* 1969;193(3):277–286.

32. Slayden SM. Risks of menopausal androgen supplementation. *Semin Reprod Endocrinol.* 1998;16(2):145–152.

33. Need AG, Durbridge TC, Nordin BE. Anabolic steroids in postmenopausal osteoporosis. *Wien Med Wochenschr.* 1993;143(14–15):392–395.

34. Petit JC, Klein T, Rodier D. Hormone therapy for advanced breast cancer with drostanolone propionate. *Bull Cancer.* 1971;58(4):511–522.

35. Wardle PG, Whitehead MI. Non reversible and wide ranging voice changes after treatment with danazol. *Brit Med J.* 1983;287:540.

36. Gelfand MM, Witta B. Androgen and estrogen-androgen hormone replacement therapy: a review of the safety literature, 1941–1996. *Clin Ther.* 1997;19(3):383–404; discussion 367–368.

37. Abitbol J, Abitbol B. [The voice and menopause: the twilight of the divas.] *Contracep Fertil Sex.* 1998;26(9):649–655.

38. Mercaitis PA, Peaper RE, Schwartz PA. Effect of danazol on vocal pitch: a case study. *Obstet Gynecol.* 1985;65: 131–135.

39. Sorgo W, Zachmann M. [Virilization caused by methandrostenoline-containing cream in prepubertal girls.] *Helv Paediatric Acta.* 1982;37(4):401–406.

40. Abitbol J, Abitbol P, Abitbol B. Sex hormones and the female voice. *J Voice.* 1999;13(3):424–446.

41. Dordain M. Étude statistique de l'influence des contraceptifs hormonaux sur la voix. *Folia Phoniatr.* 1972;24: 86–96.

42. Pahn V, Goretzlehner G. Stimmstörungen durch hormonale Kontrazeptiva. *Zentralb Gynakol.* 1978;100:341–346.

43. Schiff M. The "pill" in otolaryngology. *Trans Am Acad Ophthalmol Otolaryngol.* 1968;72:76–84.

44. Brodnitz F. Medical care preventive therapy. In Lawrence V, ed. *Transcripts of the Seventh Annual Symposium: Care of the Professional Voice.* New York, NY: The Voice Foundation; 1978:3:86.

45. Bausch J. Effects and side-effects of hormonal contraceptives in the region of the nose, throat and ear. [In German]. *HNO.* 1983;31(12):409–414.

46. Could contraceptives with progestational effect cause voice change? [In Dutch]. *Ned Tijdschr Geneeskd.* 1975;119(44):1726–1727.

47. Krahulec I, Urbanova O, Simko S. Voice changes during hormonal contraception. [In Czech]. *Cesk Otolaryngol.* 1977;26(4):234–237.

48. Wendler J. Cyclicly dependent variations in efficiency of the voice and its influencing by ovulation inhibitors. [In German]. *Folia Phoniatr* (Basel).1972;24(4):259–277.

49. Ramsey BW, Astley SJ, Aitken ML, et al. Efficacy and safety of short-term administration of aerolized recombinant human deoxyribonuclease in patients with cystic fibrosis. *Am Rev Respir Dis.* 1993;148:145–151.

50. James IM, Griffith DN, Pearson RM, Newbury P. Effect of oxprenolol on stage-fright in musicians. *Lancet.* 1977;2:952–954.

51. Brantigan CO, Brantigan TA, Joseph N. Effect of beta blockade and beta stimulation on stage fright. *Am J Med.* 1982;72(1):88–94.

52. Lyskowski JC, Dunner FJ. Hoarseness and tricyclic antidepressants. *Am J Psychiatry.* 1980;137:636.

53. Rhoads JH, Lowell SH, Hedgepeth EM. Hoarseness and aphonia as a side effect of tricyclic antidepressants. *Am J Psychiatry.* 1979;136:1599.

54. Vogel D, Carter J. *The Effects of Drugs on Communication Disorders.* San Diego, Calif: Singular Publishing Group, Inc; 1995:29–135.

55. Schatzberg A, Cole J. *Manual of Clinical Psychopharmacology* 2nd ed. Washington, DC: APA Press; 1991:40, 50, 55, 58, 66, 68, 69, 72, 73–77, 110–125, 158–165, 169–177, 185–227, 313–348

56. Sataloff RT, Mandel S, Caputo Rosen D. Neurological disorders affecting the voice in performance. In: Sataloff RT. *Professional Voice: The Science and Art of Clinical Care.* 2nd ed. San Diego, Calif: Singular Publishing Group, Inc; 1997:479–498.

57. US Food and Drug Administration. FDA proposes labeling and manufacturing standards for all dietary supplements. *FDA News.* March 7, 2003. Available at: http://www.fda.gov/bbs/topics/NEWS/2003/NEW 00876.html

58. Ernst E, Pittler MH. Herbal medicine. *Med Clin North Am.* 2002;86(1)149–161.

59. Pittler MH, Ernst E. Efficacy of kava extract for treating anxiety: systemic review and meta-analysis. *J Clin Psychopharymacol.* 2000;20(1):84–89.

60. Volz HP, Kieser N. Kava-kava extract. WS 1490 vs. placebo in anxiety disorders—a randomized placebo-controlled 25-week outpatient trial. *Pharmacopsychiatry.* 1997;30(1):1–5.

61. Escher N, Desmeules J, Giostra E, Gilles M. Hepatitis associated with Kava, an herbal remedy for anxiety. *Br Med J.* 2001;322:139.

62. Shaver K. Liver toxicity with Kava. *Pharm Lett/Prescrib Lett.* 2001;18:180115. [Online journals available at: http://www.pharmacistsletter.com and http://www.prescribersletter.com]

63. Murray MT. *The Healing Power of Herbs.* Rocklin, Calif: Prima Publishing; 1995.

64. Gilbert J. Ginkgo biloba. *Neurology.* 1997;48:1137.

65. Rowin J, Lewis SL. Spontaneous bilateral subdural hematomas with chronic Ginkgo biloba ingestion. *Neurology.* 1996;46:1775–1776.

66. Fesseden JN, Wittenborn WW, Clarke L. Ginkgo biloba: a case report of herbal medicine and bleeding postoperatively from a laparoscopic cholecystectomy. *Am Surg.* 2001:67:33–35.

67. Kudolo GB. The effect of 3-month ingestion of Ginkgo biloba extract on pancreatic beta-cell function in response to glucose loading in normal glucose tolerant individuals. *J Clin Pharmacol.* 2000;40(6):647–654

68. Gregory BJ. A seizure associated with Ginkgo biloba? *Ann Internal Med.* 2001;134(4):324.

69. Ondrizek RR, Chan PJ, Patton WC, King A. Inhibition of human sperm motility by specific herbs used in alternative medicines. *J Assist Reprod Genet.* 1999;16:87–91.

70. Jellin MJ, Gregory BJ, Patz S, Hitchens K, et al. *Natural Medicine Comprehensive Data Base.* 4th ed. Stockton, Calif: Therapeutic Research Factory; 2002:589.

71. Brinkeborn RN, Shah DV, Degenring FH. Echinaforce and other Echinacea fresh plant preparations in the treatment of the common cold. A randomized, placebo controlled, double-blind clinical trial. *Phytomedicine.* 1999;6:1–6.

72. Giles JT, Palat CT III, Chien SH, et al. Evaluation of echinacea for the treatment of the common cold. *Pharmacotherapy.* 2000;20(6):690–697.

73. Bruss K, ed. *The American Cancer Society Guide to Complimentary and Alternative Cancer Methods Handbook.* Atlanta, Ga: American Cancer Society; 2000:273.

74. Kim HL, Streltzer J, Goebert D. St. John's wort for depression: a meta-analysis of well-defined clinical trials. *J Nerv Ment Dis.* 1999;187:532–538.

75. Brown TM. Acute St. John's wort toxicity. *Am J Emerg Med.* 2000;18:231–232.

76. Miller LG. Herbal medicinals: selective clinical considerations focusing on known or potential drug-herb interactions. *Arch Int Med.* 1998;158:2200–2201.

77. Doyle H, Kargin N. Herbal stimulant containing ephedrine has also caused psychosis. *Br J Med.* 1996;313 (7059):756.

78. Haller CA, Benowitz ML. Adverse cardiovascular and central nervous system events associated with dietary supplements containing ephedra alkaloids. *N Eng J Med.* 2000;343(25):1833–1838.

79. Sabar R, Kaye AD, Frost, EA. Perioperative considerations for the patient taking herbal medicines. *Heart Dis.* 2001;3(2):87–96.

80. Surow JB, Lovetri J. "Alternative medical therapy" use among singers: prevalence and implications for the medical care of the singer. *J Voice.* 2000;14(3):398–409.

81. Blumenthal M, Busse W, Golberg A, et al, eds. *The Complete German Commission E Monographs: Therapeutic Guide to Herbal Medicines.* Austin Tex: American Botanical Council; 1998.

82. Kuhlmann J., Berger W, Podzuweit H, Schmidt U. The influence of valerian treatment on "reaction time, alertness, and concentration" in volunteers. *Pharmacopsychiatry*. 1999;32(6):235–241.

83. Sorensen H, Sonne J. A double-masked study of the effects of ginseng on cognitive function. *Curr Ther Res*. 1996;57(12):959–68276.

84. Sotaniemi EA Haapkoski E, Rautio A. Ginseng therapy in non-insulin-dependent diabetic patients. *Diabetes Care*. 1995;18(10):1373–1375.

85. Wilt TJ, Ishani A, Stark G, et al. Saw palmetto extracts for treatment of benign prostatic hyperplasia: a systematic review. *JAMA*. 1998;200:1604–1609.

86. Jellin MJ, Gregory BJ, Patz S, Hitchens K, et al. *Natural Medicine Comprehensive Data Base*. 4th ed. Stockton, Calif: Therapeutic Research Center. 2002:695.

87. Pittler MH, Ernst E: Horse-chestnut seed extract for chronic venous insufficiency: *Arch Dermatol*. 1998;134: 1356–1360.

88. Arcangeli P. Pycnogenol in chronic venous insufficiency *Fitoterapia*. 2000;71:236–244.

89. Sunter WH. Warfarin and Garlic. *Pharm J*. 1991;246:722

90. Pittler MH, Ernst E. Efficacy of kava extract for treating anxiety: systematic review and meta-analysis. *J Clin Psychopharmacol*. 2000;20:84–89.

17

Botulinum Toxin in Otolaryngology

Michael C. Neuenschwander, Edmund A. Pribitkin, and Robert Thayer Sataloff

Botulinum toxin (BT) is of interest to otolaryngologists for several reasons. First, it is becoming increasingly popular as a treatment for several otolaryngologic disorders including spasmodic dysphonias, hemifacial spasms, facial wrinkles, and cricopharyngeal spasms. Second, although its neurotoxic properties have been known about for 100 years, it is only in the last 15 years or so that we have begun to understand its structure and mechanism of action. Still, there is much we do not know about this substance, and we are in the infancy phase of its use as a diagnostic and therapeutic agent.[1] Ongoing research is helping to clarify some of the less understood biochemical aspects of BT as well as addressing the problems we face in using it as a chemical denervator.[2] Areas of investigation include the long-term effects, optimal treatment regimens, and reasons for treatment failure. We review the development of this interesting biological agent to clarify its importance in otolaryngology and its potential for future clinical uses.

History and Epidemiology

Botulism results from consumption of contaminated foods, and it can lead to muscle paralysis, suffocation, and death. The disease was first described in the late 1700s, but the toxin itself was not purified until the 1940s.[3] Interest in BT was high during World War II when reports were circulated that the Axis countries had developed the capability to use certain toxins against humans. This spurred the United States Army to study BT and other biologic toxins. Research continued until 1972, when the United States and several other nations signed the Biological and Toxins Weapons Convention agreement, which called for the ter-

mination of research on biologic agents that could be used in warfare. The study of BT for therapeutic purposes was carried on by Schantz at the University of Wisconsin and by Scott at the Smith-Kettlewell Eye Institute in San Francisco.[3]

In the United States alone, more than 100,000 persons experience some form of involuntary muscle spasm.[3] BT has been used successfully for over 25 years to treat the pain, disfigurement, and embarrassment that result from dystonias. In 1978, Scott received approval from the Food and Drug Administration (FDA) to use BT to treat patients with strabismus.[4,5] In 1989, the FDA approved the substance for use in patients with blepharospasm and hemifacial spasm. To date, these are the only FDA-approved indications.[6]

Botulinum Toxin

Structure

BT is a neurotoxin produced primarily by *Clostridium botulinum*, an anaerobic bacterium. There are seven immunologic types of BT, types A through G. Type A is the most useful clinically, but other types such as B, E, and F are being studied as potential alternatives.[7-9] In this chapter, unless otherwise indicated, we are referring to BT type A. The gene that encodes the toxin has been isolated and sequenced.[8] The toxin is synthesized as a weakly active, single chain polypeptide. When exposed to a protease, it becomes fully active in the form of a dichain molecule. The dichain is made up of a heavy chain that is responsible for binding to the end-terminal at the neuromuscular junction (NMJ), and a light chain that is responsible for blocking transmitter release. Purified toxin is unstable and loses biologic activity over time.[7] Therefore, hemagglutinin must be added to form the mixture that is intended for human therapeutic use.

Sites of Action

BT binds with high affinity to cholinergic nerve endings, including motor nerves and autonomic nerves. Motor nerves are the most sensitive to the toxin. Small quantities of BT can undergo retrograde axonal transport to the central nervous system, but there is no evidence that this has any effect in humans.[8] To exert its effect when injected into muscle, the toxin relies on cell surface receptors to become internalized. In the laboratory, however, BT can be injected directly into cells, including non-neural cells, to block acetylcholine release.Because different serotypes of BT do not share the same receptor, they can have slightly different actions inside cells. These differences may be advantageous for clinical medicine. The possibility exists that some patients will respond better to one serotype than another, and a combination of serotypes (chimeras) might be more efficacious than any single one. A combination of serotypes might also permit us to use smaller doses and thus lessen the likelihood of antibody production.[6]

Mechanism of Action

BT blocks the release of acetylcholine from cholinergic nerve endings. Three steps are involved in neuromuscular blockade. First, binding is mediated by the toxin's heavy chain. The receptors are unique and localized to the neuromuscular junction (NMJ). By itself, this step does not result in transmission blockade. The toxin is internalized by receptor-mediated endocytosis, where it resides in an endosome. In the second step, the toxin is released into the cytosol. In step three, the light-chain enzymatically blocks exocytosis and release of acetylcholine at the NMJ. The toxin does not morphologically change the nerve ending and does not lead to cell death.[8]

Recovery of Function

BT's blockage of transmission is reversible. Recovery from the neurotoxin's effects is partly mediated by the cell body's ability to synthesize and transport material to the nerve ending.[8] Two well-documented effects of paralysis are the sprouting of new nerve terminals and an increase in the number of post-junctional receptors. Experimental evidence in soleus and gastrocnemius muscles indicates that nerve sprouts begin approximately 10 days after neuromuscular blockade and that most nerve terminals demonstrate sprouting

after 3 weeks.[10,11] At first, sprouting is not functional, but some sprouts may make contact over an area outside the neuromuscular junction and do become functional. Abnormalities in the pattern of reinnervation are not uniform and can be prolonged. Evidence also indicates that there is an increase in the number of post-junctional receptors.[8,12] Muscle atrophy occurs during the initial period of denervation, stabilizes, and then recovers over several months, although microscopic abnormalities may still be seen.[11] Studies confirming the long-term microscopic changes in muscles injected with BT are lacking in humans.

There may be other reasons for the variability in treatment response. Muscle fibers can be affected differently by the same dose of toxin. Experimental evidence suggests that fast-twitch muscle fibers remained functionally denervated longer than slow-twitch fibers.[11] This is in contrast to evidence that suggests that fast-twitch fibers in the thyroarytenoid and lateral cricoarytenoid muscles are reinnervated more rapidly and to a greater degree than slow-twitch fibers.[13] The thyroarytenoid and lateral cricoarytenoid muscles have a high proportion of fast-twitch fibers, which are involved in glottic sphincteric action and fewer slow-twitch fibers, which are used in phonation. This might partially explain why the side effects of breathiness and aspiration following BT injections are transient; whereas the relief from spasticity is long lasting. Finally, we do not know what effect muscle activity has on the duration of muscle paralysis. Wong et al demonstrated that responses to BT treatment for spasmodic dysphonia were superior and longer lasting when patients underwent a period of post-injection voice rest.[14] The relationships between BT response and muscle type and activity are only now being elucidated.

There are also differences in the duration and degree of response to BT that cannot be explained by the aforementioned observations. Some patients who have a good initial response might need larger doses over the duration of treatment. Others experience a reduction in relief from spasm and a shorter duration of response over time. One possible explanation for these diminished responses might be the formation of antibodies to BT. However, Biglan et al were unable to identify any antibody response to small doses of Botox A.[15] Perhaps larger doses, in the range of 300 mouse units (MU) during a 30-day period, might lead to an antibody response.[2] The total cumulative dose might also be a factor in antibody production. Finally, some drugs (eg, aminoglycoside antibiotics) can potentiate and prolong the effect of BT; whereas others (eg, guanidine and aminopyridines) can limit its effect.[8] The roles of antibody formation and drug potentiation have not been proven, either clinically or in the laboratory; and they remain incompletely understood.

Botulinum Preparations

Two forms of BT, Botox and Dysport, are available commerically. In the United States, Botox is supplied by Allergan, Inc (Irvine, Calif). A new batch prepared in 1998 contains less albumin than the original batch, which was prepared in 1979. BT is packaged in vials of 100 MU. Dysport is supplied by Speywood (Wrexham, Wales). It is packaged in vials of 500 MU. The two formulations are not equivalent. Furthermore, either brand's potency can vary among the individual vials in each package, which must be kept in mind when reading the literature and treating patients. The dose required to kill 50% of a group of mice is 1 MU. The lethal dose for humans has been extrapolated from monkey experiments and is thought to be 2500 to 3000 MU, which is well above the usual doses used in otolaryngology (usually 1.25–75 MU).

The toxin is marketed in a lyophilized form, which must be diluted with normal saline to obtain the desired concentration. For example, a 100-MU vial that is diluted with 2 ml of saline yields 5 MU/0.1 ml. Different concentrations and different volumes are used for various purposes. For example, because the concentrations are different, a smaller volume can be used for injecting 10 MU into a thyroarytenoid muscle than for 10 MU into the orbicularis oculi.

The FDA recommends that the toxin be used within 4 hours of reconstitution, and it suggests that refreezing leads to a loss of activity. Among the valid concerns about storing toxin for later use are the alteration of its molecular structure, the development of antibodies, inconsistent responses, and irregular dosing patterns.[16] Even so, one study of forearm injections showed that there was no difference in paralysis between patients who had received fresh toxin and those who received toxin that had been refrozen or refrigerated for 2 weeks.[17]

Uses of Botulinum Toxin in Otolaryngology

BT is being administered for the treatment of at least a dozen conditions in otolaryngologic practice. Among them are two types of spasmodic dysphonia, adductor laryngeal breathing dystonia, blepharospasm, hemifacial spasm, oromandibular dystonia, torticollis, facial nerve paresis with synkinesis, hyperkinetic facial lines, and cricopharyngeal spasm.

Spasmodic Dysphonia

Spasmodic dysphonia is probably the most well-known use for BT in otolaryngology. Much work in this area has been done by Blitzer and Brin,[18,19] Woodson and colleagues,[20,21] Ford and colleagues,[22,23] and Ludlow and colleagues.[24] Spasmodic dysphonia is believed to be a disorder of central motor processing. It is a focal dystonia, and it is classified as one of two main types. The more common adductor type is characterized by involuntary spasms of the thyroarytenoid (TA) and other adductor muscles, which cause a strained or strangled voice. The abductor type is characterized by intermittent hyperabduction of the vocal folds, which gives the patient a breathy, whispered voice. Although, speech therapy may be helpful and should be attempted, most noninvasive therapies are ineffective in controlling symptoms.

A correct diagnosis is essential in the management of patients with laryngeal dystonias. Spasmodic dysphonia must be differentiated from other neurologic disorders that cause voice dysfunction.[21,25] An incorrect diagnosis can result in treatment without effect, worsening symptoms, or even life-threatening complications. Moreover, treatment of a misdiagnosed patient with psychogenic dysphonia might result in a placebo effect that could incorrectly support the inaccurate diagnosis and delay proper treatment.

Adductor Spasmodic Dysphonia

Injection of BT into the thyroarytenoid muscle has been used since 1984 to treat adductor spasmodic dysphonia and is considered the treatment of choice. Injections can be administered percutaneously or perorally. Most authorities, including Sataloff,[25] Blitzer and Brin,[19] Woodson,[20] and Adams,[26] use a percutaneous technique. A hollow, Teflon-coated, 27-gauge electromyographic (EMG) needle is used to penetrate the cricothyroid membrane. The needle is then directed superiorly and laterally toward the TA muscle, and the laryngeal lumen is avoided. Confirmation that the proper position has been reached occurs when EMG shows a sharp increase in electrical activity as the patient phonates. The disadvantage of this technique is that it requires an EMG machine and a person who is familiar with the performance and interpretation of laryngeal electromyography.

Other authors prefer the peroral technique.[22,27] Because motor end-plates are thought to be distributed throughout the muscle, the proponents of peroral injections argue that this technique allows them to more easily diffuse the toxin over the entire muscle.[20] Prior to injection, the larynx is anesthetized topically and visualized by indirect laryngoscopy or flexible nasolaryngoscopy. A syringe fitted to a curved laryngeal injection needle is used to deliver BT to two sites through the superior surface of the true vocal folds.

This technique yields a high rate of success, and patients tolerate it well. Furthermore, Ford suggests that the peroral approach requires smaller doses than the percutaneous technique because localization is more precise, [22,23] although this idea is controversial. The peroral approach also has the advantage of being a technique with which otolaryngologists are already familiar. Finally, it does not require EMG guidance. Its disadvantages are the need for special needles, the greater amount of time needed to deliver the toxin, and that some of it remains unused in the catheter.[27]

The size of the dose varies among patients and physicians. Blitzer and Brin first began injecting 2.5 MU of BT unilaterally in patients with adductor spasmodic dysphonia, but they eventually came to believe that this amount had little effect.[19] Once they began injecting 7.5 MU, they noted the onset of vocal fold paresis and prolonged breathiness and a 90% improvement in function. They also obtained successful results with bilateral injections of 3.75 MU. Blitzer and Brin have since modified their technique and now start with 1.25 MU bilaterally and titrate the dose upward until optimal function is achieved. They note that complete paralysis is not required to achieve good outcome. The author (RTS) reported similar findings.[25]

One of the most useful aspects of BT is that it can be titrated to achieve the best possible result for each individual. Doses can range from as low as 1.25 MU to as high as 30 MU, depending on response, degree of side effects, and technique. Larger doses can lead to greater improvement in vocal function; but, of course, they are also associated with a greater degree of side effects. George et al reported that dose-related responses were seen with doses up to 7.5 MU, and complete paralysis was obtained with 10 MU.[28] They concluded that doses of 10 MU are sufficient for clinical paralysis.

In general, patients with adductor spasmodic dysphonia who receive BT for the first time should receive a low-dose, approximately 1.25 to 2.5 MU bilaterally. They should be followed up within 2 weeks, and the dose should be adjusted as needed. Patients with a paralyzed vocal fold and those who have undergone a nerve section might also benefit from low-dose injection, although their improvement might not be as dramatic. Clinically, results vary among patients; and treatment patterns need to be individualized. Results also vary from treatment to treatment on the same patient.

Injections may be administered unilaterally or bilaterally in patients with adductor spasmodic dysphonia, although there is some controversy over the efficacy and degree of side effects with the two techniques.[19,26,29-31]

Nevertheless, both techniques result in significant improvements in voice quality and fluency and normally cause only minimal and transient side effects. The most common side effects are a short period, usually 1 to 2 weeks, of breathiness or hypophonia, dysphagia, choking, pain at injection site, and edema of the vocal folds if too much volume is injected. Excessive weakness or more severe side effects can occur if the toxin spreads to other adductor muscles, such as the lateral cricoarytenoid.[28] No significant or long-term side effects have been reported.

Microscopic changes in motor units and prolonged disorganization of motor units have been described, and the process of reinnervation can take as long as 3 years.[24] Longer follow-up is needed to understand the long-term effects of BT.

Bilateral injections are usually administered because weakening or paralyzing only one vocal fold theoretically stresses the other fold and can exaggerate dystonic symptoms.[17] Also, bilateral injections expose the patient to less botulinum toxin; because they can be given in smaller cumulative doses than unilateral injections. Response can be minimal or quite dramatic. Studies have shown a high success rate.[19,20,25,26,32] It has been postulated that by paralyzing laryngeal muscles and possibly altering a feedback loop, BT might modify the inappropriate timing of phonatory muscles in the speech-motor loop,[20,33] but the significance of this has not been fully studied. Although BT therapy might not always result in normal speech, it is safe and reasonable treatment to restore fluency. Its effect usually becomes evident in 24 to 72 hours; maximum effectiveness is seen in about 2 weeks; and it lasts on average 3 to 6 months, occasionally longer. Some patients have gone into remission. The reasons for this are not clear, but such instances raise questions about the accuracy of the diagnosis.

Abductor Spasmodic Dysphonia

For patients with abductor spasmodic dysphonia, injections are delivered to the posterior cricoarytenoid (PCA) muscle, although cricothyroid (CT) injections have also been used.[19,34] These injections usually require EMG guidance. When injecting the PCA muscle, the larynx is rotated away from the side of injection; and a needle is placed percutaneously into the skin over the lateral aspect of the thyroid ala below its midpoint. EMG confirmation can be achieved by having the patient sniff. The PCA can also be reached through the cricothyroid membrane, especially in females and some young adult males. Peroral injections can also be performed. The CT muscle is approached through the midline in a lateral and superficial direction. Confirmation of proper needle position is obtained by having the patient sing an ascending scale or slide (glissando) and observing an increase in EMG activity as the pitch is increased.

The PCA is injected with an initial dose usually of 3.75 MU, and this amount can be titrated as necessary.[19] Higher initial doses of 5 MU or even 7.5 MU may be used. If symptoms persist and the PCA has already been completely paralyzed, the contralateral PCA can be injected cautiously with very small increments of toxin. However, the patient must be willing to accept the risk of airway compromise. In patients who fail this technique, injections into the CT muscle can be performed.[34,35] Some patients benefit from injections into the CT muscle in addition to, or occasionally instead of, into the PCA muscle.[36]

Blitzer et al studied 32 patients with abductor spasmodic dysphonia and found that after subjective pre- and postoperative evaluations by patients, physicians, and speech pathologists, the patients' percentage of normal function improved on average from 31% to 70%.[35] Most of these patients received bilateral PCA injections. The authors did not comment on the duration of response. In another study, Ludlow et al treated 10 patients with abductor spasmodic dysphonia with cricothyroid hyperactivity.[34] They found that 6 of 10 patients responded with CT injections and experienced an increase in sentence duration (the length of time during which they could speak without breaks or breaths) and their proportion of voiced speech. Patients returned for reinjection at 4- to 6-month intervals.

As is the case with patients who have adductor spasmodic dysphonia, results in patients with abductor spasmodic dysphonia vary; but many do obtain benefit from BT injections. The most worrisome adverse effects seen with PCA injections, especially bilateral injections, are stridor and airway compromise, but they are not common. When stridor does occur, it usually manifests itself during exertion. Two other fairly common adverse effects are transient dysphagia and aspiration of fluids.

Special Laryngeal Applications

BT has been used by one of the authors (RTS) and others (Andrew Blitzer, MD, oral communication, 1996; Michael Rontal, MD, oral communication, 1997; and Steven Zeitels, oral communication, 1998) for a variety of special laryngeal problems. The toxin can be used for the treatment of recurrent laryngeal granulomata, as an adjunctive treatment for arytenoid dislocation, and for the management of laryngeal synkinesis associated with reinnervation after recurrent nerve paralysis. We have also considered its use in selected cases

of bilateral vocal fold paralysis. BT has also been used by several authors for the treatment of laryngeal tremor, as reviewed by Warrick et al.[37] The author (RTS) has found that most patients with significant laryngeal tremor experience only limited improvement (if any) in tremor symptoms and signs through treatment with BT.

Respiratory Dystonia (Adductor Laryngeal Breathing Dystonia)

The treatment of respiratory dystonia (adductor laryngeal breathing dystonia) with BT was described by Grillone et al in 1994.[38] This condition is characterized by paradoxical adduction of the vocal folds during inspiration, which leads to stridor. The stridor usually disappears during sleep and worsens with exertion. The voice is normal. Many patients experience a respiratory dysrhythmia, and many complain of severe fatigue, which may interfere with work. These patients can be treated with BT injections into each thyroarytenoid muscle, usually requiring up to 3.75 MU, depending on severity of the condition. Treatment can significantly alleviate stridor and fatigue for up to 3 or 4 months. The most common complications are a transient breathy voice and mild aspiration of liquids.

Blepharospasm

Blepharospasm is a disabling condition that may cause functional blindness. It involves the involuntary activity of the orbicularis oculi, procerus, and corrugator supercilii muscles. Its symptoms include lower facial spasms and oromandibular spasms. Blepharospasm can occur in isolation or as part of other conditions such as Meige's syndrome. BT has been used to successfully treat blepharospasm since 1982, and it is now the treatment of choice.[39-41]

The injections can be given with or without EMG guidance. Without EMG guidance, injection sites are determined by palpating the affected muscle groups. A 30-gauge needle is used to inject small doses at several sites laterally, medially, and inferiorly. Patients who do not respond might benefit from brow injections. Injections delivered outside the orbital rim have the shortest duration of action and the least effect, but they also cause fewer side effects.[42,43] Initial doses range from 2.5 to 5.0 MU per site and are titrated upward to 12.5 to 30 MU per eye. Effects are seen in 2 or 3 days and generally last 3 or 4 months.

Regardless of technique, the central part of the upper eyelid should not be injected to avoid levator palpebrae superioris paralysis and subsequent ptosis. Diplopia can occur if the toxin enters into the extraocular muscles. Other side effects include epiphora, ocular irritation, lagophthalmos and exposure keratitis. On rare occasions ectropion, entropion, or blurred vision may occur.[39,41,42,44] Side effects can occur because of diffusion of toxin, but they can be minimized by injecting smaller volumes and avoiding massage of the region.

Hemifacial Spasm

Hemifacial spasm usually begins in the orbicularis oculi, and it can spread to involve muscles of the brow, lower face, and neck. Patients with hemifacial spasm (like those with blepharospasm) might have an underlying neurologic disorder or other condition that is causing their spasm. For example, hemifacial spasm can be caused by vascular loop compression of the facial nerve or might be associated with Parkinsonism or other neurologic disorders characterized by involuntary muscle spasms. Regardless of the etiology, BT provides temporary relief of symptoms.

Before considering BT therapy, it is necessary to conduct a complete evaluation, which can include magnetic resonance imaging, EMG, angiography, neurological consultation, selected blood tests, and other studies.

Injections can be guided with EMG, but many experienced physicians feel comfortable without it. Patients usually receive 12 to 30 MU distributed in 2.5 to 5.0 MU doses. The toxin is typically injected into the zygomaticus major and minor, the levator angularis, and risorius. Improvement has been reported to occur in 92 to 100% of patients.[41,43,45] The duration of symptom relief extends beyond 4 months on average; but some patients require a reinjection after 10 weeks, sometimes sooner. A few patients have been found to go into remission.[38] There is long-term variability in treatment doses among patients, the reasons for which are not known.

Side effects include those seen with blepharospasm. Substantial facial weakness is noted occasionally. Facial asymmetry, drooling, and chewing problems can also occur.[39,41,42,44] But for many patients, these side effects are inconsequential when compared with the disabling spasms of their disease.

Oromandibular Dystonia

Oromandibular dystonia can occur alone or with other focal or generalized dystonias. Spasms of the muscles of mastication can lead to pain, abnormal jaw positioning, temporomandibular joint dysfunction, and trismus. The diagnosis can be difficult. In addition to BT, treatment includes anticholinergics and benzodiazepines.[46]

BT injections are delivered to those muscles that appear to be the most spasmodic, usually the temporalis, masseter, or medial and lateral pterygoid muscles. Injections into the pterygoid muscles must be made with EMG guidance. Toxin is delivered with one or more injections of 10 MU distributed over the muscle. Doses range from 10 to 40 MU[46] and can be titrated as necessary. The effects of BT in oromandibular dystonia are seen in 24 to 72 hours and generally last 10 weeks to 4 months.[46] Patients show significant improvement and are able to return to normal eating and speaking habits without pain.

Torticollis

BT can be used to treat torticollis due to sternocleidomastoid spasm. Larger doses are usually needed, sometimes 100 to 300 MU per sternocleidomastoid muscle. Local complications include dysphagia, neck weakness, and systemic complications including pruritis, nausea, flulike symptoms, fatigue, generalized weakness, and distant, unrelated muscle weakness.[46,47]

Dysphagia is thought to occur by toxin diffusion into the constrictor muscles. Toxin diffusion has been shown to be dose-dependent. The toxin can spread over a large area and even cross fascial planes. Symptom relief lasts 11 weeks on average.[42] Concerns over the long-term use of such large doses must be kept in mind, particularly the risk of developing antibodies against BT.[48]

Facial Nerve Paralysis

The management of patients with facial paresis can be very difficult. Involuntary eyelid closure or other facial movements associated with facial paralysis can be disfiguring. The signs are associated with aberrant regeneration of the facial nerve. Among the other treatments for facial nerve paralysis are ptosis repair, selective myectomy, and selective neurectomy. However, these procedures have their drawbacks, including weakening of an already denervated muscle, their irreversibility, and the difficulty encountered in achieving optimal results. Borodic et al studied 12 patients with synkinesis following facial nerve paralysis who received a mean dose of 22 MU of BT and found that improvement lasted about 5 months.[49] The authors noted significant improvement in synkinetic movements; but periocular injections increased facial asymmetry. Minimizing the dose can limit diffusion.

Patients with facial paralysis often do not regain complete function. Techniques used to reanimate the face improve facial symmetry; but they fail to do anything about the pull of the normal contralateral face, which can be very deforming. In these patients, BT can be injected into the contralateral zygomaticus major and risorius to improve symmetry at the nasolabial fold and oral commisure. For patients with facial nerve paralysis, the uses of BT in rehabilitation, surgical reanimation, and temporary relief of spasm, synkinesis, and asymmetry are evolving.[50]

Hyperkinetic Facial Lines

BT has been helpful in treating the aging face. Glabellar lines, crow's feet, deep forehead lines, and deep nasolabial folds have all been treated successfully. Hyperkinetic lines are a result of pull on the skin by the underlying muscles. The procerus and corrugator supercilii muscles create deep lines in the glabella when frowning. Crow's feet are created by the lateral orbicularis oculi muscle when squinting. In the forehead, lines are created by the frontalis muscle. Nasolabial folds are created by the zygomaticus, levator superioris, orbicularis oris, and levator superioris alaeque nasi. Carruthers et al first noted that patients treated for blepharospasm, hemifacial spasm, or Bell's palsy displayed a loss of their wrinkles.[51] Since then, BT has been used to lessen or eliminate the degree of hyperfunctional lines of the face.[52-55]

EMG can be used to guide placement of the needle into the corrugator supercilii and procerus muscles in the treatment of glabellar lines; but once a physician becomes familiar with the technique, EMG guidance may not be necessary. As is the case in the treatment of other muscle spasms, the advantage of using EMG is that, if a patient does not respond to the initial injection, specific sites of persistent activity can be identified; and subsequent injections can be made with greater precision. If there is absence of activity after the treatment of corrugator hyperfunction, injections can be placed in accessory muscles, such as the orbicularis oculi and frontalis. It is important to remember that injections must be placed into the *muscles*, not the *wrinkles*. Treatment usually begins with 10 MU into each corrugator supercilii and can be repeated as necessary.[52]

Crow's feet are treated in a similar fashion, usually with EMG guidance. Smaller doses (5 MU) are used to treat each eye. Forehead lines and nasolabial folds are treated with various amounts of BT. In each region, treatment can render a graded weakening of the underlying musculature with partial or complete resolution of the hyperkinetic lines. When treating these areas, small doses are delivered to several injection sites. Results can be seen in 5 to 7 days and the treatment effects last from 2 to 6 months.[51-55]

Patients are generally satisfied with their results and return for further BT therapy.[53] Complications include temporary ptosis, upper lip droop, mild swelling, ecchymosis, or local discomfort.

BT can also be an excellent alternative or adjunctive treatment to topical agents, chemical peel, laser resurfacing, soft-tissue augmentation, or surgery. No major or long-term complications have been reported following cosmetic BT injections. The maximum degree of expected improvement can be simulated by spreading apart the wrinkle to be treated with two fingers.[52] However, because improvement is only temporary, some patients opt to discontinue BT injection treatment and undergo a permanent but more invasive procedure.

Patients who are most likely to fail BT injection therapy are those who have thick, sebaceous skin, deep dermal scarring, extraordinarily deep lines, excess skin laxity as a result of aging, incomplete denervation, and accessory muscle function that is contributing to the wrinkles.[52,53]

Cricopharyngeal Spasm

BT can be used for voice failure following tracheoesophageal puncture (TEP) and dysphagia secondary to cricopharyngeal spasm. Cricopharyngeal spasm has been reported to be a cause of failure or voice restoration following TEP in as many as 12% of laryngectomy patients.[56] It is sometimes difficult to make this diagnosis; but a barium swallow, esophageal manometry, and EMG showing persistent spasm on swallow can be helpful. Injection of BT into the cricopharyngeus can be used diagnostically or therapeutically in patients with voice failure or dysphagia secondary to cricopharyngeal hyperactivity.[56,57] Under EMG guidance, the cricopharyngeus is injected at 2 to 3 sites on each side, superior and lateral to the laryngectomy stoma. The cricopharyngeus is identified by electrical activity at rest that diminishes or stops when the patient swallows. The cricopharyngeus can also be injected endoscopically. Blitzer et al studied six patients who had voice failure secondary to cricopharyngeal spasm and found that all six benefited from BT injections, including two who already had had myotomies.[56] From 1997 to date, we have also found temporary benefits in a small number of patients. Doses average 30 to 40 MU, and effects last about 3 months. This technique is also useful for patients with dysphagia secondary to cricopharyngeal spasm as a result of a neurologic impairment such as stroke, for those who have discoordinated swallowing, and for those who have undergone laryngectomy. Blitzer and Brin reported improvement in six patients with 10 MU spread over four injection sites.[57] In another study, Annese et al compared pneumatic dilatation with BT injection for 16 patients with achalasia and elevated lower esophageal sphincter tone and found that the toxin was comparable to dilatation with regard to symptom scores, even though dilatation led to a significantly lower sphincter pressure.[58] There are no published studies comparing dilatation and BT in cricopharyngeal spasm.

Typically, treatment effects become evident after a few days and can last up to 5 months. No major side effects have been reported. Some patients may prefer BT injections as an alternative to myotomy or dilatation. Patient selection is important and clinical trials are lacking, but this may become an indication for which BT might prove to be beneficial.

Antibodies to Botulinum Toxin

Published literature suggests that less than 5% of patients who receive BT type A develop demonstrable neutralizing antibodies. Hatheway and Dang found that 29 patients who tested positive for antibodies had received an average of 1,051 MU in the preceding year, compared with 59 patients without demonstrable antibodies who had received an average of 301 MU during the preceding year.[59] Greene et al studied 76 patients and found that higher doses of BT and more frequent injections were risk factors for developing antibodies that impaired botulinum toxin effect.[60] Jankovic and Schwartz compared 20 patients who tested positive for antibodies with 22 who tested negative using the mouse protection assay (MPA).[60] The antibody-positive patients had higher cumulative doses (1,709 ± 638 MU) and higher mean doses per visit (249.2 ± 32.5 MU) than the antibody-negative patients (1,066 ± 938 MU cumulative dose; 180.8 ± 68.7 MU per visit). The MPA is currently considered the most relevant test for detection of antibodies, particularly with regard to correlation with clinical response to treatment.[60] Patients with measurable levels of anti-botulinum toxin Type A antibodies in the MPA are, by definition, patients with toxin-neutralizing antibodies. In-vitro assessments of anti-botulinum toxin antibodies have not been shown to distinguish consistently between binding antibodies and neutralizing antibodies, so far.

The author's experience (RTS, unpublished data) suggests that antibodies may form after exposure to much lower doses and that not only IgG antibodies, but also IgA antibodies are formed. Additional research is in progress to clarify factors affecting the development of antibodies, their clinical implications, and to reassess the value of other assay techniques.

Botulinum Toxin Type B

Treatment of laryngeal dystonia with BT type A (BTXA) has become the standard of care for this troublesome disorder. However, some patients develop resistance to BTXA.[61] The first laryngeal use of BT type B (BTXB) was presented in June 2001 at The Voice Foundation Symposium in Philadelphia, Pennsylvania, and published thereafter.[62]

Although BTXA has been used extensively to treat a variety of disorders, [63] including many otolaryngologic problems as noted above, it is well recognized that some patients do not respond to BTXA; and some patients respond initially but cease responding, presumably due to a blocking or neutralizing antibody.[64] For patients with laryngeal dystonia, resistance to BTXA has led to either unremitting spasmodic dysphonia or to surgical procedures such as recurrent laryngeal nerve section and more recently thyroarytenoid neurectomy. BTXB may represent an alternative to neurolytic surgery in patients who do not respond to BTXA.

In 1995, Tsui et al reported a pilot study using BTXB for treatment of cervical dystonia.[65] They used an increasing-dose treatment schedule starting with 100 MU and increasing to a total cumulative dose of 1,910 MU. Injections were performed in the two most dystonic neck muscles, with the dose divided between the two muscles. Six of eight patients noted improvement after injection even with no single session utilizing more than 1,200 MU. The authors reported that a single injection of up to 1,200 MU and cumulative dosing of up to 1,910 MU of BTXB was effective, safe and well tolerated with minimal side effects (two patients with increased head tremor, one hematoma, and two patients experienced neck pain). They noted a dose-response relationship at the doses studied and estimated that a doubling of the dose led to a 40% improvement in response. Prior to the report on laryngeal use, BTXB had been used in humans but not in the larynx. In 1997, Sloop et al studied 17 different doses of BTXB (from 1.25 to 480 MU) in 17 healthy volunteers, establishing a dose-response curve that could be compared to the BTXA dose-response curve.[66] They found that maximal paralysis 2 weeks after injection with 320 to 480 MU of BTXB was 50 to 75%, measured using nerve conduction studies. Maximal paralysis with 7.5 to 10 MU of BTXA was 70 to 80%. Seven weeks after injection, paralysis from BTXB had improved by 66%; with BTXA it had improved by only 6%. By 11 weeks after injection, BTXA-induced paralysis had resolved completely. In contrast, 57 weeks after injection, 22% of the original paralysis was still present after BTXB injection.

In 1999, Brin et al studied the safety and efficacy of BTXB in patients with cervical dystonia resistant to

BTXA.[67] The authors studied 77 patients, giving 38 placebo and 39 10,000 MU of BTXB. They found BTXB to be safe and effective. The effect lasted 12 to 16 weeks with the doses they administered. A second study by many of the same authors reported similar findings on 122 patients with idiopathic cervical dystonia, comparing BTXB and placebo.[68] In this study, patients received placebo or BTXB in doses of 2,500 MU, 5,000 MU, or 10,000 MU. The authors again found BTXB to be safe, well-tolerated, and efficacious for the treatment of cervical dystonia. They also found that response time was shorter in patients who received placebo or 2,500 MU than it was among patients who received 5,000 or 10,000 MU.

In 1999, a 16-week, multicenter, randomized, double-blinded, placebo-controlled study using BTXB in patients with cervical dystonia who were still responding to BTXA was published.[69] Patients received placebo, 5,000 MU, or 10,000 MU of BTXB. The best response occurred in those receiving 10,000 MU, and the lowest cervical dystonia scores were recorded in the placebo group. BTXB injection treatment duration was 12 to 16 weeks for both doses. The authors found BTXB to be safe and effective. This study did not compare the safety and efficacy of BTXB with BTXA, even though this patient population consisted of patients who still responded to BTXA.

Although conclusions must be considered preliminary, the available data regarding safety and efficacy of BTXB for the treatment of cervical dystonia, along with the author's (RTS) initial experience using BTXB for spasmodic dysphonia, suggest that BTXB may be useful for the treatment of laryngeal disorders in patients resistant to BTXA. Additional studies are recommended.

Conclusion

Botulinum toxin has proven extremely helpful in the treatment of a variety of otolaryngologic disorders. It is particularly valuable for management of laryngeal and respiratory dystonia. Antibodies can develop and interfere with the efficacy of BTXA; and patients with such antibodies may be candidates for treatment with BTXB or other serotypes. However, additional research, including careful documentation and the reporting of results of otolaryngologic applications of botulinum toxin, should be encouraged to help answer the remaining questions and clarify the roles of botulinum toxin in otolaryngology.

References

1. Neuenschwander MC, Pribitkin EA, Sataloff RT. Botulinum toxin in otolaryngology: a review of its actions and opportunities for use. *Ear Nose Throat J.* 2000;79: 788–801.
2. Blitzer A, Sulica L. Botulinum toxin: basic science and clinical uses in otolaryngology. *Laryngoscope.* 2001;111: 218–226.
3. Schantz EJ, Johnson EA. Botulinum toxin: the story of its development for the treatment of human disease. *Perspect Biol Med.* 1997;40:317–327.
4. Scott AB, Rosenbaum A, Collins CC. Pharmacologic weakening of extraocular muscles. *Invest Ophthalmol.* 1973;12:924–927.
5. Scott AB. Botulinum toxin injection into extraocular muscles as an alternative to strabismus surgery. *Ophthalmology.* 1980;87:1044–1049.
6. NIH Consensus Development Panel on Clinical Use of Botulinum Toxin. Botulinum toxin. *J Voice.* 1992;6:394–400.
7. Tsui JK. Botulinum toxin as a therapeutic agent. *Pharmacol Ther.* 1996;72:13–24.
8. Simpson LL. Clinically relevant aspects of the mechanism of action of botulinum neurotoxin. *J Voice.* 1992;6: 358–64.
9. Mezaki T, Kaji R, Kohara N, et al. Comparison of therapeutic efficacies of Type A and F botulinum toxins for blepharospasm. *Neurology.* 1995;45:506–508.
10. Holland RL, Brown MC. Nerve growth in botulinum toxin poisoned muscles. *Neuroscience.* 1981;6:1167–1179.
11. Duchen LW. Changes in the electron microscopic structure of slow and fast skeletal muscle fibres of the mouse after local injection of botulinum toxin. *J Neurol Sci.* 1971; 14:61 74.
12. Duchen LW, Strich SJ. The effects of botulinum toxin on the pattern of innervation of skeletal muscle in the mouse. *Q J Exp Physiol.* 1968;53:84–89.
13. Castellanos PF, Gates GA, Esselman G, et al. Anatomic considerations in botulinum toxin Type A therapy for spasmodic dysphonia. *Laryngoscope.* 1994;104:656–662.
14. Wong DL, Adams SG, Irish JC, et al. Effect of neuromuscular activity on the response to botulinum toxin injections in spasmodic dysphonia. *J Otolaryngol.* 1995; 24:209–216.
15. Biglan AW, Gonnering R, Lockhart LB, et al. Absence of antibody production in patients treated with botulinum A toxin. *Am J Ophthalmol.* 1986;101:232–235.
16. Sloop RR, Cole BA, Escutin RO. Reconstituted botulinum toxin Type A does not lose potency in humans if it is refrozen or refrigerated for 2 weeks before use. *Neurology.* 1997;48:249–253.
17. Gartlan MG, Hoffman HT. Crystalline preparation of botulinum toxin Type A (Botox): Degradation in potency with storage. *Otolaryngol Head Neck Surg.* 1993;108: 135–140.
18. Blitzer A, Brin MF. Laryngeal dystonia: A series with botulinum toxin therapy. *Ann Otol Rhinol Laryngol.* 1991; 100: 85–89.
19. Blitzer A, Brin MF. Treatment of spasmodic dysphonia (laryngeal dystonia) with local injections of botulinum toxin. *J Voice.* 1992;6:365–369.
20. Zwirner P, Murry T, Swenson M, Woodson GE. Effects of botulinum toxin therapy in patients with adductor

spasmodic dysphonia: Acoustic, aerodynamic, and video-endoscopic findings. *Laryngoscope.* 1992;102:400–406.

21. Woodson GE, Zwirner P, Murry T, Swenson MR. Functional assessment of patients with spasmodic dysphonia. *J Voice.* 1992;6:338–343.

22. Ford CN, Bless DM, Lowery JD. Indirect laryngoscopic approach for injection of botulinum toxin in spasmodic dysphonia. *Otolaryngol Head Neck Surg.* 1990;103:752–758.

23. Ford CN, Bless DM, Patel NY. Botulinum toxin treatment of spasmodic dysphonia: techniques, indications, efficacy. *J Voice.* 1992;6:370–376.

24. Davidson BJ, Ludlow CL. Long-term effects of botulinum toxin injections in spasmodic dysphonia. *Ann Otol Rhinol Laryngol.* 1996;105:33–42.

25. Deems DA, Sataloff RT: Spasmodic dysphonia. In: Sataloff RT. *Professional Voice: The Science and Art of Clinical Care.* 2nd ed. San Diego, Calif: Singular Publishing Group, Inc; 1997:499–505.

26. Adams SG, Hunt EJ, Irish JC, et al. Comparison of botulinum toxin injection procedures in adductor spasmodic dysphonia. *J Otolaryngol.* 1995;24: 345–351.

27. Rhew K, Fiedler DA, Ludlow CL. Technique for injection of botulinum toxin through the flexible nasolaryngoscope. *Otolaryngol Head Neck Surg.* 1994;111:787–794.

28. George EF, Zimbler M, Wu BL, et al. Quantitative mapping of the effect of botulinum toxin injections in the thyroarytenoid muscle. *Ann Otol Rhinol Laryngol.* 1992;101: 888–892.

29. Maloney AP, Morrison MD. A comparison of the efficacy of unilateral versus bilateral botulinum toxin injections in the treatment of adductor spasmodic dysphonia. *J Otolaryngol.* 1994;23:160–164.

30. Liu TC, Irish JC, Adams SG, et al. Prospective study of patient's subjective responses to botulinum toxin injection for spasmodic dysphonia. *J Otolaryngol.* 1996;25:66–74.

31. Adams SG, Hunt EJ, Charles DA, Lang AE. Unilateral versus bilateral botulinum toxin injections in spasmodic dysphonia: acoustic and perceptual results. *J Otolaryngol.* 1993;22:171–175.

32. Troung DD, Kontal M, Rolnick M, et al. Double-blind controlled study of botulinum toxin in adductor spasmodic dysphonia. *Laryngoscope.* 1991;101:630–634.

33. Brin MF, Stewart C, Blitzer A, Diamond B. Laryngeal botulinum toxin injections for disabling stuttering in adults. *Neurology.* 1994;44:2262–2266.

34. Ludlow CL, Naunton RF, Terada S, Anderson BJ. Successful treatment of selected cases of abductor spasmodic dysphonia using botulinum toxin injection. *Otolaryngol Head Neck Surg.* 1991;104:849–855.

35. Blitzer A, Brin MF, Stewart C, et al. Abductor laryngeal dystonia: a series treated with botulinum toxin. *Laryngoscope.* 1992;102:163–167.

36. Sataloff RT, Deems DA. Spasmodic dysphonia. In: Sataloff RT. *Clinical Assessment of Voice.* San Diego, Calif: Plural Publishing Inc; 2005:241–256.

37. Warrick P, Dromey C, Irish J, et al. Botulinum toxin for essential tremor of the voice with multiple anatomical sites of tremor: a crossover design study of unilateral versus bilateral injection. *Laryngoscope.* 2000;110:1366–1376.

38. Grillone GA, Blitzer A, Brin MF, et al. Treatment of adductor laryngeal breathing dystonia with botulinum toxin Type A. *Laryngoscope.* 1994;104:30–32.

39. Mauriello JA Jr, Dhillon S, Leone T, et al. Treatment selections of 239 patients with blepharospasm and Meige syndrome over 11 years. *Br J Ophthalmol.* 1996;80: 1073–1076.

40. Jordan DR, Patrinely JR, Anderson RL, Thiese SM. Essential blepharospasm and related dystonias. *Surv Ophthalmol.* 1989;34:123–132.

41. Taylor JD, Kraft SP, Kazdan MS, et al. Treatment of blepharospasm and hemifacial spasm with botulinum A toxin: a Canadian multicentre study. *Can J Ophthalmol.* 1991;26:133–138.

42. Price J, Farish S, Taylor H, O'Day J. Blepharospasm and hemifacial spasm: randomized trial to determine the most appropriate location for botulinum toxin injections. *Ophthalmology.* 1997;104:865–868.

43. Brin MF, Fahn S, Moskowitz C, et al. Localized injections of botulinum toxin for the treatment of focal dystonia and hemifacial spasm. *Mov Disord.* 1987;2:237–254.

44. Jankovic J, Schwartz K, Donovan DT. Botulinum toxin treatment of cranial-cervical dystonia, spasmodic dysphonia, other focal dystonias and hemifacial spasm. *J Neurol Neurosurg Psychiatry.* 1990;53:633–639.

45. Biglan AW, May M, Bowers RA. Management of facial spasm with Clostridium botulinum toxin, Type A (Oculinum). *Arch Otolaryngol Head Neck Surg.* 1988;114: 1407–1412.

46. Blitzer A, Brin MF, Greene PE, Fahn S. Botulinum toxin injection for the treatment of oromandibular dystonia. *Ann Otol Rhinol Laryngol.* 1989;98:93–96.

47. Borodic GE, Joseph M, Fay L, et al. Botulinum A toxin for the treatment of spasmodic torticollis: dysphagia and regional toxin spread. *Head Neck.* 1990;12:392–398.

48. Dutton JJ. Botulinum-A toxin in the treatment of craniocervical muscle spasms: short- and long-term, local and systemic effects. *Surv Ophthalmol.* 1996;41:51–65.

49. Borodic GE, Pearce LB, Cheney M, et al. Botulinum A toxin for treatment of aberrant facial nerve regeneration. *Plast Reconstr Surg.* 1993;91:1042–1045.

50. May M, Croxson GR, Klein SR. Bell's palsy: management of sequelae using EMG rehabilitation, botulinum toxin, and surgery. *Am J Otol.* 1989;10:220–229.

51. Blitzer A, Brin MF, Keen MS, Aviv JE. Botulinum toxin for the treatment of hyperfunctional lines of the face. *Arch Otolaryngol Head Neck Surg.* 1993;119:1018–1022.

52. Keen M, Blitzer A, Aviv J, et al. Botulinum toxin A for hyperkinetic facial lines: results of a double-blind, placebo-controlled study. *Plast Reconstr Surg.* 1994;94:94–99.

53. Pribitkin EA, Greco TM, Goode RL, Keane WM. Patient selection in the treatment of glabellar wrinkles with botulinum toxin Type A injection. *Arch Otolaryngol Head Neck Surg.* 1997;123:321–326.

54. Carruthers A, Kiene K, Carruthers J. Botulinum A exotoxin use in clinical dermatology. *J Am Acad Dermatol.* 1996;34:788–797.

55. Lowe NJ, Maxwell A, Harper H. Botulinum A exotoxin for glabellar folds: a double-blind, placebo-controlled study with an electromyographic injection technique. *J Am Acad Dermatol.* 1996;35:569–572.

56. Blitzer A, Komisar A, Baredes S, et al. Voice failure after tracheoesophageal puncture: management with botulinum toxin. *Otolaryngol Head Neck Surg.* 1995;113:668–670.

57. Blitzer A, Brin MF. Use of botulinum toxin for diagnosis and management of cricopharyngeal achalasia. *Otolaryngol Head Neck Surg.* 1997;116:328–330.

58. Annese V, Basciani M, Perri F, et al. Controlled trial of botulinum toxin injection versus placebo and pneumatic dilation in achalasia. *Gastroenterology.* 1996;111:1418–1424.

59. Hatheway CH, Dang C. Immunogenicity of the neurotoxins of Clostridium botulinum. In: Jankovic J, Hallett M, eds. *Therapy with Botulinum Toxin.* New York, NY: Marcel Dekker; 1994:93–107.

60. Greene P, Fahn S, Diamond B. Development of resistance to botulinum toxin type A in patients with torticollis. *Mov Disord.* 1994;9:213–217.

61. Jankovic J, Schwartz K. Response and immunoresistance to botulinum toxin injections. *Neurology.* 1995;45:1743–1746.

62. Sataloff RT, Heman-Ackah YD, Simpson et al. Botulinum toxin Type B for treatment of spasmodic dysphonia: a case report. *J Voice.* 2002;16:422–424.

63. Jancovic J, Brin M. Therapeutic uses of botulinum toxin. *N Engl J Med.* 1991;324:1186–1194.

64. Borodic G, Johnson E, Goodnough M, Schantz E. Botulinum toxin therapy, immunologic resistance and problems with available materials. *Neurology.* 1996;46:26–29.

65. Tsui JK, Hayward M, Mak EK, Schulzer M. Botulinum toxin type B in the treatment of cervical dystonia: a pilot study. *Neurology.* 1995;45:2109–2110.

66. Sloop RR, Cole BA, Escutin RO. Human response to botulinum toxin injection: type B compared with type A. *Neurology.* 1997;49:189–194.

67. Brin MF, Lew MF, Adler CH, et al. Safety and efficacy of NeuroBloc (botulinum toxin type B) in type A-resistant cervical dystonia. *Neurology.* 1999;53:1431–1438.

68. Lew MF, Adornato BT, Duane DD, et al. Botulinum toxin type B: A double-blind, placebo-controlled, safety and efficacy study in cervical dystonia. *Neurology.* 1997;49:701–706.

69. Brashear A, Lew MF, Dykstra DD, et al. Safety and efficacy of NeuroBloc (botulinum toxin type B) in type A-responsive cervical dystonia. *Neurology.* 1999;53:1439–1446.

18

Voice Surgery

Robert Thayer Sataloff

Laryngeal surgery may be performed endoscopically or through an external approach. To provide optimal care, laryngologists must be familiar with the latest techniques in both approaches. Modern microsurgery of the voice is referred to widely as *phonosurgery*, although von Leden introduced that term originally in 1963 for procedures designed to alter vocal quality or pitch.[1] *Voice surgery* is a better term for delicate, precise laryngeal surgery in general, although phonomicrosurgery has also become widely used. It is usually performed using the microscope, small, modern instruments, and with great respect for the induplicatable anatomic complexity of the vibratory margin of the vocal fold.

Most surgical procedures for voice disorders can be performed endoscopically, obviating the need for external incisions and minimizing the amount of tissue disruption. Although endoscopic microsurgery seems intuitively more "conservative," this supposition holds true only when the equipment provides good exposure of the surgical site and the abnormality can be treated meticulously and thoroughly with endoscopic instruments. When endoscopic visualization is not adequate because of patient anatomy, disease extent, or other factors, the surgeon should not compromise the results of treatment or risk patient injury by attempting to complete an endoscopic procedure. In such patients, it may be safer to leave selected benign lesions untreated or to treat the pathology through an external approach.

Patient Selection and Consent

Prior to performing voice surgery, it is essential to be certain that patient selection is appropriate and that the patient understands the limits and potential complications of voice surgery. Appropriate patients for voice surgery not only have voice abnormalities, but also really want to change their voice quality, effort, and/or endurance. For example, not all people with "pathological" voices are unhappy with them. Sports announcers, female trial attorneys with gruff, masculine voices, and others sometimes consult a physician only because of fear of cancer. If there is no suspicion of malignancy, restoring their voices to "normal" (eg, by evacuating Reinke's edema) may be a disservice and even jeopardize their careers. Similarly, it is essential to distinguish accurately between organic and psychogenic voice disorders before embarking on laryngeal surgery. Although breathy voice may be caused by numerous organic conditions, it is also commonly found in people with psychogenic dysphonia. The differentiation may require a very skilled voice team.

Although all reasonable efforts should be made to avoid operative intervention in professional voice users, particularly singers, there are times when surgery is appropriate and necessary. Ultimately, the decision depends on a risk-benefit analysis. If a professional is unable to continue his or her career, and if surgery may restore vocal function, surgery certainly should not be withheld. Sometimes, making such judgments can be challenging. A rock or pop singer with a vocal fold mass may have satisfactory voice quality with only minimal technical adjustments. Pop singers perform with amplification, obviating the need to sing loudly and project the voice in some cases (depending on the artist's style). Such a patient may be able to "work around" pathology safely for many years. However, even much more minor pathology may be disabling in some classical singers. For example, if a high soprano specializing in Baroque music develops a mild to moderate superior laryngeal nerve paresis, she may experience breathiness and instability. If she gives in to the temptation to compensate by slightly retracting her tongue and lowering her larynx, the breathiness will be controlled because of increased adductory forces, but she will lose the ability to perform rapid, agile runs and trills. Similar problems may occur from compensatory maladjustments in response to other lesions such as vocal fold cysts. In such instances, the artist may be served better by surgical correction of the underlying problem than by long-term use of hyperfunctional compensation (bad technique) that can itself cause other performance problems, as well as vocal fold pathology. The patient must understand all of these considerations clearly, including the risks of surgery. He or she needs to acknowledge the risk that any voice surgery may make the voice worse permanently, and the patient must consider this risk acceptable in light of ongoing vocal problems.

Even in the best hands, an undesirable scar may develop, resulting in permanent hoarseness. Also, the patient must be aware that there is a possibility that the voice may be worse following surgery. Naturally, other complications must also be discussed including (among others) complications of anesthesia, dental fracture, recurrence of laryngeal lesions, airway compromise, vocal fold webbing, and other untoward occurrences. In addition to the hospital's standard surgical consent, the author provides patients with additional written information prior to surgery. The patient keeps one copy of the "Risks and Complications of Surgery" document, and one signed copy remains in the chart. Specialized informed consent documents are used also for other selected treatments such as injection of cidofovir, topical application of mitomycin-C, injection of collagen, and injection of botulinum toxin, even though such documents are not really required. If medications are used for treatment purposes (rather than research purposes) and are off-label uses of medicines approved by the FDA for other purposes, their use does not necessarily require institutional review board (IRB) approval. However, this author believes it is helpful and prudent to provide patients with as much information as possible and to document that they have been so informed.

It is often helpful for the laryngologist, speech-language pathologist, singing voice specialist and patient to involve the patient's singing teacher in the decision-making process. Everyone must understand not only the risks of surgery, but also the risk involved in deciding against surgery and relying upon technical maladjustments. In many cases, there is no "good" or "right" choice; and the voice care team must combine great expertise with insight into the career and concerns of each individual patient to help the voice professional make the best choice.

Documentation

As has been noted elsewhere in this book, preoperative objective voice assessment and documentation are essential in addition to routine documentation of informed consent discussions. As a bare minimum, a high-quality tape recording of the patient's voice must be done before surgery. Auditory memories of physicians and patients are not good in general, and both the doctor and postoperative professional voice user are often surprised when they compare postoperative and preoperative recordings. Frequently, the preoperative voice is worse than either person remembers. In addition, such documentation is invaluable for medical-legal purposes. Photographs or videotapes of the larynx obtained during strobovideolaryngoscopy are extremely helpful. Ideally, complete objective laboratory voice assessment and evaluation by a voice team should be performed. Proper documentation is essential for assessing outcomes, even for the physician who is not interested in research or publication.

Timing of Voice Surgery

The time of voice surgery is important and can be particularly challenging in professionals with demanding voice commitments. Many factors need to be taken into account including the menstrual cycle, pre- and postoperative voice therapy, concurrent medical conditions, psychological state, professional voice commitments, and others.

Hormonal considerations may be important, especially in female patients with symptomatic laryngopathia premenstrualis. In patients who have obvious vocal fold vascular engorgement, or those who have a history of premenstrual vocal fold hemorrhages, it may be better to avoid elective surgery during the premenstrual period (unless the surgery is intended to treat vessels that have hemorrhaged repeatedly and that are only prominent prior to menses). In such patients, it may be best to perform surgery between approximately days 4 and 21 of the menstrual cycle. Although it appears unnecessary to time surgery in this way for all patients, the issue has not been fully studied.

Timing of surgery with regard to voice therapy and performance commitments can be especially difficult in busy voice professionals. The surgeon must be careful to avoid letting the patient's professional commitments and pressures dictate inappropriate surgery or surgical timing that is not in the patient's best interest. For example, some professional voice users will push for early surgery for vocal nodules and promise to appear for voice therapy after a busy concert season ends. This is not appropriate, because therapy may cure the nodules and avoid surgical risks altogether. However, professional commitments often require that appropriate surgery be delayed until a series of concerts or the run of a play is completed. In treating vocal fold cysts, polyps, and other conditions, such delays are often reasonable. They are made safer through ongoing voice therapy and close laryngologic supervision. Sometimes individualized treatments may help temporize. For example, aspiration of a cyst as an office procedure can provide temporary relief from symptoms, although the cyst is likely to return and require definitive surgery eventually.

At least a brief period of preoperative voice therapy is also helpful. Even when therapy cannot cure a lesion, it ameliorates the abuses caused by compensatory hyperfunction; and good preoperative therapy is the best postoperative voice therapy. It is also invaluable in educating the patient about vocal function and dysfunction and in making sure that he or she is fully informed about surgery and other options. Following surgery, voice therapy is medically necessary for many conditions. It is extremely important to long-term surgical outcome to time surgery so that the patient will be able to comply with postoperative voice rest and postoperative rehabilitation.

Many other conditions must be taken into account when deciding the timing of voice surgery. Concurrent medical conditions such as allergies that produce extensive coughing or sneezing (which may injure vocal folds following surgery), a coagulopathy (even temporary coagulopathy from aspirin use), and other physical factors may be important contributors to voice results. Psychological factors should also be considered. The patient must not only understand the risks and complications of surgery, but also be as psychologically prepared as possible to accept them and to commit to the therapeutic and rehabilitation process. Sometimes psychological preparation requires a delay in surgical scheduling to allow increased time for the patient to work with the voice team. There are very few indications for benign voice surgery that contraindicate a delay of several weeks. It is generally worth taking the time to optimize the patient's comfort and preparedness. Indeed, in the author's opinion, the patient is the most important part of the voice rehabilitation team. Realistic, committed collaboration by the patient is invaluable in achieving consistent, excellent surgical results.

Voice Cosmesis: The "Voice Lift"

In the modern communication age, the voice is critical in projecting image and personality and establishing credibility. Until very recently, voice has not received enough attention from the medical profession or from the general public. In fact, most people (doctors and the general public) do not realize anything can be done to improve a voice that is unsatisfactory or even one that is adequate but not optimal.

Historically, some techniques for voice improvement date back centuries. Singers, actors, and public speakers have sought out "voice lessons" for centuries. However, recently techniques for voice improvement have expanded and improved; and they have become practical for a great many more people.

Vocal weakness, breathiness, instability, impaired quality, and other characteristics can interfere with social and professional success. Many problems (particularly breathiness, softness, instability, tremor, and change in habitual pitch) are associated commonly with aging. For most people, these vocal characteristics, which lead people to perceive a voice (and its owner) as "old" or "infirm," can be improved or eliminated.

The first step for anyone seeking voice improvement is a comprehensive voice evaluation. Often, voice problems that people ascribe to aging, or even to their natural genetic makeup, are caused or aggravated by medical problems. The possibilities are numerous and include such conditions as reflux, low thyroid function, diabetes, tumors, and many others. Sometimes, voice deterioration is the first symptom of a serious medical problem, so comprehensive medical evaluation is essential before treating the voice complaints.

Once medical problems have been ruled out or treated, the next step for vocal habilitation or restoration is a program of therapy or exercise provided by a multidisciplinary team that incorporates the skills of not only a laryngologist, but also a speech-language pathologist and an acting-voice specialist. The training involves aerobic conditioning to strengthen the power source of the voice. In many cases, neuromuscular retraining (specific guided exercise) is sufficient to improve vocal strength and quality, eliminate effort, and restore youthful vocal quality. Doing so is important not only for singers, and other voice professionals (teachers, radio announcers, politicians, clergy, salespeople, receptionists, etc), but also really for almost everyone. This is especially true for the elderly. It is ironic but true that, as we age, voices get softer and weaker and at the same time our spouses and friends lose their hearing. This makes not just professional communication, but also social interaction, difficult, especially in noisy surroundings such as cars and restaurants. When people have to work too hard to communicate, it is often related to vocal deficiencies. Therefore, it is not surprising that, when exercises and medications alone do not provide sufficient improvement, many patients elect voice surgery in an attempt to strengthen their vocal quality and endurance and to improve their quality of life.

Several different procedures can be used to strengthen weak or injured voices. The selection of the operation depends on the individual's vocal condition as determined by a voice team evaluation, physical examination including strobovideolaryngoscopy, and consideration of what the person wants. Care must be taken to ensure that patient expectations are realistic. In most cases, surgery is directed toward bringing the vocal folds closer together so that they close more firmly. This eliminates the air leak between the vocal folds that occurs as a consequence of vocal aging (atrophy or wasting of vocal nodules or other tissues) or as a result of paresis or paralysis (partial injury to a nerve from a viral infection or other causes). In some cases, the operation is done by injecting a material through the mouth or neck into the tissues adjacent to the vocal folds, to "bulk up" the vocal tissues and bring the vocal folds closer together. This is called injection laryngoplasty and is performed usually using fat, collagen, or hydroxyapatite. This operation is sometimes done in the operating room under local anesthesia and, in selected patients, in the office with only local anesthesia. Alternatively, the problem can be corrected by performing a thyroplasty. This operation involves making a small incision in the neck. The skeleton of the voice box is entered, and the laryngeal tissues are compressed slightly using Gore-Tex or Silastic implants. This procedure is generally done under local anesthesia with sedation. All of these procedures usually are performed on an outpatient basis.

Recovery usually takes days to weeks (depending on the procedure). Any operation can be associated with complications. Rarely, the voice can be made worse. The most likely complication is that voice improvement is not quite sufficient or that it does not hold up completely over time. When this problem occurs, it usually can be corrected easily by "fine tuning" through additional injections or surgical adjustment of the implants. However, most of the time, satisfactory results are achieved the first time.

Voice rehabilitation through medical intervention and therapy/exercise training is appropriate for anyone unhappy with his or her vocal quality (so called "voice lift surgery") and is suitable for almost anyone who does not have major, serious medical problems such as end-stage heart disease and is not on blood thinner medication that cannot be stopped safely for surgery, so long as that person has realistic vocal goals and expectations. However, "voice lift" surgery should be thought of as a comprehensive program stressing medical diagnosis and physical rehabilitation not as surgery alone.

Indirect Laryngoscopy

Laryngoscopic surgery is generally performed through direct laryngoscopy, as discussed below. However, indirect laryngoscopic surgery has been performed for many years and still has value in some circumstances. It permits gross biopsy of lesions under local anesthesia, removal of selected foreign bodies, and injection of fat, collagen, and other substances. In patients whose neck will not flex or extend enough to permit rigid direct laryngoscopy (cervical arthritis, fracture, fusion), indirect laryngoscopic surgery may provide a safe alternative to external surgery.

For indirect laryngoscopic surgery, the patient is generally seated. Topical anesthesia is applied and may be augmented by regional blocks. The larynx is visualized either with a laryngeal mirror, laryngeal telescope, or flexible fiberoptic laryngoscope. When surgery is performed solely for injection (eg, fat or collagen), either an external or transoral technique may be used. External injection may be performed by passing the needle through the cricothyroid membrane and into the desired position lateral to the vocal fold or through the thyroid lamina usually near the midpoint of the musculomembranous vocal fold, about 7 to 9 mm above the inferior border of the thyroid cartilage. Transoral injection has been used more commonly (Fig 18–1), and the transoral technique is also suitable for biopsy and other procedures. Assistance is required. The patient's tongue is held with gauze, as for routine indirect laryngoscopy. Cooperative patients may be asked to hold the tongue themselves. Angled instruments designed specifically for indirect laryngoscopic surgery are passed through the mouth and guided visually. Only a surgeon who is skilled in the necessary maneuvers should perform the procedure. The advantages of this technique include relatively easy access in anyone whose larynx can be visualized with a mirror, avoidance of the need for an operating room procedure, and ready availability when delays in getting to a hospital and waiting for an operating room might cause serious problems (eg, a chicken bone perched above the laryngeal inlet). However, the procedure also has distinct disadvantages. Precise control is not as good as that accomplished with microlaryngoscopy under sedation or general anesthesia, intraoperative loss of patient cooperation may result in injury, and the ability to handle complications such as bleeding and edema is limited. Nevertheless, at times the procedure is invaluable, and it should be in the armamentarium of the laryngological surgeon.

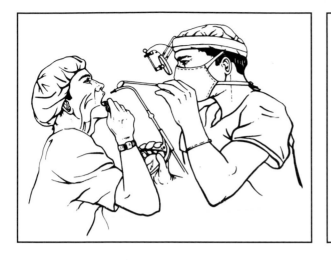

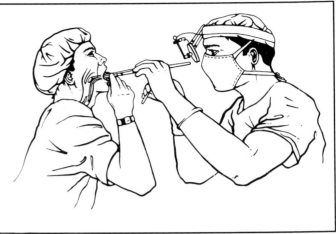

Fig 18–1. (*Left*) After topical anesthesia, the patient firmly holds his tongue extended while the mirror and indirect needle are positioned. (*Right*) The patient phonates a falsetto /i/ as the needle is inserted for injection. Similar positions may be used for biopsy and foreign body removal.

Direct Laryngoscopy

Suspension microlaryngoscopy is now the standard technique for endoscopic laryngeal surgery. The concept of direct laryngoscopy was introduced by Horace Green in 1852[2] using sunlight and supported later by Brünings.[3] The most common light source used later with laryngoscopes was a headlight worn by the examiner. Light carriers built into laryngoscopes were first developed by Chevalier Jackson in 1915.[4] He utilized a light carrier with a tiny incandescent light bulb. Jackson's laryngoscope design included a flat, removable blade that permitted introduction of a bronchoscope. A fiberoptic version of this instrument is still in common use (Fig 18–2). Holinger modified Jackson's laryngoscope by eliminating the removable, sliding component and adding a slight lift near the tip[5] (Fig 18–3). This lifted the epiglottis, improving visualization of the anterior commissure. Holinger's design is still in common use. Kleinsasser popularized the idea of using the microscope as a light source.[6] Since that time, the use of microscope magnification has become an essential, routine part of laryngeal surgery (Fig 18–4). The microscope provides excellent stereoscopic vision and light and magnification that enhances diagnosis and helps refine surgical technique. It should be used in nearly all cases. The Holinger and Jackson laryngoscopes have such small internal diameters that stereoscopic vision cannot be obtained using the microscope. Jako solved these problems by developing a larger laryngoscope and adding two fiberoptic

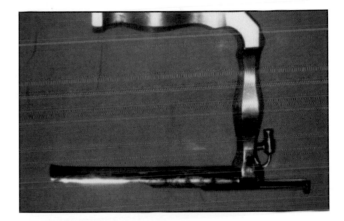

Fig 18–2. Jackson laryngoscope.

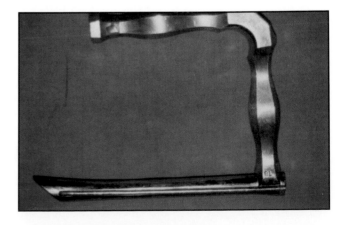

Fig 18–3. Holinger laryngoscope.

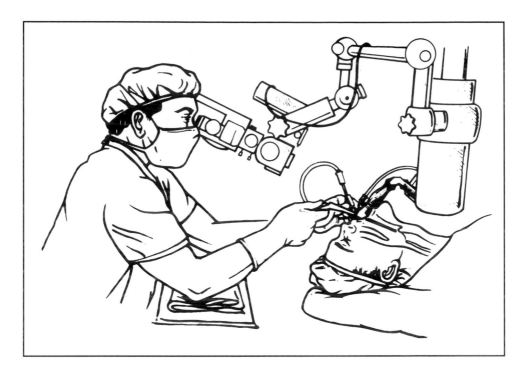

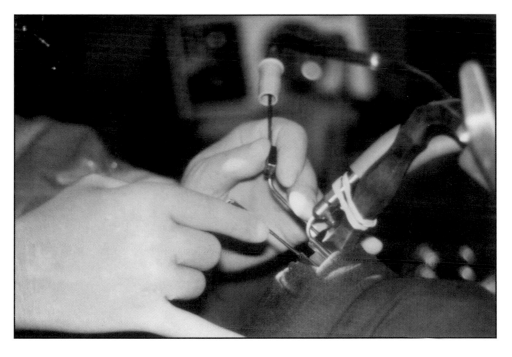

Fig 18–4. Direct microlaryngoscopy. (*Top*) Note the use of the operating microscope and the suspension device. A Mayo stand is placed under the surgeon's arms for stability, and towels cushion the elbows. (*Bottom*) Laryngoscope suspension permits bimanual surgery.

light bundles to improve illumination, especially for photography.[7] Jako's design was a great improvement, but it was too wide and thick to permit good visualization in many patients. Dedo designed a laryngoscope that incorporated many of the advantages of the Jako and of the Holinger laryngoscopes,[8] permitting better visualization of the anterior commissure (Fig 18–5), and stereoscopic vision, as long as the surgeon is at least 61 cm from the patient. Using an operating microscope with a 400-mm objective lens

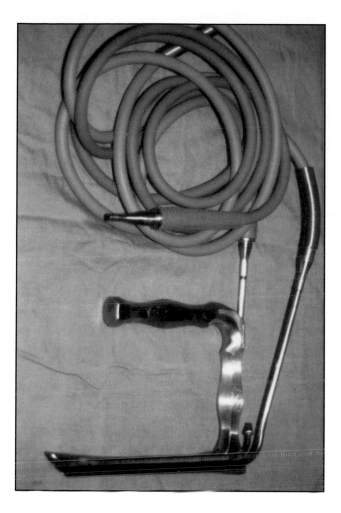

Fig 18–5. Dedo laryngoscope.

larynx to be pulled toward the ceiling (with the patient in supine position)—rather than necessitating a lever action that might fracture teeth, and that works well with the laryngoscope and head position preferred by the surgeon. It should be remembered that the suspension system should be used as a stabilizing device. That is, the surgeon should place the laryngoscope in the desired position and use the "suspension" device to keep it there, rather than using the suspension system to generate the forces necessary to obtain exposure. Adherence to this principle allows safe use of leverage systems such as the Lewy device, as well as lifting systems such as Killian's gallows or the Boston "Window Crank" (Pilling Company, Fort Washington, Pa) suspension systems. In general, the best view of the vocal folds can be obtained with the patient in "sniffing" position, with the neck flexed and the head extended (Fig 18–7). This is also the position used most commonly by anesthesiologists for intubation. When the laryngoscope is placed and suspended, the teeth must be protected from trauma by the laryngoscope; and it is essential that the patient's head be held still. Sudden motion or biting on the laryngoscope may result in patient injury. Direct laryngoscopy may be performed using local anesthesia with sedation, or general anesthesia.

In addition to choosing an appropriate laryngoscope, it is important to understand the principles not only of suspension, but also of internal distention and external counterpressure. In most cases, the laryngoscope should not only provide visualization of the entire vocal fold, but also should distend the false vocal folds and larynx in a way that optimizes visualization. Rarely, this is not desirable; and a laryngoscope positioned in the vallecula (such as the Lindholm, Karl Storz, Culver City, Calif) provides an alternative. However, this is the exception rather than the rule. In addition to internal distention, external counterpressure is important. Gentle pressure over the thyroid cartilage often can produce dramatic improvement in laryngeal visualization through the laryngoscope. Traditionally, a resident, nurse, or anesthetist has been asked to provide the counterpressure. It is better to use 1-inch tape that extends from one side of the headrest of the bed to the other and holds steady pressure on the larynx, maintaining the desired position. It is also important to realize that there can be a disadvantage to counterpressure. Although it improves visibility (especially anteriorly), it also introduces laxity in the vocal folds that may distort slightly the relationships between pathology and normal tissue. Hence, an appropriate compromise much be achieved in each case to optimize visibility of the area of interest without introducing excessive distortion.

permits these conditions to be met and provides adequate working room for the long instruments necessary for endolaryngeal surgery. Numerous modifications of these laryngoscopes have been designed since Jako and Dedo introduced their laryngoscopes, including the Gould laryngoscope[9] and numerous other thoughtfully designed laryngoscopes, a few of which are pictured in Figure 18–6, A-F. It is important for the surgeon to have a choice of laryngoscopes available and to select the one best suited to the patient's anatomy. The surgeon must choose an instrument that minimizes tissue damage while optimizing exposure and facilitating the manipulation of instruments.

Killian introduced the first laryngoscope suspension system in 1910.[10] Numerous suspension systems were invented subsequently. The choice is a matter of personal preference. However, in selecting a suspension system, one should look for a device that allows for two-handed surgery, that permits the tongue and

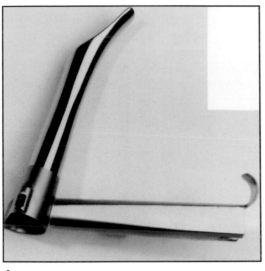

A

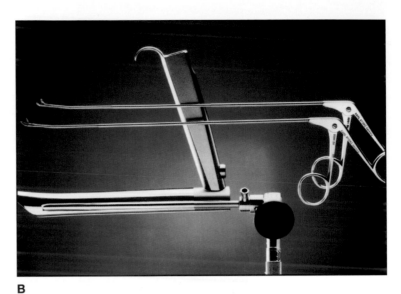

B

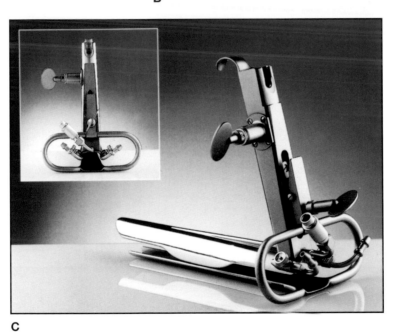

C

Fig 18–6. A. Lindholm laryngoscope (Storz), which fits in the vallecula, is ideal in combination with a Benjamin light clip and is particularly good for photography with 10 mm and other Storz telescopes. **B.** Kantor/Berci video-laryngoscope (Storz). **C.** Weerda distending operating laryngoscopes (Storz). *(continues)*

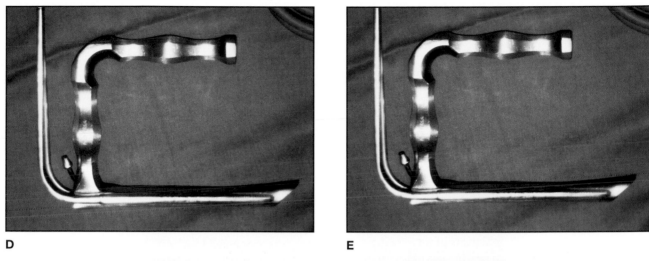

D

E

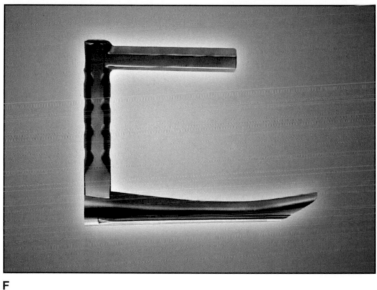

F

Fig 18–6. *(continued)* **D.** Fragen laryngoscope. **E.** Ossoff-Pilling laryngoscope, lateral view. The tip of this laryngoscope is identical to the Holinger anterior commissure laryngoscope. However, the proximal end of the larger male and even the smaller female laryngoscope is just large enough to permit binocular vision and effective laser use. This scope is invaluable for patients who are difficult to visualize, and who ordinarily would have required surgery through the Holinger laryngoscope. **F.** The Sataloff laryngoscope (Medtronics-Xomed, Jacksonville, Fla) has a triangular distal end that approximates the shape of the glottis, and enough lift near the tip to permit good exposure of the anterior commissure. It is available in large, medium (most commonly used), and pediatric sizes, as well as in a small adult anterior commissure form for patients who are particularly difficult to visualize.

Readers interested in additional information regarding counterpressure and the forces involved in laryngoscopy are advised to consult other literature.[11,12]

Anesthesia

Local Anesthesia

Local anesthesia with sedation is desirable in some cases for endoscopic laryngeal surgery, especially if fine adjustments of vocal quality are to be made, as during injection for vocal fold paralysis or reduction of a dislocated arytenoid cartilage. Many techniques of local anesthesia are used. They involve a variety of systemic, topical, and regional medications. The technique described below has proven most effective in the author's hands but should be considered only one of many options. In rare instances, direct laryngoscopy may be performed without operating room support and with topical anesthesia alone.

Generally, procedures are performed in the operating room with monitoring and sedation. Intravenous sedation is administered prior to anesthetic applica-

tion. The author prefers a sedative that produces amnesia, such as midazolam. The oral cavity is sprayed with a topical anesthetic. Cetacaine, 10% Xylocaine, 0.5% Pontocaine, cocaine, and others have all given satisfactory results. Topical anesthetic is routinely supplemented with regional blocks and local infiltration. Bilateral superior laryngeal nerve blocks are achieved using 1% Xylocaine with epinephrine 1:100,000. Superior laryngeal nerve block is accomplished by injecting 1 to 2 cc of Xylocaine into the region where the nerve penetrates the thyrohyoid membrane, anterior to a line between the greater cornu of the thyroid cartilage and the greater cornu of the hyoid bone (Fig 18–8). Glossopharyngeal nerve blocks are placed using 2 cc of Xylocaine in the lateral oropharyngeal wall, a few millimeters medial to the midportion of the posterior tonsillar pillar on each side. The tongue base is then infiltrated with 2 to 4 cc, using a curved tonsil needle and metal tongue depressor. Anesthesia is concluded with intratracheal application

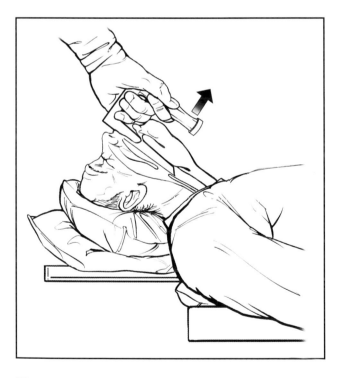

Fig 18–7. "Sniffing position," ideal for visualization during direct laryngoscopy. Note that the neck is flexed and the head is extended. Often the neck must be flexed considerably more than illustrated. The occiput is approximately 15 cm above the bed, supported by a pillow. The arrows indicate correct direction of pull during laryngoscopy.

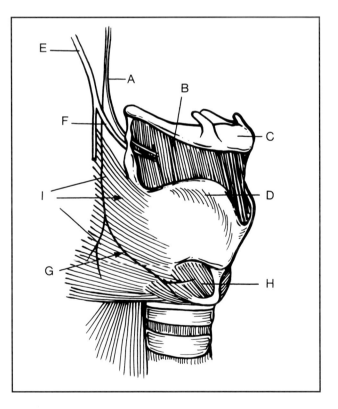

Fig 18–8. Lateral view of the larynx showing penetration of the internal branch of the superior laryngeal nerve (**A**) as it passes through the thyrohyoid membrane (**B**) between the hyoid bone (**C**) and the thyroid cartilage (**D**). Also illustrated are the superior thyroid artery (**E**), superior laryngeal artery (**F**), external branch of the superior laryngeal nerve (**G**), cricothyroid muscle (**H**), and the inferior constrictor (**I**).

of 4 cc of 4% topical xylocaine, administered through a midline injection in the cricothyroid membrane (after anesthetizing the skin with 1% of xylocaine with epinephrine 1:100,000 or by spraying topical anesthetic between the vocal folds if they can be visualized easily using a metal tongue blade). Although this anesthetic procedure can be performed very rapidly, patients frequently have difficulty managing secretions by the time the anesthesia has been applied. Suction should be available.

The adequacy of anesthesia application can be tested by placing a metal tongue depressor against the tongue base and lifting it anteriorly and inferiorly, simulating laryngoscope pressure and placement, while the hypopharynx is suctioned. If anesthesia is adequate, these maneuvers should not disturb the patient. Throughout the application of anesthesia, the physician and anesthesiologist should maintain verbal contact with the patient, carefully control the airway, and monitor vital signs including blood oxygen saturation. If adequate topical and regional anesthesia cannot be established, or if adequate sedation cannot be achieved safely, the procedure either should be discontinued or general anesthesia should be induced. Both the patient and the anesthesia team should be prepared for possible use of general anesthetic in all cases.

Most laryngeal procedures can be performed safely under local anesthesia. This choice provides not only the opportunity to monitor voice during the procedure, but also protection from the risks of endotracheal intubation. However, there are also disadvantages. When maximal precision is necessary, the motion present during local anesthesia may be troublesome. Greater accuracy is enhanced by general anesthesia with paralysis. The safety of local anesthesia during some cases of endolaryngeal surgery is questionable. In addition to mechanical surgical problems, in some patients with cardiac or pulmonary problems, the respiratory suppression caused by sedation may be more hazardous than general anesthesia. In addition, local anesthetics themselves may produce side effects. These may include mucosal irritation and inflammation (contact dermatitis) that may cause not only erythema and pruritus, but also vesiculation and oozing; dehydration of mucosal surfaces or an escharotic effect (especially from prolonged contact); hypersensitivity (rash); generalized urticaria (edema); methemoglobinemia; and anaphylaxis. Safety for use during pregnancy has not been established for most topical anesthetics used commonly in laryngology; and they should be utilized only under pressing clinical circumstances, if at all, during the first trimester of pregnancy. Methemoglobinemia may be a particularly frightening complication of local anesthesia. Methemoglobin is also called ferric protoporphyrin (IX globulin), ferrihemoglobin, and hemiglobin; because the iron in methemoglobin is trivalent (or ferric) instead of divalent (ferrous). Methemoglobinemia produces cyanosis, although skin discoloration is usually the only symptom or sign of acquired methemoglobinemia. This condition can be induced by any amine-type local anesthetic. Prilocaine and benzocaine are the drugs implicated most commonly.[13] Infants may be somewhat more susceptible, but the condition may occur in patients of any age. Methemoglobinemia is actually a misnomer because the pigment is intracellular and is not found in the plasma. Methemoglobincythemia would be more accurate; but methemoglobinemia is used commonly. Methemoglobinemia is treated by intravenous administration of methylene blue, although the condition is not life threatening and will resolve spontaneously. The notion that local anesthesia is always preferable to general anesthesia should be viewed with skepticism. The choice depends on the patient, the lesion, the surgeon, and the anesthesiologist.

General Anesthesia

Probably the most important consideration in general anesthesia for voice patients is the choice of the anesthesiologist. Laryngologists performing voice surgery must insist on the collaboration of an excellent anesthesiologist who understands vocal fold surgery and the special needs of voice patients. Those of us who work in teaching institutions recognize that medical students and first-year anesthesia residents need to practice intubation. However, this need should not be met on patients undergoing surgery for voice improvement, especially professional voice users. When a gentle, skilled, well-informed anesthesiologist and laryngologist collaborate, the choice of anesthetic depends solely on the patient and lesion, and safe effective surgery can be carried out. Such teamwork benefits the laryngologist, anesthesiologist, hospital, and especially the patient; and every effort should be made to establish the necessary professional collaboration.

The choice of agents for general anesthesia is beyond the scope of this chapter. However, in general, the regimen includes use of a short-term paralytic agent to avoid patient motion or swallowing. Intubation and extubation should be accomplished atraumatically, using the smallest possible tube. Most laryngeal endoscopic procedures are short in duration, and a 5-0 tube is generally sufficient even for most moderately obese patients. The laser may be used during many procedures, and it is best to employ a laser-resistant endotracheal tube unless the surgeon is absolutely certain that the laser will not be activated. Laser precautions are discussed in *Professional Voice*.[15]

Antireflux medications are prudent especially in patients with symptoms and signs of reflux, but reflux may occur under anesthesia even in patients who do not have significant clinical reflux. The combination of acid exposure and direct trauma from the endotracheal tube can lead to laryngeal mucosal injury. Intravenous steroids (eg, 10 mg of dexamethasone) may be helpful in minimizing inflammation and edema and possibly in protecting against cellular injury; and intravenous steroids should be used at the surgeon's discretion, if there is no contraindication.

Endotracheal intubation provides the safest, most stable ventilation under general anesthesia; and it generally provides adequate visibility. However, in some cases, even a small endotracheal tube may interfere with surgery. Alternatives include general anesthesia without intubation and with jet ventilation. Laryngeal microsurgery without intubation was reported by Urban.[14] The technique involves intravenous thiopental, 100% oxygen by mask initially, and manually controlled oxygen insufflation. Few anesthesiologists are comfortable with this technique, and the oxygen insufflation can be an inconvenience during surgery.

Venturi jet ventilation can be a useful technique. Anesthetic and oxygen can be delivered through a needle placed in the lumen of the laryngoscope, through a ventilation channel in specially designed laryngoscope channels, through a catheter just above or below the vocal folds, such as the Hunsicker catheter (Medtronics-Xomed, Jacksonville, Fla) used by the author Fig 18–9A) or through a Carden tube (Fig 18–9B).[16] The author uses the Hunsicker catheter because of its easy placement, security, laser resistance, and the fact that the jet ventilation initiates below the vocal folds. This seems to cause less mechanical interference at the vibratory margin during surgery. However, the catheter must be placed between the vocal folds carefully by an expert anesthesiologist or the laryngologist and removed carefully, to avoid intubation and extubation trauma as might be caused by placement of any endotracheal tube. During any surgery that employs jet ventilation, it is essential that the surgeon be a knowledgeable, cooperative part of the anesthesia team. The airway must remain unobstructed for expiration. If the laryngoscope moves or is removed obstructing the airway without a warning to the anesthesia team, pneumothorax may result.

All the care exercised in gentle intubation may be for naught unless similar caution is exercised during extubation. The most common error during extubation is failure to fully deflate the endotracheal tube cuff. This may result in vocal fold trauma or arytenoid cartilage dislocation. The anesthesia team should be aware of these problems. The surgeon should be present and attentive during intubation and extubation to help minimize the incidence of such problems.

Anesthesia is also a prime concern during surgery outside the head and neck. Laryngologists are frequently called on for guidance by professional voice users, surgeons, and anesthesiologists. The anesthesiologist must appreciate that the patient is a voice professional, and ensure that intubation and extubation are performed by the most skilled anesthesiologist available. In addition, anesthesiologists must temper their tendency to use the largest possible tube. There are very few procedures that cannot be performed safely through a size 6.5 or smaller endotracheal tube, and many can be performed with mask anesthesia or a Brain laryngeal mask without intubating the larynx at all. When possible, alternatives to general anesthesia should be considered, such as spinal blocks, regional blocks, and acupuncture. Many procedures commonly done under general anesthesia with intubation can be performed equally well using another technique. After surgery, postoperative voice assessment by the anesthesiologist, patient, and operating surgeon is essential. If voice abnormalities are present (other than very mild hoarseness that resolves within 24 hours), prompt laryngological examination should be arranged.

Instrumentation

Microlaryngeal surgery utilizes magnification, usually provided by an operating microscope, which is used through a laryngoscope (laryngoscope placement is discussed above). Many surgeons are not familiar with formulas that determine accurately the amount of magnification used, and it is often recorded incorrectly in operative reports. It is not unusual for surgeons to assume that the number on the indicator on the zoom control correlates with the number of times the image is magnified; but accurate determination is more complex than that. This author usually works with a Zeiss operating microscope (Oberkochen, Germany), and the information in this discussion refers specifically to Zeiss instruments. However, the principles are the same for microscopes manufactured by other companies. To determine the amount of magnification, the focal length of the binocular tube is divided by the focal length of the objective lens, and then multiplied by the magnification of the eyepieces.[17] That number is then multiplied by the indicator on the magnification (zoom) control of the microscope, on a modern microscope. The focal length of the binocular tube is usually a number such as F125,

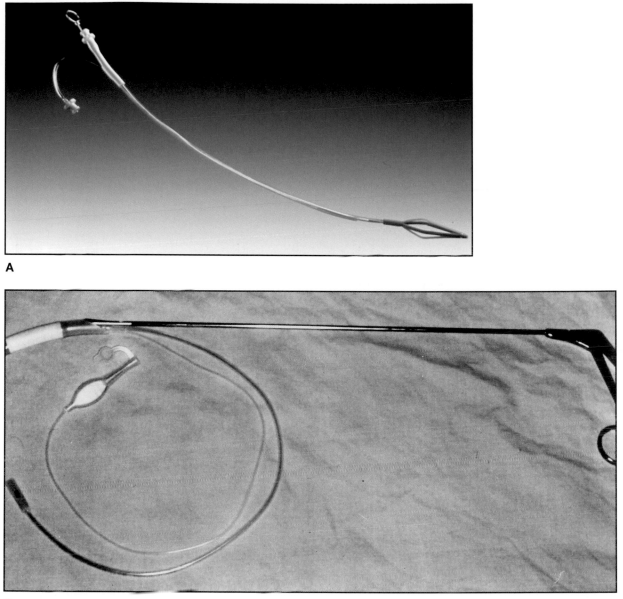

Fig 18–9. **A.** The Hunsicker Jet Ventilation Catheter (Medtronics-Xomed, Jacksonville, Fla). **B.** Carden tube grasped in forceps in preparation for insertion. Except for the ventilating and inflation tubes, the entire device will be positioned below the vocal folds before the cuff is inflated.

F160, or F170. For example, the Zeiss OPMI-6 microscope has a binocular tube with a focal length of F160, and the newer design with the wider angle of view has a focal length of F170. The focal length of the objective lens varies depending on the surgeon's preference. For ear surgery, it is usually 250 or 300 mm. For laryngeal surgery, a 400-mm lens is used most commonly. The usual eyepiece magnification is either 10× or 12.5×. The indicator number on a modern Zeiss operating microscope can be read through a small window next to the zoom control knob, and the number ranges from 0.4 to 2.4. The OPMI-6-S, for example, provides a continuous magnification range of 1:4. Older Zeiss operating microscopes (such as the OPMI-1) have magnification changes that are steplike rather than continuous and have numbers that range from 6 to 40 next to the dial. These provide five magnification steps in a range of 1:6. These numbers should not be used in the formula noted above, but can be converted as follows: 40 corresponds to 2.5; 25 corresponds to 1.6; 16

corresponds to 1.0; 10 corresponds to 0.6; 6 corresponds to 0.4. So, for example, if a surgeon is using an OPMI-1 microscope with 10× eyepieces, a 400-mm objective lens, and the magnification set at 40 (maximum), image magnification is 7.8× ($^{125}/_{400}$ × 25 × 10 = 7.8×), not 40×, as misstated commonly.

Simply changing the eyepieces from 10× to 12.5× increases the magnification from 7.8× to 9.8× and using 20× eyepieces increases the magnification to 15.6. Utilizing an objective lens with a shorter focal length also increases magnification but brings the microscope closer to the operating field. Although this approach is used during ear surgery, it is not suitable for laryngeal surgery because the decreased space between the microscope and direct laryngoscope is not sufficient to permit unimpeded manipulation of long-handled laryngeal instruments. It is important for surgeons to be familiar with these principles to optimize surgical conditions for each specific case and to document surgery accurately.

Magnifying laryngeal telescopes are also invaluable for assessing vocal fold pathology and mapping lesions for surgery. Most commonly, the author uses 10-mm 0° and 4-mm 70° telescopes (Karl Storz, Culver City, Calif); and 30° and 120° telescopes are useful in some circumstances. Laryngeal telescopes allow the surgeon to visualize lesions in great detail, to appreciate the limits of lesions in three dimensions better than can be accomplished through a microscope, and to visualize obscure areas such as the laryngeal ventricle (Fig 18–10).

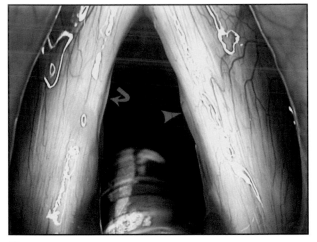

B

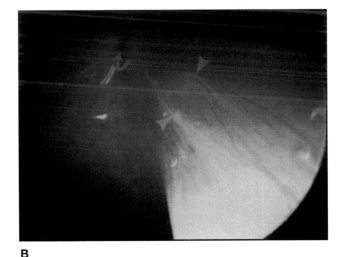

B

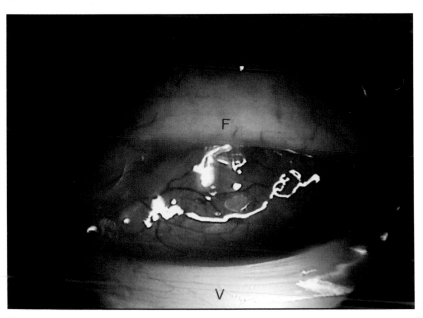

C

Fig 18–10. A. Vocal folds visualized through 10-mm 0 degree telescope (Karl Storz, Culver City, Calif.) showing a right vocal fold cyst (*arrowhead*) and left reactive swelling (*curved arrow*). **B.** Vocal folds visualized through a 70° telescope, allowing better evaluation of the vertical surface of the vibratory margin. This view shows that the cyst (*arrowheads*) involves only the superior one-third to one-half of the vibratory margin. The anterior commissure can be seen, as well (*curved arrow*). **C.** The laryngeal ventricle visualized above the true vocal fold and below the false vocal fold through a 70° telescope.

A technique known as *contact endoscopy* has been used by gynecologic surgeons for many years. Its value in microlaryngeal surgery was recognized by Dr. Mario Andrea.[18] This technique uses a vital staining agent such as methylene blue. Contact endoscopy permits visualization of the cellular nature and integrity of vocal fold epithelium at any given point along the vocal fold. Cell nuclear characteristics are visible, and specific borders between pathologic, transitional, and normal epithelium can be defined, permitting precise surgical intervention. (Fig 18–11, A–F). Although this technique is relatively new and requires additional study and experience, it appears extremely valuable in selected cases.

Delicate microsurgery requires sharp, precise, small instruments. The few heavy cupped forceps and scissors that constituted a laryngoscopy tray through the early 1980s are no longer sufficient. It is now possible to obtain microlaryngeal instruments that look like ear instruments on long handles. Instruments should be long enough to be manipulated easily in the laryngoscope, but not so long that they bump into the microscope. They should include scissors (straight up, up-biting, curved left, and curved right), small grasping cupped forceps (straight, up-biting, right, and left), larger cupped forceps (straight and up-biting, at least), alligator forceps (straight, right, and left), scalpel, right-angle and oblique blunt ball-tipped dissectors, spatula, scalpel, retractors, mirrors for reflecting lasers, and suctions (Fig 18–12 and 18–13A–Z). Cutting instruments should be sharp at all times. Suctions should be thumb controlled, of several sizes, and should include both open tip and velvet eye designs. A suction/cautery tip may be valuable occasionally and should be available, as should cotton carriers. Nonreflective instruments with laser-resistant coating may be advantageous in some situations. The selection and use of lasers are discussed in *Professional Voice*.[15]

Powered laryngeal surgery is a relatively new concept, although powered surgery for other areas of the body has been utilized for many years.[19] Acoustic neuroma surgeons have used powered instruments such as the House-Urban Rotary Dissector (Urban Engineering, Burbank, Calif) for 3 decades; arthroscopic knee surgeons use powered instruments regularly; and powered instruments have been important to functional endoscopic sinus surgery. Their role in laryngeal surgery is not defined completely; but powered laryngeal surgery is clearly useful in the treatment of some conditions such as selected papillomas and neoplasms. The author uses the Medtronics-Xomed XPS Power System (Jacksonville, Fla) with disposable laryngeal shaver blades. To use powered instruments safely, it is important to understand the blades and instrument settings. For example, to debulk a large, exophytic or fibrous lesion, the tri-cut laryngeal blade is utilized at 3,000 rpm. To remove papilloma near the vibratory margin or anterior commissure in a controlled fashion, it is more appropriate to use a 3.5-mm laryngeal skimmer blade at a speed of 500 rpm in the "oscillate" mode. Although some surgeons prefer using powered instruments under endoscopic control rather than using a microscope (Fig 18–14), this author generally prefers using a microscope to permit binocular vision and bimanual manipulation. However, surgeons should have endoscopes available and be comfortable with their use. In some cases, difficult anatomy precludes visualization of certain regions of the larynx, especially at and above the anterior commissure. In such cases, the best way to remove pathology may be through the use of a 70° telescope for visualization and a powered skimmer blade for resection. Although delicate microdissection is still the most controlled and appropriate technique for removing most benign lesions such as cysts and polyps from the vibratory margin of the vocal fold and remains this author's preferred technique for most lesions, powered instruments used properly allow surprising precision and may be helpful especially for selected papillomas and neoplasms.

Laryngeal Microsurgery

Submucosal Infusion; Hemorrhage Control; Steroid Injection

The concept of laryngeal infusion was introduced in the 1890s for the purpose of anatomic studies.[20-21] The technique has been used intermittently over the years for a variety of purposes including infusion of steroids to disrupt adhesions in vocal fold scar, placement of collagen along the vibratory margin, and for separating benign and malignant lesions from underlying structures. The technique has been become more popular among clinicians since the 1990s.[22-24]

Submucosal infusion may be appropriate for a variety of vocal fold masses, but it has disadvantages as well as advantages. Infusion usually is performed utilizing a solution made by combining 9 cc of sterile saline with 1 cc of epinephrine 1:1,000 (a 1 to 10,000 dilution). A small amount of this mixture is infused submucosally using a 30-gauge needle to increase the fluid content of the superficial layer of the lamina propria, to separate the undersurface of the lesion more clearly from the vocal ligament, and to help define the

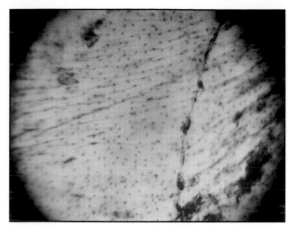

A

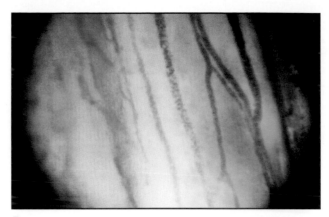

B

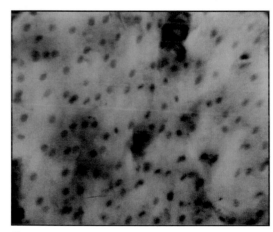

C

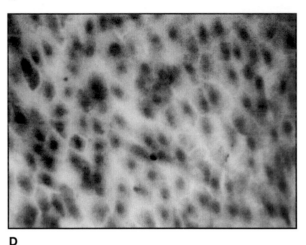

D

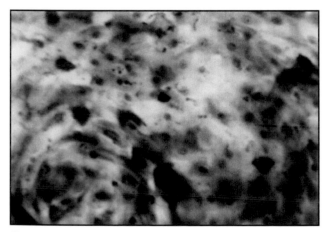

E

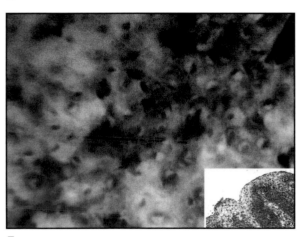

F

Fig 18–11. A. Contact endoscopy of the vocal folds (60×) revealing regular cellular characteristics, and epithelial folds. **B.** Contact endoscopy (60×) showing the normal pattern of the microvascular of the vocal fold. **C.** Contact endoscopy of normal vocal fold epithelium (150×) showing nuclear characteristics in greater detail. **D.** Contact endoscopy revealing dysplasia (150×) illustrated by the heterogeneous appearance of the epithelium, and the increased dimensions and irregular staining of the nuclei. **E.** Contact endoscopy (150×) of carcinoma, illustrating marked irregu- larity in the epithelial cellular pattern and nuclei with abnormalities of shape, size, staining characteristics, and nucleus/cytoplasmic ratio. **F.** Contact endoscopy (150×) of papilloma showing ballooning of the cells and cytoplasmic vacuoles pushing the nuclei toward the periphery of the cells. Also seen are inflammatory cells with regular, large nuclei. The insert shows a histological section of papilloma. Contact endoscopy may be helpful in identifying the boundary between papilloma and normal mucosa. (Reprinted from Andrea and Dias,[17] with permission.)

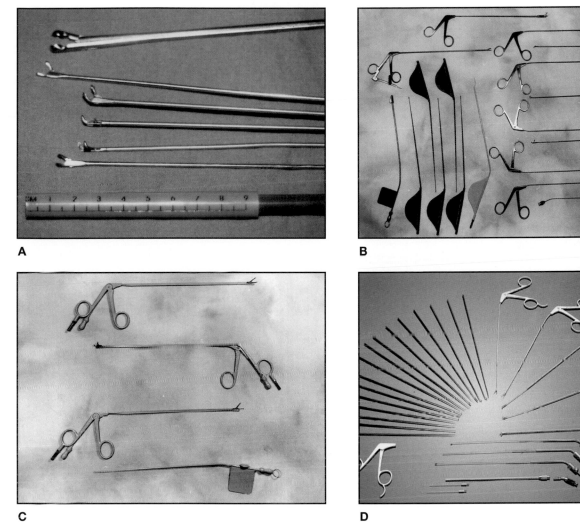

A

B

C

D

Fig 18–12. A. Traditional laryngeal cupped forceps (*top*), compared with more modern instruments designed by Dr Marc Bouchayer (Medtronics-Xomed, Jacksonville, Fla). **B.** Additional delicate Medtronics-Xomed instruments used routinely by this author. **C.** Extremely useful Medtronics-Xomed (Jacksonville, Fla) suction cautery instruments designed by J Abitbol. **D.** Selected instruments designed by the author (RT Sataloff), manufactured by Medtronics-Xomed, Jacksonville, Fla.

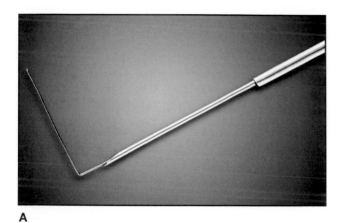

A

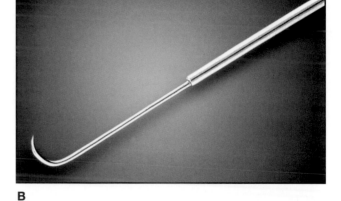

B

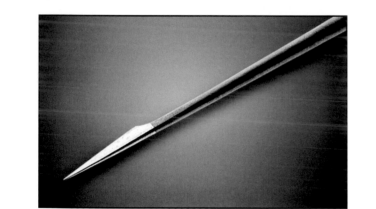

C

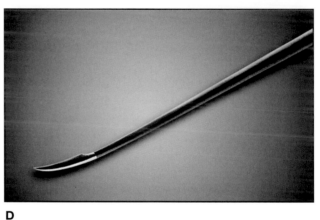

D

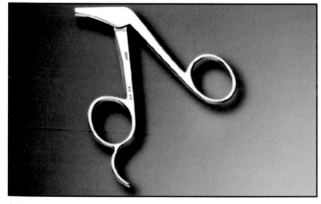

E

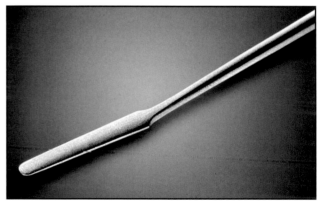

F

Fig 18–13. Selected microlaryngeal instruments (A-W are Sataloff Instruments, Medtronics-Xomed, Jacksonville, Fla). **A.** 30-gauge straight disposable needle (with cleaning stylet in place) for submucosal infusion or collagen injection. **B.** 30-gauge right-angle disposable needle with cleaning stylet in place. **C.** Sharp microknife. This and the sickle knife are disposable and screw into a handle. The vascular knife and selected other sharp instruments are designed similarly. They are intended for single use so the instruments are optimally sharp for each patient. **D.** Sickle knife. **E.** Universal scissor handle. All of the straight-handle Sataloff instruments are designed to fit in the universal scissor handle. This not only allows the instrument tip to be positioned at any angle, but it also permits case-by-case adjustments of instrument length from the handle to the tip. This allows the tip of the instrument to be on the vocal fold, while the handle is close enough to the laryngoscope to permit the surgeon's fingers to be placed against the head or laryngoscope for stabilization. **F.** Straight spatula. *(continues)*

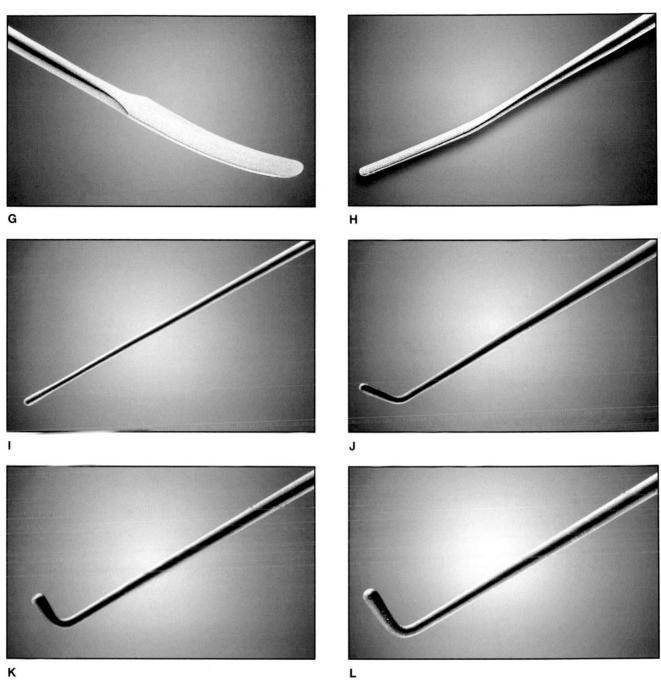

Fig 18–13. *(continued)* **G.** Curved spatula. **H.** Fine angled spatula. **I.** Straight blunt ball dissector. **J.** Oblique blunt ball dissector. **K.** Small right angle blunt ball dissector. **L.** Long right-angle blunt ball dissector. *(continues)*

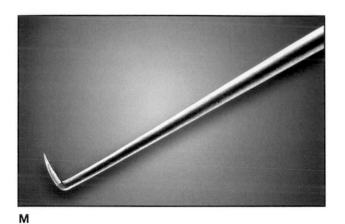

M

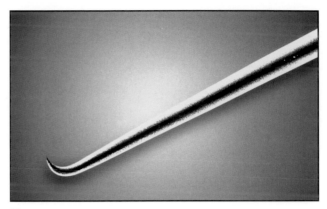

N

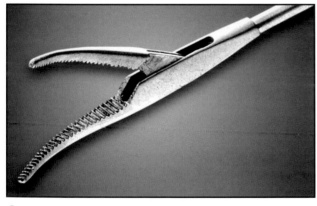

O

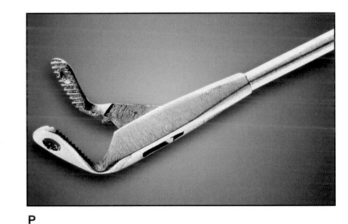

P

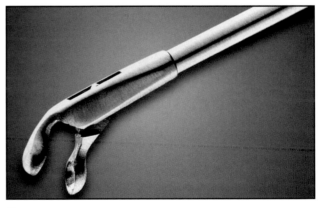

Q

R

Fig 18–13. *(continued)* **M.** Sharp right-angle hook. **N.** Vascular knife. This 1-mm instrument is sharp on the point and blunt on the bottom. It is used for dissecting varicose blood vessels off the vocal fold. It is essential that it not be confused with the mini-microflap knife. **O.** The mini-microflap knife is similar to the sharp right-angle hook, except the mini-microflap knife is sharpened on the bottom, as well as the tip. This allows it to be placed within a mucosal pocket and to cut tissue sharply through a small access incision. If it is inadvertently confused with the vascular knife and used for vascular dissection, the sharp inferior surface of the microknife can damage the vocal fold. **P.** Small heart-shaped grasper (comes in right and left directions, left only shown). **Q.** Left alligator forceps. **R.** Down-biting forceps. *(continues)*

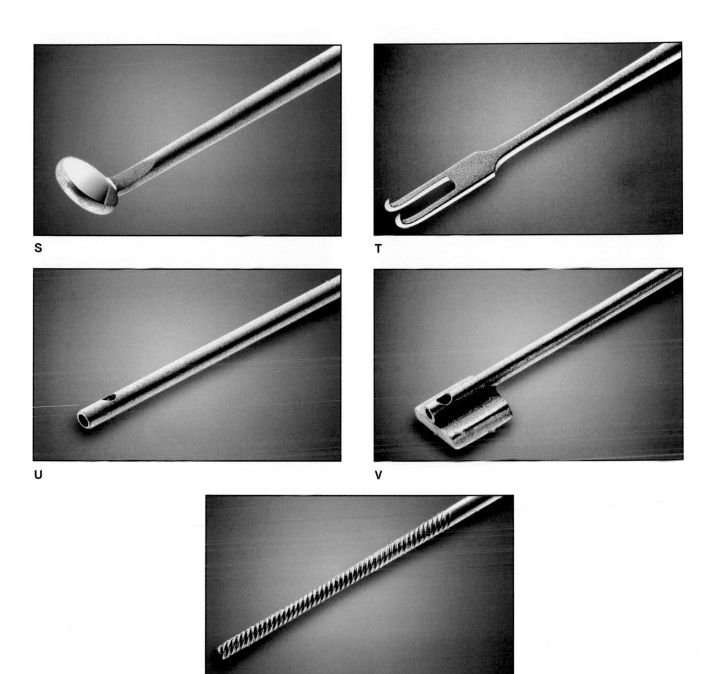

Fig 18–13. *(continued)* **S.** Polished mirror for reflecting and redirecting laser light (small and large mirrors are available). **T.** Fine double hook for retracting laryngeal flaps and large lesions. **U.** 3-French velvet eye suction used during microflap dissection. **V.** 3-French velvet eye suction with metal surface to retract tissue and to prevent tissue prolapse into the surgical field. **W.** Cotton carrier. *(continues)*

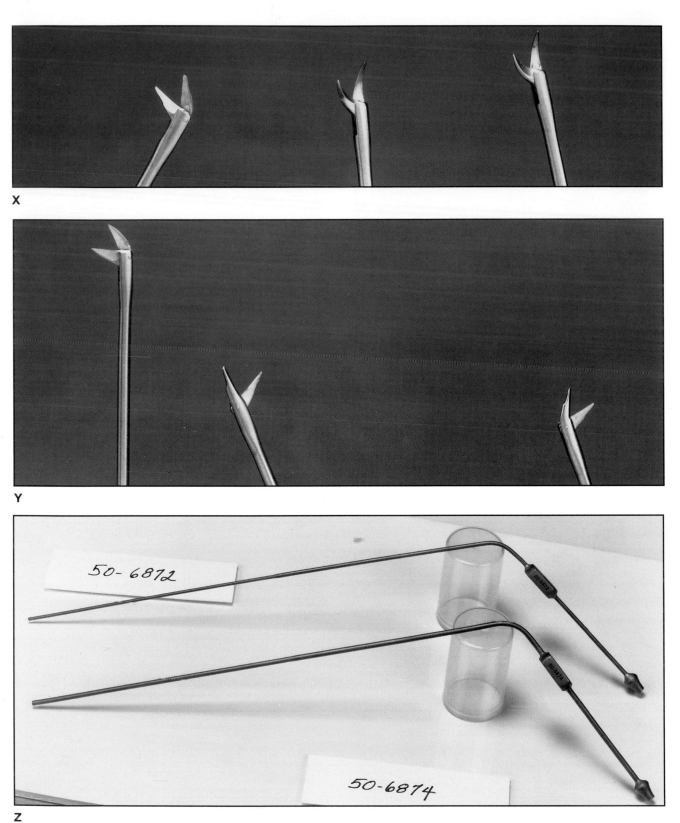

Fig 18–13. *(continued)* **X.** Blunt scissors, vertical action, angled down; blunt scissors, horizontal action, curved blades, open left; sharp scissors, horizontal action, curved blades, open left. **Y.** From left to right, sharp scissors, vertical action, angled down; blunt scissors, vertical action, straight blades; blunt scissors, vertical action, angled up (numerous other variations are available). **Z.** Suctions, 5 French and 7 French diameter.

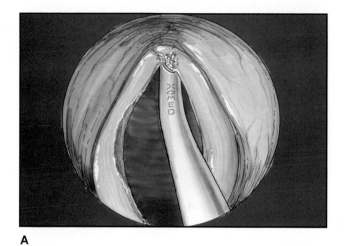

A

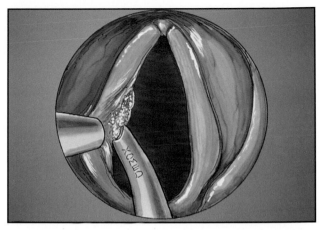

B

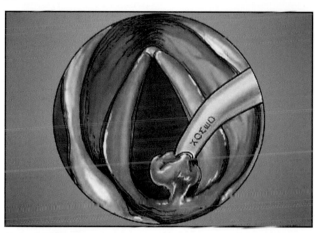

C

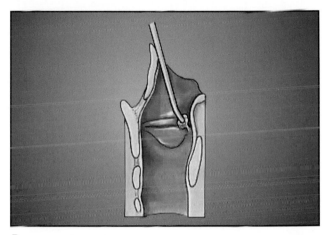

D

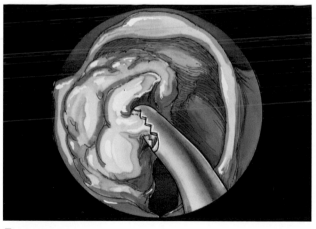

E

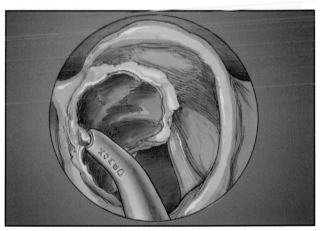

F

Fig 18–14. Powered laryngeal surgery using a skimmer blade in the right hand, endoscope in the left hand, and video monitor for visualization. **A.** 3.5-mm skimmer blade at 500 rpm, visualized through a laryngeal telescope, being used to remove papilloma from the anterior commissure. **B.** 3.5-mm skimmer blade removing papilloma from the under-surface of the left vocal fold. An operating microscope is being used, allowing use of a suction in the left hand to retract the vocal fold. **C** and **D.** 3.5-mm skimmer blade is used to remove a posterior laryngeal polyp. A collection system is placed in line with the suction tubing to collect the pathological specimen **E.** A 4-mm tri-cut blade is used at 3,000 rpm to debulk a large tumor. **F.** After most of the tumor mass has been removed, a 4-mm, angle-tip laryngeal blade can be used at 500 to 1,000 rpm to remove tumor from the margins more delicately. *(continues)*

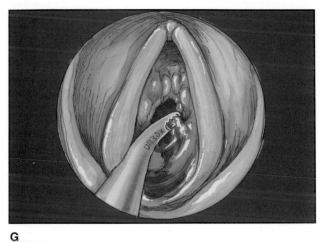

G

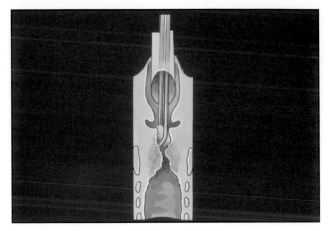

H

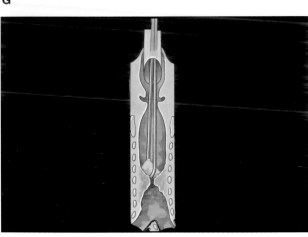

I

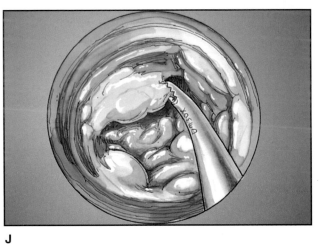

J

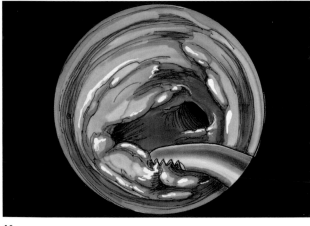

K

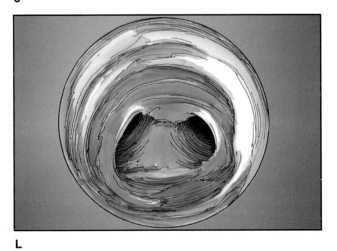

L

Fig 18–14. *(continued)* **G** and **H.** An angle-tip blade at 500 to 1,000 rpm or subglottic blade 4.0 mm or 3.5 mm in diameter can be used to remove subglottic granulation tissue. A tri-cut blade at 3,000 rpm would be more appropriate for a densely fibrotic, stenotic lesion in this region. **I–L.** A 4-mm angle-tip tri-cut subglottic blade at 3,000 rpm can be invaluable for treating tracheal stenosis endoscopically.

The laryngeal shaver can remove tissue that is difficult to treat with cold instruments and difficult to reach with a laser. Visualization can be provided through a microscope, or utilizing an endoscope, as illustrated in **I.** Removal of tissue (**J** and **K**) generally allows reestablishment of an appropriate tracheal lumen (**L**) with good visual and technical control. *(continues)*

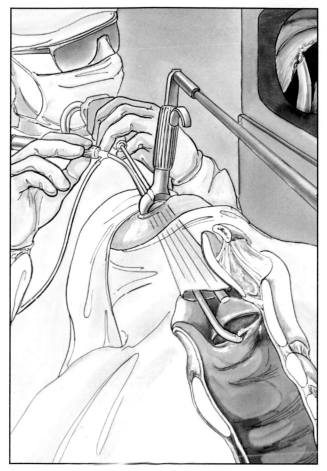

M

Fig 18–14. *(continued)* **M.** Although this author prefers to use a microscope permitting use of powered instrumentation in one hand and a suction or other instrument in the opposite hand, some surgeons prefer to operate while looking at a monitor and using an endoscope in one hand and a powered instrument in the other hand. (Courtesy of Medtronics-Xomed, Jacksonville, Fla.)

vocal ligament more clearly. In lesions such as sulcus vocalis, vocal fold scar, and papilloma, this technique is extremely helpful. In other lesions such as small vocal fold cysts, it may actually obscure the pathology making surgery more difficult. When utilized in appropriate cases, the epinephrine also causes vasoconstriction and helps minimize bleeding. When bleeding does occur, in most cases, it can be controlled with topical application of epinephrine 1:1,000 on a small cottonoid. Rarely, cauterization with a laser or cautery is required. Infusion of saline and epinephrine does not have to be limited to the vocal fold itself. Infusion also can be performed in the false vocal fold and lateral to the ventricle. This infusion technique can be successful in everting the ventricle into the surgical field, providing direct access to lesions that involve the deep recesses of the laryngeal ventricle.

In some cases, submucosal infusion may be performed with a substance other than saline with epinephrine. For example, if the surgeon plans to inject steroid in a patient with scar or sulcus, the steroid may be used for infusion initially. It is as effective as saline and epinephrine in defining the lesion and tissue planes, but it does not provide an equally good hemostatic effect. The efficacy of steroid injection in the vocal folds is unknown. Some surgeons use it regularly. Others are concerned that it may result in muscle atrophy. If used, it is important for the surgeon to utilize an aqueous solution, not an oil-based preparation. Moreover, the author recommends against using milky-colored preparations such as Kenalog (Westwood Squibb, Buffalo, NY). Occasionally, the white suspended particles can precipitate and form a plaque that takes months to resolve.[24] *This* problem has not been encountered with clear solutions such as dexamethasone. Cidofovir can also be used sparingly as the infusion material in patients with papilloma.

Vocal Fold Cysts (with an Overview of the Evolution of Voice Microsurgery)

When submucosal cysts cause symptoms sufficient to warrant surgery, it is essential to resect them without damaging adjacent normal tissue. At the time the first edition of this book was published, the author recommended laryngeal microflaps to accomplish this goal. By the time the second edition was published, that recommendation had changed. Management of vocal fold cysts provides a particularly good window on the evolution of voice surgery.

Vast improvements in surgical care of vocal fold abnormalities occurred in the 1980s and 1990s. These changes have resulted largely because of advances in knowledge of the anatomy and physiology of the vocal tract, technological developments that have improved our ability to examine and quantify voice function, and the availability of better surgical instruments.[25-30] Because the human is the only species with a vocal ligament, there is no experimental animal for vocal fold surgery. Therefore, surgical advances have been based largely on anecdote and common sense. Consequently, it is essential to reevaluate results continually and to consider changing pronouncements about optimal techniques, especially when research provides important new information.

Through the mid-1970s (and later in some centers), the operation of choice for benign vocal fold pathology was "vocal cord stripping," an operation now abandoned except perhaps in selected cases of laryngeal cancer. However, until the mid-1970s, the available facts led us to believe that the operation made sense. Not knowing the complexity of the anatomy of the vibratory margin, we reasoned that the mucosa of the vocal fold edge had become deranged. If we removed it, it seemed probable that the healing process would replace diseased mucosa with new, healthy mucosa. Mucosal healing in the oral cavity and elsewhere in the upper respiratory tract was rarely a problem; so, why should there be a problem on the vocal folds? We had no explanation for the patients who appeared to have normal vocal folds but terrible voices after this operation and we tended to diagnose their persistent dysphonia as psychogenic. In retrospect, knowing what we do now about vocal fold anatomy and physiology, we have no explanation for the fact that so many of those patients were not permanently hoarse. Nevertheless, the beginning of the end of vocal fold stripping came in 1975 when Hirano described the anatomy of the vocal fold (Fig 18–15), which led to a better understanding of vocal fold scar formation and the development of surgical techniques to try to avoid it.[26]

Hirano demonstrated that the vocal fold consisted of an epithelium; superficial, intermediate, and deep layers of the lamina propria; and thyroarytenoid muscle. Further, he pointed out that fibroblasts capable of producing scar were numerous, primarily in the intermediate and deep layers of the lamina propria and the muscle. Most benign vocal fold pathology (nodules, polyps, etc) is superficial. Moreover, research from numerous centers highlighted the importance of the complex mucosal wave created during phonation.[28-34] Consequently, although delicate microsurgery had been advocated by a small number of farsighted laryngologists in the past, the need for this approach to voice surgery quickly became generally accepted.[35] Eventually, surgeons began to think of the anatomy and function of the vocal fold in layers, of pathology in layers, and to conceptualize surgery in layers. This paradigm resulted in the current concepts and techniques of phonomicrosurgery that are designed to remove the pathology without disturbing any adjacent normal tissue.

Vocal fold microsurgery developed rapidly in the 1980s and became the new standard of care. It was based on the notion that surgery should be designed

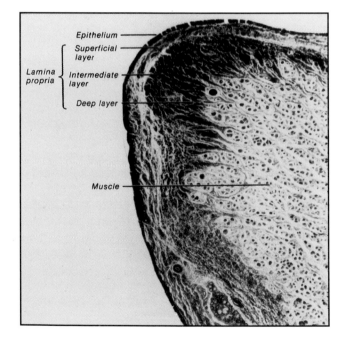
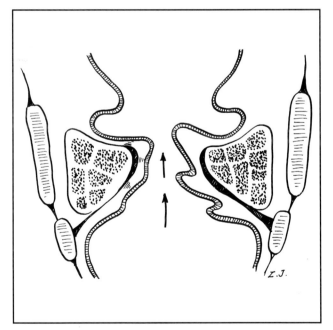

Fig 18–15. The structure of the vocal fold. The vocal fold on the right shows normal free mobility of the cover over the body of the vocal folds as air flows (*arrows*) through the glottis. The drawing on the left illustrates scarring of the epithelium to the deeper layers of the lamina propria, resulting in restriction of the mucosal wave and stiffness, as seen during stroboscopy. When the scarring is severe enough to stop vibration, the nonvibrating portion is known as an adynamic segment. Minimizing trauma to fibroblast-containing layers helps avoid this complication. (From Hirano M. *Clinical Examination of Voice*. New York, NY: Springer-Verlag, 1981:5, with permission.)

to remove pathology without provoking scar formation, that is, without stimulating fibroblasts in the intermediate layer of the lamina propria, or deeper. With this goal in mind, it seemed reasonable to protect the intermediate layer of lamina propria by preserving mucosa along the vibratory margin. If mucosa were absent, then the intermediate layer of lamina propria would be traumatized directly by contact with the contralateral vocal fold during phonation or swallowing. This contact trauma was prevented by elevating a microflap, resecting submucosal lesions, and replacing the mucosa (Fig 18–16). This technique was proposed first by the author in about 1982 and was published and illustrated in 1986.[36] It has been recommended by numerous other authors since that time.[25,35-40] This technique was attractive because the vocal folds *looked* "healed" almost immediately. However, this surgical

concept was based entirely on reasoning, not on research. Although this is unfortunate, in many ways it is unavoidable. In the absence of an animal model with a layered lamina propria, we have little alternative. Nevertheless, although it may not be reasonable to perform prospective, randomized human research on microsurgical techniques, at the very least we are obligated to look closely and critically at our results to see whether our common sense is producing consistently favorable outcomes in our patients. To be sure, laryngeal microflap surgery was a great improvement over vocal fold stripping. Since laryngologists began operating with delicate, small instruments and handling tissues gently, we have seen far fewer cases of permanent dysphonia from extensive vibratory margin scar. Nevertheless, the author was not universally happy with the results of microflap surgery. Many

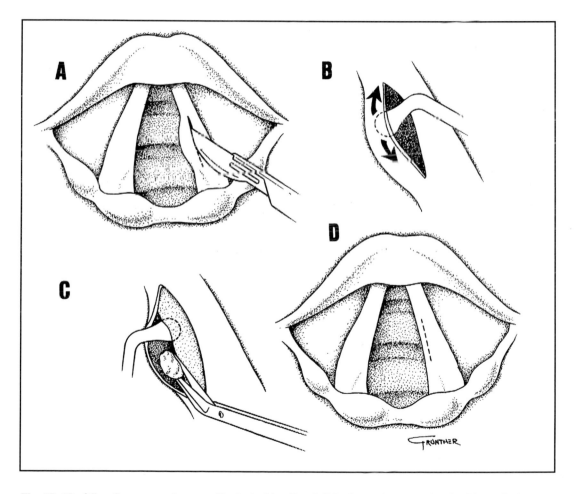

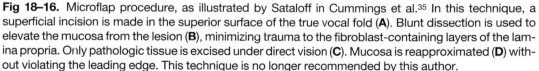

Fig 18–16. Microflap procedure, as illustrated by Sataloff in Cummings et al.[35] In this technique, a superficial incision is made in the superior surface of the true vocal fold (**A**). Blunt dissection is used to elevate the mucosa from the lesion (**B**), minimizing trauma to the fibroblast-containing layers of the lamina propria. Only pathologic tissue is excised under direct vision (**C**). Mucosa is reapproximated (**D**) without violating the leading edge. This technique is no longer recommended by this author.

were excellent (as were the results of some vocal fold strippings years ago), but careful strobovideolaryngoscopic analysis and voice assessment showed too many cases in which the final outcome was inexplicably not perfect. In fact, despite what appeared to be technically flawless operations, a small number of patients had severe, prolonged stiffness for many months after vocal fold surgery; and critical analysis revealed permanent stiffness even in some patients who were happy with their voice results. Moreover, some of this stiffness was located anterior and posterior to the region of the mass, in areas that had been normal preoperatively. This critical assessment of surgical results led the author to the uneasy feeling that we were still doing something wrong. The problem became clear immediately upon reading the basement membrane research of Dr Stephen Gray.[41]

Before Gray's landmark discovery, microflap surgery made sense. Now, it usually does not. Gray demonstrated a complex basement membrane structure between the epithelium and superficial layer of the lamina propria. Moreover, he illustrated that the epithelium and basement membrane are attached to the superficial layer of the lamina propria through an intricate series of type VII collagen loops. These loops emanate from and return to basement membrane cells. Type III collagen fibers of the superficial layer of the lamina propria pass through them. This highly sophisticated architectural arrangement is probably variable from person to person, and perhaps from family to family. Basement membrane structures and the integrity of their attachments are probably related to numerous vocal fold functions, including wound healing, if we can extrapolate from basement membrane behavior elsewhere in the body. Hence, when we elevate microflaps, we are not simply manipulating structurally insignificant tissue. Rather, we are ripping apart delicate, functionally important anatomic structures.

Armed with this new anatomic knowledge and evidence that previous surgical results had not been consistently as good as desired, revised common sense suggested that the destruction of normal tissue structures involved in elevating microflaps probably rendered this technique counterproductive. Consequently, in the latter part of 1991, "traditional" microflap surgery was abandoned by this author. Since that time, the author has limited surgery strictly to the region of pathology, without elevating or disturbing any surrounding tissue. Masses are either excised with the smallest possible amount of their overlying mucosa or a mini-microflap is elevated directly over the lesion (Fig 18–17).[42] In this technique, a small mucosal incision is made anteriorly, superiorly, and

posteriorly underlying the vocal fold mass. Gentle retraction is accomplished with a small suction on the surface of the lesion; and blunt dissection is used to separate the mass from the lamina propria, reflecting it medially. The mass is then excised either with all of its overlying mucosa or, preferably, retaining a small inferiorly based medial flap of mucosa. This is generally easy to do once the mass has been reflected medially, because the mucosa is already stretched because of the lesion. The micro-miniflap is a small, medially based pedicled flap. It should not be confused with Dedo and Sooy's much larger "micro-trap-door flap" for use in supraglottic stenosis[43] or with Ossoff and colleague's larger "serial micro-trap-door flaps" used for subglottic stenosis.[43-45]

Unfortunately, for the reasons stated above, good, prospective scientific data comparing vocal fold stripping and microflap and mini-microflap surgery are not available. The author's initial anecdotal impressions, and the data presented on excision of 96 vocal fold masses in 60 patients (49 of them singers)[42] provide convincing evidence that mini-microflap surgery and limited mass excision with overlying mucosa (without disturbing any adjacent tissue) (Fig 18–18) provide substantially better results than the microflap surgery advocated originally by this author. Since abandoning microflap surgery, the author has not encountered the kind of extensive and prolonged postoperative stiffness encountered after some cases of microflap surgery. Mini-microflap is currently recommended for excision of vocal fold submucosal cysts and similar lesions. When a mini-microflap cannot be created, resection of the mass with the smallest possible amount of overlying mucosa should be performed.

Vocal Fold Polyps and Nodules

Like the vocal fold masses discussed above, vocal fold polyps and nodules should be removed conservatively, preserving normal mucosa and remaining superficial to the intermediate layer of the lamina propria. This is accomplished best by excising the lesion entirely with sharp instruments, rather than by tearing the mucosa using cupped forceps. Nodules rarely require surgery. If they are diagnosed correctly, more than 90% will resolve or become asymptomatic through voice therapy alone. However, those that persist in causing symptoms despite voice therapy should be removed with little or no trauma to the subjacent superficial layer of the lamina propria. Many vocal fold polyps are accompanied by an obvious central blood vessel that extends from the superior surface of the vocal fold. Occasionally, feeding vessels may course along the vibratory margin or originate below

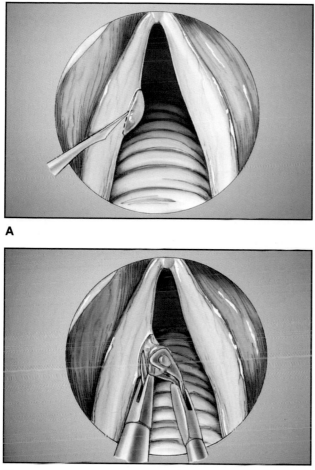

A

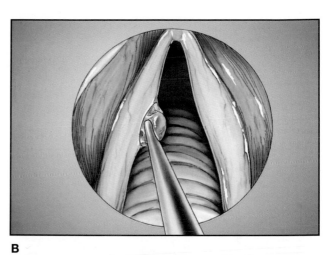

B

C

D

Fig 18–17. A. In elevating a mini-microflap, an incision is made with a straight knife at the junction of the mass and normal tissue. Small vertical anterior and posterior incisions may be added at the margins of the mass if necessary, usually using a straight scissors. **B.** The mass is separated by blunt dissection, splitting the superficial layer of the lamina propria and preserving it as much as possible. This dissection can be performed with a spatula, blunt ball dissector (illustrated), or scissors (as illustrated in **A**). **C.** The lesion is stabilized and a scissors (straight or curved) is used to excise the lesion, preserving as much adjacent mucosa as possible. The lesion itself acts as a tissue expander, and it is often possible to create an inferiorly based mini-microflap. **D.** The mini-microflap is replaced over the surgical defect, establishing primary closure and acting as a biological dressing.

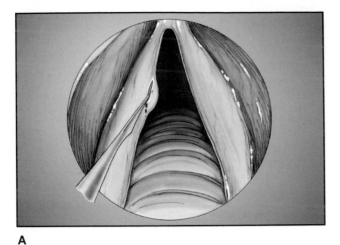

A

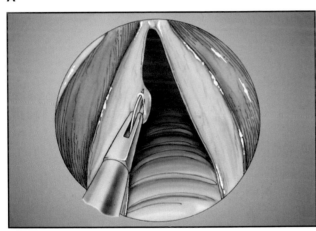

B

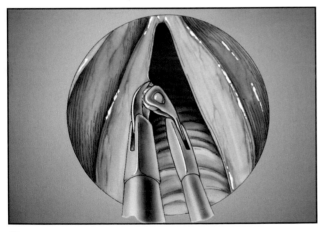

C

Fig 18–18. **A.** An incision is made on the superior surface of the vocal fold at the junction of the lesion and normal mucosa. **B.** Blunt dissection with the scissors is used to split the superficial layer of lamina propria. Note that the force of the side of the scissors is directed toward the base of the lesion and the glottis, not laterally toward the vocal ligament. **C.** The lesion is stabilized (not retracted) with heart-shaped forceps and excised, without adjacent normal tissue. A small mucosal gap results, but this usually heals well.

the vocal fold edge. Prominent feeding vessels should be vaporized with a carbon dioxide laser (at 1 watt, 0.1 second, defocused) or resected to help prevent recurrent hemorrhage and polyp formation (Fig 18–19). The author prefers resection in most cases. The polyp can then be removed from the vibratory margin with traditional instruments (Fig 18–20) or laser (Fig 18–21). The author uses cold instruments, but the laser can be used safely, as discussed in *Professional Voice*.[15]

Varicosities and Ectatic Vessels and Vocal Fold Hemorrhage

Ectatic blood vessels and varicosities are usually asymptomatic. However, occasionally, they require treatment. Usually, this is due to repeated submucosal hemorrhage emanating from the enlarged, weakened blood vessel. More rarely, it is due to dysphonia caused by engorgement of the blood vessel following the exercise of voice use (just like the veins that pump up in arms following exercise), which changes the mass of the vocal fold. This is a proven but uncommon cause of voice fatigue (Fig 18–22).

In patients with recurrent hemorrhage from a varicose or ectatic vessel, or with voice dysfunction resulting from small vessel enlargement, vaporization of the abnormal vessels used to be the treatment of choice

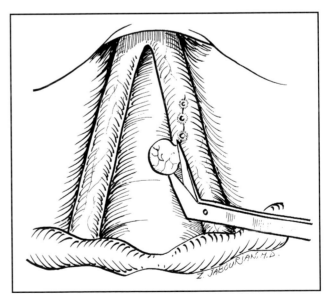

Fig 18–19 The feeding vessel of a hemorrhagic polyp may be treated with a 1-watt defocused laser burst of short duration to cauterize the vessel and prevent recurrent hemorrhage. The polyp can then be removed from the leading edge with scissors, avoiding the risk of laser injury to the vibratory margin.

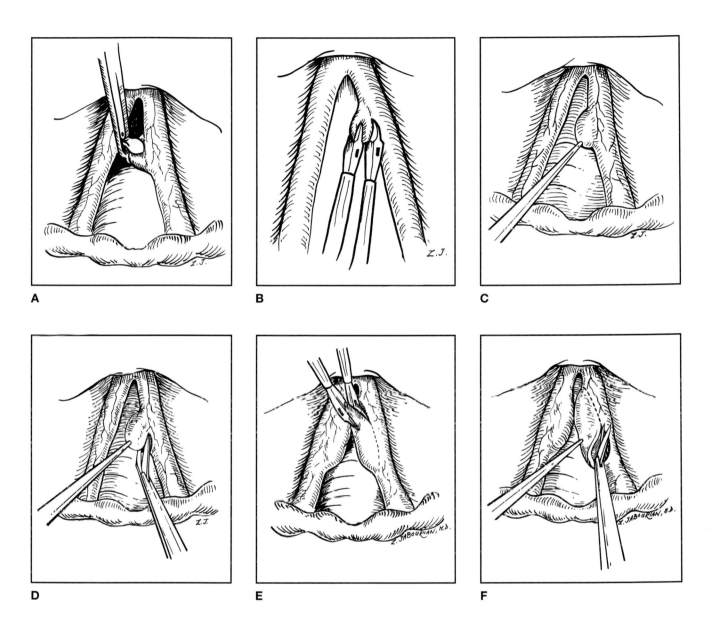

Fig 18–20. A. The old technique of grasping the lesion with a cupped forceps and evulsing the lesion from the vocal fold is not sufficiently precise. It allows for tearing of the mucosa beyond the necessary area of excision. Instead, the lesion may be grasped with a delicate forceps (**B**), or preferably stabilized with a fine suction (**C**). The lesion should not be retracted medially with forceps, as this will tent the mucosa and often result in excessive excision. The mucosa is cut sharply rather than ripped (**D**), limiting resection strictly to the area of pathology. Even with small lesions, but especial-ly with larger lesions, it is often helpful to bluntly separate the lesion from the underlying lamina propria with a blunt dissector (**E**), or spreading with scissors (**F**). This must be done superficially, and any pressure should be directed medially (toward the portion being resected), taking care not to traumatize the intermediate layer of the lamina propria. Reinke's space is not rich in fibroblasts (although it contains some), and utilizing this technique permits resection of the diseased tissue only, while minimizing the chance of scarring.

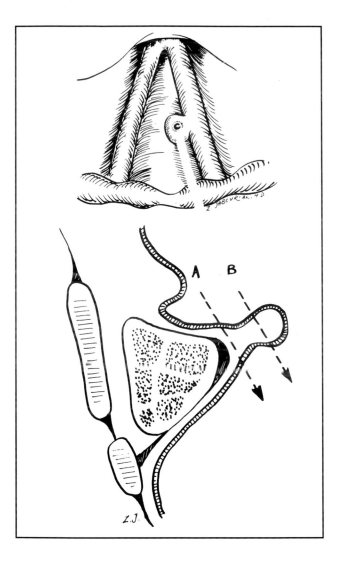

Fig 18–21. (*Top*) When a lesion on the vibratory margin is resected with laser, the center of the laser beam must be located in the body of the mass. Thus, the zone of destruction (rather than center of the laser beam) is approximately even with the vibratory margin. (*Bottom*) A cross-section of the vocal fold illustrates the same principle. Arrow B represents the center of the laser beam, and arrow A represents the outermost region of the zone of destruction around the laser beam. The zone of destruction should be superficial to the intermediate layer of the lamina propria to help prevent scar formation.

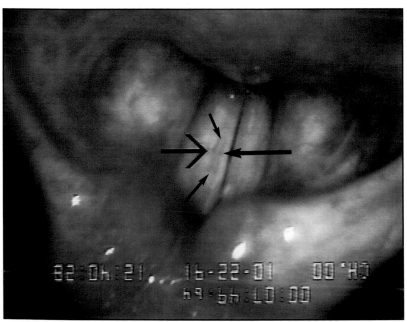

Fig 18–22. Video print revealed a prominent varicosity on the left vocal fold. The large black arrow marks the lateral margin of the varicosity, the smaller arrow marks the medial margin, and the smallest arrows mark the anterior and posterior extent of the varicosity. This vein pumped up during the singing exercises much the same as extremity veins become prominent during other forms of exercise. This added to the mass effect of the left vocal fold causing interruptions in the vibratory pattern, voice fatigue, loss of upper range, increased vocal effort, and slight hoarseness. These symptoms resolved after vaporization of the vessel. (From *Ear Nose Throat J.* 73(7):445, with permission.)

and still may be indicated in some cases. This is performed using a carbon dioxide laser, using defocused 1-watt laser bursts interrupted with single pulses at 0.1 second, and icing the vocal fold. Care should be taken not to permit heat transfer to the intermediate or deep layers of the lamina propria. Protection may be accomplished by submucosal infusion and by directing the laser beam tangentially for blood vessels directly on the vibratory margin, so that the direct impact of the laser beam is not aimed at the vibrating surface. In some cases, the mucosa may be gently retracted using alligator forceps with a cottonoid along the superior surface, stretching blood vessels onto the superior surface where they may be vaporized more safely over the body of the thyroarytenoid muscle. If the vessel is positioned over the lamina propria such that laser vaporization cannot be performed safely, delicate resection of the vessel with preservation of adjacent mucosa has proven successful in the author's hands[46] (Fig 18–23). This approach is similar to that used for symptomatic varicose vessels elsewhere in the body, and its rationale, technique and results were reviewed by Hochman, Sataloff, Hillman, et al in 1999.[46] Thirty-four of the 42 patients we reported were female, 84% of the patients with documented hemorrhages were female, and 39 of 42 of the patients were singers. Most ectasias and varices are located in

the middle of the musculomembranous vocal fold, usually on the superior surface. This observation has been reported previously.[47,48] We noted that 66% of the varices and ectasias occurred in the region of the superior and lateral extent of the mucosal wave. This is probably the point at which maximum shearing forces are generated in the superficial layer of the lamina propria, as the mucosal wave reaches its superior/lateral endpoint, decelerates quickly, and reverses direction to begin the closing phase of the oscillatory cycle. We speculate that this whiplashlike effect and the limitation of the microvasculature by the basement membrane of the epithelium are probably responsible for the preponderance of hemorrhages, ectasias, and varices that occur on the superior and lateral surfaces near the middle of the musculomembranous portion of the vocal fold. The middle segment of the musculomembranous portion of the vocal fold is now referred to as the striking zone, a term coined by Zeitels and introduced in our article on ectasias and varices.[46] We believe that chronic mechanical trauma to the microvasculature is responsible for the development of varicosities and ectasias and that direct collision forces are responsible for most of the vascular abnormalities that occur on the medial surface of the vocal fold. The fact that so many such abnormalities are actually on the superior surface rather than on the

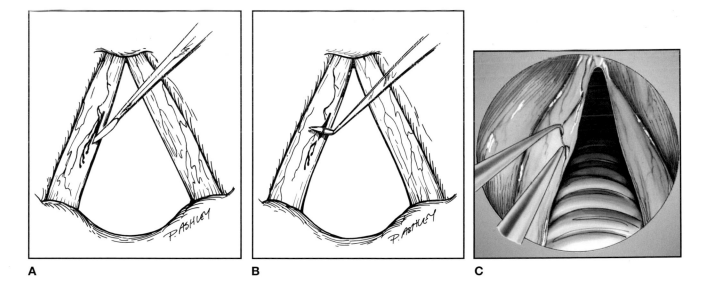

A   **B**   **C**

Fig 18–23. Ectasia. **A.** This figure illustrates the technique for elevating and resecting a varicose vessel. A superficial incision is made in the epithilium adjacent to the vessel using the sharp point of the vascular knife, or using a microknife (illustrated). **B.** The 1-mm right-angle vascular knife is inserted under the vessel and used to elevate it. It may be necessary to make more than one epithelial incision in order to dissect the desired length of the vessel. **C.** Once the pathologic vessel has been elevated, it is retracted gently to provide access to its anterior and posterior limits. These can be divided sharply with a scissors or knife (bleeding stops spontaneously) or divided and cauterized with a laser, as long as there is no thermal injury to adjacent vocal ligament.

vibratory margin probably is due to the fact that the maximum shearing stresses during oscillation are on the superior surface. Because of the whiplashlike mechanism of injury, superficial vessels are more likely to be injured than deeper vessels. This is convenient, because their superficial nature facilitates surgical management. In our reported series of 42 patients for whom sufficient pre- and postoperative data were available, mucosal vibration remained the same or improved in all patients who underwent excision of ectasias or varices using cold instruments. This had not been the author's (RTS) experience with laser management of similar lesions in earlier years, prior to developing this technique. Although the author (RTS) prefers resection of vessels in most cases, laser cauterization should still be considered an acceptable option, particularly for lesions far lateral to the vibratory margin. However, regardless of location, the importance of avoiding trauma to adjacent tissues cannot be overstated.

In patients with very extensive hemorrhage distorting a vocal fold, an incision along the superior surface with evacuation of the hematoma may speed healing. In general, this is not necessary. However, if the bulging vocal fold has not flattened satisfactorily through resorption of the hematoma within a few days after the hemorrhage, evacuation may be considered. Surgery involves suction evacuation of the hematoma through a small incision on the superior surface.

Reinke's Edema

When surgery is performed for Reinke's edema, in this author's opinion, only one vocal fold should be operated on at a sitting in most cases, although this practice remains controversial. The vocal fold may be incised along its superior surface, and the edematous material removed with a fine suction (Fig 18–24). Redundant mucosa may be trimmed, and mucosa should be reapproximated. Care must be exercised to avoid resecting too much mucosa. The second vocal fold may be treated similarly after the first vocal fold has healed. However, the voice improvement that follows unilateral evacuation of Reinke's edema is often surprisingly good, and patients frequently elect to leave the other vocal fold undisturbed.

In addition, there is a more important reason for staging surgery for Reinke's edema. Occasionally, surgical treatment for this condition results in a stiff vocal fold, sometimes even adynamic, even though this complication theoretically should be rare with the technique advocated. Nevertheless, it can occur even when surgery has been performed well. If it occurs on one side and there is still Reinke's edema on the other side, the polypoid side usually compensates. Voice quality is generally satisfactory, and (most importantly) phonation is not effortful. If stiffness occurs bilaterally, the voice is not only hoarse, but moreover requires high phonation pressures. Patients are unhappy not only with voice quality, but especially with the fatigue that accompanies increased effort required to initiate and sustain phonation. Under these circumstances, they often feel that they are worse than they were with untreated Reinke's edema. If surgery is staged so that healing can be observed on one vocal fold before surgery is performed on the second vocal fold, this situation can be avoided in nearly all cases.

Granulomas and Vocal Process Ulcers

Prior to surgical excision, causative and contributing factors should be addressed. Reflux should be treated,

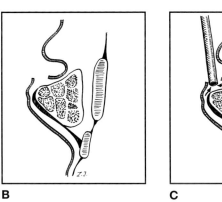

A   **B**   **C**   **D**

Fig 18–24. A. Bulky vocal fold showing Reinke's edema (*small dots*) in the superfical layer of the lamina propria. **B.** Incision in the superior surface opens easily into Reinke's space. **C.** Using a fine needle suction, the edema fluid is aspirated (*arrows*). **D.** The mucosal edges are reapproximated, trimming redundant mucosa if necessary.

and voice therapy instituted. If the lesions do not resolve within a few weeks, they should be excised. The laser may be helpful in removing these lesions because they are generally not on the vibratory margin. Therefore, scarring is unlikely to cause hoarseness. In addition, they are often friable; and laser excision helps minimize bleeding. However, although lasers are convenient in controlling hemorrhage in vocal fold granuloma surgery, it must be remembered that we are treating a nonhealing area. Like other thermal injury, laser burns cause substantial tissue damage. Any surgeon who has accidentally struck his or her finger with a laser beam knows that the effect is more traumatic than a sharp cut of similar size with a knife. Consequently, to minimize tissue trauma and promote healing, this author prefers to minimize or avoid laser use at the base of these lesions. The underlying perichondrium should not be traumatized. In all cases, a generous specimen should be removed for biopsy to rule out carcinoma and other possible etiologies.

In patients with recurrent granulomas, botulinum toxin injection may be considered. This can be performed as an outpatient or during surgical resection of granulomas in the operating room. In general, only a small amount of botulinum toxin is required, and it is best to place it in the lateral cricoarytenoid muscle (LCA) for recurrent granulomas near the vocal process. In these patients, there appears to be dominance of LCA activity during the adduction process, causing point-contact near the tip of the vocal process rather than the broader contact that results from a different balance of activity between the lateral cricoarytenoid and interarytenoid muscles, as noted initially by Zeitels (Steven Zeitels, MD, personal communication, 1997) and confirmed by this author's (RTS) experience. Both LCA muscles are injected usually with only 1.25 to 2.5 mouse units of Botox (Allergan, Irvine, Calif) or the equivalent, as discussed in chapter 17.

Papillomas

Laryngeal papillomatosis has been recognized as a problem for more than a century. Papilloma was described by Czermak in 1861.[49] It also was illustrated by Mackenzie, Türck, and Elsberg.[50-52] Sixty-seven of Mackenzie's first 100 mirror-guided laryngeal procedures were for papillomatous lesions.[53] Nevertheless, optimal treatment continues to elude us.

When papillomas interfere with voice quality or airway patency, surgery is the standard treatment. To minimize the risk of seeding the lower airway with virus, intubation must be accomplished under direct vision, with a small tube that does not traumatize the papillomas as it passes through the larynx. . In general, resection of laryngeal papillomas has been performed with a carbon dioxide laser, and this instrument offers great advantages. However, it can also cause problems. When used, a smoke evaporator should be employed to avoid the risks of infecting the surgeon or other operating room personnel with viruses in the laser smoke. Only one side of the larynx should be operated on at a sitting; in many cases, multiple procedures are often necessary.

Early discouraging experience with recurrent juvenile papillomatosis, and general agreement that laser surgery is called for in papillomas, have led to a somewhat indelicate approach to laser surgery, in this author's opinion. For many surgeons, laser surgery for papilloma means directly vaporizing all the areas of papillomatous involvement on one vocal fold; this invariably means injury to underlying tissues. This produces permanent dysphonia in many patients. Moreover, recurrences tend to involve deeper structures (vocal ligament and muscle) that were not involved initially.

Anecdotally, the author believes that adult-onset laryngeal papilloma may behave differently from the virulent, juvenile papillomatosis many of us are accustomed to treating. Consequently, a method has been employed to attempt cure, rather than simply palliation, and to preserve underlying structures. The method works best when the papillomas have not been operated on previously, but it has been used effectively in recurrent cases, as well[54] (Fig 18–25). An incision is made on the superior surface of the vocal fold with the laser, leaving a small margin of grossly normal tissue around the papilloma. A microflap is then elevated in the superficial layer of the lamina propria under the papilloma. The flap and papillomas are generally retracted medially, and anterior and posterior margin incisions are made with scissors or a laser. Contact endoscopy may be helpful in determining the optimal incision site. The inferior margin can then be divided with the laser under direct vision, and the mucosa and papillomas are resected en bloc. Although elevation of a microflap does not ensure preservation of good vocal quality (as discussed above), the odds of a good result are certainly better with this technique than they are with indiscriminately "cooking" the vocal ligament. This technique appears to produce acceptable voice results, and some apparent cures in patients who have gone 5 years or more without recurrent papillomas. More research is needed, but the author continues to use this approach and recommends its consideration. In cases of frequently recurrent papilloma in which only debulking is planned, powered laryngeal instruments can be help-

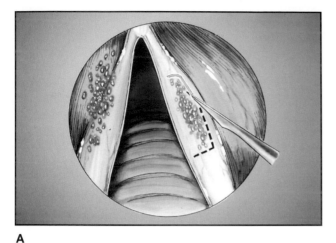

A

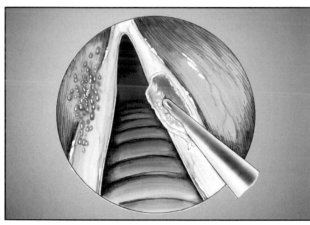

B

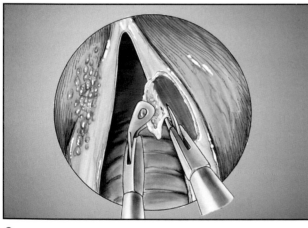

C

ful and provide surprisingly good control of the limits of tissue removal (Fig 18–26).

The use of cidofovir for laryngeal papillomatosis is promising. This antiviral agent can be injected directly into the papillomatosis lesions; and some patients respond dramatically. The use of this substance was pioneered by Wellens.[55] Although cidofovir is approved by the United States Food and Drug Administration (FDA) for other uses, laryngeal injection is an off-label use. The medication may have serious side effects, but they are not likely to occur in the doses used commonly for laryngeal surgery. Concentrations recommended most commonly for laryngeal use are in the range of 2.5 to 5 mg per ml, but higher concen-

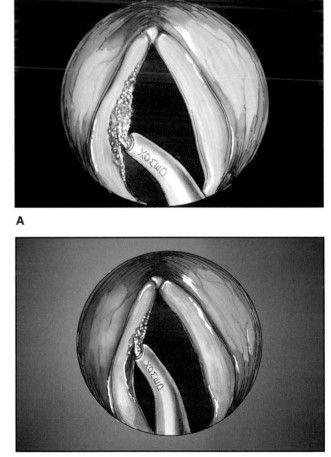

A

B

Fig 18–25. A. An incision is made around the area of papilloma with a sharp knife, approaching it as one might approach an area of carcinoma in situ. **B.** A microflap is elevated bluntly, sparing the underlying superficial layer of lamina propria. **C.** The region of papilloma is resected. (Courtesy of Medtronics-Xomed, Jacksonville, Fla.)

Fig 18–26 A. Papilloma is debulked with a 3.5- or 4.0-mm angle-tip laryngeal blade at 5,000 rpm. **B.** Final removal is performed with limited trauma to the mucosa and underlying tissues using a 3.5-mm angle-tip laryngeal skimmer blade at 500 rpm. (Courtesy of Medtronics-Xomed, Jacksonville Fla.)

trations in the range of 15 mg per cc have been used frequently without apparent adverse affect. In a few cases, concentrations as high as 75 mg per cc have been used without any adverse consequences; but there are questions about long-term effect including (oncogenicity). So, patients need to be informed fully, and this antiviral material should be used with caution in adults and children.

Ventricular Fold Cysts

Ventricular fold (false vocal fold) cysts are uncommon mucous retention cysts, frequently lined with cuboidal cells, which generally are seen in patients over 50 years of age. They occur generally anteriorly along the ventricular fold. They must be differentiated from other lesions such as Hürthle cell tumor and oncocytoma arising from thyroid remnants and from other lesions such as laryngoceles and cancer. Multiple cysts may occur. Surgical removal involves grasping the cyst with a cupped forceps and dissecting the base with a scissors or laser. The cyst may extend to the floor of the ventricle. If bilateral lesions are present, especially anteriorly, both sides should not be operated on at the same sitting.

Epiglottic Cysts

Epiglottic cysts occur on the lingual surface of the free edge of the epiglottis or in the area of the epiglottic folds. They may become large and cause muffling of the voice. Whenever possible, they should be removed completely. If they rupture and complete removal is not possible, they should be marsupialized.

Laryngoceles

The ventricle of Morgagni is located between the true and false vocal folds. The appendix of the ventricle of Morgagni is a blind pouch called the saccule in the anterior superior section. Laryngoceles are abnormal dilations or herniations of the laryngeal saccule.[55] They communicate with the laryngeal lumen and generally are filled with air. They become apparent clinically when they are distended after air is forced into them or when they are filled with fluid. They are connected to the ventricle by a narrow stalk and form a sac lined with pseudostratified, ciliated columnar epithelium. The appendix of the ventricle is considered abnormal if it extends above the upper border of the thyroid cartilage.

Laryngoceles limited to the interior of the larynx are called internal; those that protrude outside the thyroid cartilage into the neck are called external. They may also be mixed (internal and external). Laryngoceles should be distinguished from pharyngoceles, which are not true pouches and which generally diminish in size in the absence of pharyngeal pressure (eg, when not whistling or playing a wind instrument).[57] Outpouchings of the laryngeal ventricle extend through the openings in the thyrohyoid membrane for the superior laryngeal vessels and nerve, and balloon outward and upward toward the submandibular triangle.[58] It should be noted that external and mixed laryngoceles are really variants of the internal laryngocele. Because laryngoceles arise from the region of the saccule within the larynx, if the lesion is a laryngocele, there must be an intralaryngeal component manifested at least as a tract connecting the lateral component with the ventricle, with or without internal dilation. Hence, pure external laryngoceles do not exist. Lesions without an intralaryngeal component should be classified differently (eg, as pharyngoceles).

There are several proposed mechanisms for laryngocele formation. In neonates, they are presumed to be remnants of the lateral air sacs seen in other primates. In adults, they can represent a congenital enlargement of the saccule or an acquired lesion associated with increased intraluminal pressure. The association of laryngoceles with laryngeal carcinoma and with occupations that involve long periods of forced expiration supports this notion.[59]

Brass and woodwind players are at risk for a variety of head and neck abnormalities as a result of increased intraluminal pressure during their musical performances.[59] Transient ischemic attacks, temporomandibular joint dysfunction, and dental malocclusion have been reported. Injury to the orbicularis oris in brass players can require surgical repair.[60] Stress velopharyngeal incompetence has been documented in trumpeters and bassoonists. Young trumpet players are at greatest risk for injury to oral and cervical tissues when they generate peak respiratory pressure averaging 151 torr.[61]

Several authors have examined laryngocele formation in woodwind players. Stephani and Tarab obtained plain x-rays on 25 wind instruments players and found laryngoceles in all of them.[62] Macfie found laryngoceles in 53 of 94 (56%) woodwind bandsman.[63] Subclinical laryngoceles are common among horn players, and they rarely require surgical intervention.

Surgery for laryngoceles in young musicians poses several problems. The literature offers no guidance regarding the timing of surgery, the healing period before playing can be resumed, and the risk of recurrence with continued performance. Furthermore, the cervical approach used commonly for the treatment of external laryngoceles can disrupt the normal function of the strap muscles, which are important for tone generation.[63] The risks of infection and progression of the defect must be balanced against a young performer's desire for musical growth.

Since Ward's early reports on this subject,[57] our understanding of laryngoceles and pharyngoceles has changed slightly. Both laryngoceles and pharyngoceles can change size and appearance with variations in internal pressure. Although the classical definitions of laryngocele remain valid, combinations of both can occur. Air-filled masses that arise in the pharynx (commonly in the region of the piriform sinuses) and lack a laryngeal component or origin should be called pharyngoceles. Those that arise in the laryngeal ventricle should be called laryngoceles. Considering the origins of pharyngeal pouches as reviewed in Ward's 1963 paper[57] as well as the forces involved, it appears likely that most lesions with a laryngeal component originated in the larynx and extended in the neck rather than vice versa; but it is not always possible to prove origin. It is also important to recognize that the therapeutic implications of the distinctions are not as clear-cut as they once were and that lesions that combine the features of laryngoceles and pharyngoceles occur[65] (Fig 18–27). The distinctions between laryngoceles and pharyngoceles were quite important when we still believed laryngoceles usually required surgery and pharyngoceles required surgery only rarely. However, as arts-medicine has evolved, experience has shown that in most cases neither lesion requires surgery. Contrary to our earlier understandings, the vast majority of laryngoceles are asymptomatic.

If surgery is necessary, it is commonly performed externally, particularly if the laryngocele produces a large bulge in the neck. When an external approach is used, a variety of thyrotomy techniques may be employed as discussed in this chapter and elsewhere in the literature.[66] However, in selected cases, endoscopic surgery may be adequate. This procedure usually is performed under general anesthesia. This type of surgery is most effective for internal laryngoceles or mixed laryngoceles with a large connecting neck between the internal and external components. The technique involves excising the false vocal fold. This effectively marsupializes the cyst into the larynx. The false vocal fold should be retracted toward the midline, and the incisions are made most effectively using the carbon dioxide laser (Fig 18–28). The removal of the false vocal folds may affect vocal resonance, especially in singers. Therefore, this procedure must be used with great caution, if used at all, in professional voice users.

Miscellaneous Masses

In some cases, both the surgeon and the patient must realize that health considerations sometimes have to take precedence over the preservation of optimal voice quality. Although every effort must be made to design a procedure that optimizes the voice result, sometimes a serious benign process or a neoplasm does not permit perfection. This situation is encountered commonly when treating papilloma (Fig 18–29) and other lesions. In the granular cell tumor seen in Figure 18–30, for example, the disease extended onto the posterior aspect of the membranous portion of the vocal fold. Endoscopic resection required removal of the posterior half of the vocal fold in this professional soprano. Although a good neovocal fold was formed and vocal quality was very acceptable for speech within a few months, she was not able to return to professional singing performance for more than a year following surgery.

Carcinoma

The surgical management of vocal fold carcinoma is discussed in chapter 23 and in other sources.[67]

Surgery for Postoperative Vocal Fold Injury and Scar

This subject is covered in chapter 19.

Sulcus Vocalis

Numerous techniques have been used to treat sulcus vocalis. The mucosa can be dissected from the deeper structures to which it is adherent and simply replaced in its original position. This technique fails frequently, however. The area of the sulcus can also be resected, and mucosa can be reapproximated. This technique seems to work a little better than simple elevation, but it also does not produce consistently satisfactory results. Collagen injection has been used to treat sulcus vocalis;[68] but it, too, has not been consistently successful. Pontes and Behlau introduced a technique involving multiple crossed incisions throughout the length of the sulcus.[69] At first glance, this technique looks as if it should cause greater scarring; but it is actually a series of multiple relaxing incisions following established, classical surgical principles. Substantial voice improvement has been achieved in a majority of patients undergoing this procedure. Autologous lipoinjection and fat implan-

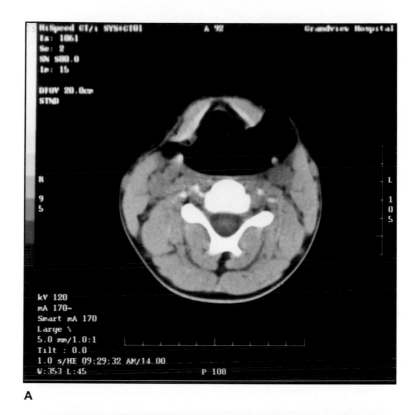

A

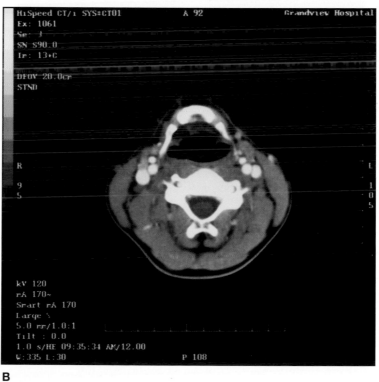

B

Fig 18–27. Laryngoceles. **A.** Bilateral dilatations that could be mistaken for pharyngoceles. **B.** Right intralaryngeal component suggesting laryngeal origin. This 16-year-old trumpet player's presentation involved features consistent with both laryngocele and pharyngocele.

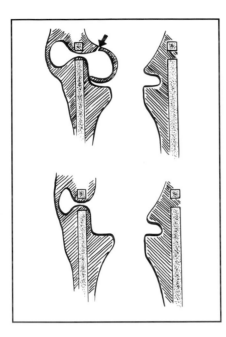

Fig 18–28. (*Top*) Depiction of a left internal laryngocele that has enlarged and displaced the false vocal fold into the glottic lumen. It has dissected through the hyothyroid space to present externally. With microsurgical techniques or a laser, the involved false vocal fold is excised. (*Bottom*) Following removal of the false vocal fold, the remaining laryngocele drains easily into the lumen of the larynx, and its external component no longer is troublesome.

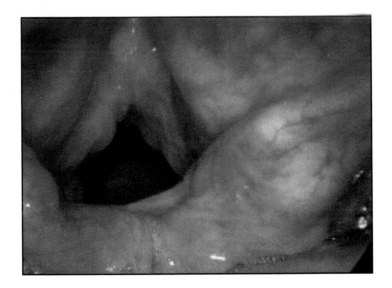

Fig 18–29. Recurrent papilloma involving the vibratory margin. Controlling the lesion and avoiding airway complications are primary treatment priorities, although it is possible to restore reasonable voice in most cases.

tation also may be efficacious. At present, the best surgical technique has not been determined. However, it is now clear that various surgical interventions provide at least partial voice improvement in many patients. The principles of management are the same as those discussed for scar in chapter 19. It is necessary to address compensatory hyperfunction through voice therapy, failure of glottic closure through medialization, and recreation of a mucosal wave through

surgery on the vibratory margin. At the time of the writing of the first edition of this book, surgical intervention was not recommended. However, developments over the last 15 years suggest that patients with significant symptoms caused by sulcus should be offered surgical options, with the clear understanding that surgical recommendations for this condition are still evolving, voice quality could be worse following voice surgery, and that there is certainly no

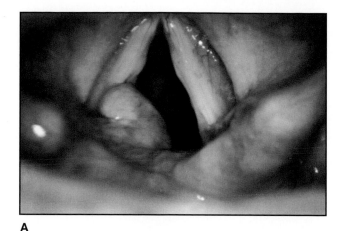

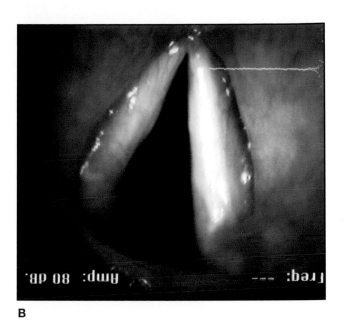

A

B

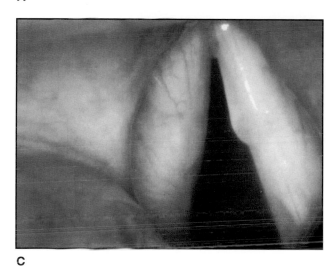

C

Fig 18–30. A. Preoperative granular cell tumor. **B.** Postoperative appearance 11 months after surgery. **C.** Appearance 5 years after surgery.

guarantee of improvement. The decision on whether the chances of achieving better voice are worth the risks should be made by the patient and physician on an individual basis. Surgical treatment is now good enough that it should not be denied to symptomatic and informed patients who elect it.

Laryngeal Webs

Before embarking on surgical repair, the laryngologist should determine whether the web is symptomatic and its longitudinal and vertical extent. Many webs cause no vocal or respiratory problems and should be left undisturbed. The selection of a surgical approach for symptomatic webs depends on their extent, especially subglottically. Complete assessment including strobovideolaryngoscopy and high-resolution CT scan is helpful in defining the lesion. The importance of stroboscopy cannot be overstated. When the voice is hoarse after trauma (surgical or otherwise), and a small web is present, it is essential to determine pre-

operatively whether the web is truly the cause of the dysphonia. Often the web is asymptomatic, and the hoarseness is caused by scarring elsewhere in the vocal folds (an adynamic segment) that cannot be diagnosed under routine light. It is extremely helpful to make such determinations before subjecting the patient to surgery that may not only fail to improve the voice, but make it worse. For relatively small, symptomatic webs, surgery may be performed endoscopically. More extensive external approaches can be used when necessary.

Endoscopic resection of a laryngeal web may be performed with traditional instruments or laser. In a small number of cases, it may be possible to treat a web successfully endoscopically without placement of a keel. This is accomplished by dividing one edge near a vocal fold, and allowing the free edge to fold in on its base on the other side. The edge may be left free, fixed with fibrin glue, or "laser welded." This technique is minimally traumatic, but recurrences appear more frequently than they do following placement of a keel.

In general, it is necessary to place a laryngeal keel to prevent reformation of the web. A tracheotomy is rarely necessary. The keel is fashioned individually out of Silastic, Teflon, metals, or other minimally reactive substances. Sutures are passed into the larynx through 16-gauge needles inserted through the cricothyroid membrane, and above the thyroid notch (Fig 18–31). The keel can be guided into position, and the sutures are fixed into the skin. Hospitalization and close observation for airway obstruction are required for the first 24 hours. The rare complications of the procedure include displacement of the keel with aspiration and obstruction and deep neck infection. Nevertheless, the procedure is less traumatic than the external approach, and frequently is effective. Whether the endolaryngeal or external approach is used, the keel should be left in position for at least 2 to 3 weeks.

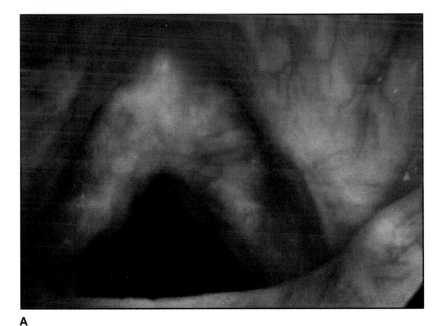

A

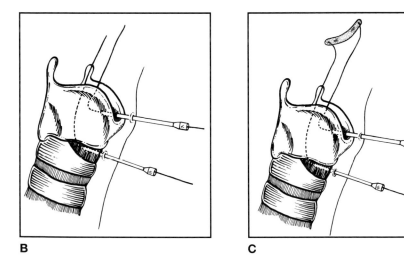

B   **C**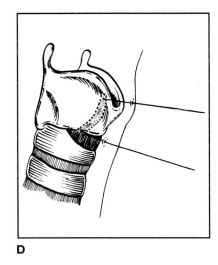

D

Fig 18–31. A. Videoprint showing a thick anterior web caused by repeated surgery for papillomas. Webs this thick often require an open procedure; but sometimes they can be repaired adequately endoscopically. **B.** Placement of 16-gauge needles above and below the thyroid cartilage in the midline, in preparation for endoscopic placement of a keel. This procedure would not generally be used in the presence of papillomas, but is useful for webs from other causes. **C.** Individually fashioned Teflon keel is attached to sutures, passed through the 16-gauge needles. **D.** The sutures are drawn through the needles in order to place the keel in final position in the anterior commissure.

A new technique was reported by Sataloff and Hawkshaw in 1998.[70] This technique permits placement of an internal laryngeal stent without external manipulation, even for placement of sutures. The original procedure was performed endoscopically using a rectangle of 0.02 inch reinforced Silastic usually used in middle ear surgery. This procedure was designed originally for a patient with aggressive, active papillomatosis and a severe web. Because of the aggressiveness of the papilloma, the author (RTS) was reluctant to create even a suture tract from the larynx through the skin to secure a keel or stent in the usual fashion, because of the risk of seeding papilloma. This entirely endoscopic, technique permits web resection without contamination of tissues outside of the endolarynx (Fig 18–32, A–D).

Postoperative management following resection of vocal fold webs can be important to ensuring success. The technique used for many years in Germany and more recently reintroduced in the United States by Stasney should be in the armamentarium of all laryngologists performing surgery for glottic web.[71] If a

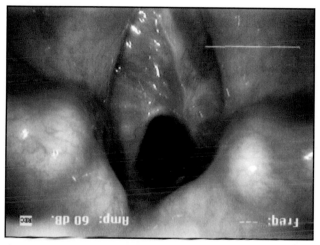

A

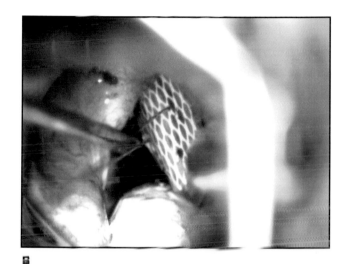

B

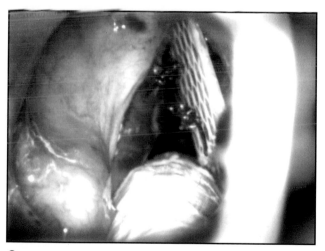

C

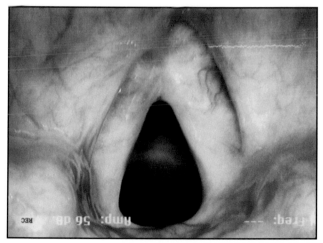

D

Fig 18–32. A. Thick anterior glottic web with significant respiratory compromise. A 38-year-old professional speaker and businesswoman with aggressive, recurrent papillomatosis developed a web severe enough to interfere with respiration. **B.** 0.02-inch Silastic was sewn endoscopically through the vocal fold, without sutures being passed through the thyroid cartilage or externally. **C.** As originally described, the knots were tied medially as shown. Now, the knots are tied lateral to the Silastic to avoid knot-induced trauma to the contralateral vocal fold. The sutures were left in place until the contralateral vocal fold appeared to be remucosalized. This took about 3 ½ weeks. **D.** Postoperative appearance, which has remained stable during 4 years following surgery.

web starts to re-form early in the postoperative period, it can be divided easily in the office. Under indirect laryngoscopy or nasal fiberoptic guidance, a curved indirect laryngoscopic instrument is used. The ideal instrument is a medicine applicator with a slight ball-like enlargement on the end, used in past years for dripping cocaine onto the vocal folds. Topical anesthetic can be applied with this instrument, after which the instrument is passed between the vocal folds and pulled forward to break up the web. The procedure can be repeated periodically, if necessary; and it is effective in preventing web re-formation in some cases.

Bowed Vocal Folds

As discussed previously, dysphonia from vocal fold bowing generally responds to expert voice therapy, especially if the bowing is due to "senile vocal fold atrophy." Occasionally, even this condition is so severe that therapy is insufficient. This problem is encountered more often when the bowing is due to neurological injury or dysfunction, particularly superior laryngeal nerve paresis or paralysis. In such cases, surgery is reasonable.

Injection of Teflon into mobile vocal folds is virtually never necessary or advisable. The potential complications of Teflon do not justify its use under these circumstances. However, injection of autologous fat or allogeneic collagen laterally (the same position as Teflon) may be useful. Type I thyroplasty may also be helpful in selected cases. If the larynx is not too severely ossified, the effects of medialization can be predicted to some extent by medial compression of the thyroid cartilage. If there is a significant height disparity, superficial collagen injection may be of value in selected cases. Approximately 0.2 cc is injected into the region of the lamina propria to increase the bulk of the vocal fold. Vocal lengthening procedures designed for pitch elevation have also been used. However, improvements are generally short-lived, and this approach is rarely indicated. Arytenoid adduction rotation will help restore a unilaterally bowed vocal fold to appropriate height, and this procedure is useful in the case of complete vocal fold paralysis. However, if the superior laryngeal nerve alone is paralyzed and the vocal fold is still mobile, this procedure is generally not a good choice.

Presbyphonia

The principles discussed above for management of severely bowed vocal folds may be applied in cases of profound presbyphonic changes. However, appropri-

ate cases are uncommon. In general, medical management and voice therapy are sufficient to restore acceptable vocal quality. Occasionally, judicious medialization procedures (fat injection, collagen injection, AlloDerm injection, or thyroplasty) may be called for. Lengthening procedures are even more rarely appropriate and are often disappointing. However, in unusual cases of severe and disturbing masculinization of a female voice, as may occur with advancing age, these procedures may have a place, in conjunction with voice therapy.

Vocal Fold Paresis/Paralysis

Unilateral vocal fold paralysis is common. It may be idiopathic, or it may occur after injury to the recurrent laryngeal nerve during neck or thoracic surgery, after neurosurgical procedures, or even following simple intubation. When the paralyzed fold remains in the partially abducted position, the functioning fold may be unable to cross the midline far enough to permit complete glottic closure. This will result in hoarseness, breathiness, ineffective cough, and, occasionally, in aspiration (especially after neurosurgical procedures if other cranial nerves have also been injured).

In some cases, surgery should not be performed for vocal fold paralysis until voice therapy has been tried. In many cases, strengthening vocal muscles and improving speaking technique result in good voice quality; and surgery is unnecessary. This is true especially if there is some recruitment response on EMG, even if the vocal fold is not mobile. When the paralysis is idiopathic, or when the nerve is not known to be cut, approximately 1 year of observation and therapy should usually be completed to allow time for spontaneous return of function before performing any irreversible operation. Traditionally, most surgical procedures have worked best for unilateral recurrent laryngeal nerve paralysis.

Many factors must be considered in selecting a surgical procedure for vocal fold repositioning (such as medialization). For example, the surgeon must assess the glottal configuration. It may be normal during soft phonation, but there may be insufficient lateral resistance to permit loud phonation. This scenario is amenable to injection techniques or thyroplasty. If there is a gap in the middle of the musculomembranous vocal fold but good closure at the vocal process, implantation of a traditional thyroplasty prosthesis with a straight inner edge (such as carved silastic block) is often less satisfactory than injection or use of a conformable prosthesis such as Gore-Tex. If there is a large posterior gap, injection techniques alone often do not work well, and arytenoid repositioning procedures should be considered. If there is a large posterior gap and a foreshortened vocal fold, arytenopexy may yield a more satisfactory result than traditional arytenoid reduction/rotation. Structural considerations should be weighed in light of the patient's vocal needs, his or her medical condition, and the surgeon's experience, as well as other factors such as vibratory function of the vocal fold (presence or absence of scar) and the person's phonatory skill and demands. Surgeons and patients must be prepared for changes in the surgical plan if intraoperative voice changes are not optimal. Staged surgery is appropriate in some cases (thyroplasty followed by injection laryngoplasty, or vice versa); and it is not rare to need to revise laryngoplastic surgery to optimize results. Patients and surgeons should be prepared for all possibilities.

Teflon Injection

Most surgeons inject materials for vocal fold paralysis endoscopically under local or general anesthesia.

Transcutaneous and transoral injection with indirect mirror, telescopic or flexible fiberoptic laryngoscopic guidance is also possible. The most common treatment used to be injection of Teflon (Dupont, Wilmington, Del) lateral to the paralyzed vocal fold. The Teflon paste pushes the paralyzed vocal fold toward the midline, allowing the nonparalyzed vocal fold to meet it more effectively (Fig 18–33). This author has used Teflon only once since 1987. Teflon has many disadvantages, and better techniques are available. However, when used, correct technique involves injecting Teflon lateral to the vocalis muscle. The quantity of Teflon should be sufficient to move the vocal fold just to the midline. Injecting too much or injecting too superficially into the vocal fold mucosa often results in worsened voice quality. When properly placed, Teflon usually produced a foreign-body reaction locally but little or no reaction in the surrounding cartilage and muscle.[72] Teflon is usually surrounded by a fibrous capsule. However, occasionally a severe foreign-body reaction and granuloma formation may occur. Pre- and postoperative functional evaluation of

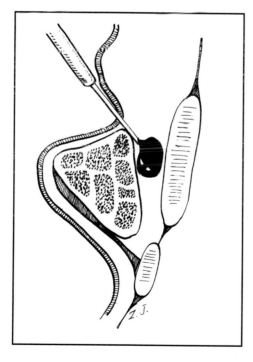
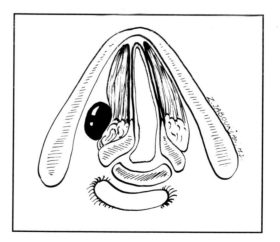

Fig 18–33. (*Left*) Injection of Teflon lateral to the vocalis muscle. (*Right*) Seen from above, the collection of Teflon lateral to the vocalis muscle displaces the vocal fold medially. Moving the vocal fold toward the median position allows the mobile vocal fold to meet it. The depth of the injected Teflon depends on the size of the larynx, but the injection is usually 3 to 5 mm. below the surface. Generally, 0.3 to 1.0 cc of Teflon paste is required. Each click of the Brünings syringe delivers approximately 0.2 cc of Teflon paste. In the author's practice, the use of Teflon injection was virtually abandoned in the mid-1980s.

the voice was advocated by von Leden et al in 1967 for all voice patients undergoing surgery for vocal fold paralysis and should now be standard practice.[73]

Gelfoam Injection

Effects of Teflon injection or other injected materials can be predicted fairly well by prior injection of Gelfoam paste, which was introduced in 1978 by Schramm et al.[74] This material is injected in the same position as Teflon, but it is temporary, resorbing in 2 to 8 weeks. In professional voice users, periodic Gelfoam injections may be appropriate early in the course of a recurrent laryngeal nerve paralysis, when recovery cannot be predicted and injection of permanent materials is not appropriate. For this technique, 1 g of sterile Gelfoam powder is mixed with 4 cc of physiologic saline. The saline must be added slowly, and the mixture should be stirred continuously. This produces 5 cc of thick paste that can be transferred to a syringe and then into the Brünings syringe. Injection technique is then identical to that of Teflon. It should be noted that, although Gelfoam injection has been used for this purpose for decades, it has never been formally approved by the FDA for this use. Gelfoam can be injected in the operating room or in the office. Office injection usually is performed per-orally, using a Brünings syringe with a curved needle. However, like injection of collagen and AlloDerm (discussed below), it also can be injected transcutaneously. Anderson and Mirza have reported success with this technique for immediate treatment of acute vocal fold immobility with aspiration.[75] Although Gelfoam is considered temporary, it usually does cause an inflammatory reaction. Scientific studies of laryngeal Gelfoam injection are wanting, and the assumption that laryngeal anatomy returns to normal following Gelfoam resorption remains unproven.

Collagen, AlloDerm, and Fascia Injection

Several other materials are still being injected to treat vocal fold paralysis, especially collagen, fat, AlloDerm (LifeCell Corporation, Branchburg, NJ), fascia and calcium hydroxyapatite (Coaptite, BioForm, Inc, Franksville, Wisc). Ford and Bless have advocated the use of collagen for many conditions including selected cases of unilateral vocal fold paralysis.[68,76,77] Collagen is in liquid form, rather than a thick paste like Teflon. These mechanical differences enhance the ease and accuracy of injection. In addition, collagen may reduce scar formation because it stimulates production of collagenase. Before injecting Bovine collagen, safety precautions such as skin testing are mandatory. However,

human autologous and allogeneic collagen are available now and appear superior to Bovine collagen for various reasons. Not only does the use of human material eliminate the severe reactions encountered occasionally with Bovine collagen (skin testing is no longer necessary), but preliminary experience suggests also that human collagen (Dermalogen, Collagenesis, Beverly, Mass) may last longer following injection,[78] potentially making it more useful for lateral injection (medialization) than Bovine collagen.[79-82] Unlike other substances, collagen is designed for superficial injection into the vocal fold margin. A special 25-, 27-, or 30-gauge laryngeal needle is inserted through the mucosa overlying the vibratory margin until the resistance of the vocal ligament is felt. Usually a 0.03 to 0.08 cc injection of collagen is injected superficially. If the standard collagen preparation (Dermalogen) is too viscous for a given clinical situation, less viscous collagen (Demalogen-lite) can be obtained from the manufacturer. However, viscosity is usually adequate with Dermalogen if it has been warmed to *body* temperature. Collagen may also be injected laterally. A peroral technique is best for superficial injection, although collagen can be injected superficially using an external approach through the cricothyroid membrane, in selected cases. For injection laterally along the vocal fold, an external approach through the thyroid lamina usually works well. The thyroid lamina is usually pierced 7 to 9 mm above its inferior border. The position of the needle can be confirmed by observing paraglottic soft tissue movement through a fiberoptic flexible laryngoscope. If the patient's gag reflex is too severe to permit peroral injection of collagen or other substances, or if the laryngeal cartilage is too ossified to allow passage of a needle through the thyroid lamina, it is often possible to inject the paraglottic space by passing a needle behind the posterior aspect of the thyroid lamina (Fig 18–34). Vocal fold injection also can be performed through the thyrohyoid membrane, using flexible nasolaryngoscopic visual guidance. This technique was developed for cidofovir injection. A 25-gauge needle is inserted into the midline at the superior border of the thyroid notch after application of topical anesthesia; and vocal injection can be performed easily (Milan R. Amin, personal communication, June 2004). Collagen injections appear to be efficacious in selected patients and are a valuable addition to the laryngologist's surgical armamentarium. Collagen is not FDA approved specifically for use in the larynx, although its use has become standard practice.

Cymetra micronized AlloDerm (LifeCell Corporation, Branchburg, NJ) is an acellular human tissue material that includes collagen, elastin, and proteogly-

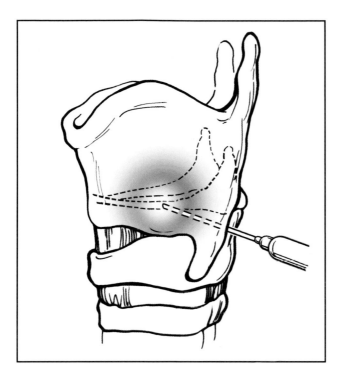

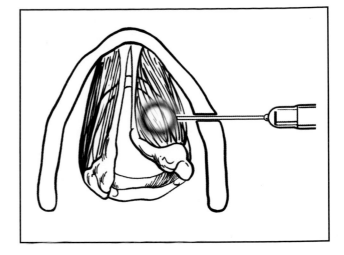

Fig 18–35. Injection of Alloderm, collagen, or other substances may be performed by passing a needle through the thyroid lamina. The point of insertion is usually about halfway between the anterior and posterior borders of the thyroid lamina and about 7 to 9 mm above the inferior border.

Fig 18–34. In most patients, the paraglottic space can be reached through a posterior approach, passing a needle behind the posterior border of the thyroid lamina and then angling it anteriorly and superiorly. Care should be taken to keep the needle close to the thyroid cartilage to help avoid injury to the piriform sinus or branches of the recurrent laryngeal nerve.

cans. Its use in the larynx was reported by Passalaqua et al.[83] They employed an external technique in which the thyroid lamina is pierced with a 22- or 24-gauge needle. Needle localization was confirmed using flexible nasolaryngoscopy, and AlloDerm was injected laterally to treat conditions such as bowing (Fig 18–35). Like collagen, AlloDerm can be injected either through this external technique, through a peroral indirect technique in the office, or through direct laryngoscopy in the operating room.

Autologous fascia also has been advocated for vocal fold augmentation. Rihkanen advised cutting fascia into small pieces and delivering it through a Brünings syringe.[84] This author (RTS) has tried this technique and variations of it over the years. We have used fascia alone in a manner similar to that described subsequently by Rihkanen and fascia mixed with fat to try to diminish the amount of reabsorption of augmentation material. The principal problem with fascia is technical. If all of it is not cut into tiny pieces, it is very difficult to pass through the injection syringe. In one instance, it obstructed the Brünings syringe so firmly that an attempt to pass it further forward resulted in

breakage of the metal syringe. However, if the fascia is prepared properly, it can be a good material. Relatively little is resorbed, and excessive overcorrection should be avoided.

Calcium hydroxyapatite (Coaptite, BioForm, Inc. Franksville, Wisc) is a slurry of calcium hydroxyapatite (CaHA) particles. It is approved by the FDA for use in the larynx, but there has not been enough experience with this substance to comment on its use and potential problems, yet.

Autologous Fat Injection

The first use of autologous fat in the larynx was reported by Dedo in 1975 for patients with laryngeal cancer.[85] He described the placement of a free fat graft under a mucosal advancement flap for creating a neovocal fold following vertical hemilaryngectomy. In many ways, the concept is analogous to the fat implantation reported here. Unfortunately, Dedo did not provide the number of patients or any form of objective assessment; but he reported postoperative voices with minimal hoarseness or breathiness in all cases. This technique has not been used widely, and there are no recent reports of its continued use. However, in appropriate cases, Dedo still employs a modification of this technique and has had continued good experience with it (personal communication, April 1995). Human autologous fat injection into the larynx was first reported by Mikaelian, Lowry, and Sataloff in 1991[86]—and subsequently by Brandenburg, Kirkham, and Koschkee.[87] These and subsequent reports dealt with autologous lipoinjection lateral to the vibratory margin, placing fat in the same position in which Teflon was used. The author has had continued excellent experience with fat injection, particularly in patients who need only minimal medialization. For patients with a wide posterior glottic gap, thyroplasty, or thyroplasty in combination with fat injection, and/or arytenoid adduction has been preferable.

There has been extensive experience with autologous fat transplantation in various areas of the body. In a particularly good review in 1989, Billings and May summarized the literature on this subject and addressed many of the problems that make the use of fat controversial.[88] In particular, the final bulk of the graft and fate of the fat are notoriously unpredictable. At present, the preponderance of evidence suggests that transplanted fat survives and that the relocated adipose tissue remains dynamic. However, observations in soft tissue sites such as the face and chest may or may not be applicable to the fate of fat transplanted to the larynx, especially to the vibratory margin.

Wexler et al studied the fate of fat implanted surgically in the vocal folds of five dogs.[89] The fat was introduced through a laryngofissure approach, not by injection. The fat was retrieved 2 months after the initial surgery, and in 4 of the 5 dogs was found still to be present. Moreover, the autograft produced good functional results, including greater vocal intensity, lower threshold pressures for phonation, and other improvements in the acoustic output. Hill, Meyers, and Harris used microinjection in canines after recurrent laryngeal nerve section.[90] They used an injection technique without laryngofissure and studied the experimental animals histologically at 3 weeks. The bulk of the fat was found to persist for at least that period of time.

An excellent study was reported by Archer and Banks.[91] They designed their study to evaluate the long-term viability of fat introduced submucosally into scarred vocal folds, a procedure very similar to the one the author developed independently for human use, as described in this chapter. Archer and Banks studied 15 canine subjects in three groups. The first group underwent mucosal excision of one vocal fold. The second group underwent mucosal excision of both vocal folds, one of which was augmented 6 weeks later with autologous fat by submucosal injection at three positions along the vocal fold. These two groups were sacrificed at 6 months. The third group was treated the same as the second group, but was sacrificed at 12 months. Each animal was used as its own control. The stripped vocal folds were thin as compared with normal and fat-augmented vocal folds. All

of the fat-augmented vocal folds revealed viable adipose cells in the superficial mucosa. The vocal folds in the fat-augmented group were statistically thicker when compared with the mucosally damaged, nonaugmented groups.

Although the studies cited above are important, their application to humans must be questioned, as with all canine research. Unfortunately, there is no better nonhuman alternative, because humans are the only species with a layered lamina propria and vocal ligament. Because dogs have no vocal ligament, extrapolations from dog research to human response must be made with great caution. Nevertheless, it is encouraging to note that autologous fat appears to be preserved and efficacious in the animal research performed so far. This is especially comforting considering the paucity of experience with fat implantation in human larynges.

The author has had continued good experience with autologous fat injections since our first report.[86] Several technical considerations are important in achieving success. The first is patient selection. The patients who do best with autologous fat injection are those who have only a small glottal gap or those who actually close the glottis during soft phonation but have insufficient resistance on the paralyzed side to permit loud phonation. Such conditions occur after spontaneous compensation for laryngeal paralysis or occasionally following Type I thyroplasty, especially when additional thyroarytenoid muscle atrophy occurs. Similar situations may be seen in patients with vocal fold bowing, as discussed elsewhere in this chapter. Second, the fat should be traumatized as little as possible, maintaining large globules. Third, fat should not be injected much more posteriorly than the middle third of the membranous portion of the vocal fold. A properly placed injection at this location provides adequate medial displacement and allows the medialized vocal fold to pull the arytenoid and vocal process into better position. Injecting too far posteriorly creates a mechanical impediment to passive arytenoid motion, often resulting in persistent vertical height disparity at the vocal processes and inferior voice results. Fourth, unlike Teflon, fat requires overinjection by approximately 30%. The vocal fold should be convex at the conclusion of the procedure to account for expected resorption (Fig 18–36). This overinjection causes moderate dysphonia. If the voice is excellent at the end of the surgical procedure, a good final result is unlikely. Initially, the author recommended performing these procedures under local anesthesia, in a manner similar to that used for Teflon injection. However, because overinjection of fat is performed routinely and there is no need to fine-tune the surgical procedure based on

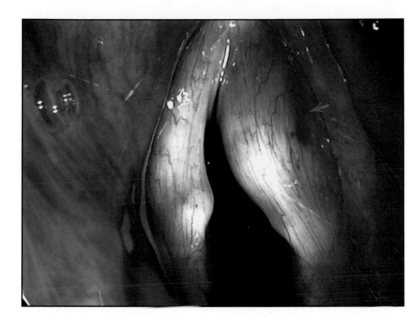

Fig 18–36. This 40-year-old marketing executive and avocational choir singer and musical theater performer had right recurrent nerve paralysis, apparently as a consequence of Lyme disease. Injection was performed near the middle of the right vocal fold (*arrow*). This intraoperative photograph shows 30 to 40% overcorrection, the desired endpoint. The apparent bowing of the left vocal fold is an artifact.

phonatory function, fat injection can be performed equally well under general anesthesia.

Until recently, it has been said that one could not inject too much fat. Although this is generally true, there are rare exceptions. After more than 10 years of utilizing the technique, the author has encountered one case in which excess fat had to be resected. Interestingly, histologically normal, viable fat was removed 1 year following the injection (Fig 18–37). However, this situation represents the exception; and surgeons tend to err by injecting too little. Overcorrection should normally be at least 30 to 40% as described above, or repeated injections will be needed in many patients. In most cases, initial fat resorption occurs fairly quickly. Patients achieve a serviceable voice within 4 to 12 weeks. Additional changes occur over 6 to 12 months. Occasionally, they may even occur later, necessitating reinjection. Such delayed changes have been observed most commonly following substantial weight loss or a severe upper respiratory infection. However, in general, if glottic closure is satisfactory, the improvement is permanent.

Removal of Teflon

One of the complications of Teflon injection is overinjection. If Teflon is injected in excessive amounts or too superficially, the voice will be substantially worse after surgery than it was before Teflon injection. Treating such complications and restoring satisfactory vocal quality are widely (and correctly) regarded as difficult. However, the otolaryngologist may be helped greatly by an accurate preoperative assessment of the problem.

Cross-sectional imaging using computed tomography (CT) of a larynx after Teflon injection documents the position of deposited Teflon easily, including its amount and depth (Fig 18–38). Although this high attenuation material (216 Houndsfield units) is seen easily, the value of radiologic assessment in these cases has been appreciated only in the later 1980s.[92]

In general, preoperative evaluation by strobovideolaryngoscopy, CT, and objective voice analysis allows for reasonably accurate definition of the problem. If the Teflon has been injected incorrectly submucosally and the vibratory margin is adynamic but fairly straight, the patient should be advised that further surgical procedures are unlikely to produce improvement, especially if the vocal fold edge is smooth. If there are multiple lumps of superficial Teflon with failure of glottic closure between them, it is usually worthwhile to remove them and smooth the vibratory margin to improve glottic closure, even if vibration is not restored. If Teflon has been injected in a correct

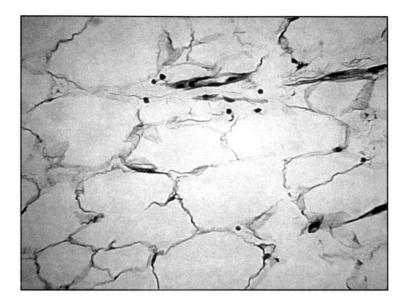

Fig 18–37. This 78-year-old corporate executive had substantial dysphonia related to bilateral superior laryngeal nerve paresis. He had undergone a fat injection 1 year previously. The usual overcorrection was performed on the right vocal fold, and a small amount of fat was injected at the same time into the left vocal fold, but without the usual excess to avoid airway obstruction. Postoperatively, he retained more fat than usual, especially anteriorly. This resulted in vocal strain and fatigue. An incision was made laterally, and the excess fat was resected 1 year following injection. The fat appeared normal and healthy grossly and microscopically, as seen above.

position, but vocal fold convexity exists because of excessive Teflon and/or granuloma formation, results are more satisfactory. It should be noted that the excess may not be due to faulty technique on the part of the surgeon. Although Teflon should not ordinarily cause a reaction, some people do form a granulomatous response or thick capsule, thus increasing mass. Consequently, the amount of Teflon may have been correct at the time of surgery but became more than was necessary after the tissue response occurred. In the author's opinion, the best way to address this problem usually is with an incision with laser laterally over the collection of Teflon. The incision should be far from the vibratory margin. When the CO_2 laser touches the Teflon, a bright white glow is noted. If there is extensive granulomatous reaction around the Teflon, it may be necessary to excise the Teflon with the laser. In other cases, exposing a small portion of the Teflon allows it to be expressed and suctioned. Gentle pressure with the side of suction against the vocal fold edge is used to milk the desired amount of Teflon out of the vocal fold and to re-establish a smooth vocal fold margin. Slight overevacuation creating a minimal concavity of the vocal fold edge seems to produce the best results. Alternatively, Teflon can be excised externally through a thyrotomy. Techniques for the external approach to resection of Teflon granuloma have been published by Netterville and coworkers.[93,94] The approach requires a thyrotomy, and the inner perichondrium is incised. In some cases, the Teflon mass can be shelled out easily. However, if Teflon and inflammatory response involve the vibratory margin, penetration into the airway can occur. If an external approach is used and it appears as if the Teflon mass has been removed safely, it may be desirable to fill part of the resulting cavity, although it is difficult to assess final phonatory outcome during these procedures. This is because Teflon often produces vocal fold stiffness and scar, and the vocal fold may not lateralize completely in the operating room. However, if a large cavity is created by the resection, some lateralization is likely to occur during healing. The cavity can be filled with a free fat graft or with a strap muscle flap. Recently, Netterville has modified his procedure (James Netterville, MD, personal communication, 2001). Rather than using a lateral cartilage flap, he approaches the paraglottic space now through a vertical thyrotomy incision made approximately 4 mm from the midline of

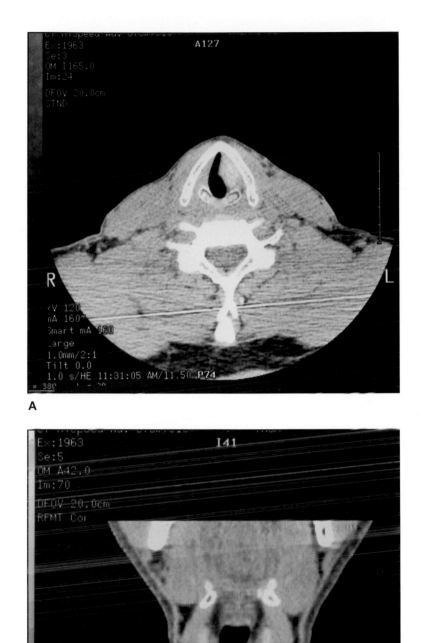

Fig 18–38. Axial (**A**) and coronal (**B**) CT scans of patient with left Teflon granuloma, illustrating the value of CT imaging in mapping the position of the Teflon prior to surgery.

the thyroid cartilage. He also has abandoned the inferiorly based strap muscle flap because of a few cases of fibrosis that produced inferior-lateral scarring of the vocal fold. Instead, he is using a platysmal flap with its attached fat. This author (RTS) has had reasonable success with inferiorly based and superiorly based strap muscle flaps, so long as they are divided at the point of origin or insertion, not in the body of the muscle. An excess amount of muscle is placed, and the muscle is sutured into position with stitches through the thyroid cartilage. If the tissue deep to the vocal fold is deficient (muscle atrophy or absence), a flap including fat or a free fat graft is used. It should be noted that total removal of Teflon is difficult (often impossible) using either the external or endoscopic approach. Unless a hemilaryngectomy is performed, small Teflon particles remain often. In some cases, they may produce recurrent symptomatic granulomas months or years after successful treatment. Such problems are the primary reasons why use of Teflon was abandoned in the late 1980s in favor of injection of fat or other materials or thyroplasty.

Thyroplasty

Another excellent approach to medialization is Type I thyroplasty. This procedure was popularized by Isshiki et al in 1975,[95] although the concept had been introduced early in the century by Payr.[96] Thyroplasty is performed under local anesthesia. Although the author rarely uses the original technique anymore, in classical thyroplasty, with the neck extended, a 4-cm to 5-cm incision is made horizontally at the midpoint between the thyroid notch and the lower rim of the thyroid cartilage. A rectangle of thyroid cartilage is cut out on the involved side. It begins approximately 5 mm to 7 mm lateral to the midline and is usually approximately 3 mm to 5 mm by 3 mm to 10 mm. The inferior border is located approximately 3 mm above the inferior margin of the thyroid cartilage. Care must be taken not to carry the rectangle too far posteriorly, or it cannot be displaced medially. The cartilage is depressed inward, moving the vocal fold toward the midline. The wedge of silicone is then fashioned to hold the depressed cartilage in proper position (Fig 18–39). Since Isshiki's original description, many surgeons have preferred to remove the cartilage. Most preserve the inner perichondrium, although techniques that involve incisions through the inner perichondrium also have been used successfully. Surgeons have also used various or other materials including autologous cartilage, hydroxyapatite, expanded polytetrafluoroethylene, and titanium.[97-103]

Various additional technical modifications were proposed as this technique has became more popular,

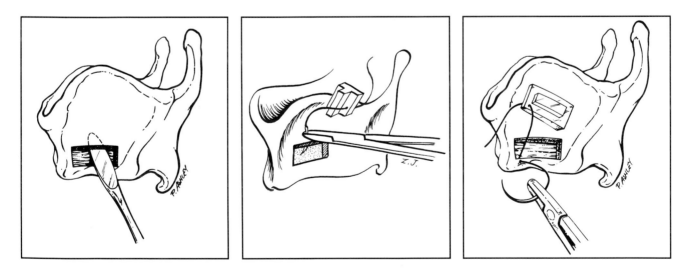

Fig 18–39. (*Left*) In Type I thyroplasty, cartilage is cut beginning 5 to 7 mm lateral to the midline. The window is about 3-5 mm × 3–10 mm. The window should be no more than 5 mm from the inferior border of the thyroid cartilage. After the cartilage cut has been completed, the inner perichondrium is elevated. This drawing illustrates correct window placement. (*Middle*) A silicone block is used to depress the cartilage into proper position, displacing the vocal fold medially. The silicone may be sutured to the cartilage. It is often necessary to taper the silicone anteriorly. This drawing also illustrates the most common errors in thyroplasty surgery, placing the window slightly too high and making the block too thick anteriorly. (*Right*) Appropriate thyroplasty window position and tapered prosthesis.

and several varieties of preformed thyroplasty implant devices have been introduced commercially. Many of these modifications have proven helpful, especially techniques that obviate the need to carve individualized silicone block implants, a technique that is often challenging for inexperienced thyroplasty surgeons. The silicone block modifications described by Dr Harvey Tucker[104] are also useful, particularly the technique of cutting out a portion of the prosthesis to allow for the placement of a nerve-muscle pedicle. However, this author has generally abandoned all of these techniques except during revision cases in favor of Gore-Tex (expanded polytetrafluoroethylene). The use of Gore-Tex in the larynx was reported initially by Hoffman and McCulloch.[101] Since then, several reports have documented its efficacy,[105-107] and others are in preparation. In our center, the author has used Gore-Tex for primary Type I almost exclusively since 1999. The material is easy to place, easy to adjust, and can be contoured to compensate for vocal fold bowing.

Our preferred technique is slightly different from procedures published previously. One of the major advantages of Gore-Tex is that it can be placed through a mini-thyrotomy, obviating the need to traumatize or transect strap muscles. A small (2 cm) horizontal incision is made centered in the midline, in a skin crease near the lower third of the vertical dimension of the thyroid cartilage. The cartilage is exposed in the midline, and the perichondrium is incised and elevated. A 4-mm diamond bur is used to drill a 4-mm mini-thyrotomy. Its anterior border is located approximately 7 mm from the midline in females and 9 mm from the midline in males; and its inferior margin is approximately 3 to 4 mm above the inferior border of the thyroid cartilage. The inner perichondrium is left intact. A fine elevator, such as a Woodson elevator or Sataloff Thyroplasty Elevator (Medtronics-Xomed, Jacksonville, Fla), is used to elevate the perichondrium posteriorly. In this author's opinion, it is very important that only minimal elevation be performed. A small pocket, only 2 to 3 mm in width, parallel to the inferior border of the thyroid cartilage is sufficient. This is substantially different from the extensive elevation performed during traditional thyroplasty. However, if the perichondrium is elevated excessively, it is difficult to control the position of the Gore-Tex. Any additional elevation necessary will be accomplished by the Gore-Tex during insertion. Gore-Tex is then layered through the thyrotomy incision and adjusted to optimize phonation (Fig 18–40). This procedure is performed under local anesthesia with sedation, and vocal fold position can be monitored by flexible laryngoscopy during the operation. We do not use continuous monitoring routinely, but ordinarily we check the final position visually at conclusion of the operation. For closure, other surgeons use perichondrial flaps that are repositioned and sutured. This author has found this maneuver unnecessary and time consuming. Once Gore-Tex has been positioned optimally, it is cut a few millimeters outside the thyrotomy. The thyrotomy is then filled with a few drops of cyanoacrylate. This glue does not react with the Gore-Tex. However, it forms a customized buttonlike seal with a small inner flange of cyanoacrylate, and with a wick of Gore-Tex in the center of the cyanoacrylate block. This prevents extrusion of the Gore-Tex; and the cyanoacrylate "button" and Gore-Tex are removed easily when revision surgery is necessary, simply by pulling on the end of the Gore-Tex that extends a few millimeters beyond the cyanoacrylate. Gore-Tex thyroplasty is so expeditious and atraumatic that it can be performed bilaterally at the same sitting. This is done commonly to treat vocal fold bowing from bilateral superior laryngeal nerve paresis and other causes and to treat presbyphonia refractory to voice therapy. Bilateral thyroplasties can be accomplished ordinarily in less than 1 hour. A small drain usually is placed at the conclusion of the procedure and removed on the first postoperative day. In many cases, the procedure is performed as an outpatient, although overnight observation is appropriate if there is vocal fold swelling or any concern about airway compromise.

There have been no studies documenting the efficacy of routine use of steroids or antibiotics in thyroplasty surgery. Many surgeons use both routinely. This author does not use either antibiotics or steroids routinely. In our practice, we have encountered only one infection following thyroplasty in over 20 years and that was believed to be due to contaminated sutures recalled by the manufacturer shortly after that operation. However, because a foreign body is implanted during thyroplasty, many surgeons prefer to give antibiotics prophylactically.

Revision thyroplasty is a more complex matter. Most thyroplasties that have required revision, so far, have been performed originally using a Silastic block or one of the preformed, commercially available implants. During these initial operations, a large thyroplasty window was created and perichondrium was elevated. Removing the Silastic block and replacing it with Gore-Tex generally does not prove satisfactory. Gore-Tex position cannot be controlled well because of the post-surgical anatomy. In general, this author prefers to revise such cases by carving a new Silastic block, or by modifying the prosthesis that had been placed originally. If revision is being performed because of insufficient medialization, it is sometimes

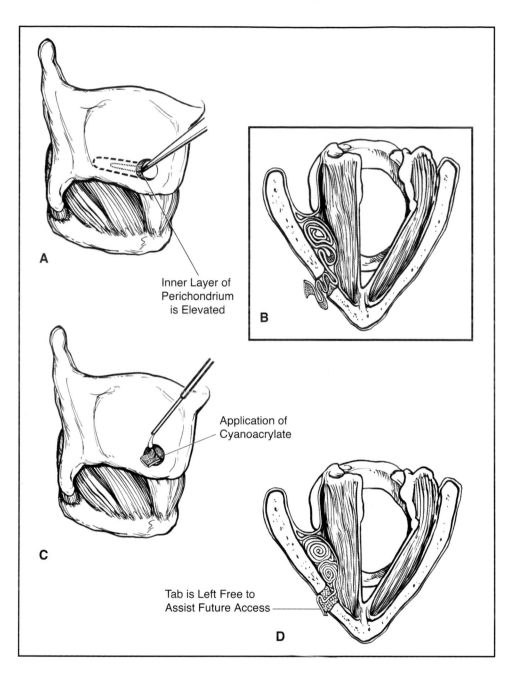

Fig 18–40. A. A mini-thyrotomy is created using a 4-mm diamond burr. Limited perichondrial elevation is performed. **B.** Gore-Tex (W.L. Gore and Associates Incorporated, Newark, Del) is layered into the space between the cartilage and perichondrium. The patient is asked to phonate, and Gore-Tex is adjusted until phonatory output is optimal. **C.** Cyanoacrylate is used to seal the thyrotomy. **D.** A small amount of Gore-Tex is left externally.

possible to elevate the anterior aspect of the prosthesis and layer Gore-Tex medial to it. However, such cases are uncommon. More often, it is necessary to incise the fibrotic capsule in the region of the inner perichondrium with an electric cautery (which often produces momentary discomfort for the patient) and to create a new prosthesis. The most common problems that

require revision are undermedialization resulting in persistent glottic insufficiency, excessive anterior medialization resulting in strained voice, excessively high placement of the original prosthesis, and inappropriate patient selection. Undermedialization can be corrected by underlaying Gore-Tex or creating a larger prosthesis as discussed above, or endoscopically by injecting fat or collagen. Excessive anterior medialization is corrected by reshaping the prosthesis. In such cases, the original implant is usually too thick and placed too far anteriorly. Excessively high placement is often associated with a cartilage window that is considerably higher than the desirable 3 to 4 millimeters above the inferior border of the thyroid cartilage. When additional cartilage is removed to place the prosthesis at the desired height, cartilage deficiency from the original operation often leaves the prosthesis unstable. In such cases, the implanted device should be secured to the thyroid cartilage by sutures. In fact, when using an implant other than Gore-Tex for primary or revision surgery, this author always secures the prosthesis to cartilage with proline suture to prevent migration or extrusion.

Another common reason for revision is inappropriate patient selection. If there is a large, symptomatic posterior glottal gap, thyroplasty alone is often insufficient. Procedures to alter arytenoid cartilage position are necessary in many such cases. Failure to recognize this need and perform the appropriate operation initially may lead to a need for revision surgery that includes arytenoid repositioning procedures. Apart from malposition of the implant, Type I thyroplasty is generally uncomplicated. Successful thyroplasty improves vibratory function.[108] However, if thyroplasty is complicated by hemorrhage with superficial hematoma along the vibratory margin, or by infection, vocal fold stiffness with permanent dysphonia can result. Hemorrhage and edema also can produce airway obstruction. Although this author has never seen a case, Weinman and Maragos[108] reported on 630 thyroplasty procedures. Seven of their patients required tracheotomy. Five of 143 patients who underwent arytenoid cartilage adduction in association with thyroplasty required tracheotomy. In the experience of Weinman and Maragos, the median interval from surgery to tracheotomy was 9 hours, with five of the seven patients requiring airway surgery within 18 hours following thyroplasty.[109] Hence, although in our experience and most other series airway obstruction has not been common, it must be recognized that this complication and the need for tracheotomy are possible.

Isshiki also described other thyroplasty techniques.[38] (Fig 18–41). The Type I thyroplasty described above was designed to medialize the vocal fold. Type II thyroplasty expands the vocal folds laterally. It is designed for patients with airway insufficiency after laryngeal trauma. The thyroid cartilage is separated anteriorly and held apart with cartilage or some other material. This uncommon procedure restores the airway at the expense of the voice. Type III thyroplasty shortens the vocal folds by incising and depressing the anterior segment of the thyroid cartilage. This may be used to lower vocal pitch. An additional decrease in fundamental frequency may be obtained by combining this procedure with vocal fold injection to increase vocal fold mass. However, it involves a fairly significant risk of dysphonia. Type III thyroplasty also has shown at least temporary efficacy in some patients with spasmodic dysphonia.

Type IV thyroplasty was designed to lengthen the vocal folds and increase their tension in order to raise vocal pitch. The cricoid and thyroid cartilages are approximated anteriorly with nylon sutures. This procedure has been used primarily for patients undergoing male to female sex-change surgery and for elderly women with excessive vocal masculinization. Unfortunately, the long-term results (beyond 6 to 12 months) have been disappointing. Sataloff et al described an alternative procedure that fuses the cricoid and thyroid (Fig 18–42), which has proven more satisfactory.[110] The position of the cricoid and thyroid cartilage can be held either with sutures as illustrated, or with miniplates. Surprisingly, these patients have maintained approximately a 1-octave frequency range despite complete cricothyroid fusion and fixation.

Pitch can also be raised by shifting the anterior commissure forward. The procedure is performed by making incisions similar to those used for Type III thyroplasty. However, the anterior segment is advanced. The advancement is maintained by interposing silastic blocks in the gaps between the cartilage edges, and fixing the cartilage with miniplates. Care must be taken not to detach the anterior commissure ligament during this procedure, and during cosmetic laryngoplasty used in sex-change patients.

If the anterior commissure tendon is detached, dysphonia usually is severe. The vocal folds become flaccid, and habitual pitch drops. The ability to change pitch diminishes and pertubation increases. Separation of the anterior commissure can occur iatrogenically, as noted above, or as a consequence of blunt trauma such as may occur from steering wheel injuries or elbow injuries during sports. Anterior commissure laryngoplasty is performed through an external approach. The technique for repair depends on the nature of the injury and the presence or absence of cartilage at the point at which the anterior commissure should be attached. If cartilage is missing following a laryngeal shave procedure or fracture, it is sometimes possible to identify the retracted anterior commissure tendon without additional trauma to the cartilage. If this is not possible, it may be necessary to perform a laryngofissure or to cut a window near the vertical midpoint of the thyroid cartilage. The vocal folds

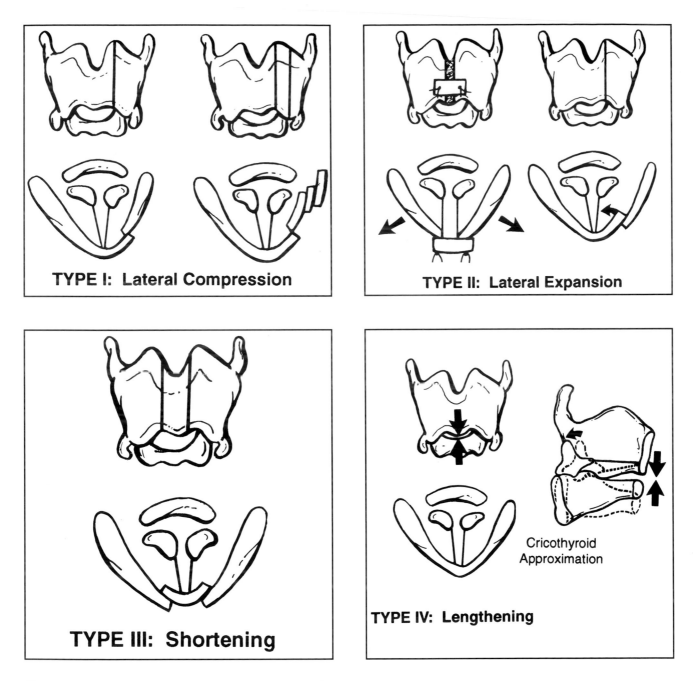

Fig 18–41. Four types of thyroplasty described by Isshiki.[37]

should be mobilized for a distance of several millimeters bilaterally. Then, the anterior commissure ligament can be drawn forward and sutured to cartilage (if present); to a piece of cartilage harvested from the lateral aspect thyroid lamina and placed external to the midline of the thyroid cartilage; or to a miniplate. In particularly difficult cases, other technical modifications may be necessary.

Occasionally, singers and actors inquire about surgery for pitch alteration. Laryngeal framework surgery has proven successful in altering pitch in specially selected patients, such as those undergoing gender reassignment (sex-change) surgery. However, these operations do not provide consistently good enough voice quality to be performed on a professional voice user for elective pitch change. In addition, con-

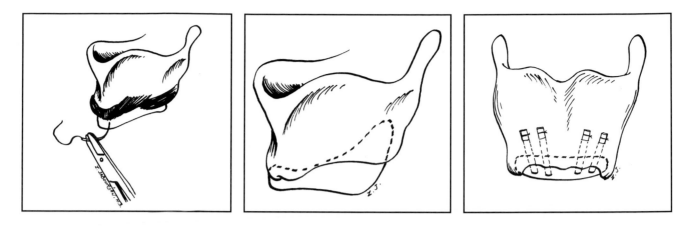

Fig 18–42. In cricothyroid approximation surgery described by Isshiki (*left*), sutures tied over bolsters are used to narrow the cricothyroid space, simulating the action of the cricothyroid muscle. In our modification (*middle*), the cricoid cartilage is subluxed behind the thyroid cartilage. It is fixed into position (*right*) using sutures and bolsters or using miniplates. Although the cricothyroid space is obliterated, the ability to vary pitch remains surprisingly good.

siderably more than habitual fundamental frequency is involved in the perception of voice classification, and important other factors (such as the center frequency of the singer's formant) are not modified by laryngeal surgery.

Nomenclature

In an effort to standardize the confusing nomenclature of laryngoplastic voice surgery (commonly called phonosurgery), the Committee on Speech, Voice and Swallowing Disorders of the American Academy of Otolaryngology—Head and Neck Surgery developed a nomenclature, which the author recommends using (see Table 18–1).[111]

Arytenoid Cartilage Adduction/Rotation, Cricothyroid Subluxation, Arytenoidectomy

All of the procedures discussed above work fairly well for recurrent laryngeal nerve paralysis but not nearly so well if the superior laryngeal nerve is involved or if the arytenoid cartilage is in abnormal position for some other reason. In these cases, arytenoid cartilage adduction/rotation or alternative techniques of arytenoid cartilage repositioning procedures are preferable.[111] Arytenoid adduction/rotation surgery is usually performed under local anesthesia. The thyropharyngeus muscle is divided, and the posterior margin of the thy-

roid cartilage is exposed. Subperichondrial elevation is carried onto the inferior surface of the thyroid ala. The cricothyroid joint is dislocated, and the piriform sinus is protected. When the piriform sinus has been elevated for arytenoid cartilage adduction/rotation or arytenopexy (discussed below), it is advisable to reattach the mucoperichondrial flap at the conclusion of the procedure. This helps prevent fibrosis and constriction that may interfere with swallowing. In addition, if extensive piriform sinus mucosa elevation is performed, the piriform sinus may prolapse producing airway obstruction, especially in the presence of a posterior thyroid cartilage window. This problem can be avoided by suturing the piriform sinus mucosa to the thyroid cartilage (Nicholas E. Maragos, MD, personal communication, 2003). The muscular process of the arytenoid cartilage is identified, and the joint is opened in the classic approach through a small incision over the cricoarytenoid muscle. However, in many cases, it is not necessary to open the joint; and it may even be better not to. Two 3-0 permanent sutures are fixed in soft tissue across the muscular process and tied in the directions of the lateral cricoarytenoid and lateral thyroarytenoid muscles, adjusting vocal fold position (Fig 18–43).

This author prefers not to divide the cricothyroid joint in most cases. When it is divided, it heals with scar. The resulting fixation may impair movement of the functioning on the contralateral side and is likely to impair passive movement of the ipsilateral side in response to contralateral cricothyroid muscle contraction. In addition, if the joint is divided and not re-

Table 18–1. Nomenclature for Laryngoplastic Voice Surgery.

A. Laryngeal framework surgery (LFS) with

Arytenoid adduction (AA)

Medialization (M)

Lateralization (L)

Anterior Commissure

Retrusion (relaxation) (ACR)

Protrusion (tensing) (ACP)

Cricothyroid approximation (CTA)

Medialization laryngoplasty can be qualified by method of medialization

Medialization laryngoplasty with

s = silicone elastoner

c = cartilage

e = expander

o = other

B. Injection laryngoscopy (IL)

D = Direct

I = Indirect

Injection laryngoplasty with

t = Teflon

g = Gelfoam

col = collagen

f = fat

o = other

Abbreviations may be used

Laryngeal framework surgery with medialization-silicone elastomer (LFS-M-s)

Laryngeal framework surgery with arytenoid adduction (LFS-AA)

Injection laryngoplasty-direct-Teflon (IL-D-t)

From Benninger et al,[111] with permission.

paired, the natural forces of the neck tend to push the inferior cornu posterior to the cricothyroid joint facet, shortening the vocal fold and aggravating the dysphonia. Traditionally, this author has prevented that problem by suturing the cricothyroid joint into its normal position, if it has been divided. This prevents retrusion, but it does not result in passive mobility of the joint in most cases.

An alternate technique called cricothyroid subluxation has been described by Zeitels.[113] This technique also does not ensure passive mobility, but it has been surprisingly successful at improving frequency range and dynamic range of phonation, at least during short-term follow-up. A suture is tied around the inferior cornu of the thyroid cartilage and passed through the midline of the cricoid cartilage (Fig 18–44). The inferior cornu is pulled gently forward and adjusted in accordance with the patient's phonatory response. In Zeitels' illustrations, the inferior cornu is pictured as

fairly far anterior to the cricothyroid joint facet. In this author's experience (RTS), it is usually unnecessary to distract it so far anteriorly. Usually, optimal results are achieved when the posterior aspect of the inferior cornu is fairly close to the anterior aspect of the cricoid joint facet.

When arytenoid cartilage adduction is combined with thyroplasty, it is not always necessary to create a thyroplasty window. The author has devised a technique in which a Silastic block is placed through a posterior approach. The arytenoid cartilage procedure is performed first (adduction/rotation or arytenoidopexy). The inner perichondrium is then elevated from posterior to anterior under direct vision. A Silastic block is carved and adjusted to the appropriate size and shape. The position of the Silastic block is noted, and the block is removed. A suture is passed through the thyroid cartilage from external to internal at approximately the position of the junction of the ante-

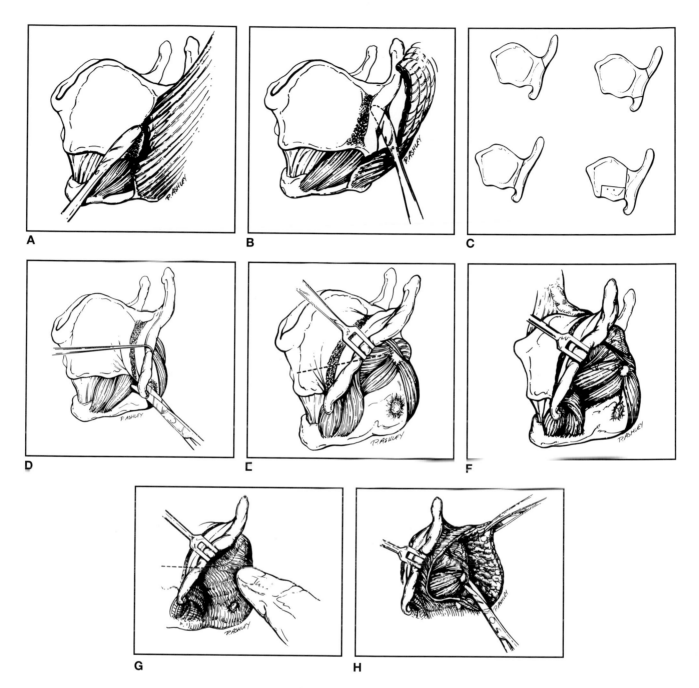

Fig 18–43. A. In arytenoid adduction/rotation surgery, the thyropharyngeus muscle is separated from the ala of the thyroid cartilage. **B.** Starting at the posterior aspect of the thyroid cartilage, the inner perichondrium is elevated to prevent entrance into the airway. **C.** Ordinarily, the procedure can continue simply with anterior retraction of the thyroid cartilage. However, especially with a large thyroid ala as encountered in some men, it is helpful to transect the thyroid cartilage in one of the patterns illustrated above by solid lines. **D.** Ordinarily, simple anterior retraction of the thyroid cartilage allows the surgeon to divide the cricothyroid joint with the scissors, exposing the cricothyroid joint surface. **E.** The muscular process of the arytenoid is located at approximately the level of the vocal fold (*dotted line*). **F.** The distance (*arrow*) between the upper margin of the cricothyroid joint and the lower margin of the cricoarytenoid joint is ordinarily less than 1 cm. The position of the muscular process (*m*) and vocal process (*v*) are also illustrated. **G.** The muscular process can often be identified by palpation. **H.** After elevating the mucosa lining the piriform sinus to avoid entering the airway, the posterior cricoarytenoid muscle fibers are divided, and the cricoarytenoid joint is entered. Entry into the joint is not necessary in every case.

(continues)

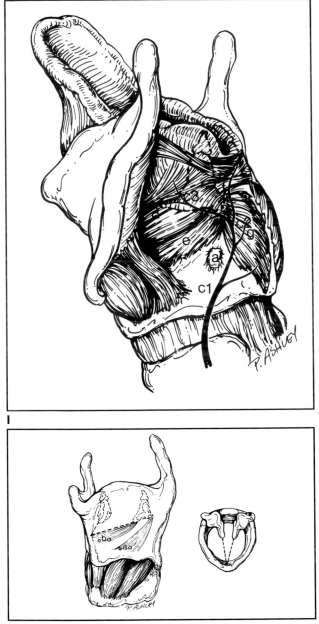

I

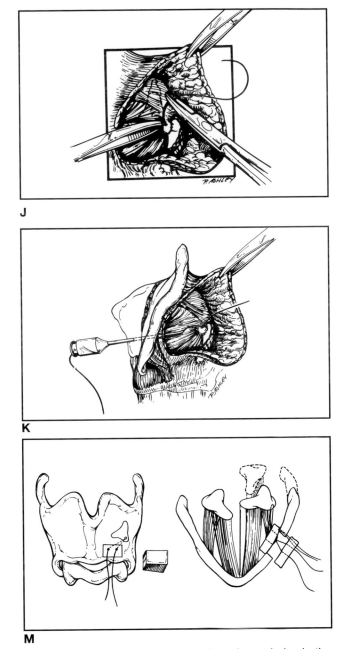

J

K

L

M

Fig 18–43. *(continued).* **I.** It is important to be familiar with the anatomic structures that may be encountered during this procedure. The most important ones include the cricothyroid joint (*a*), cricoarytenoid joint (*b*), recurrent laryngeal nerve (*c-1*), one with its abductor branches (*c-2*) and adductor branches (*c-3*); thyroarytenoid muscle (*d*), laterocricoarytenoid muscle (*e*), interarytenoid muscle (*f*) and posterior cricoarytenoid muscle (*g*). **J.** A 4-0 nylon suture is placed through the muscular process of the arytenoid. The tip of the needle is visible in the joint space. **K.** After the suture is tied to the muscular process, it is passed through the thyroid ala. An injection needle may be used if the suture cannot be passed easily using suture needles. **L.** Left, one or two sutures may be used, pulling the vocal fold in the direction of the lateral cricoarytenoid (*a*) and the direction of the thyroarytenoid (*b*). Adjusting tension between these two sutures permits proper positioning of the vocal fold. Often, only the cricoarytenoid suture is necessary. Each suture is passed through two holes in the thyroid cartilage (*circles*) and tied externally on the thyroid cartilage. Suture placement (*right*) in the arytenoid is important. If the suture is placed posteriorly (*black dot*) on the muscular process, more adduction is possible than if the suture is placed more anteriorly (*open circle*). **M.** (*Left*) Arytenoid adduction/rotation can be combined with Type I thyroplasty. Suture is passed first through the region of the intended window using either a needle, or small holes created with a drill. The suture is left untied. (*Right*) After the inner perichondrium is elevated, the cartilage may be depressed medially, and the suture can be tied. Alternatively, the suture can be passed through a Silastic block and tied over the prosthesis. The suture is then passed through another implant placed lateral to the window and tied again to maintain secure position and prevent the internal prosthesis or cartilage from pulling medially away from the inner aspect of the thyroid lamina.

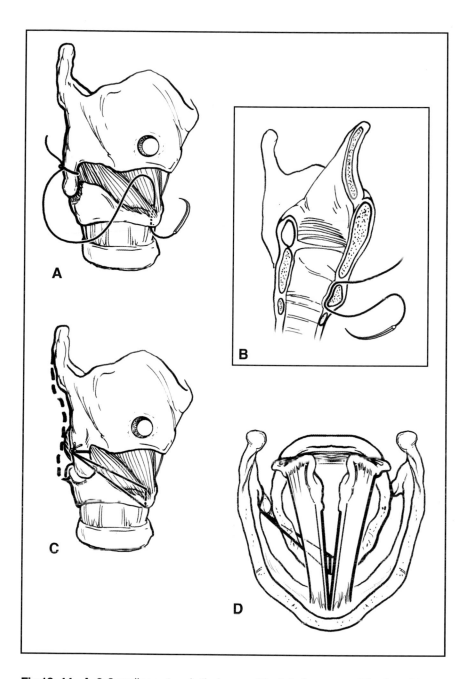

Fig 18–44. A. 2-0 proline suture is tied around the inferior cornu of the thyroid cartilage and (**B**) passed circumferentially around the cricoid arch in the midline. **C** and **D.** The suture is adjusted to pull the inferior cornu forward, lengthening the vocal fold. The patient is asked to phonate. When frequency and dynamic range are optimal, it is best to overcorrect slightly (approximately 1 mm) and fix the inferior cornu in that position.

rior and middle thirds of the final position of the Silastic block. The needle is then passed through the outer surface of the junction of the anterior and middle thirds of the Silastic block near its upper border and brought back through the Silastic block from medial to lateral near its lower border. It is then passed from the inner surface of the thyroid lamina through the outer surface, below the initial suture entry point. The suture is then tied on the outside of the thyroid cartilage. As the suture is tightened, the Silastic block is reinserted and anchored into position. If the position is not completely stable, a second suture can be used.

This procedure has proven extremely fast and effective. Gore-Tex (Newark, Del) has not been used in this scenario, because the Gore-Tex would probably extrude through the posterior opening unless it were sutured into position; and, even then, maintaining optimal Gore-Tex position would be challenging. When Gore-Tex is preferred in combination with an arytenoid cartilage procedure, it is performed in the usual fashion through an anterior mini-thyrotomy.

Zeitels also introduced adduction arytenopexy (Fig 18–45) as an alternative to classical arytenoid cartilage adduction/rotation.[114] This is an interesting and effective procedure, although it can be challenging technically for inexperienced laryngeal framework surgeons. It often is necessary to divide the cricothyroid joint to obtain adequate exposure, so that the procedure is combined routinely either with suture repair of the joint or cricothyroid subluxation. In adduction arytenopexy, it is easiest to exposure the cricoid cartilage at the cricothyroid joint, follow the cartilage from the joint to the superior surface of the cricoid, and dissect along the superior surface of cricoid cartilage. This allows easy identification of the cricoarytenoid joint, particularly after the lateral cricoarytenoid and posterior cricoarytenoid muscles have been divided from the muscular process. The cricothyroid joint is opened during this procedure, a maneuver not always necessary in classic arytenoid cartilage adduction/rotation. A suture is placed initially through the medial aspect (near the midline) of the posterior face of the cricoid cartilage and through the medial aspect of the cricoarytenoid joint. The suture is then passed through the arytenoid cartilage, looped around the lateral aspect of the arytenoid, and then brought back through the joint and posterior face of the cricoid cartilage where it is tied. This technique pulls the arytenoid cartilage up the cricoid facet, closing the posterior glottic gap. It also eliminates sutures that extend anteriorly and, in some cases, may interfere with thyroplasty. In addition, this technique tends to pull the vocal process posteriorly, lengthening the vocal fold. However, optimizing vocal process height can be difficult. To facilitate vocal process alignment, the patient should be asked to phonate at his or her habitual pitch (not at high pitch, as used commonly during mirror examination). This author (RTS) sometimes finds it necessary to place an additional proline suture or two to stabilize the arytenoid cartilage in the positioned desired.

Woodson et al have also recognized the problem of controlling the vertical position of the vocal process and have proposed a technique to help control this variable factor during arytenoid cartilage adduction/rotation surgery.[115] Their technique works better with arytenoid cartilage adduction/rotation (for which it was designed) than with arytenopexy because of the degree of joint instability created during arytenopexy and because of the final position of the inferior cornu of the thyroid cartilage when arytenoidopexy is combined with cricothyroid subluxation. However, the principle can be applied during either operation. Woodson noted that, in flaccid laryngeal paralysis, the vocal process often is displaced superiorly and laterally. She observed correctly that arytenoid cartilage adduction tends to move the vocal process medially and caudally, but that its position often ends up more caudal than normal. She hypothesized that this was due to the absence of the normal action of the posterior cricoid arytenoid muscle and proposed a posterior anchoring suture to replace posterior cricoarytenoid support. She used sutures from the arytenoid cartilage to the inferior cornu of the thyroid cartilage or to the posterior midline of the cricoid cartilage. Tension on these sutures decreased caudal displacement, but the sutures anchored near the midline widened the glottic gap. Consequently, anchoring the sutures to the inferior cornu of the thyroid cartilage is preferable when using this approach. Although classical arytenoid adduction/rotation is substantially easier and provides excellent results in some cases, adduction arytenoidopexy has clear advantages in selected cases and should be used especially in patients with complete unilateral vocal fold paralysis when there is a large posterior glottic gap and the arytenoid cartilage is tipped far laterally.

Iwamura has described yet another procedure for arytenoid cartilage repositioning called the lateral cricoarytenoid muscle pull procedure.[116,117] This operation is performed under local anesthesia through a 10 × 8 mm thyrotomy window. The window is placed immediately in front of the oblique line, over the lateral cricoarytenoid muscle (Fig 18–46). Sutures are passed through several points along the atrophic lateral cricoarytenoid (LCA) muscle bundle and tied first around the muscle, and then to the thyroid cartilage. The sutures are adjusted according to intraoperative voice improvement.

Nerve Anastomosis

Reanastomosing divided or injured recurrent laryngeal nerves has not resulted in the restoration of normal motion in most cases and traditionally has been considered not helpful. Failures may be due to abnormal intermingling of abductor and adductor fibers or to other causes. Attempts have been made to improve the results, optimizing abduction by dividing intralaryngeal adductor nerve branches.[117] However, this

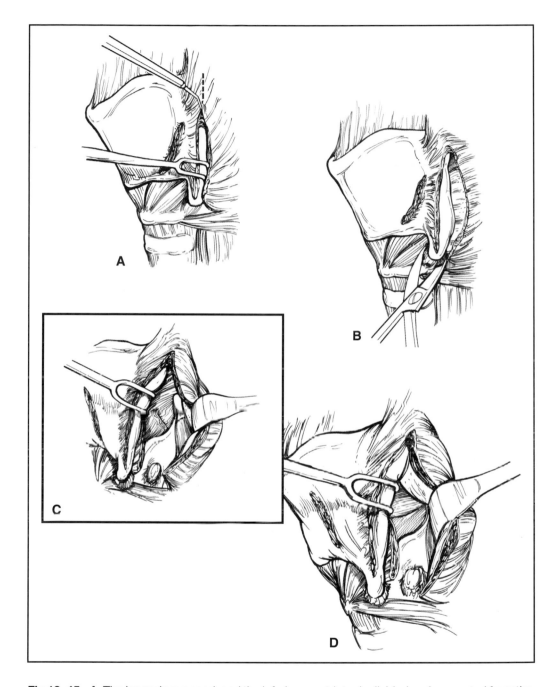

Fig 18–45. A. The larynx is exposed, and the inferior constrictor is divided and separated from the thyroid lamina. **B.** The cricothyroid joint is separated with scissors. **C.** Dissection follows the cricoid cartilage from the cricothyroid joint facet to the superior rim of the cricoid cartilage. The piriform sinus is dissected gently posteriorly. The cricothyroid muscle is cut during this dissection. **D.** The lateral cricoarytenoid and posterior cricoarytenoid muscles are divided from the muscular process.

(continued)

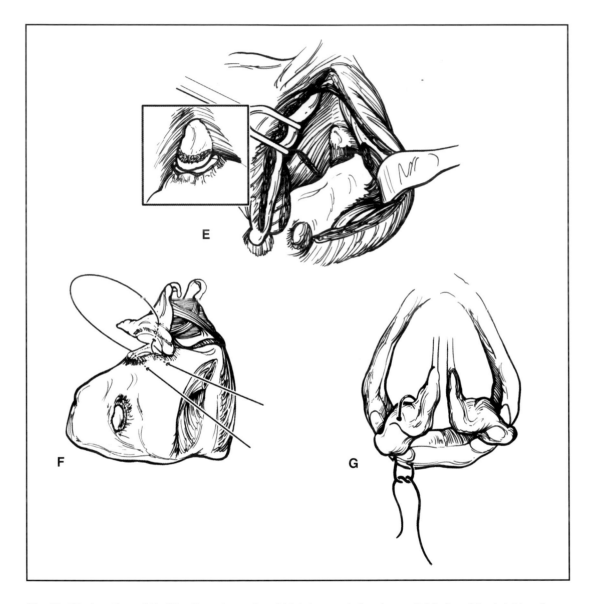

Fig 18–45. *(continued)* **E.** After the cricoarytenoid joint capsule has been divided and the joint has been opened widely, the posterior cricoarytenoid muscle is dissected off of the posterior aspect of the cricoid cartilage. **F.** 4-0 proline suture on a cutting needle is passed through the posterior face of the cricoid cartilage and through the cricoarytenoid joint. It is then wrapped around the anterolateral aspect of the arytenoid and brought back through the joint and posterior cricoid plate. **G.** Arytenoid position is adjusted by the tension on the suture as it is tied along the posterior face of the cricoid cartilage. In some cases, additional simple sutures through the arytenoid and cricoid may be necessary to adjust vocal process position optimally.

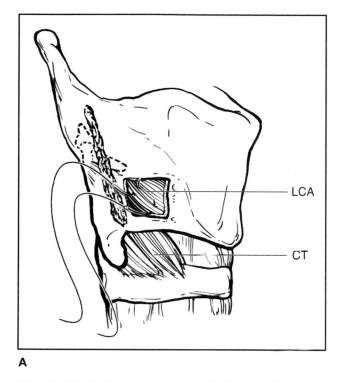

A

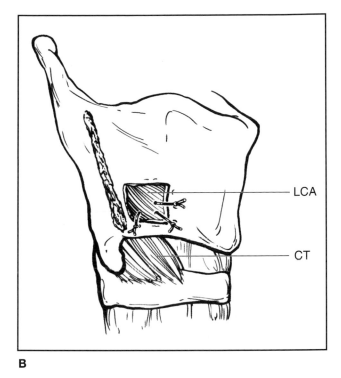

B

Fig 18–46. A. Sutures are placed through the lateral cricoarytenoid muscle. **B.** The tension on the sutures is adjusted to optimize phonatory output, and they are fixed to the thyroid cartilage anteriorly and inferiorly.

technique has limited applicability. Procedures using various other nerves, including vagus nerve bypass, split vagus nerve, phrenic nerve, and other nerves in the region, have been tried. Results have been variable.

However, research on reinnervation suggests that the technique may be much more valuable than previously appreciated. In at least some patients with vocal fold paralysis, there appears to be some degree of vocal fold atrophy after long-term denervation. Although some vocal folds show return of normal function even after complete recurrent laryngeal nerve section, reestablishing neural supply may be important to maintain vocal fold bulk (hence the effectiveness of medialization surgery) and to help control vocal fold pitch.[118-121] If a recurrent laryngeal nerve is known to have been cut during surgery, it is worthwhile for the surgeon to suture the cut ends, even though this is not likely to result in normal abduction and adduction (Fig 18–47). This subject is discussed at greater length elsewhere.[122]

Nerve Muscle Pedicle Surgery

Nerve muscle pedicle surgery involves implanting a portion of the omohyoid or other muscle with its intact motor branch from the ansa hypoglossi into a paralyzed laryngeal abductor muscle (Fig 18–48A-D) or a

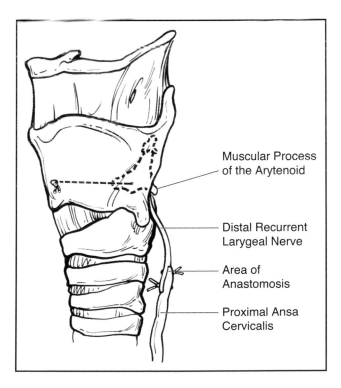

Fig 18–47. Anastomosis between ansa cervicalis and distal recurrent laryngeal nerve. Primary end-to-end recurrent laryngeal nerve reanastomosis may be performed when both portions of the severed nerve are available

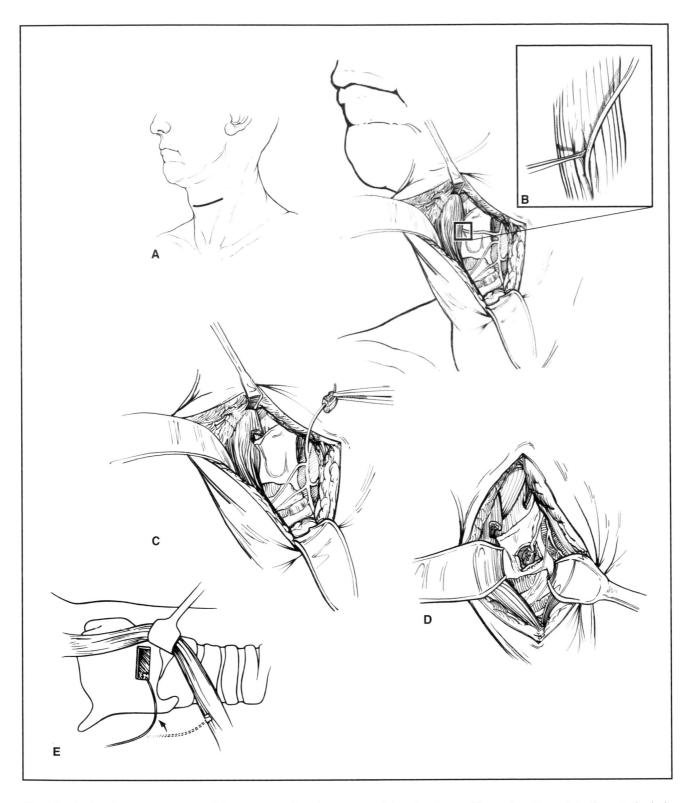

Fig 18–48. B. The ansa hypoglossi is seen entering the omohyoid muscle. **C.** The nerve is followed 2 to 3 cm into the muscle to the point at which it branches and is included in a muscle block that leaves the nerve-muscle junctions untraumatized. **D.** The nerve-muscle pedicle is sutured to the desired intrinsic laryngeal muscle. **E.** Nerve-muscle pedicle using the ansi hypoglossi branch to the anterior belly of the omohyoid muscle. After using Tucker's technique of rotating the nerve-muscle pedicle and suturing it to the exposed thyroarytenoid muscle through a thyroplasty window, the thyroplasty prosthesis must then be notched in order to prevent injury to the nerve-muscle pedicle.

portion of the cricothyroid muscle with its motor branch of the superior laryngeal nerve into a paralyzed adductor muscle. The concept was originally reported by Takenouchi and Sato in 1968,[124] and was popularized by Tucker et al in 1970,[125] and described in numerous publications thereafter. Success rates have varied, and the operation certainly has not been universally satisfactory. Probably, the small improvement that is often seen results more from change in mass or position than from return of mobility. Avoidance of atrophy may occur also. This subject is discussed later in this chapter in the section in bilateral vocal fold paralysis. Failure of reinnervation after this procedure has been demonstrated histochemically in some patients. This procedure is often most effective when it is combined with a medialization procedure such as Type I thyroplasty that can be performed through the same incision (Fig 18–48E).

Other Techniques

Numerous other techniques have been tried to restore voice quality in patients with vocal fold paralysis. They include switching of intact muscles, implantation of artificial muscles, cartilage implantation, and other methods. None of the techniques available is entirely satisfactory, although interest in laryngeal pacing is particularly encouraging.[126,127] It shows promise for management of both unilateral and bilateral vocal fold paralysis along with other exciting advances undergoing research.

Treatment of Cricoarytenoid and Cricothyroid Subluxation

Treatment of cricoarytenoid and cricothyroid joint injuries is discussed in chapter 21.

Arytenoidectomy

Arytenoidectomy remains the most reliable technique for reestablishing a good airway in patients with bilateral vocal fold paralysis or arytenoid fixation. Unfortunately, it generally does so at the expense of voice quality. However, it results in voice quality superior to the operation it replaced, which was total cordectomy.[126] Traditionally, arytenoidectomy has been performed through an external incision. The procedure was introduced initially in 1946 by Woodman. He described removing the arytenoid cartilage with preservation of the vocal process.[128] Endoscopic arytenoidectomy was described 2 years later by Thor-

nell.[129] Endoscopic arytenoidectomy has been successful and effective, and has proven a particularly satisfactory approach since use of the carbon dioxide laser was introduced for this operation.[130-133]

The procedure is performed using suspension microlaryngoscopy. A 400-mm objective lens is usually optimal. Lasers with a spot size of 0.4 mm are generally used at 6 to 10 watts in repeat mode with 0.1-second pulses. The corniculate cartilage and mucosa over the apex of the arytenoid are vaporized, as is the mucoperiosteum of the apex and body of the arytenoid cartilage. The upper portion of the body of the arytenoid is ablated using continuous mode. Repeat mode is then used to vaporize the mucoperichondrium of the lower body, which is then vaporized from lateral to medial. The lateral ligament is transected, and the cricoid cartilage is exposed. The vocal process is vaporized, as is the muscular process preserving the attachment of the arytenoideus muscle (Fig 18–49). Vaporization is continued lateral to the vocalis muscle to create a scar that will assist in lateralization of the vocal fold (Fig 18–50). Because of cartilage exposure, antibiotics are generally recommended. If there is no tracheotomy in place, intraoperative corticosteroids are also used by many surgeons. There are no data proving the efficacy of either antibiotics or steroids during this procedure. Their use at present depends on the surgeon's judgment. There are various modifications of arytenoidectomy procedures. Many surgeons (including this author) preserve a mucosal flap, suturing it over the resection site. Closing mucosa helps avoid granuloma formation, a troublesome complication of arytenoidectomy. Arytenoidectomy patients also should be treated prophylactically for la-

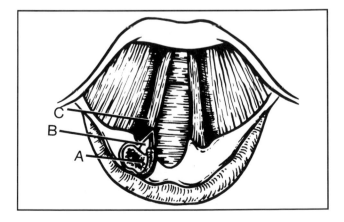

Fig 18–49. Intermittent step during laser arytenoidectomy, showing exposure of the cricoid cartilage (*A*), vocal process of the arytenoid cartilage (*B*), and vocalis muscle (*C*).

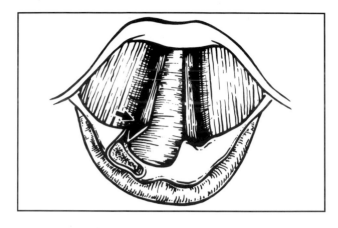

Fig 18–50. Completed arytenoidectomy with remnant of muscular process and arytenoideus attachment, and laser-induced trauma lateral to the vocal muscle to help lateralization (*arrow*).

rynogopharyngeal reflux. This appears to expedite healing and does not appear to interfere with formation of lateralizing scar.

It also is possible to resect only portions of the arytenoid cartilage. Medial arytenoidectomy (preserving a thin, lateral shell of arytenoid cartilage) often provides an adequate airway and minimizes collapse of the posterior laryngeal anatomy. Medial arytenoidectomy was popularized by Crumley.[132] This procedure may be advantageous particularly in patients who are likely to aspirate after complete arytenoidectomy. Medial arytenoidectomy also has been used in unusual circumstances, such as bilateral pseudoparalysis.[133]

Other Techniques for Bilateral Vocal Fold Paralysis

Bilateral vocal fold paralysis still places the patient and surgeon in a most difficult position. No good treatment is available, yet. Arytenoidopexy is an alternative to arytenoidectomy. In this procedure, no tissue is removed; but the arytenoid cartilage is sutured into the abducted position.[135,136] Unfortunately, this procedure is less consistent than arytenoidectomy in producing a good airway. However, suture lateralization (passing a stitch through the skin in the lateral neck, around the vocal fold, and back out through the skin) can be a useful adjunct to arytenoidectomy, helping to lateralize the posterior aspect of the vocal fold.

An interesting alternative to placement of a suture or arytenoidectomy was proposed by Cummings et al[137] (Fig 18–51). They developed a double-helix, double-cam, stainless steel/polythene device that is

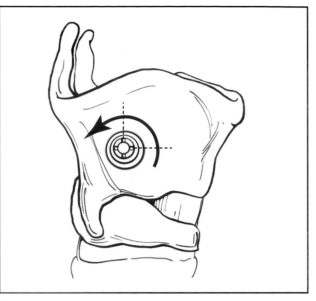

A

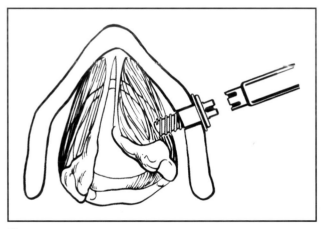

B

Fig 18–51. A. The Cummings device is snapped into a 1-cm hole cut in the thyroid cartilage, which stabilizes the device and provides access for adjustment. **B.** Once the device is attached to the region of the vocal process, the outer cam is retracted lateralizing the true vocal fold. The double-helix, double-cam, stainless steel/polythene device is attached to the vocal process through a 1-cm window in the thyroid cartilage. This screwlike device can be adjusted incrementally to lateralize the vocal fold precisely, establishing an optimal balance between airway and voice.

attached to the vocal process through a 1-cm window in the thyroid cartilage. This screwlike device can be adjusted incrementally to lateralize the vocal fold precisely, establishing an optimal balance between airway and voice. This minimally invasive technique was reported after studies in sheep; and human efficacy studies are pending. However, the technique appears promising.

Although arytenoidectomy provides a good airway, as discussed above, it usually results in a breathy, somewhat hoarse voice. The better the airway is, the worse the voice. However, if the vocal folds are near the midline, producing good voice, a tracheotomy is usually required for active individuals. Another technique proposed to reestablish adequate airway is posterior cordotomy, as described by Dennis and Kashima.[138] This procedure involves removal of the posterior third of the vocal fold. This may produce better voice quality than arytenoidectomy alone.[138] Many surgeons combine this principle with arytenoidectomy with a lateral, wedgelike resection of thyroarytenoid muscle anterior to the vocal process (posterior cordotomy).

If bilateral vocal fold paralysis presents with good voice and borderline airway, reinnervation may be worth trying; reinnervation may be worthwhile even when the vocal folds are in midline. In order to undergo reinnervation of the posterior cricoarytenoid muscles, patients must have mobile arytenoids and intact cricoarytenoid joints. Ascertaining the condition of the cricoarytenoid joints may require palpation during direct laryngoscopy with paralysis. It is advisable to palpate the arytenoid cartilages routinely on all patients, so that the surgeon knows the degree of pressure required to move a normal arytenoid cartilage. Palpation should be accomplished with the side of a suction or with a spatula placed against the medial or lateral face of the arytenoid cartilage. Pressure directly on the vocal process or its junction with the body of the arytenoid cartilage should be avoided to prevent fracturing the vocal process off the arytenoid body.

A nerve muscle pedicle 2 to 3 mm square is created from any of the strap muscles,[139,140] although the omohyoid is used most commonly. The posterior cricoarytenoid muscle is exposed by retracting the posterior aspects of the cricoid cartilage and separating the inferior constrictor muscle near the base of the inferior cornu of the thyroid cartilage. Care must be taken to reflect rather than transgress the piriform sinus. The posterior cricoarytenoid muscles are recognized easily because they run at right angles to the inferior constrictor. The nerve-muscle pedicle is sutured into the cricoarytenoid muscle. When the procedure works, there is usually a 4- to 6-month delay between surgery and active abduction and abduction. Further details are provided elsewhere.[123]

This author occasionally has used botulinum toxin for bilateral vocal fold paralysis. Although this seems counterintuitive, it should be remembered that at least a small amount of reinnervation is common following vocal fold paralysis. When reinnervation occurs, there is synkinesis. That is, both abductors and adductors are innervated. Consequently, if a borderline airway is present, injecting botulinum toxin into the adductor muscles may allow enough unopposed abductor function to result in an extra millimeter or two of glottic space. If this is sufficient for the patient, it is certainly less traumatic than arytenoidectomy; and usually it results in better voice quality.

Vocal Process Avulsion

Vocal process avulsion may occur with internal or external laryngeal trauma. Examination findings may be subtle. Highly magnified strobovideolaryngoscopic evaluation is helpful. Endoscopic evaluation with palpation under general anesthesia may be necessary. Voice therapy should be administered initially. Surgical options include the use of injectable materials for closed reduction, chemical tenotomy with botulinum toxin, endoscopic open reduction of the fracture via a cordotomy approach, or open reduction using a laryngofissure.

Vocal process avulsion can result from intubation or from external trauma to the larynx. These are also the most common etiologies of arytenoid dislocation, which should be included in the differential of dysphonia after such events. Discrepancy in the heights of the vocal processes may be seen with either vocal process avulsion or arytenoid dislocation. Close examination of movement of the body of the arytenoid cartilage in relation to the vocal process may help distinguish between the two. Of note, when reducing an anterior arytenoid cartilage dislocation, one should take care not to insert the laryngoscope too deeply into the laryngeal inlet so as to place the vocal process at risk for avulsion. External laryngeal trauma is a potentially life-threatening injury. Dysphonia is an ominous sign and should alert the physician to a possible laryngeal fracture or vocal fold injury.

In the author's experience, patients with vocal process avulsion have presented with persistent dysphonia weeks to months after the initial insult.[141] Some structure injury was suspected from examination and EMG results. Other symptoms in the acute setting may include pain and dysphagia. Findings of a vocal process avulsion can be subtle, and close examination of the larynx with both flexible laryngoscopy and rigid videostroboscopy is critical in the evaluation of these injuries. Signs of avulsion may include an apparent separation of the vocal process from the arytenoid body, abnormal angle or position of the vocal process, overlapping of the avulsed vocal process with the contralateral process, mobility of the vocal process independent from the body of the arytenoids, and foreshortening and decreased stretch of the vocal fold during glissando.

Treatment of the vocal process avulsion must be geared toward the severity of the injury and the expectations of the patient. A trial of voice therapy usually is warranted, as this may provide a satisfactory voice for some patients. If one proceeds with surgery, several options are available. Endoscopic open reduction of the fracture may be performed.

Laryngofissure and Lateral Thyrotomy

In some situations, it is necessary to operate on the vocal folds or paraglottic tissue through an external approach. In addition to laryngeal framework procedures discussed elsewhere in this chapter, laryngofissure and thyrotomy can be used to provide access to the area of interest.

Laryngofissure is performed through a horizontal incision in the anterior neck, centered near the vertical midpoint of the thyroid cartilage. Laryngofissure was performed initially in 1788 by Pellatone to remove a laryngeal foreign body, although it had been suggested early by Desault.[142] In 1834, Brauers in Belgium was the first surgeon to use laryngofissure to remove a neoplasm.[141] The operation also was utilized by Billoff

for eight patients between 1870 and 1884, and by many others in the later 19th and early 20th centuries.[141] Before the end of the first quarter of the 20th century, it had become the standard approach for surgical treatment of early carcinoma of the vocal folds. It is sometimes still used for that indication; but now it is used more commonly to repair vocal fold trauma, to resect other neoplasms, and in combination with other procedures such as anterior and/or posterior cricoid cartilage split. Soft tissues are divided and strap muscles are retracted, exposing the cartilage in the midline. An incision is made in the anterior midline of thyroid cartilage with a knife or saw, taking care not to damage the underlying soft tissue (Fig 18–52). Ordinarily, an incision is then made through the cricothyroid membrane. As this incision is carried superiorly, the vocal folds are visualized so that they can be divided exactly in the midline. Dissection can be performed with a knife or with straight scissors placed between the vocal folds and pulled gently forward to ensure proper position. If the cricothyroid membrane is not amenable to surgery because of pathology or previous injury, a superior approach can be used, although it is slightly more difficult because of the additional thickness of tissue that must be traversed before entering the airway. Once the cartilage, vocal folds, and soft tissue above and below the anterior commissure have been divided, the thyroid cartilage is retracted laterally to expose the interior of the larynx. When closing, it

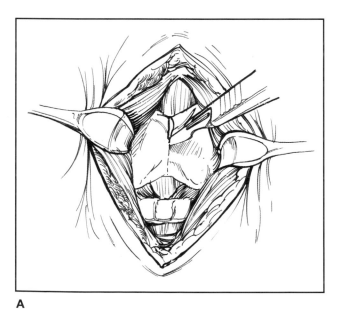

A

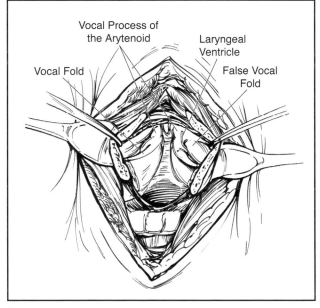

B

Fig 18–52. A. An incision is made vertically through the midline of the thyroid cartilage. **B.** After the thyroid cartilage and soft tissues have been exposed, the interior of the larynx can be visualized.

is essential to reattach the anterior commissure tendon and to suture both vocal folds at the same level. Ideally, suture (and especially suture knots) should be in the soft tissues anteriorly, not in the airway. This precaution helps avoid granuloma formation. The cartilages can be reapproximated with miniplates, but the author has found figure-of-eight sutures entirely satisfactory. If miniplates are used, it is preferable to use absorbable miniplates, which do not interfere with future imaging studies as do metal miniplates.

Lateral thyrotomy permits access to the paraglottic space and is useful for removing Teflon, excising laryngoceles, and for approaching similar lesions. Entry can be made through the thyroid cartilage using a variety of approaches. The inner perichondrium is then incised, and the operation is individualized depending on the pathology (Fig 18–53). Lateral thyrotomy was introduced in 1914 by Lewis, who divided the thyroid cartilage vertically anterior to the superior and inferior cornu of the thyroid cartilage.[143] He used the

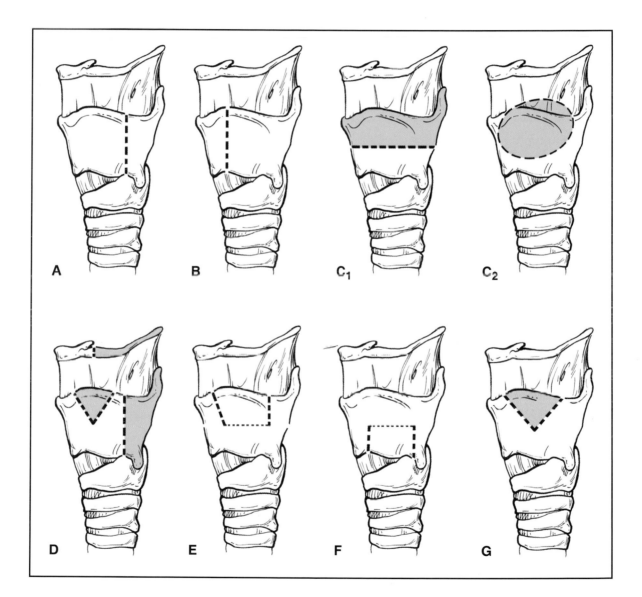

Fig 18–53. A. A vertical lateral thyrotomy incision near the junction of the posterior and middle thirds. **B.** Vertical thyrotomy near the junction of the anterior and middle thirds. **C₁.** Exposure also can be obtained through a horizontal incision with removal of the superior portion of the thyroid cartilage or (**C₂**), by biting away a portion of the thyroid cartilage; **D,** by creating a triangular thyrotomy along with removing the posterior third of the laryngeal cartilage and the greater cornu of the hyoid bone; **E,** by creating an superiorly-based trapped-door flap which can be folded inferiorly; **F,** by creating a inferiorly-based trap-door flap which can be folded superiorly; or **G,** by using a V-shaped resection of thyroid lamina.

procedure to resect a congenital cyst in the paraglottic space. Other authors have modified the position of the cartilaginous incision, using a vertical incision at the junction of the anterior and middle third,[144,145] a horizontal incision with resection of thyroid lamina,[146-150] biting away a portion of the thyroid cartilage,[151] using a rectangular "fold down trap-door flap,"[152] or a superiorly-based trap-door fold-up flap,[153] and using a triangular resection of thyroid cartilage superiorly.[66] Keim and Livingstone enlarged the exposure by resecting a triangular segment of thyroid lamina superiorly, along with the posterior third of the thyroid lamina and the greater cornu of the hyoid bone.[154] These and other variations are useful for a variety of paraglottic lesions.

Thyroarytenoid Neurectomy

When Dedo introduced recurrent laryngeal nerve section as a treatment for spasmodic dysphonia in 1976,[155] the procedure was greeted with great enthusiasm. However, it quickly became clear that there were problems associated with this approach[156,157]; and it was abandoned by most surgeons in the 1980s. Disappointment and controversy surrounding recurrent laryngeal nerve section may be responsible in part for the delay in recognizing the value of selective thyroarytenoid neurectomy. This procedure was developed by Shinobu Iwamura in 1978 and introduced to the United States in 1979.[158] This procedure involves creating a window similar to a thyroplasty window but placed more posteriorly. The posterior aspect of the window is adjacent to the oblique line. The window should be approximately 8 × 10 mm in size. The inner perichondrium is incised, and blunt dissection is used to identify the thyroarytenoid branch of the recurrent laryngeal nerve (Fig 18–54). Iwamura describes dividing the nerve to paralyze the thyroarytenoid muscle. The procedure is actually slightly more complex, as described below.

Iwamura's procedure was reintroduced by Berke and coworkers in 1991. Their initial report described bilateral thyroarytenoid denervation in dogs, with anastomosis of the ansa cervicalis to the distal, cut end of the thyroarytenoid nerve, thereby preventing reinnervation from the proximal stump of the thyroarytenoid nerve.[159] This procedure was also believed to limit atrophy and fibrosis of the thyroarytenoid muscle. Since that time, Berke has used this approach in humans and continues to advocate anastomosis of the ansa cervicalis with the distal end of the cut thyroarytenoid nerve to prevent recurrence of symptoms.[160]

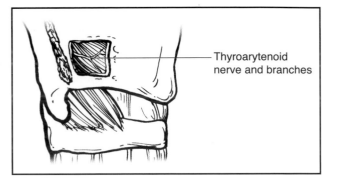

Fig 18–54. A window approximately 10 mm by 8 mm is created in the thyroid lamina, just anterior to the oblique line. Usually, after opening the inner perichondrium, the thyroarytenoid nerve can be exposed easily with blunt dissection. However, occasionally it may branch prior to this point and be more difficult to find.

Initially, the procedure advocated by Berke seems superior to Iwamura's operation because reinnervation should occur in some patients if the thyroarytenoid nerve is merely cut or even if it is cut, avulsed, and clipped. This author is familiar with cases in which that problem has occurred. Interestingly, Iwamura reports that he has not had problems with recurrence of symptoms (Shinobu Iwamura, MD, personal communication, 2000); but it was not clear to this author why the discrepancy existed until Dr. Iwamura visited Philadelphia and we had an opportunity to discuss his procedure in detail and review videotapes of the operation. In addition to performing a thyroarytenoid neurectomy, Iwamura routinely removes a large amount of thyroarytenoid muscle. The myomectomy not only helps ensure that all branches of the thyroarytenoid nerve are cut, but also removes so much muscle that normal activity cannot occur even if the residual fibers are reinnervated. In our experience with laryngeal electromyography in patients with adductor spasmodic dysphonia following botulinum toxin injection, we have found that many patients remain fluent with as little as 30 to 40% reduced recruitment in the thyroarytenoid muscle. Having observed the amount of muscle that Dr. Iwamura removes, it seems likely that muscle loss and fibrosis would result in substantially diminished TA muscle function, even if substantial reinnervation from the proximal end of the cut nerve were to occur. So, ansa anastomosis is unnecessary if the procedure is performed in this fashion. Dr. Iwamura usually operates on one side, proceeding to surgery on the contralateral side if control is insufficient (a minority of cases). This author has utilized Iwamura's approach and had similar results. Although the operation results in some dysphonia, in most patients, generally after 3 to 6 months, it is minimal and comparable to voice quality noted during successful treatment with botulinum toxin injection.

This author has been pleased with results of thyroarytenoid neurectomy and myomectomy, but both this procedure and the procedure described by Berke (ansa cervicalis anastomosis) are reasonable options. However, in this author's opinion, it is unwise to simply divide the thyroarytenoid nerve without performing either simultaneous myomectomy or nerve anastomosis.

Laryngeal Transplantation

Laryngeal transplantation is a major surgical procedure that is extremely important but has few indications. The first successful laryngeal transplantation was performed by Strome.[161] Like other transplantation procedures, laryngeal transplant requires long-term use of immunosuppressive medications. Hence, at present it is not advocated for patients with a history of malignancy. Currently, it is considered most suitable for patients with little or no voice who are dependent on tracheotomy for respiration. This scenario is most likely to occur following trauma, as in Strome's patient. The patient achieved a human-sounding voice with inflection, range, and qualities unique to him; and he was able to swallow normally. He has a tracheostoma; and at 36 months, the characteristics of his speech were considered within the normal range. He has been able to work as a motivational speaker. Laryngeal transplantation requires substantially more study and experience but represents an important option for a small, select group of patients.

Other Considerations

Voice Rest

The efficacy of voice rest as therapy is unproven. Its wide standard is based on anecdotal experience and common sense, which may or may not turn out to be correct. Voice rest may be indicated after vocal fold hemorrhage, mucosal tear, and vocal fold surgery, especially if the mucosa of the leading edge of the vocal fold has been removed. The rationale is attractive, even though it is unsubstantiated. Microsurgical techniques are designed to minimize scar formation. A scar forms when fibroblast proliferation is initiated in the intermediate and deep layers of the lamina propria. If vibratory margin mucosa has been removed,

then the lamina propria is exposed. Therefore, it seems reasonable to minimize contact trauma to this region through voice rest until the mucosal cover is restored (sometimes within 2 to 3 days, rarely more than 1 week). Although some vocal fold contact will occur inevitably because of swallowing and coughing, more (avoidable) contact occurs during speech. When a patient phonates at a pitch of A below middle C, the vocal folds make contact 220 times per second. This is close to the normal fundamental frequency of the female speaking voice. In addition, these contacts may be abusive if the patient attempts to achieve voice quality and volume after surgery. Consequently, the author recommends voice rest routinely after surgery, unless the vibratory margin mucosa has been left intact. Absolute voice rest is maintained until the vocal fold has remucosalized (rarely more than 1 week). The author's patients' first utterance is the /i/ in the examining chair approximately 1 week after surgery. Patients then have a short session with the speech-language pathologist to assist in the transition from silence to limited voice use. Relative voice rest and good vocal hygiene under the supervision of speech-language pathologists are maintained until complete healing has occurred. Details of voice rest technique are discussed in chapter 5. Preoperative voice therapy is extremely helpful in preparing patients for voice rest and voice conservation.

Related Surgery

Velopharyngeal insufficiency has also been suggested as a cause of problems for singers, actors, and instrumentalists. Damsté[161] has described push-back surgery for "congenital short palate" in a professional singer who presented with nodules and voice fatigue. The prevalence and importance of this problem await further clarification, and most of us who care for large numbers of singers and actors do not encounter it frequently.

Obstructive Sleep Apnea Syndrome

Obstructive sleep apnea syndrome in professional voice users is discussed elsewhere.[162]

Miscellaneous Laryngeal Procedures

Many laryngeal procedures are not included in detail in this chapter. They include operations for recreating new vocal folds, readjusting vocal fold height, and many other purposes. This chapter is not intended to be all-inclusive, and the reader is encouraged to consult other chapters, and other literature for additional information about laryngeal surgery.[26,36,37]

References

1. von Leden H. The history of phonosurgery. In: Sataloff RT. *Professional Voice: The Science and Art of Clinical Care.* 2nd ed. San Diego, Calif: Singular Publishing Group, Inc; 1997:561–580.

2. Green H. Morbid growths within the larynx. In: *On the Surgical Treatment of Polypi of the Larynx, and Oedema of the Glottis.* New York, NY: GP Putnam; 1852:56–65.

3. Brünings W. Direct laryngoscopy: criteria determining the applicability of autoscopy. In: *Direct Laryngoscopy, Bronchoscopy, and Esophagoscopy.* London, England: Bailliere, Tindall, Cox; 1912:93–95.

4. Jackson C. *Peroral Endoscopy and Laryngeal Surgery.* St Louis, Mo: Laryngoscope Co; 1915.

5. Holinger P. An hour-glass anterior commissure laryngoscope. *Laryngoscope.* 1960;70:1570–1571.

6. Kleinsasser O. [Microlaryngoscopy and endolaryngeal microsurgery. II: A review of 2500 cases.] *HNO.* 1974; 22(3):69–83.

7. Jako G. Laryngoscope for microscopic observation, surgery, and photography. *Arch Otolaryngol.* 1970;91:196–199.

8. Dedo HH. A fiberoptic anterior commissure laryngoscope for use with the operating microscope. *Trans Sect Otolaryngol Am Acad Ophthalmol Otolaryngol.* 1976;82:91–92.

9. Gould WJ. The Gould laryngoscope. *Trans Sect Otolaryngol Am Acad Ophthalmol Otolaryngol.* 1973;77:139–141.

10. Killian G: Suspension laryngoscopy—a modification of the direct method. *Trans 3rd Internat Laryngol Congr.* Germany. (Part II) Transactions; 1911:12.

11. Zeitels SM, Vaughan CW. "External counterpressure" and "internal distention" for optimal laryngoscopic exposure of the anterior glottal commissure. *Ann Otol Rhinol Laryngol.* 1994;103(9):669–675.

12. Hochman II, Zeitels SM, Heaton JT. Analysis of the forces and position required for direct laryngoscopic exposure of the anterior vocal folds. *Ann Otol Rhinol Laryngol.* 1999;108(8):715–724.

13. Adriani J, Naraghi M. Drug induced methemoglobinemia: local anesthetics. *Anesthesiol Rev.* 12(1):54–59.

14. Urban GE. Laryngeal microsurgery without intubation. *South-Med J.* 1976;69:828–830.

15. Abitbol J, Sataloff RT. Laryngeal laser surgery. In: Sataloff RT. *Professional Voice: The Science and Art of Clinical Care.* 3rd ed. San Diego, Calif: Plural Publishing Inc; 2005:1227–1252.

16 Carden E, Becker G, Hamood H. Percutaneous jet ventilation. *Ann Otol Rhinol Laryngol.* 1976;85:652–655.

17. Hoerenz P. The operating microscope: I. optical principles, illumination systems, and support systems. *J Microsurg.* 1980;1:364–369.

18. Andrea M, Dias O. *Atlas of Rigid and Contact Endoscopy in Microlaryngeal Surgery.* Philadelphia, Pa: Lippincott Williams and Wilkins; 1995:1–112.

19. Flint PW. Powered surgical instruments for laryngeal surgery. *Otolaryngol Head Neck Surg.* 2000;122(2):263–266.

20. Hajek M. Anatomische Untersuchungen uber das Larynxodem. *Arch Klin Chir.* 1891;42:46–93.

21. Reinke F. Uber die Funktionelle Struktur Menschlichen Stimmlippe mit Besonderer Berucksichtigung des Elastischen Geweber. *Anat Heft.* 1897;9:103–117.

22. Pressman J, Dowdy A, Libby R, Fields M. Further studies upon the submucosal compartments and lymphatics of the larynx by the injection of dyes and radioisotope. *Ann Otol Rhinol Laryngol.* 1956;65:963–980.

23. Welsh LW, Welsh JJ, Rizzo TA Jr. Laryngeal spaces and lymphatics: current anatomic concepts. *Ann Otol Rhinol Laryngol Suppl.*1983;105:19–31.

24. Kass ES, Hillman RE, Zeitels SM. Vocal fold submucosal infusion technique in phonomicrosurgery. *Ann Otol Rhinol Laryngol.* 1996;105(5):341–347.

25. Rosen C. Kenalog laryngoscope.

26. Hirano M. Phonosurgery. Basic and clinical investigations. *Otologia Fukuoka.* 1975;21:239–442.

27. Sataloff RT. *Professional Voice: The Science and Art of Clinical Care.* New York, NY: Raven Press; 1991.

28. Gould WJ, Sataloff RT, Spiegel JR. *Voice Surgery.* Chicago, Ill: Mosby Year Book; 1993.

29. Sataloff RT. The human voice. *Sci Am.* 1992;267(6):108–115.

30. Sundberg J. *The Science of the Singing Voice.* DeKalb, Ill: Northern Illinois University Press; 1987.

31. Titze IR, Strong WJ. Normal modes in vocal cord tissues. *J Acoustic Soc Am.* 1975;57(3):736–744.

32. Titze IR, Talkin DT. A theoretical study of the effects of various laryngeal configurations on the acoustics of phonation. *J Acoustic Soc Am.* 1979;66(1):60–74.

33 Titze IR. Comments on the myoelastic-aerodynamic theory of phonation. *J Speech Hear Res.* 1980;23(3):495–510.

34. Titze IR. The physics of small-amplitude oscillation of the vocal folds. *J Acoustic Soc Am.* 1988;83(4):1536–1552.

35. von Leden H. The history of phonosurgery. In: Gould WJ, Sataloff RT, Spiegel JR eds. *Voice Surgery.* Chicago, Ill: Mosby Year Book; 1993:65–96.

36. Sataloff RT: The professional voice. In: Cummings CW, Frederickson JM, Harker LA, et al, eds. *Otolaryngology— Head and Neck Surgery.* St. Louis, Mo: CV Mosby; 1986; 3:2029–2056.

37. Gould WJ, Lawrence VL: Surgical care of voice disorders. In: Arnold GE, Winckel F, Wyke BD, eds. *Disorders of Human Communication.* New York NY: Springer-Verlag; 1984.

38. Isshiki N. *Phonosurgery—Theory and Practice.* New York, NY: Springer-Verlag; 1989.

39. Ford CN, Bless DM. *Phonosurgery: Assessment and Surgical Management.* New York, NY: Raven Press; 1992.

40. Sataloff RT. Endoscopic microsurgery. In: Gould WJ, Sataloff RT, Spiegel JR, eds. *Voice Surgery.* Chicago, Ill: Mosby Year Book; 1993:227–267.

41. Gray S. Basement membrane zone injury in vocal nodules. In: Gauffin J, Hammarberg B, eds. *Vocal Fold Physiology.* San Diego, Calif: Singular Publishing Group; 1991.

42. Sataloff RT, Spiegel JR, Heuer RJ, et al. Laryngeal mini-microflap: a new technique and reassessment of the microflap saga. *J Voice.* 1995;9(2):198–204.

43. Dedo HH, Sooy CD. Endoscopic laser repair of posterior glottic, subglottic, and tracheal stenosis by division or micro-trap-door flap. *Laryngoscope.* 1984;94:445–450.

44. Duncavage JA, Ossoff RH, Toohill RJ. Carbon dioxide laser management of laryngeal stenosis. *Ann Otol Rhinol Laryngol.* 1985;94:565–569.

45. Werkhaven J, Ossoff RH. Surgery for benign lesions of the glottis. *Otolaryngol Clin North Am.* 1991;24(5):1179–1199.

46. Hochman I, Sataloff RT, Hillman R, Zeitels S. Ectasias and varices of the vocal fold: clearing the striking zone. *Ann Otol Rhinol Laryngol.* 1999;108(1):10–16.

47. Baker DC Jr. Laryngeal problems in singers. *Laryngoscope.* 1962;72:902–908.

48. Feder RJ. Varix of the vocal cord in the professional voice user. *Otolaryngol Head Neck Surg.* 1983;91:435–436.

49. Czermak JN. On the laryngoscope and its employment in physiology and medicine. *N Sydenham Soc.* 1861:11:1–79.

50. Mackenzie M. *The Use of the Laryngoscope in Diseases of the Throat with an Appendix on Rhinoscopy.* London, England: J & A Churchill; 1865.

51. Turck L. *Atlas zur Klinik der Kehlkopfkrankheiten.* Wien, Austria: Willhelm Braumuller; 1860.

52. Elsberg L. *Laryngoscopal Surgery Illustrated in the Treatment of Morbid Growths Within the Larynx.* Philadelphia, Pa: Collins; 1866.

53. Mackenzie M. *Growths in the Larynx.* London, England: J & A Churchill; 1871.

54. Zeitels SM, Sataloff RT. Phomicrosurgical resection of glottal papillomatosis. *J Voice.* 1999;13:123–127.

55. Wellens W, Snoeck R, Desloovere C, et al. Treatment of severe laryngeal papillomatosis with intralesional injections of Cidofovir® [(S)-1-(3-Hydroxy-Phosphonylmethoxypropyl) Cytosine, HPMPC Vistide®] Transactions of the XVI World Congress of Otorhinolaryngology—Head and Neck Surgery; March 2–7, 1997; Sydney, Australia.

56. Holinger LD, Barnes DR, Smid LJ, Holinger PH. Laryngocele and saccular cysts. *Ann Otol Rhinol Laryngol.* 1978; 87:675–685.

57. Ward PH, Frederickson J, Strandjord NM, Valvessori GE. Laryngeal and pharyngeal pouches. Surgical approach and the use of cinefluorographic and other radiologic techniques as diagnostic aids. *Laryngoscope.* 1963;73:564–582.

58. DeSanto LW. Laryngocele, laryngeal mucocele, large saccules, and laryngeal saccular cysts: a developmental spectrum. *Laryngoscope.* 1974;84:1291–1296.

59. Norris CW. Pharyngoceles of the hypopharynx. *Laryngoscope.* 1979;89:1788–1807.

60. Papsin BC, Maaske LA, McGrail JS. Orbicularis oris muscle injury in brass players. *Laryngoscope.* 1996; 106:757–760.

61. Fiz JA, Aguilar J, Carreras A, et al. Maximum respiratory pressure in trumpet players. *Chest.* 1993;104:1203–1204.

62. Stephani A, Tarab S. [Obscure and ventricular laryngocele.] *Schweiz Rundsch Med Prax.* 1972;61:1520–1523.

63. Macfie DD. Asymptomatic laryngoceles in wind-instrument bandsmen. *Arch Otolaryngol.* 1966;83:270–275.

64. Backus J. The effect of the player's vocal tract on woodwind instrument tone. *J Acoust Soc Am.* 1985;78:17–20.

65. Isaacson G, Sataloff RT. Bilateral laryngoceles in a young trumpet player: case report. *Ear Nose Throat J.* 2000;4:272–274.

66. Thome R, Thome DC, De La Cortina RA. Lateral thyrotomy approach on the paraglottic space for laryngocele resection. *Laryngoscope.* 2000;110:447–450.

67. Stern SJ, Sven JY. Conservation surgery of the larynx and its relationship to voice result. In: Rubin JS, Sataloff RT, Korovin GS, Gould WJ, eds. *Diagnosis and Treatment of Voice Disorders.* New York, NY: Igaku-Shoin; 1995:445–467.

68. Ford CN, Bless DM, Loftus JM. The role of injectable collagen in the treatment of glottic insufficiency: a study of 119 patients. *Ann Otol Rhinol Laryngol.* 1992;101(3):237–247.

69. Pontes P, Behlau M. Treatment of sulcus vocalis: auditory perceptual and acoustic analysis of the slicing mucosa surgical technique. *J Voice.* 1993;7(4):365–376.

70. Sataloff RT, Hawkshaw MJ. Endoscopic internal stent: a new procedure for laryngeal webs in the presence of papilloma. *Ear Nose Throat J.* 1998;77(12):949–950.

71. Stasney CR. Laryngeal webs: a new treatment for an old problem. Presented at the 22nd Annual Symposium: Care of the Professional Voice; June 12, 1993; The Voice Foundation, Philadelphia, Pa.

72. Stone JW, Arnold GE. Human larynx injected with Teflon paste. Histological study of innervation and tissue reaction. *Arch Otolaryngol.* 1967;86:550–561.

73. von Leden H, Yanagihara N, Kukuk-Werner E. Teflon in unilateral vocal cord paralysis. *Arch Otolaryngol.* 1967; 85(6):666–674.

74. Schramm V, May M, Lavorato AS, Gelfoam paste injection for vocal fold paralysis: temporary rehabilitation of glottic incompetence. *Laryngoscope.* 1978;88:1268–1273.

75. Anderson TD, Mirza N. Immediate percutaneous medialization for acute vocal fold immobility with aspiration. *Laryngoscope.* 2001;111:1318–1321.

76. Ford CN, Bless DM. Collagen injected in the scarred vocal fold. *J Voice.* 1988;1:116–118.

77. Ford CN, Bless DM. Selected problems treated by vocal fold injection of collagen. *Am J Otolaryngol.* 1993;14(4):257–261.

78. Cendron M, DeVore DP, Connolly R, et al. The biological behavior of autologous collagen injected into the rabbit bladder. *J Urol.* 1995;154:808–811.

79. Ford CN, Staskowski PA, Bless DM. Autologous collagen vocal fold injection: a preliminary clinical study. *Laryngoscope.* 1995;105(9):944–948.

80. DeVore DP, Hughes E, Scott JB. Effectiveness of injectable filler materials for smoothing wrinkle lines and depressed scars. *Med Prog Technol.* 1994;20:243–250.

81. Burstyn DG, Hagerman TC. Strategies for viral removal and inactivation. *Dev Biol Stand.* 1996;88:73–79.

82. DeVore DP, Kelman C, Fagien S, Casson P. Autologen: autologous, injectable dermal collagen. In: Bosniak S, ed. *Ophthalmic Plastic and Reconstructive Surgery.* vol 1. Philadelphia, Pa: WB Saunders Company; 1996:670–675.

83. Passalaqua P, Pearl A, Woo P, Ramospizarro CA. Direct transcutaneous translaryngeal injection laryngoplasty with AlloDerm. Presented at the 30th Annual Symposium: Care of the Professional Voice; June 16, 2001; Philadelphia, Pa.

84. Rihkanen H. Vocal fold augmentation by injection of autologous fascia. *Laryngoscope.* 1998;108(1):51–54.

85. Dedo H. A technique for vertical hemilaryngectomy to prevent stenosis and aspiration. *Laryngoscope.* 1975;85:978–984.

86. Mikaelian D, Lowry LD, Sataloff RT. Lipoinjection for unilateral vocal cord paralysis. *Laryngoscope.* 1991;101:465–468.

87. Brandenburg J, Kirkham W, Koschkee D. Vocal cord augmentation with autologenous fat. *Laryngoscope.* 1992;102:495–500.

88. Billings E Jr, May JW Jr. Historical review and present status of free fat graft autotransplantation in plastic and reconstructive surgery. *Plast Reconstr Surg.* 1989;83;368–381.

89. Wexler D, Jiang J, Gray S, et al. Phonosurgical studies: fat-graft reconstruction of injured canine vocal cords. *Ann Otol Rhinol Laryngol.* 1989;98:668–673.

90. Hill DP, Meyers AD, Harris J. Autologous fat injection for vocal cord medialization in the canine larynx. *Laryngoscope.* 1991;101:344–348.

91. Archer SM, Banks ER. Intracordal injection of autologous fat for augmentation of the mucosally damaged canine vocal fold: a long-term histological study. Presented at the Second World Congress on Laryngeal Cancer; February 24, 1994; Sydney, Australia.

92. Sataloff RT, Mayer DP, Spiegel JR. Radiologic assessment of laryngeal Teflon injection. *J Voice.* 1988;2(1):93–95.

93. Netterville JL, Coleman JR Jr, Chang S, et al. Lateral laryngotomy for the removal of Teflon granuloma. *Ann Otol, Rhinol Laryngol.* 1998;107:735–744.

94. Coleman JR, Miller FR, Netterville JL. Teflon granuloma excision via a lateral laryngotomy. *Oper Techn Otolaryngol Head Neck Surg.* 1999;10(1):29–35.

95. Isshiki N, Okamura H, Ishikawa T. Thyroplasty type I (lateral compression) for dysphonia due to vocal cord paralysis or atrophy. *Acta Otolaryngol.* 1975;80:465–473.

96. Payr E. Plastik am schildknorpel zur Behebung der Folgen einseitiger Stimmbandlahmung. *Dtsch Med Wochensch.* 1915;43:1265–1270.

97. Cummings CW, Purcell LL, Flint PW. Hydroxylapatite laryngeal implants for medialization: preliminary report. *Ann Otol Rhinol Laryngol.* 1993;102:843–851.

98. Montgomery WW. Montgomery SK, Warren MA. Thyroplasty simplified. *Operat Techn Otolaryngol Head Neck Surg.* 1993;4:223–231.

99. Montgomery WW. Montgomery SK. Montgomery thyroplasty implant system. *Ann Otol Rhinol Laryngol Suppl.* 1997;170:1–16.

100. Flint PW, Corio RL, Cummings CW. Comparison of soft tissue response in rabbits following laryngeal implantation with hydroxylapatite, silicone rubber, and Teflon. *Ann Otol Rhinol Laryngol.* 1997;106:339–407.

101. McCulloch TM, Hoffman HT. Medialization laryngoplasty with expanded polytetrafluoroethylene. Surgical technique and preliminary results. *Ann Otol Rhinol Laryngol.* 1998;107:427–432.

102. Friedrich G. Titanium vocal fold medializing implant: introducing a novel implant system for external vocal fold medialization. *Ann Otol Rhinol Laryngol.* 1999;108:79–86.

103. Giovanni A, Vallicioni JM, Gras R, Zanaret M. Clinical experience with Gore-Tex for vocal fold medialization. *Laryngoscope.* 1999;109:284–288.

104. Tucker HA. External laryngeal surgery for adjustment of the voice. In: Gould WJ, Sataloff RT, Spiegel JR, eds. *Voice Surgery.* St. Louis: CV Mosby Co; 1993:275–290.

105. Zeitels SM, Jarboe J, Hillman RE. Medialization laryngoplasty with Gore-Tex for voice restoration secondary to glottal incompetence, Presented at the Voice Foundation's Annual Symposium, Care of the Professional Voice; July 2, 2000; Philadelphia, Pa.

106. Zeitels SM. New procedures for paralytic dysphonia: adduction arytenopexy, Gore-Tex medialization laryngoplasty, and cricothyroid subluxation. *Otolaryngol Clin North Am.* 2000;33:841–854.

107. McCulloch TM, Hoffman HT, Andrews BT, Karnell MP. Arytenoid adduction combined with Gore-Tex medialization thyroplasty. *Laryngoscope.* 2000;110:1306–1311.

108. Omori K, Slavit D, Kacker A, et al. Effects of thyroplasty type I on vocal fold vibration. *Laryngoscope.* 2000;110:1086–1091.

109. Weinman EC, Maragos NE. Airway compromise in thyroplasty surgery. *Laryngoscope.* 2000;110:1082–1085.

110. Sataloff RT, Spiegel JR, Carroll LM, Heuer RJ. Male soprano voice: a rare complication of thyroidectomy. *Laryngoscope.* 1992;102(1):90–93.

111. Benninger MS, Crumley RL, Ford CN, et al. Evaluation and treatment of the unilateral paralyzed vocal fold. *Otolaryngol Head Neck Surg.* 1994;111(4):497–508.

112. Isshiki N, Tanabe M, Sawada M. Arytenoid adduction for unilateral vocal cord paralysis. *Arch Otolaryngol.* 1978;104:555–558.

113. Zeitels SM. Adduction arytenoidopexy with medialization laryngoplasty and cricothyroid subluxation: a new approach to paralytic dysphonia. *Oper Techn Otolaryngol Head Neck Surg.* 1999;10(1):9–16.

114. Zeitels SM, Hochman I, Hillman RE. Adduction arytenopexy: a new procedure for paralytic dysphonia and the implications for medialization laryngoplasty. *Ann Otol Rhinol Laryngol Suppl.* 1998;107:2–24.

115. Woodson JE. Picerno R, Yeung D, Hengesteg A. Arytenoid adduction: controlling vertical position. *Ann Otol Rhinol Laryngol.* 2000;109:360–364.

116. Iwamura S, Curita N. A newer arytenoid adduction technique for one-vocal-fold paralysis: a direct pull of

the lateral cricoarytenoid muscle. *Otolaryngol Head Neck Surg.* 1996;6(1):1–10.

117. Iwamura S, Murakawa Y. Tomographic assessment of the arytenoid body and unilateral vocal fold paralysis before and after lateral cricoarytenoid muscle-pull surgery. *Jpn J Broncoesophagol.* 1997; 48(4):310–320.

118. Murakami Y, Kirchner JA. Vocal cord abduction by regenerated recurrent laryngeal nerve. *Arch Otolaryngol.* 1971;94:64–68.

119. Tucker HM. Reinnervation of the unilaterally paralyzed larynx. *Ann Otol Rhinol Laryngol.* 1977;86:789–794.

120. Tucker HM, Rusnov M. Laryngeal reinnervation for unilateral vocal cord paralysis: long-term results. *Ann Otol Rhinol Laryngol.* 1981;90:457–459.

121. May M, Berry Q. Muscle-nerve pedicle laryngeal reinnervation. *Laryngoscope.* 1986;96:1196–1200.

122. Crumley R. New perspectives in laryngeal reinnervation. In: Bailey BJ, Biller HF, eds. *Surgery of the Larynx.* Philadelphia, Pa: WB Saunders; 1985:135–147.

123. Rubin AD, Sataloff RT. Vocal fold paresis and paralysis. In: Sataloff RT. *Professional Voice: The Science and Art of Clinical Care.* 3rd ed. San Diego, Calif: Plural Publishing Inc; 2005:871–886

124. Takenouchi S, Sato F. [Phonatory function of the implanted larynx.] *Jpn J Bronchoesophagol.* 1968;19:280–281.

125. Tucker HM, Harvey J, Ogura JH. Vocal cord remobilization in the canine larynx. *Arch Otolaryngol.* 1970;92:530–533.

126. Goldfarb D, Keane WM, Lowry LD. Laryngeal pacing as a treatment for vocal fold paralysis. *J Voice.* 1994; 8(2):179–185.

127. Lundy DS, Casiano RR, Landy HJ, Gallo J, et al. Effects of vagal nerve stimulation on laryngeal function. *J Voice.* 1993;7(4):359–364.

128. Woodman D. A modification of the extralaryngeal approach to arytenoidectomy for bilateral abductor paralysis. *Arch Otolaryngol.* 1946;43:63–65.

129. Thornell WC. Intralaryngeal approach for arytenoidectomy in bilateral abductor vocal cord paralysis. *Arch Otolaryngol.* 1948;47:505–508.

130. Eskew JR, Bailey BJ. Laser arytenoidectomy for bilateral vocal cord paralysis. *Otolaryngol Head Neck Surg.* 1983;91:294–298.

131. Strong MS, Jako GJ, Vaughan CW. The use of the CO_2 laser in otolaryngology: a progress report. *Trans Sect Otolaryngol Am Acad Ophthalmol Otolaryngol.* 1976;82:595–602.

132. Ossoff RH, Duncavage JA, Shapshay SM, et al. Endoscopic laser arytenoidectomy revisited. *Ann Otol Rhinol Laryngol.* 1990;99:764–771.

133. Crumley RL. Endoscopic laser medial arytenoidectomy for airway management in bilateral laryngeal paralysis. *Ann Otol Rhinol Laryngol.* 1993;102:81–84.

134. Cantarella G, Neglia CB, Marzano AV, Ottaviani A. Bilateral laryngeal pseudocoparalysis in xanthoma disseminatum treated by endoscopic laser medial arytenoidectomy. *Ann Otol Rhinol Laryngol.* 2001;110:263–268.

135. Ejnell H, Mansson I, Hallen O, et al. A simple operation for bilateral vocal cord paralysis. *Larynogoscope.* 1984; 94:954–958.

136. Geterud A, Ejnell H, Stenborg R, Bake B. Long-term results with simple surgical treatment of bilateral vocal cord paralysis. *Laryngoscope.* 1990;100:1005–1008.

137. Cummings CW, Redd EE, Westra WH, Flint PW. Minimally invasive device to effect vocal fold lateralization. *Ann Otol Rhinol Laryngol.* 1999;108(9):833–836.

138. Dennis DP, Kashima H. Carbon dioxide posterior cordectomy for treatment of vocal cord paralysis. *Ann Otol Rhinol Laryngol.* 1989;98:930–934.

139. Tucker HM. Human laryngeal reinnervation: long-term experience with nerve-muscle pedicle technique. *Laryngoscope.* 1978;88:598–604.

140. Tucker HM. *The Larynx.* 2nd ed. New York, NY: Thieme Medical Publishers; 1993:255–265.

141. Rubin AD, Hawkshaw M, Sataloff RT. Vocal process avulsion. *J Voice.* 2005: in press.

142. Willemot J, Naissance et developpement de l'oto-rhino-laryngologie dans l'histoire de la medicine. *Acta Otorhinolaryngol Belg.* 1981;35 (suppl 2,3,4):1–1622.

143. Lewis DD, Discussion on ventricle of larynx. *Ann Otol Rhinol Laryngol.* 1914;24:129–138.

144. New GB, Erich JB. Congenital cysts of the larynx: report of a case. *Arch Otolaryngol.* 1939;30:943–949.

145. New GB. Treatment of cysts of the larynx. *Arch Otolaryngol.* 1942;36:687–690.

146. Alonso JM, Caubarrere NL. The laryngocele. *Ann Otorinolaringol Urug.* 1944;14:38–44.

147. Schall LA. An extralaryngeal approach for certain benign lesions of the larynx. *Ann Otol Rhinol Laryngol.* 1959;68:346–355.

148. Thawley SE, Bone RC. Laryngopyocele. *Laryngoscope.* 1973;83:362–368.

149. Stell PM, Maran AG. Laryngocele. *J Laryngol Otol.* 1975;89:915–924.

150. Gil Tutor E. [Laryngoceles: a clinical and therapeutic study.] *An Otorinolaringol Ibero Am.* 1991;18:451–464.

151. Montgomery WW. *Surgery of the Upper Respiratory System.* Vol. 2. Philadelphia: Pa: Lea & Febiger; 1971:467–479.

152. Malis DJ, Seid AB. Fold-down thyroplasty: a new approach for congenital lateral saccular cysts. *Laryngoscope.* 1998;108:941–943.

153. Netterville JL, Coleman JR Jr, Chang S, et al. Lateral laryngotomy for removal of Teflon granuloma. *Ann Otol Rhinol Laryngol.* 1998;107:735–744.

154. Keim WF, Livingstone RG. Internal laryngocele. *Ann Otol Rhinol Laryngol.* 1951;60:39–50.

155. Dedo HH. Recurrent laryngeal nerve section for spastic dysphonia. *Ann Otol Rhinol Laryngol.* 1976;85:451–459.

156. Aronson AE, DeSanto LW. Adductor spastic dysphonia: three years after recurrent laryngeal nerve resection. *Laryngoscope.* 1983;93:1–8.

157. Dedo HH, Izdebski K. Problems with surgical (RLN section) treatment of spastic dysphonia. *Laryngoscope.* 1983;93:268–271.

158. Iwamura S: Comments in spastic dysphonia: state of the art. In: Lawrence VL, ed. *Transcripts pf the Symposium: Care of the Professional Voice.* New York, NY: The Voice Foundation; 1979:26–32.

159. Sercarz JA, Berke GS, Ming YE, et al. Bilateral thyroarytenoid denervation: a new treatment for laryngeal hyperadduction disorders studied in the canine. *Head Neck Surg.* 1992;107(5):657–668.

160. Berke GS, Blackwell KE, Gerratt BR, et al. Selective laryngeal adductor denervation-reinnervation: a new surgical treatment for adductor spasmodic dysphonia. *Ann Otol Rhinol Laryngol.* 1999;108:227–231.

161. Strome M, Stein J, Esclamado R, et al. Laryngeal transplantation and 40-month follow-up. *N Engl J Med.* 2001; 344(22):1676–1679.

162. Damsté PH. Shortness of the palate: a cause of problems in singing. *J Voice.* 1988;2(1):96–98.

163. Courey MS. Sleep-disordered breathing: considerations in surgical management for the professional voice user. In: Sataloff RT. *Professional Voice: The Science and Art of Clinical Care.* 3rd ed. San Diego, Calif: Plural Publishing Inc; 2005:1409–1414.

19

Vocal Fold Scar

Robert Thayer Sataloff

Vocal fold scar poses great therapeutic challenges in treatment of voice professionals. Unfortunately, laryngologists frequently are confronted with patients who have remained or become dysphonic after laryngeal surgery. Occasionally, a cause such as arytenoid dislocation can be found and treated. More often, however, the problem is scar producing and adynamic segment, decreased bulk of one vocal fold following "stripping," bowing caused by superior laryngeal nerve paralysis, or some other serious complication in a mobile vocal fold. None of the surgical procedures available for these conditions is effective consistently. If surgery is considered at all in such patients, it should be discussed pessimistically. The patient should be aware that the chances of returning the voice to normal or professional quality are slight and there is a chance of making it worse. However, advances in the management of vocal fold scar have increased our therapeutic options.

Symptomatic vocal fold scarring alters phonation by interfering with the mucosal wave. This may be due to the obliteration of the layered structure of the vibratory margin, as seen commonly after vocal fold stripping, or, to a limited extent, after other vocal fold surgery trauma. Similar disruption of the layered structure and mucosal wave function may also occur congenitally, as in some cases of sulcus vocalis. Scarring may also cause dysphonia by mechanical restriction of vibration or glottic closure, as seen in some cases of dense vocal fold web, or fibrotic masses on the membranous vocal fold, as may form subsequent to vocal fold hemorrhage. It is also necessary to distinguish raised scar that causes failure of glottic closure by mass effect from the more common scar that effectively thins the vocal fold edge and causes failure of glottic closure by adhering the epithelium to the vocal ligament or muscle. In the former case, treatment must include resection of the scar tissue mass to reestablish a straight vocal fold edge. However, most of this chapter will discuss the even more challenging problem of vocal scar that has obliterated the layered structure and mucosal wave. A scar involving the posterior, subglottic, and arytenoid regions may also be troublesome, but this discussion will be limited to scarring involving membranous portion of the vocal folds.

Reliable, valid, objective voice assessment is essential in diagnosing vocal fold scar, as well as in the assessment of other voice disorders. Accurate assessment of vibration is critical, and strobovideolaryngoscopy is virtually indispensable to proper diagnosis and management of vocal fold scar.[1,2] Integrity of the vibratory margin of the vocal fold is essential for the complex motion required to produce good vocal quality. Under continuous light, the vocal folds vibrate approximately 250 times per second while phonating at middle C. Naturally, the human eye cannot discern necessary details during such rapid motion. Assessment of the vibratory margin may be performed through high-speed photography, strobovideolaryngoscopy, electroglottography, or photoglottography. Only strobovideolaryngoscopy provides the necessary clinical information in a practical fashion. For example, in a patient with poor voice following laryngeal surgery and a normal looking larynx, stroboscopic light reveals adynamic segments (scar) that explain the problem even to an untrained observer (such as the patient). In most instances, stroboscopy provides all of the clinical information necessary to assess vibration. However, objective voice analysis, particularly aerodynamic and acoustic assessment, is extremely valuable for diagnosis, therapy, and evaluation of treatment efficacy.

Therapy for Vocal Fold Scar

Therapy for vocal fold scar depends on the size, location, and severity of the scar; the vocal needs of the individual patient, the patient's motivation; and the skill of the voice team. In general, once the vibratory margin of the vocal fold has been scarred (the layered structure obliterated), it is not possible to return the voice to normal. However, several options are available to improve the voice.

Voice therapy is essential for anyone interested in obtaining optimal results. Most patients do not use their vocal mechanisms optimally. Consequently, even in the presence of vocal fold scar, teaching the individual to make effective use of the support and resonator systems generally improves vocal intensity and ease and helps diminish fatigue. Nearly everyone with significant vocal fold injury develops compensatory behaviors. These gestures are usually hyperfunctional, counterproductive, and in some cases dangerous. Such unconscious adjustments are seen even in the most skilled voice professionals after sustaining a vocal fold injury and scar. Expert voice therapy eliminates this compensatory muscular tension dysphonia, further decreasing fatigue and allowing a more accurate assessment of vibratory margin function. After voice technique has been optimized, and the vocal fold scar has matured (usually about 6 to 12 months), judgments can be made about the acceptability of the final voice result. If voice function is not satisfactory to the patient, then surgery may be considered. However, it is essential for the laryngologist to be sure that the patient's expectations are reasonable. These do not include restoration to normalcy. However, in some cases, it is possible to decrease hoarseness and breathiness substantially.

Surgery for Vocal Fold Scar

Vocal fold scar causes dysphonia by disrupting or obliterating the mucosal wave and by interfering with glottic closure. Clear understanding of these facts is necessary if one is to design rational surgical intervention. At present, there is no generally accepted, highly successful surgical treatment for vocal fold scar. However, numerous procedures have been tried, and some are useful in selected cases. Although there is very little information published on older attempts at surgical procedures to correct vocal fold scar, anecdotally, many experienced voice surgeons admit to having attempted surgery in a very small number of patients. Procedures to restore the mucosal wave have included injection of steroids into the vibratory margin, elevation of a microflap to "lyse adhesions," followed by simply replacing the microflap, elevation of microflap with the placement of steroids under the flap, and other procedures. Although none of these procedures produces consistently excellent results, they may help

somewhat. Microflap elevation with steroids is sometimes helpful and is still used (M. Bouchayer, personal communication, April 1995); but the results are not consistently excellent. Pontes and Behlau have suggested a unique approach to the treatment of sulcus vocalis that essentially involves multiple releasing incisions.[3] The voice results have been surprisingly good, considering the limited success achieved by previous procedures for this condition. These principles have been applied to iatrogenic vocal fold scar and appear to have some merit in severe, extensive scarring (P. Pontes, personal communication, April 1995).

The problem of glottic incompetence is generally addressed through medialization surgery. Most medialization procedures in the past have involved injection of Teflon. Because this substance can itself cause profound scarring, many otolaryngologists have abandoned its use in most cases since the mid- to late 1980s. At present, the medialization techniques of choice are generally thyroplasty or injection of a substance other than Teflon. For extensive failure of glottic closure, the author has found Type I thyroplasty with Gore-Tex to be the most effective. For limited medialization, lateral injection of autologous fat (in the same place where Teflon used to be injected) has proven successful.[4] Approximately 30% overinjection is necessary to account for resorption. Other injection materials are discussed in chapter 18. Techniques to manage vibratory margin scar are worthy of more complete discussion.

Collagen injection was investigated most-extensively by Ford and coworkers.[5-7] Long-term results from skin injections of collagen have shown a reduction of scar tissue in the treated areas. Collagen is a thin liquid that can easily be injected in small quantities. Consequently, collagen injections are ideally suited for small adynamic segments. The ease and accuracy of injection allow for attempts at augmentation in areas of scar, as well as for managing difficult problems such as persistent posterior glottic incompetence and combined recurrent and superior laryngeal nerve paralysis. Former concerns about efficacy and safety of this material[8] seem to be less warranted, and experience using collagen has been most encouraging. When used, collagen is injected into the region of the vocal ligament and appears particularly appropriate for treating limited vocal fold scarring. Such cases are common, for example, after laser resection of vocal nodules. For more extensive scarring, as may be seen following stripping of an entire vocal fold, collagen appears less effective. However, since autologous and allogeneic human collagen have come into use, results appear to have been better than they were with allogeneic collagen, as discussed in chapter 18. The author

(RTS) uses collagen more frequently than he did at the time of the last edition of this book; but it is still generally not satisfactory as the sole treatment for severe, extensive scarring.

In 1995, the author introduced a technique for autologous fat implantation into the vibratory margin of the vocal fold as a treatment for vocal fold scar.[9] The technique involves implantation into the vibratory margin, not injection.

To recreate a mobile vibratory margin, a mucosal pocket is created and filled with fat in order to prevent readherence of the mucosa to the vocal ligament and vocalis muscle. An incision is made on the superior surface (Fig 19–1A), and a small access tunnel is elevated toward the vibratory margin. The superior incision is placed in a position that will permit angled instruments to be passed through the tunnel to reach the anterior and posterior limits of the vocal fold scar.

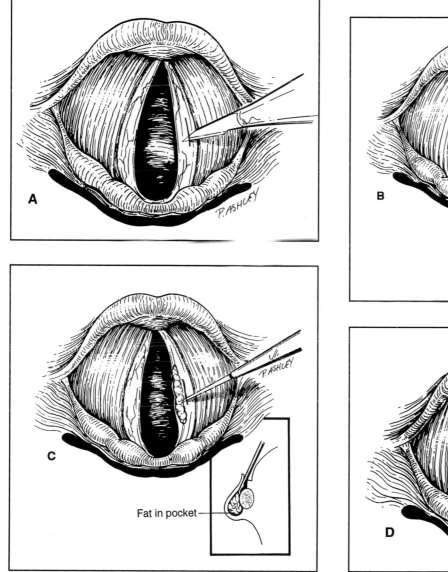

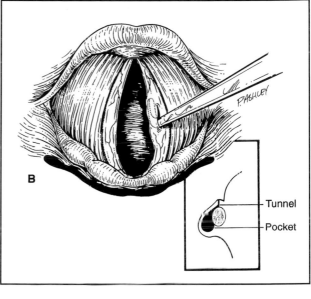

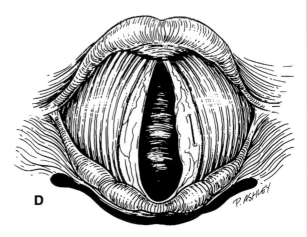

Fig 19–1. **A.** A small incision is made on the superior surface of the scarred vocal fold, and a narrow access tunnel is excavated to provide access to the medial edge. **B.** Through the access tunnel, an angled instrument is used to elevate a pocket. It is essential that the mucosa along the medial and inferior margins be kept intact. **C.** A Brünings syringe with the largest needle is passed through the tunnel and used to deposit fat in the pocket. **D.** When the needle is removed, the small access tunnel closes spontaneously, preventing extrusion of the fat. Fat should not extrude even when pressure is placed against the medial margin. If fat extrusion occurs, a suture can be placed.

Although working through a small access tunnel is technically more difficult than elevating a large flap, we believe that it is advantageous because it closes spontaneously upon removal of instruments and prevents fat extrusion from the surgically created pocket. If a larger incision is made along the superior surface, sutures are necessary to prevent fat extrusion; and even small sutures create additional tissue trauma.[10] A pocket is created along the medial margin using a right-angle dissector and an angled knife or scissors, as needed (Fig 19–1B). The pocket extends to the superior aspect of the vibratory margin and inferiorly for at least 3 to 5 mm to encompass all of the medial surface ordinarily involved in creating the mucosal wave vertical phase difference during phonation. Fat harvested at the beginning of the surgery to fill the tunnel (Fig 19–1C). Instruments are then withdrawn, and the access tunnel closes and provides sufficient resistance against fat extrusion (Fig 19–1D). The procedure is performed under local anesthesia. At the conclusion of the procedure, the patient is asked to phonate briefly and to cough in order to be certain that the implant is secure. Although no problems preventing closure of the mucosal flap have occurred to date, if extrusion occurred, fibrin glue would be tried (if available) or a suture would be placed.

Previous experience with lipoinjection has provided convincing evidence that it is important to avoid extensive manipulation or trauma to the fat. The fat is harvested in large globules either by resecting a small amount of fat (usually from the abdomen) with traditional instruments or by harvesting it with the largest available liposuction cannula. The fat is gently rinsed with saline, but it is not morselized. Packing the fat through the access tunnel with microinstruments has been attempted, but it is technically difficult to pack the fat tightly and evenly; and this method appears to cause more trauma to the access tunnel, flap, and fat than delivering the implant through a Brünings syringe. At present, the fat globules are loaded into the Brünings syringe and the largest Brünings needle is used to deliver the fat into the preformed vibratory margin pocket. Gross examination with a microscope indicates that passing the fat through the Brünings syringe certainly elongates the fat globules and must traumatize them to some degree, but they appear to be largely intact and not too badly traumatized. At present, this seems to be the best available method, although technical improvements are tested regularly. In a recent review, Neuenschwander, Sataloff, Abaza, et al[11] reported on the first eight patients who had undergone vocal fold fat implantation for severe scar and dysphonia. Their mean follow-up time was 23 months. Analysis of strobovideolaryngoscopy revealed statistically significant improvement in glottic closure, mucosal wave,

and stiffness. In perceptual studies, there was statistically significant improvement in all five parameters of the GRBAS rating scale. All eight patients had undergone more than one surgical procedure, including fat injection in all eight, thyroplasty in one, scar excision in two, lysis of adhesions in two, and steroid injection in two. The senior author (RTS) continues to utilize this procedure. However, it should still be considered one among various options for the treatment of dysphonia caused by vocal fold scar.[12]

Occasionally, surgeons are faced with extreme cases of vibratory margin scar. These are especially common after major trauma or extensive cancer surgery. When a nonvibrating scarred vocal fold is lateralized so that glottic closure is impossible, and when the involved hemilarynx is so densely scarred that the vocal fold cannot be adequately medialized even with thyropasty, occasionally more extensive surgery for vocal fold scar may be appropriate. For example, some such cases may be improved through resection of the scarred hemilarynx and creation of a pseudovocal fold using modifications of strap muscle techniques employed routinely for cordectomy or vertical hemilaryngectomy.[13] Certainly, this is an unusual and extreme approach for the treatment of vocal fold scar, but it is an option that should be in the surgeon's armamentarium for the rare, appropriate patient.

Familiarity with the latest concepts in vocal fold anatomy and physiology is essential in understanding the consequences of vocal fold scar.

References

1. Sataloff RT, Spiegel JR, Carroll LM, et al. Strobovideolaryngoscopy in professional voice users: results and clinical value. *J Voice.* 1988;1:359–364.
2. Sataloff RT, Spiegel JR, Hawkshaw MJ. Strobovideolaryngoscopy: results and clinical value. *Ann Otol Rhinol Laryngol.* 1991;100:725–757.
3. Pontes P, Behlau M. Treatment of sulcus vocalis: auditory perceptual and acoustic analysis of the slicing mucosa surgical technique. *J Voice.* 1993;7(4):365–376.
4. Mikaelian D, Lowry LD, Sataloff RT. Lipoinjection for unilateral vocal cord paralysis. *Laryngoscope.* 1991;101:465–468.
5. Ford CN, Bless DM, Loftus JM. The role of injectable collagen in the treatment of glottic insufficiency: a study of 119 patients. *Ann Otol Rhinol Laryngol.* 1973;101(3):237–247.
6. Ford CN, Bless DM. Collagen injected in the scarred vocal fold. *J Voice.* 1988;1:116–118.
7. Ford CN, Bless DM. Selected problems treated by vocal fold injection of collagen. *Am J Otolaryngol.* 1993;14(4):257–261.

8. Spiegel JR, Sataloff RT, Gould WJ. The treatment of vocal fold paralysis with injectable collagen. *J Voice*. 1987;1:119–121.

9. Sataloff RT, Spiegel JR, Hawkshaw M, et al. Autologous fat implantation for vocal fold scar: a preliminary report. *J Voice*. 1997;11(2):238–246.

10. Feldman MD, Sataloff RT, Epstein G, Ballas SK. Autologous fibrin tissue adhesive for peripheral nerve anastomosis. *Arch Otolaryngol Head Neck Surg*. 1987;113:963–967.

11. Neuenschwander MC, Sataloff RT, Abaza M, et al. Management of fold scar with autologous fat implantation: perceptual results. *J Voice*. 2001;15(2):295–304.

12. Benninger MS, Alessi D, Archer S, et al. Vocal fold scarring: current concepts and management. *Otolaryngol Head Neck Surg*. 1996;115(5):474–482.

13. Spiegel JR, Sataloff RT. Surgery for carcinoma of the larynx. In: Gould WJ, Sataloff RT, Spiegel JR, eds. *Voice Surgery*. St. Louis, Mo: CV Mosby Co; 1993:307–338.

20

Laryngotracheal Trauma

Yolanda D. Heman-Ackah and Robert Thayer Sataloff

The incidence of laryngotracheal trauma is estimated to be 1 in 14,000 to 30,000 emergency department visits yearly in the United States.[1,2] Trauma to the laryngotracheal complex can be classified as blunt, penetrating, caustic, thermal, and iatrogenic injuries. The morbidity associated with these injuries ranges from chronic airway obstruction to voice compromise, with complication rates as high as 15 to 25%.[3-5] Because of their potential for airway compromise, these injuries can be lethal, with mortality rates of 2 to 15%.[3,5] Injuries to the larynx and trachea often accompany other severe injuries, and the neck can appear to be deceptively normal even in cases of serious laryngotracheal disruption.

Laryngotracheal injuries can be caused by external or internal trauma. External insults include blunt and penetrating injuries. In the past, most external laryngeal trauma was the result of motor vehicle accidents. Studies have shown that, due to improved car safety features such as seat belts, shoulder harnesses, child safety seats, padded dashboards, and reduced speed limits, laryngeal trauma is seen less frequently. Many laryngeal injuries still occur, however, in other types of accidents and in sports. Baseball bats, hockey sticks, and lacrosse sticks, hockey pucks, elbows, shoulders, and knees have all been sources of blunt laryngeal trauma. In addition, penetrating injuries are becoming more prevalent due to increasing urban violence.[6-8]

The majority of internal laryngeal injuries are iatrogenic. Intubation and flexible and rigid endoscopy can lead to injuries of the upper airway.[9,10] Noniatrogenic internal injuries can result from foreign-body aspiration, caustic ingestion and toxin inhalation, and, occasionally, voice abuse or trauma (including phonation, coughing, and sneezing).

Despite some excellent retrospective reviews and ongoing studies with animal models, many points of controversy remain in the surgical treatment of laryngeal trauma.[2,4,7,11-15] This chapter focuses on the state-of-the-art methods for evaluation and surgery that seem to lead to the most consistently acceptable results: a stable airway with good vocal quality.

Blunt Injury

Blunt injury to the larynx and trachea is the most common cause of laryngotracheal injury in the United States today, accounting for 60% of all injuries to the laryngotracheal complex.[2,4] These injuries result from motor vehicle collisions in the adult population and from accidents involving all-terrain vehicles, bicycles, contact sports, and hanging type injuries in the young adult, adolescent, and pediatric populations. Adults and children differ not only in the mechanisms of injury, but also in the types of injuries experienced. These differences can be accounted for, at least in part, by differences in the relative size, position, and degree of calcification of the larynx and trachea.

Adult Framework Injuries from Blunt Trauma

In the adult, the inferior border of the cricoid cartilage sits at the level of the sixth and seventh cervical vertebrae.[16] Thus, in the normal upright position, the larynx is relatively protected from trauma by the overhang of the mandible superiorly, the bony prominence of the clavicles and sternal manubrium inferiorly, and by the mass of the sternocleidomastoid muscles laterally. Laryngeal injuries are relatively rare except when there is a direct blow to the neck. The usual victim of laryngotracheal trauma in a motor vehicle collision is an unbelted front seat passenger or driver in a vehicle without protective airbags. Upon collision, the front seat

263

passenger or driver is propelled forward with the neck in extension, eliminating the mandible as a protective shield. The laryngotracheal complex hits the dashboard or steering wheel with a posterior-superiorly based vector of force, and the thyroid and cricoid cartilages are crushed against the cervical vertebrae (Fig 20–1).[17,18] Direct blows to the larynx can also occur during athletic competition, while falling forward onto a blunt object, or with hanging of the neck from a suspended rope or wire.

A wide spectrum of predictable injuries occurs. The thyroid and cricoid cartilages interact dynamically to protect the airway from blunt injury.[18] Forces to the anterior larynx often are encountered first by the thyroid prominence, which bends against the cervical vertebrae on impact. The thyroid cartilage eventually

reaches a point of maximal flexibility, and a single median or paramedian fracture occurs (Fig 20–2).

The force then impacts the cricoid ring, which was previously shielded by the anterior projection of the thyroid cartilage. In a patient with a marked laryngeal prominence, multiple fractures of the thyroid cartilage in both the vertical and horizontal planes may occur prior to the distribution of force onto the cricoid cartilage (Fig 20–3).[18] The cricoid has a relatively thin anterior arch that blends laterally into rigidly buttressed tubercles. Lower level impacts result in a single median fracture or multiple paramedian vertical fractures. The airway is maintained by the lateral buttresses (Fig 20–4). With higher impact forces, secondary lateral arch fractures can occur in the cricoid cartilage, resulting in airway collapse and possible injury to the recur-

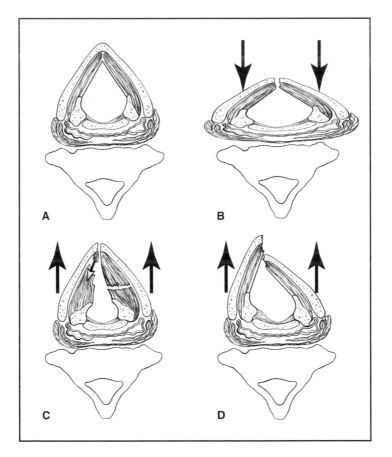

Fig 20–1. Mechanism of blunt laryngeal trauma. **A.** Normal laryngeal position; **B.** Posteriorly directed force crushing thyroid ala against cervical vertebrae, resulting in a midline fracture; **C.** Recovery of larynx from force resulting in detachment of the vocal ligament on the left, tear in the right thyroarytenoid muscle, and bilateral arytenoid dislocation; **D.** Recovery of larynx from force resulting in overlapping, displaced thyroid lamina fracture and malposition of the vocal fold. (Illustrations courtesy of Sabrina M. Heman-Ackah.)

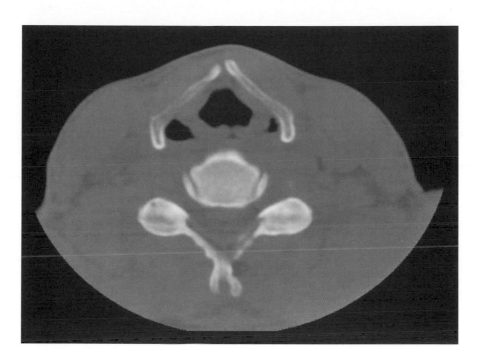

Fig 20–2. Axial CT scan of the thyroid ala. There is a midline thyroid ala fracture with diastasis of fracture segments.

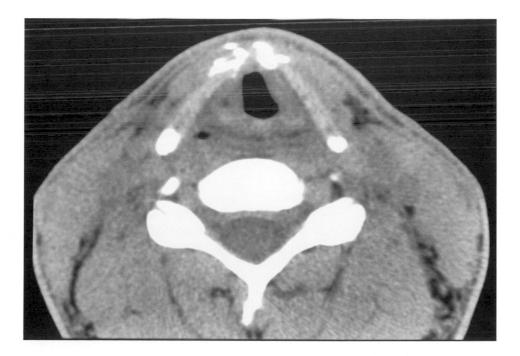

Fig 20–3. Axial CT scan of the thyroid ala demonstrating an anterior comminuted thyroid ala fracture sustained by the patient in a motor vehicle collision.

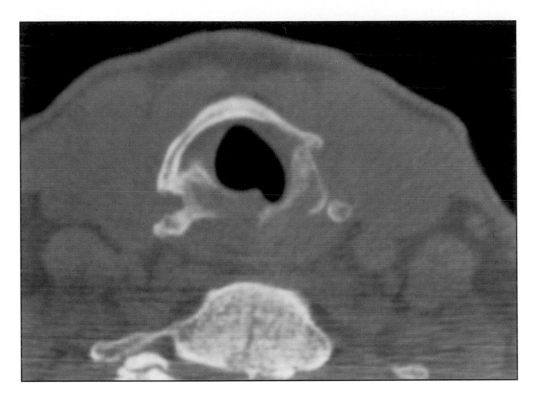

Fig 20–4. Axial CT scan at the level of the thyroid and cricoid cartilages. There is a vertical, displaced posterior cricoid lamina fracture with fusion of the right cricothyroid joint. The airway is maintained by the lateral buttresses.

rent laryngeal nerve due to impingement at the level of the cricothyroid joint (Figs 20–5 and 20–6).

If the force is severe or low in the neck, complete laryngotracheal separation may occur.[19] Separation usually occurs between the cricoid cartilage and the first tracheal ring, resulting in displacement of the trachea inferiorly and soft tissue collapse into the airway, with consequent airway obstruction.[19-22] The strap musculature and surrounding cervical fascia can serve as a temporary conduit for air until edema and hematoma formation result in obstruction of this temporary airway.

Pediatric Framework Injuries from Blunt Trauma

Fractures of the thyroid and cricoid cartilage from blunt trauma are uncommon in the pediatric population. The pediatric larynx sits higher in the neck than in the adult, and depending on age, can lie between the second and seventh cervical vertebrae. The mandible serves more as a protective shield in the child than it does in the adult.[23] The greater elasticity of the pediatric cartilaginous framework makes it more resilient to external stresses, and the mobility of the supporting tissues tends to protect the laryngotracheal

complex more effectively. Children are likely to sustain soft tissue injuries resulting in edema and hematoma formation.[22,23] This is of particular concern in a child because of the relatively smaller diameter of the pediatric airway.

The pediatric patient is more likely than an adult to sustain transection and telescoping injuries. An individual who falls onto the handlebar of a bicycle may suffer a telescoping injury in which the cricoid cartilage is dislocated superiorly underneath the thyroid lamina (Fig 20–7).[22-25] With more forceful blows, complete laryngotracheal separation may occur. The adolescent and young adult riding a snowmobile or an all-terrain vehicle may sustain a "clothes-line" type injury to the neck upon collision with a cable or wire. A horizontal, linear force is applied low in the neck, compressing the cricotracheal complex against the anterior cervical vertebrae and resulting in cricotracheal separation.[25] The elasticity of the intercartilaginous ligaments contributes to substernal retraction of the trachea. These are often fatal injuries, but occasionally there is enough fascial stenting to maintain an adequate airway until an artificial airway can be established. There may be an associated injury and possibly transection of both recurrent laryngeal nerves, which

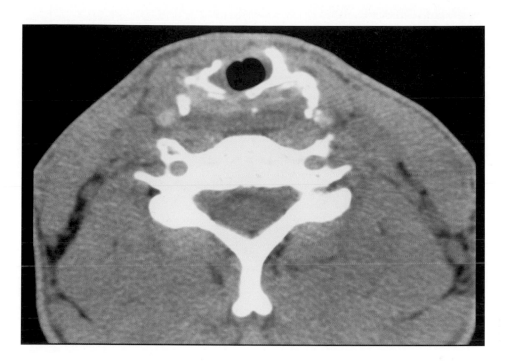

Fig 20–5. Axial CT scan of the cricoid cartilage. The airway is narrowed secondary to anterior and posterior vertical, displaced cricoid lamina fractures.

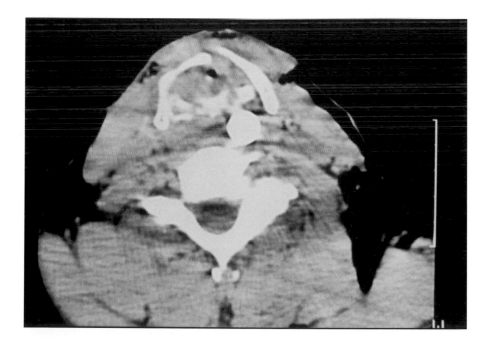

Fig 20–6. Axial CT scan at the level of the thyroid and cricoid cartilages. There are midline and left lateral fractures of the thyroid ala and comminuted fractures of the posterior cricoid lamina with loss of the airway space. The airway was secured below the fracture segments with tracheostomy.

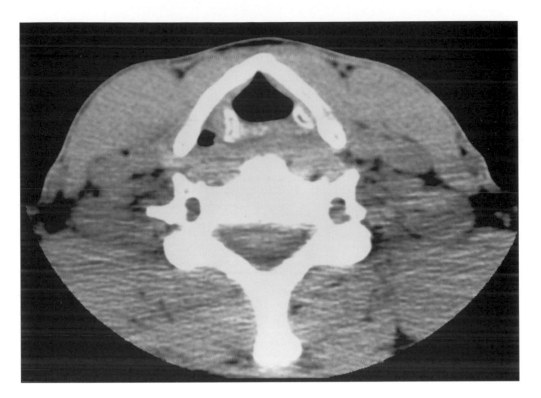

Fig 20–7. Axial CT scan at the level of the thyroid and cricoid cartilages. There is subluxation of the cricoid cartilage under the thyroid ala after the patient sustained an elbow injury to the neck while playing basketball.

are also compressed against the cervical vertebrae during the injury.[22,25]

Young children may accidentally hang themselves while playing, and adolescents may do so intentionally in suicide attempts. In these instances, the fall to hanging position is usually less than 1 to 2 feet. The rope around the neck tightens usually in the region of the thyrohyoid membrane, resulting in airway obstruction as the epiglottis closes over the glottis. The distinction between this and the injury that results from hanging inflicted by a second party is that in self-inflicted or accidental injuries, death is not necessarily imminent; and in those who survive, there is usually injury, possibly avulsion, at the level of the thyrohyoid membrane. In homicidal hanging (professional execution), the victim is usually dropped a distance of several feet, resulting in death secondary to tracheal transection or spinal cord injury from C1–C2 dislocation.[25]

Soft Tissue Injuries from Blunt Trauma

Blunt trauma to the larynx may result in soft tissue injuries with or without associated framework injuries. Rupture of the thyroepiglottic ligament can be associated with either horizontal or vertical fractures of the thy-

roid cartilage. Narrowing of the laryngeal lumen can occur secondary to herniation of pre-epiglottic tissue or posterior displacement of the epiglottic petiole.[17,21]

Vocal fold injuries result from vertical fractures of the thyroid ala (see Fig 20–1). As the thyroid cartilage snaps back from its compression against the cervical vertebrae, the thyroarytenoid muscle and ligament may tear, resulting in a separation at any point along its length. This may be evident as mucosal lacerations or hemorrhage of one or both vocal folds. The mucosa on the arytenoids may be denuded or avulsed. Because of the traction on the arytenoids from this springlike motion of the thyroid cartilage, the arytenoid cartilages may also become displaced from the cricoarytenoid joint into a more posterior and lateral or anterior position (Fig 20–8). If one segment of the thyroid cartilage fails to return to its normal position, an overlapping fracture may occur, resulting in malposition of the vocal fold (Figs 20–9 and 20–10). Lacerations of the piriform sinus and upper esophagus may occur as the thyroid cartilage rubs against the cervical vertebrae.[17,21]

Soft tissue injuries associated with cricoid, tracheal, and cricotracheal separation injuries within the cartilaginous framework usually involve crushed or lacerated mucosa. Both recurrent laryngeal nerves are fre-

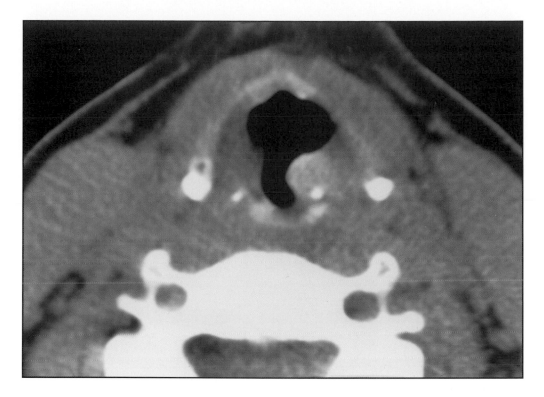

Fig 20–8. Axial CT scan of the larynx at the level of the arytenoids demonstrating anterior dislocation of the right arytenoid cartilage.

quently injured and can be severed by blunt trauma that results in cricoid fractures and/or cricotracheal separation. The phrenic nerve can also be injured, especially in cases of cricotracheal separation.[17,19,21,22,25] Associated esophageal lacerations and perforations are common.

Assessment of Blunt Injuries

Initial evaluation and assessment of the blunt trauma patient is similar for adults and children. It is important to obtain an understanding of the mechanism of injury. A high index of suspicion for blunt neck injury should be maintained in motor vehicle collisions, even without obvious external signs. Knowledge of the speed of the vehicle at the time of collision, the use of seatbelts by the trauma victim, and the presence and deployment of airbags can also be helpful in estimating the amount of force involved. In the patient with short stature, the force of deceleration against a locking "shoulder" strap that is draped over the neck may also produce significant injury. Assessment of the patient begins with evaluation and stabilization of the airway, paying particular attention to the status of the cervical spine. Assessment then proceeds with evaluation and stabilization of respiratory, cardiovascular,

cervical spine, neurologic, and other emergent organ system injuries. Management of aerodigestive tract injuries varies depending upon the presence of acute airway distress (Fig 20–11).

Evaluation of the Blunt Trauma Patient Without Airway Distress

In the patient without immediate signs of upper airway compromise, the evaluation can proceed with a complete examination, including palpation of the neck, assessment of voice quality, and flexible fiberoptic evaluation of the larynx and upper airway. Fiberoptic laryngoscopy allows assessment of the mobility of the vocal folds, patency of the upper airway, and integrity of the mucosa. If there is an adequate airway, intubation is not necessary. Because of the potential for the development of worsening laryngeal edema and airway compromise, serial examinations of the airway should be performed during the first 24 to 48 hours after injury if intubation is initially deemed unnecessary.

Adequate visualization of the endolarynx is imperative in completing the physical examination. Indirect laryngoscopy is the easiest method but can be dangerous in a patient with airway compromise. Flexible

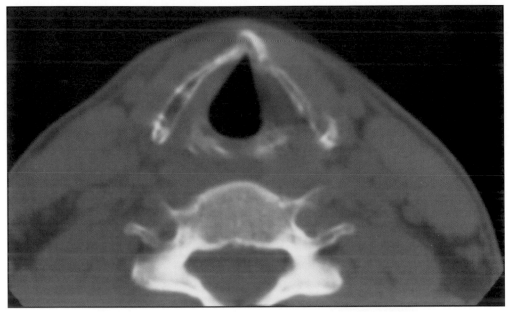

A

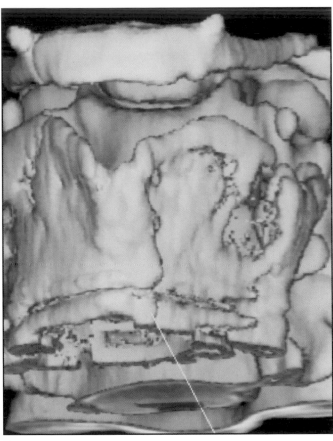

B

Fig 20–9. A. Axial CT scan of the subglottic larynx demonstrating a displaced, paramedian fracture of the left thyroid ala. The vocal folds (not shown) are malpositioned. **B.** Three-dimensional CT reconstruction of the left paramedian thyroid ala fracture demonstrating overlapping of the fracture segments.

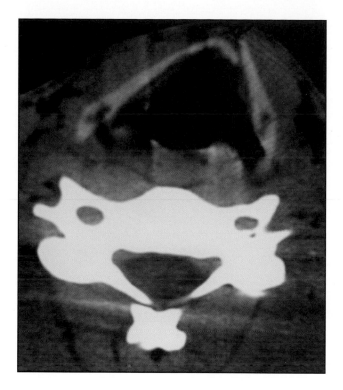

Fig 20–10. Axial CT of the supraglottic larynx. There is a displaced paramedian fracture of the right thyroid ala.

laryngoscopy has almost completely obviated this risk and is currently the preferred method of initial laryngeal examination. In patients with concomitant facial trauma or severe airway trauma, a flexible bronchoscope is sometimes preferred due to the presence of a suction channel. Strobovideolaryngoscopy can be invaluable in assessing injuries involving vocal fold mobility and integrity. Microscopic direct laryngoscopy continues to provide the most detailed evaluation of the larynx (except for determinations of dynamic function, which must be made by stroboscopy). However, advances in flexible endoscopy and the availability of stroboscopy have limited the use of direct laryngoscopy to the last step in assessment, usually at the time of the operative repair.

Management is based on the severity of the initial signs and symptoms.[7]

Patients with any sign of endolaryngeal injury (Table 20–1) should undergo radiologic imaging to evaluate for possible laryngeal framework injury.[7,24,26] Minimally displaced fractures of the thyroid cartilage can be present with very mild endolaryngeal signs and should be evaluated to determine the likelihood of fracture stability. Radiologic evaluation is best preformed by high-resolution CT scanning in multiple planes.[24] Thyroid and cricoid cartilage integrity,

cricoarytenoid joint status, cricothyroid joint status, and even soft tissue laryngeal injuries can all be assessed by an experienced radiologist if fine-cut, 1-mm, multiplanar techniques are used. MRI scanning may provide additional information about the degree of soft-tissue injury, but the CT scan remains the study of choice in laryngeal trauma.

When exposed cartilage is noted on endolaryngeal examination, or when the CT scan reveals a multiply comminuted thyroid cartilage fracture, the need for open reduction and stabilization is unquestioned (Fig 20–12) Studies by Hirano et al and Stanley et al also have shown that reduction of a single, linear, even minimally displaced, thyroid cartilage fracture is important in obtaining an adequate post-injury voice.[27,28] Although no comparative studies are available, the authors believe that only stable, nondisplaced thyroid cartilage fractures with normal endolaryngeal architecture should be treated without operative intervention. Table 20–2 lists CT findings that suggest fracture stability and instability.

Fractures that appear to have the potential for instability should be evaluated further with direct laryngoscopy and open exploration for repair. Patients with minimally displaced fractures that are associated with significant endolaryngeal injuries also require direct laryngoscopy, open exploration, and repair of the soft tissue injuries (Table 20–3). Because of the high potential for concomitant cervical spine injuries, assessment of the cervical spine is always performed prior to operative intervention of the laryngeal injuries. The presence of a cervical spine injury may preclude the ability to perform a direct laryngoscopy, and repair is begun based on findings on CT scan and flexible endoscopic examination (Fig 20–13).

Dislocation of the cricoarytenoid joint is now being recognized as a fairly common component of laryngeal trauma.[29,30] It can be seen as the only significant lesion after blunt neck trauma, in combination with nondisplaced laryngeal fractures, or as part of a complex laryngeal surgery. It must be suspected by the laryngologist if proper diagnosis and treatment are to be obtained. If a posterior dislocation is present, the involved side may appear to be paralyzed, and the involved vocal process is high. In anterior dislocations, the involved vocal process is below the normal side, and the vocal fold may appear to be short. In many acute cases, edema prohibits good assessment by indirect laryngoscopy. Stroboscopic assessment may reveal asymmetry of the mucosal wave or level of vocal fold apposition, particularly during pitch sliding maneuvers. The "jostle sign" is often absent on the dislocated side, helping to differentiate arytenoid dislocation from vocal fold paralysis. However, arytenoid

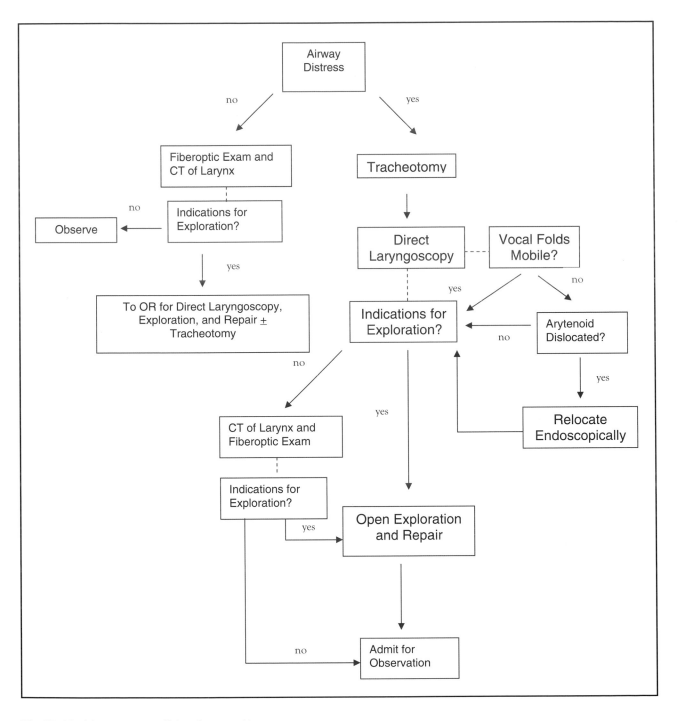

Fig 20–11. Management of blunt laryngeal trauma.

Table 20–1. Signs and Symptoms of Laryngeal Injury.

Hoarseness/dysphonia	Dyspnea
Stridor	Endolaryngeal edema
Endolaryngeal hematoma	Subcutaneous emphysema
Endolaryngeal laceration	Neck pain/point tenderness
Dysphagia	Loss of laryngeal landmarks
Odynophagia	Impaired vocal fold mobility
Hemoptysis	Arytenoid dislocation
Ecchymosis/abrasions of anterior neck	Exposed endolaryngeal cartilage

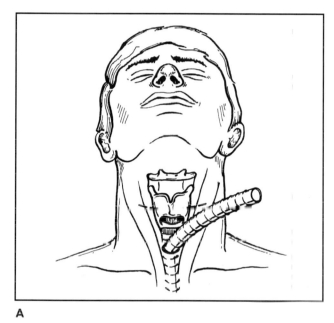

A

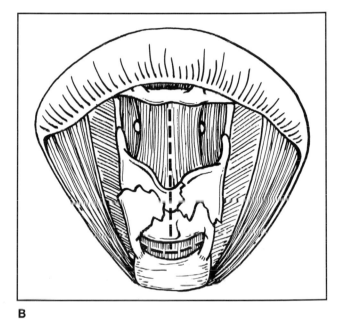

B

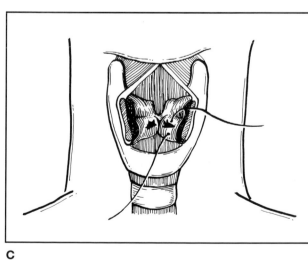

C

Fig 20–12. A. Surgical access for repair of laryngeal trauma is best obtained through a transverse incision superior to the tracheotomy site. **B.** In cases of comminuted thyroid cartilage fractures, the larynx must be entered through the thyrohyoid or cricothyroid membranes so the mucosal incision can be made accurately under direct vision at the anterior commissure. **C.** Mucosal lacerations are meticulously closed using fine absorbable sutures.

Table 20–2. CT Findings That Suggest Fracture Stability.

Fracture Type	Displacement	Stable	Suggested Management
Single Vertical, Unilateral	Nondisplaced	yes	Observe, fixate if symptoms or exam worsen
	Minimally displaced (<1 cartilage width)	yes	Fixate if immediate or delayed voice change, otherwise observe
	Displaced (>1 cartilage width)	no	Reduce and fixate
Single Horizontal, Unilateral	Nondisplaced	yes	Observe, fixate if symptoms or exam worsen
	Minimally displaced	yes	Observe, fixate if symptoms or exam worsen
	Displaced	no	Reduce and fixate
Multiple Unilateral	Nondisplaced	no	Reduce and fixate
	Displaced	no	Reduce and fixate
Multiple Bilateral	Nondisplaced	no	Reduce and fixate
	Displaced	no	Reduce and fixate

Table 20–3. Indications for Operative Repair After Blunt Laryngeal Trauma.

Laceration of vibrating edge of true vocal fold

Laceration of anterior commissure

Deep laceration of thyroarytenoid muscle

Exposed cartilage

Impaired vocal fold mobility

Arytenoid dislocation

Epiglottis displacement

Herniation of pre-epiglottic contents

Unstable/displaced laryngeal fractures

Airway compromise

Extensive endolaryngeal edema

dislocation does not necessarily imply immobility, especially acutely. A recently dislocated arytenoid may still be mobile, but close observation reveals abnormal speed, smoothness, and direction of arytenoid motion. Stroboscopic assessment may reveal asymmetry of the mucosal wave or level of vocal fold apposition. A laryngeal EMG may be useful in distinguishing between cricoarytenoid subluxation and recurrent laryngeal nerve paralysis. Diagnosis is facilitated by noting the asymmetric position of the arytenoid on laryngoscopy and on CT scan.

In the case of severe injury, inspection and palpation of the arytenoid at the time of surgery is necessary to determine joint integrity. Anterior dislocations occur most commonly and usually result from blunt external trauma compressing the larynx against the cervical spine or from traumatic intubations. Posterior dislocations occur from prolonged intubation, traumatic intubation and extubation, and traumatic endoscopy. Arytenoid dislocations should be reduced as soon as possible. Even when they are discovered long after the initial injury, reduction should be attempted because improve-

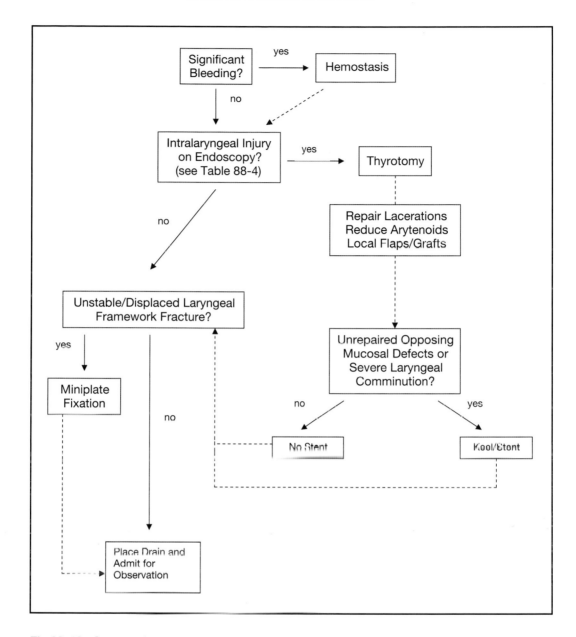

Fig 20–13. Open exploration of laryngeal trauma.

ment in vocal quality can be obtained in most cases.[30]

Patients without fractures on CT scanning and those with minimally displaced, stable fractures can be observed closely. Soft tissue injuries that consist of isolated mucosal lacerations of the supraglottic larynx, superficial lacerations of the nonvibrating edge of the true vocal fold, small hematomas of the true vocal fold, and/or mild mucosal edema may also be observed. Management of these patients includes the use of antibiotics, antireflux medications, reflux precautions, elevation of the head of bed, voice rest, and humidity. The use of antireflux medications and reflux

precautions, including elevation of the head of the bed, helps to limit additional inflammation and delays in wound healing caused by laryngopharyngeal reflux. Humidity helps to maintain lubrication of the vocal folds, which aids in the re-epithelialization process. The benefit of steroids in this scenario is controversial. The disadvantage of corticosteroids is that their anti-inflammatory action may interfere with and prolong the natural process of wound healing. The advantage of using steroids is that they may minimize the formation of granulation tissue and decrease laryngeal edema.[7,11,13,28,29,31] In the patient with mild to moderate mucosal edema, high dose steroids are given during the first 24 to 48 hours to minimize mucosal edema acutely.

Evaluation of the Blunt Trauma Patient with Airway Distress

Signs of upper airway distress include stridor, sternal retraction, and dyspnea. The patient should be examined for signs of upper aerodigestive tract injury. In the presence of immediate post-traumatic airway distress, significant laryngotracheal injury is likely. The neck is stabilized to prevent worsening of unrecognized cervical spine injuries, and the airway is secured with a tracheotomy fashioned at least two rings below the injured segments or through the distal transected segment under local anesthesia.[1,2,15,17,19,22,32-36] Tracheotomy prevents further laryngeal injury, and may expose an unnoticed laryngotracheal separation. Orotracheal and/or nasopharyngeal intubation in the presence of severe laryngotracheal trauma can lead to further laryngeal injury and airway compromise.

In the child with upper airway distress, the airway is secured in the operating room if time permits. General anesthesia is induced using an inhalational agent that is unlikely to cause laryngospasm. During spontaneous respiration, a rigid bronchoscope is passed gently through the injured larynx and trachea to a point distal to the sites of injury. Tracheotomy is performed over the bronchoscope followed by repair of the injuries.[20,23]

Operative evaluation of the larynx with direct laryngoscopy is performed after securing the airway. If direct laryngoscopy reveals significant endolaryngeal injuries (see Table 20–3), open exploration and repair are performed. The presence of palpable laryngeal fractures is also an indication for open exploration and repair. If direct laryngoscopy does not reveal a need for open exploration, then a postoperative CT of the larynx is obtained to complete the evaluation.

Surgical Evaluation

Full evaluation and determination of the need for surgical intervention should begin as soon as a laryngeal injury is suspected. Schaefer and Leopold both have reported better results when treatment is initiated in the first 24 hours.[2,11] Although many patients who suffer multiple trauma must have the evaluation delayed, it should still proceed as soon as their general condition allows. Indications for surgery can be divided into three groups: the need to restore cartilaginous integrity, the need to restore mucosal integrity, and the need to restore normal cricoarytenoid joint function.

Intraoperative evaluation begins with direct laryngoscopy to assess the extent of endolaryngeal injury, esophagoscopy to assess for esophageal lacerations, and bronchoscopy to assess for subglottic and tracheobronchial injuries. The arytenoid cartilages are palpated for possible dislocation. In the patient with isolated cricoarytenoid joint dislocation, reduction can usually be accomplished endoscopically, especially if the dislocation is noted early. With delays in diagnosis beyond even a week, joint ankylosis can begin, making reduction more difficult. Nonetheless, an attempt should be made to relocate the arytenoid cartilage back to its normal position on the cricoid regardless of the interval from the time of injury. In cases of posterior dislocation, this can be accomplished by inserting the anterior lip of an intubating laryngoscope into the posterior aspect of the cricoarytenoid joint while exerting a lifting motion in an antero-medial direction on the arytenoid cartilage. Anterior dislocations can be reduced by exerting a posteriorly directed force on the cricoarytenoid joint using the tip of a rigid laryngoscope.[33,37] Anterior dislocations can also be reduced by direct manipulation of the arytenoid body or with a blunt right-angle hook or right-angle cup forceps placed under the anteriorly displaced arytenoid body. Care must be taken not to fracture the vocal process during this maneuver. If no other injuries that require repair are noted on CT scan or on direct laryngoscopy, then open exploration is not necessary.

Open Exploration and Repair

Open exploration is performed to repair mucosal lacerations involving the anterior commissure and/or the vibratory edge of the vocal fold; to repair deep lacerations of the thyroarytenoid muscle; to restore mucosal cover over exposed cartilage; to reposition the vocal ligament and anterior commissure; to reposition a displaced epiglottis or herniated pre-epiglottic contents; to reanastomose separated segments; and to reduce and fixate displaced and/or unstable fractures (Fig 20–13). If not previously done, tracheotomy is performed to allow intraoperative access to the larynx and postoperative airway management.

Principles of Repair

The basic principles of repair follow the primary principles of wound healing elsewhere in the body. Repair within the first 24 hours after injury is most desirable to prevent granulation tissue formation from occurring prior to closure.[7,19] An attempt should be made to repair all mucosal lacerations and defects to promote healing by primary intention. Healing by secondary intention predisposes to a greater deposition of collagen and an increased likelihood of granulation tissue and scar formation, which may result in vibratory dysfunction, stenosis, or webbing of the vocal folds. All de-epithelialized areas that cannot be closed primarily without tension should be covered with local mucosal flaps to minimize scar formation. Free mucosal grafts can be used to cover de-epithelialized areas when local flaps cannot be fashioned; however, these are rarely needed. Fine, absorbable suture on an atraumatic needle seems to help minimize granulation tissue formation also.

Exposure

For open exploration, a horizontal neck incision is made and subplatysmal skin flaps are elevated. To expose the thyroid and cricoid cartilages, the strap muscles may be divided in the midline and retracted laterally. When endolaryngeal repair of soft tissue injuries is necessary, entry into the larynx is gained through fractures of the thyroid cartilage that are median or those that are paramedian and less than 0.5 cm from the midline. In patients with lateral or horizontal fractures of the thyroid cartilage, a midline thyrotomy is performed. A midline cut is then made through the anterior commissure under direct visualization, with care not to further disrupt the architecture of the vocal fold. Above the level of the glottis, the endolaryngeal incision is curved lateral to the epiglottis on one side to avoid cutting through its cartilage or mucosa. Care is taken during the exposure to avoid further injury to the recurrent and superior laryngeal nerves.

Endolaryngeal Repair

The functional goal of repair is to realign glottic tissues to their premorbid anteroposterior and transverse planes, beginning posteriorly and proceeding in an anterior direction to maximize exposure. The arytenoid is repositioned with meticulous closure of overlying mucoperichondrial defects. If the arytenoid mucosa is damaged badly, local rotation flaps can be developed from the piriform sinus or postcricoid region. Regardless of the extent of the injuries, an attempt should be made to repair severe unilateral and bilateral arytenoid injuries. Consideration of arytenoidectomy as a secondary procedure can be made at a later date after healing has occurred, and the wounds have matured.[17] This approach allows for the possibility of vocalization and respiration if at least one of the arytenoids retains some function.

Lacerations in the thyroarytenoid muscle or mucosa may be repaired with fine, absorbable suture. Avascular and crushed mucosal injuries are debrided prior to closure. If primary closure of mucosal disruptions is difficult, local advancement or rotational flaps should be performed. Local advancement or rotational flaps from the piriform sinus or postcricoid region usually provide adequate coverage of the arytenoid and its vocal process. A sternohyoid muscle flap can fill small defects, but does not provide cartilaginous support (Fig 20–14). Adequate mucosa for coverage of the anterior commissure region usually can be obtained from the epiglottis. If an extensive amount of mucosa is needed, the epiglottic mucosa can be elevated off the laryngeal and lingual surfaces of the epiglottis with removal of the cartilage to allow for a large superiorly based epiglottic flap (Fig 20–15).[38] It is important to ensure meticulous closure and re-epithelialization of the anterior commissure region, as this is the region most likely to develop a web or stenosis as a late complication.

Mucosal defects on the false vocal fold and epiglottis are less likely to pose significant problems with stenosis. If primary repair or a local flap cannot be accomplished, this area can be left open to granulate and mucosalize by secondary intention. A ruptured thyroepiglottic ligament should be reattached anteriorly to reposition the epiglottis to its more anatomical position. Herniated contents of the pre-epiglottic space should be removed or replaced anterior to the epiglottis and the thyroepiglottic ligament.

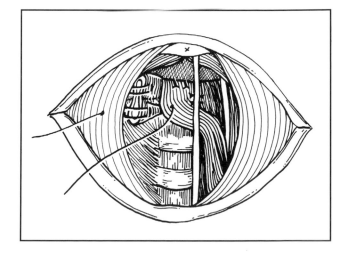

Fig 20–14. An inferiorly based sternohyoid muscle flap is utilized to cover a posterior mucosal defect.

The attachment of the vocal ligament at the anterior commissure is inspected. If torn, it is repaired by placing a slow-absorbing monofilament suture through the anterior aspect of the ligament and bringing it through a midline fracture to secure to the thyroid cartilage. If the fracture is paramedian, the suture is brought through the midline of the cartilage and secured. It is important to re-establish the appropriate height of the vocal fold as well as the appropriate midline placement for optimal post-operative voice results. Proper placement of the vocal ligament helps to ensure the proper position of the remainder of the vocal fold.

Endolaryngeal Stenting

Questions regarding when and how to utilize stents in acute trauma repair have not yet been answered adequately. However, there are some definitive and relative guidelines. Definitive indications for stenting include severely comminuted fractures where direct fixation is inadequate (to maintain) cartilaginous integrity; severe disruption of the anterior commissure; severe endolaryngeal mucosal disruption; and large mucosal defects that require application of skin or mucosal grafts. If bilateral mucosal lacerations produce webbing or if a web has been resected, a stent may also be employed. Although stenting may seem to promote a more consistent restoration of the laryngeal airway, it may also be harmful. Stents have been shown to cause local inflammatory reaction in almost all cases.[39] The wires and sutures used to fix the stent to the cervical skin also produce chronic irritation from the shearing caused by vertical laryngeal motion during swallowing (Fig 20–16).

Thus, in cases where the anterior commissure is the major problem, a keel that will prevent anterior webbing while not having contact with most of the endolaryngeal mucosa is preferred. The keel can be formed of Silastic, Teflon, or tantalum (Fig 20–17).[40,41]

Keels can be placed through an open incision or endoscopically. In cases where a patient has normal vo-

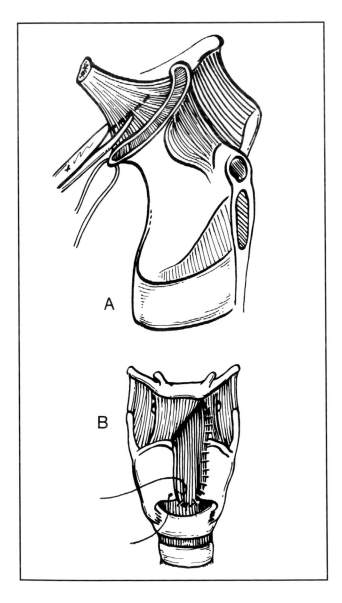

Fig 20–15. A. The epiglottis is grasped and its anterior attachments are severed so that it can be advanced inferiorly into the laryngeal defect. **B.** The epiglottic flap is sutured in the laryngeal defect using interrupted, permanent sutures.

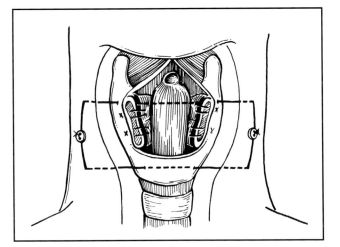

Fig 20–16. Wires sutured over buttons on the external skin hold a soft stent in place. The wires also restrict vertical laryngeal motion in the neck.

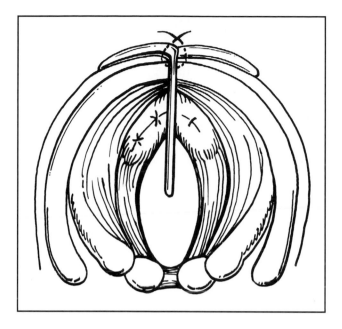

Fig 20–17. A tantalum keel is utilized to reduce scarring at the anterior commissure.

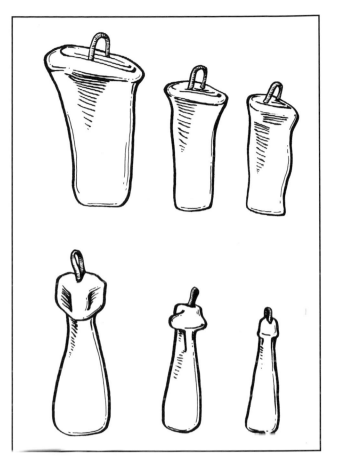

Fig 20–18. Montgomery premolded laryngeal stents come in male, female, and pediatric sizes.

cal fold motion or undergoes cricoarytenoid reduction, stents are avoided if at all possible. Whenever stents are utilized, they are removed as soon as possible. Two weeks is adequate for most patients unless other medical problems that may delay healing (eg, diabetes, malnutrition, or advanced age) coexist. Stents are rarely left in place longer than 4 weeks. Both prefabricated molded stents and soft stents have been used with success. Molded stents are available in varying sizes and conform to the endolaryngeal surfaces, presumably reducing frictional trauma (Fig 20–18).

Both Silastic and Gore-Tex varieties are available. Soft stents, usually a latex finger cot filled with gauze or a rubber sponge, allow for mucosal swelling and may be less traumatic than molded materials. Mucosal or split-thickness skin grafts can be fixed circumferentially to either type of stent with the epidermis away from the laryngeal mucosa as a biological dressing (Fig 20–19).

Laryngeal Fixation

Reduction and fixation of the cartilaginous framework is performed after all mucosal injuries have been addressed. If a stent is deemed necessary, it is placed prior to repair of the framework injuries. The fractures are reduced and fixated to ensure a stable reduction. Traditionally, stabilization has been achieved using

stainless steel wire or nonabsorbable suture. However, because these provide only two-dimensional fixation, there can be some movement of the laryngeal fragments with head turning, flexion, and swallowing. The recent availability of titanium and absorbable miniplates has allowed more rigid fixation of the laryngeal framework in three-dimensional planes (Fig 20–20). This has the advantage over wire or suture fixation in that it allows for immediate immobility of the fracture segments, can be used effectively in most comminuted fractures and can decrease the need for endolaryngeal stenting.[42,43] The miniplates can be bent to conform to the geometry of the laryngeal framework, thus preserving the anteroposterior and transverse dimensions of the larynx. Usually, low profile plates in the 1.2 mm to 1.4 mm size range provide adequate fixation of the laryngeal framework and are less prominent than larger profile systems. In patients without significant ossification of the thyroid cartilage, it is often necessary to use drill bits that are two sizes smaller than the screw in order to prevent prob-

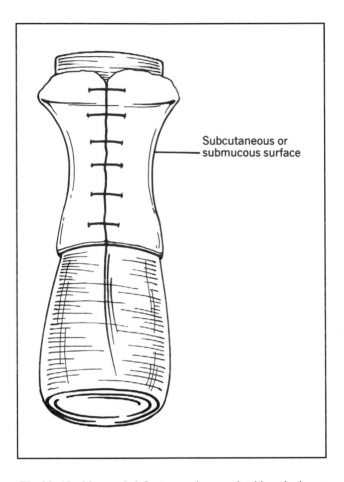

Fig 20–19. Mucosal defects can be repaired by placing a skin graft circumferentially around the laryngeal stent with the dermis facing out.

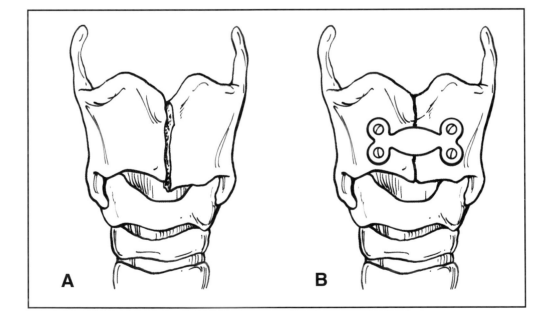

Fig 20–20. Miniplate fixation of a vertical thyroid lamina fracture. (Ilustrations courtesy of Sabrina M. Heman-Ackah.)

lems with overdrilling of the soft cartilage.[42-44] For example, if one were to use a 1.3-mm plating system, the hole would be drilled with a 0.8-mm drill bit instead of the usual 1.0-mm drill bit. Alternatively, one may use the 1.0-mm drill bit with the wider threaded "emergency" screws (1.5-mm diameter) from the 1.3 mm-plating set or self-drilling screws.

Laryngotracheal Reanastomosis

In patients with cricotracheal separation, initial intubation is through the distal segment. Any avulsed or badly bruised mucosa or cartilage is resected prior to reanastomosis to decrease the incidence of granulation tissue formation. Repair is begun with placement of sutures from the posterior tracheal mucosa to the inner cricoid perichondrium using 3-0 absorbable suture or fine wire. The repair then proceeds anteriorly, tying all knots extraluminally. The cricoid and tracheal perichondria and cartilages are then repaired using a 2-0 or 3-0 absorbable suture.[17] The use of absorbable suture decreases the incidence of anastomotic granulation tissue formation and late stenosis.[45] In the presence of cricoid injury and/or in patients in whom post-operative edema seems likely, a T-tube may be placed as a temporary stent. Post-operatively, the neck is kept in flexion for 7 to 10 days to prevent traction on the anastomotic closure.

Recurrent Laryngeal Nerve Repair

Laryngotracheal separation injuries may be accompanied by bilateral recurrent laryngeal nerve injuries. An attempt should be made to locate the nerves if the vocal folds exhibit evidence of immobility preoperatively. Crushed or otherwise damaged but intact nerves should be left alone to regenerate on their own. If a severed nerve is found, the severed ends should be freshened; and an attempt should be made to reanastomose the epineurium using a fine monofilament suture under tension-free closure. If a tension-free closure cannot be obtained or if the proximal end cannot be located and the opposite nerve is intact, unilateral ansa-cervicalis to recurrent laryngeal nerve transfer is an option. Recurrent laryngeal nerve repair is unlikely to restore full abductor or adductor function to the vocal fold, but it should provide enough tone to the thyroarytenoid muscle for long-term vocalization purposes.[46,47] If soft-tissue injury in the neck is extensive and ansa cervicalis to recurrent laryngeal nerve transfer cannot to be performed, hypoglossal to recurrent laryngeal nerve transfer or cable grafting using a greater auricular or sural nerve graft are other possibilities for nerve repair. In general, better results are obtained with nerve transfer than with cable grafting procedures.

Post-operative Management

The goal of post-operative management is to promote wound healing and limit granulation tissue formation. Patients who undergo mucosal repair of the vocal folds should exercise strict voice rest for the first few days to allow the initial phases of epithelialization to occur. Consideration should be given to the placement of a small flexible nasogastric feeding tube intraoperatively to allow enteral feeding in the early post-operative period. All patients with mucosal injuries are placed on an aggressive antireflux protocol, even in the absence of a history of gastroesophageal reflux, to minimize delays in wound healing associated with reflux-induced laryngeal injury. Prophylactic antibiotics are given to patients with open wounds to minimize the risk of chondritis. Routine tracheotomy care is performed gently to minimize excessive coughing.

Penetrating Injuries

Penetrating injuries are the second most common cause of laryngotracheal injuries in adults and the most common cause in the pediatric population.[1,4,22] These injuries result from accidental or deliberate stab wounds and from gunshot wounds. It is important to understand the mechanism of the injury, the direction of the force, as well as the instrument used to create the injury. If the path has traversed the midline, an injury to the upper aerodigestive tract is likely.

In victims of gunshot wounds, in addition to noting both the entry and exit wounds, it is also helpful to know the caliber and velocity of the weapon used. The kinetic energy ($KE = \frac{1}{2} mv^2$, where KE is kinetic energy, m is mass of the projectile, and v is projectile velocity) released from the bullet on impact determines the degree of tissue damage. Thus, small caliber, high velocity bullets tend to produce greater tissue damage than do larger caliber, low velocity bullets. The long bullet of the shotgun produces a different type of injury than the short bullet of the pistol or handgun. Because of their shorter length, handgun bullets fly with a straight trajectory, resulting in tissue damage at the site of impact. The bullets of the shotgun are longer and unstable in their trajectory. They, thus, tumble as they leave the barrel of the weapon. This "tumbling" produces significant circumferential "shock wave" damage to surrounding tissue that may extend several centimeters from the site of impact.[48]

In victims of stab wounds, the location and direction of the entrance wound are particularly important to note. Long penetrating objects can create injuries to structures at a significant distance from the entrance wound. As in the blunt trauma patient, victims of penetrating injuries to the larynx and trachea can appear to be comfortable; however, complications from airway compromise, vascular injuries, and esophageal perforations can result in mortality rates as high as 19%.[5,40,50] Therefore, a high index of suspicion coupled with a thorough physical examination is necessary.

Assessment of Penetrating Injuries

The initial concerns in evaluating and treating patients with penetrating injuries are the assessment and establishment of a patent airway and the evaluation and control of vascular and cervical spine injuries, as these are often major contributing factors to early morbidity and mortality in penetrating neck injuries.[49] In patients who require emergent airway control, the decision to perform orotracheal intubation versus tracheotomy must be individualized. The patient with a minor injury

is less likely to have an occult laryngotracheal separation, making attempts at intubation less problematic.[49]

Examination of the patient who has sustained a penetrating neck injury involves assessment of all of the neck structures. Signs and symptoms of disruption of the upper aerodigestive tract are the same as in the blunt trauma patient (see Table 20–1). If they are stable, patients with penetrating neck injuries that cross the midline should have a flexible laryngoscopic examination and CT scan of the neck and larynx to evaluate for possible endolaryngeal injury (Fig 20–21). The patient without any symptoms or signs on flexible endoscopic examination or CT scan of laryngeal injury may be observed closely for development of airway, voice, or esophageal abnormalities. Patients with mild laryngeal inflammation and no other signs of endolaryngeal injury may also be observed. Because of the potential for esophageal injuries, an esophagram with water-soluble contrast should be obtained in patients with minor injuries who do not require rigid endoscopy. The false negative rate with esophagrams has been reported as high as 21%.[50,51] Thus, patients with a negative esophagram who begin to develop

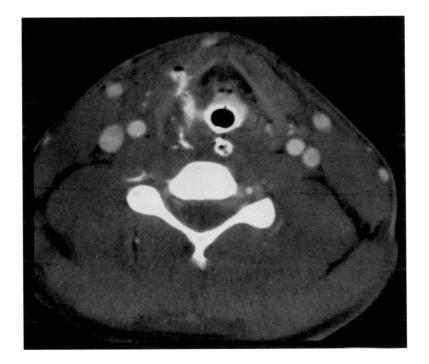

Fig 20–21. Axial CT of the larynx at the level of the false vocal folds after gunshot wound to the left neck. There is shrapnel debris along the trajectory of the bullet from the soft tissues of the left neck anterior to the sternocleiodmastoid muscle, through the left thyroid ala, and within the soft tissues of the endolarynx. An endotracheal tube is surrounded by significant endolaryngeal soft tissue edema.

odynophagia, fever, or back or chest pain should be evaluated for possible esophageal perforation with flexible or rigid esophagoscopy.

Patients who are noted to have signs and symptoms of a significant aerodigestive tract injury (Table 20–4) should undergo rigid direct laryngoscopy with consideration for possible open neck exploration and repair.[49] Because associated esophageal injuries have been reported in as many as 20 to 50% of the patients with laryngeal injuries, esophagoscopy should also be performed at the time of rigid endoscopy.[5,49]

Repair of Penetrating Injuries

Repair of penetrating laryngeal injuries and postoperative management is accomplished in a similar fashion as would be done with the blunt trauma patient. In patients with combined esophageal and posterior tracheal wall injuries, consideration should be given to placing a muscle interposition flap between the trachea and esophagus to prevent the formation of a tracheoesophageal fistula. This can be accomplished with the use of a nearby pedicled strap or sternocleidomastoid muscle flap.

Caustic and Thermal Injuries

Caustic and thermal injuries to the larynx can cause significant acute and chronic airway compromise as well as late vocal complications. Caustic injuries occur in both the adult and pediatric populations. Caustic injuries can result from ingestion of bases, acids, or bleaches. The most severe injuries are caused by bases,

which produce a liquefaction necrosis of muscle, collagen, and lipids with progressively worsening injury over time. Acids cause a coagulation necrosis that occurs more rapidly and tends to damage superficial structures only. In children under age 5, these tend to be accidental ingestions. Adolescent and adult ingestions usually are suicide attempts and thus tend to produce the most severe injuries.[53,54]

Caustic ingestions most often affect the oral cavity, pharynx, and esophagus, but can occasionally contact the larynx and result in edema and mucosal disruption secondary to burn injury. Because the epiglottis and false vocal folds are the initial barriers in preventing aspiration, the laryngeal edema typically seen in caustic ingestions involves the epiglottis and supraglottic larynx, often sparing the true vocal folds.[53,55] The larynx is examined in all caustic ingestions. Of particular concern is the ingestion of low phosphate or nonphosphate detergents. Ingestions of even small amounts of these may cause severe upper airway edema and airway compromise 1 to 5 hours after ingestion and warrant admission to the hospital for airway observation even in the absence of other significant injuries.[55] If significant edema or stridor is present, the airway should be stabilized with tracheotomy. Because of the potential for exacerbating the laryngeal injuries, nasotracheal and orotracheal intubation are avoided; tracheotomy is the preferred method of airway stabilization. The mouth, pharynx, and laryngeal inlet should be irrigated with water to remove any remnants of the offending agent. The use of steroids and antibiotics remains common but controversial. Further evaluation and management of esophageal injuries should then proceed. A discussion of the protocol for evaluation and treatment of esophageal injuries is beyond the scope of this chapter but can be found elsewhere.[53,54,56,57]

Thermal laryngeal injuries are usually encountered in patients who have experienced significant burn injuries from closed-space fires.[58] The laryngeal injuries most often result from thermal insult to the supraglottic and glottic larynx.[59] Because inhalational injuries may affect the larynx, tracheobronchial tree, or the lung parenchyma, all patients experiencing significant inhalational injuries should undergo flexible laryngoscopy and bronchoscopy. The diagnosis of laryngeal or tracheal injury is made by the presence of carbonized materials with inflammation, edema, or necrosis.[58] In patients with hypovolemic shock, as commonly occurs in patients with significant burn injuries, there may be severe injury to the larynx or trachea without signs of edema initially. The edema usually ensues with cardiovascular resuscitation.[60] The

Table 20–4. Indications for Operative Evaluation of Penetrating Laryngeal Injury.

Endolaryngeal lacerations

Expanding neck hematoma

Subcutaneous emphysema

Audible air leak from neck wound

Hemoptysis

Laryngeal framework disruption

Impaired vocal fold mobility

Endolaryngeal edema

Dysphagia/odynophagia

Stridor/dyspnea

epiglottis, aryepiglottic folds, and hypopharynx are most prone to edema, which is usually progressive in the first few hours after injury.[60]

The primary concern is protection of the airway. The decision to perform tracheotomy versus orotracheal intubation is controversial. Orotracheal and nasotracheal intubation carry the risk of causing further mucosal injury. Several studies have suggested that tracheotomy in the burn patient places the patient at increased risk of long-term sequelae such as tracheal stenosis and sepsis.[59,61,62] In general, tracheotomy is recommended in patients who cannot be endotracheally intubated due to significant laryngeal injury, those who fail extubation, and/or those in whom prolonged respiratory support will be necessary.[58,60,62]

Late complications associated with thermal and caustic injuries include stenosis and webbing. Scar formation may continue for several months following the initial insult.[58] Thus, the larynx and trachea should be serially evaluated over the course of several months. Repair is delayed until scar formation has stabilized. This helps to minimize the incidence of recurrent scar formation and enhances the likelihood for successful repair.[58,60]

Iatrogenic Injuries

Iatrogenic injuries to the larynx include radiation injuries and injuries that result from intubation. Doses of radiation used to treat head and neck cancer (6000 cGy–7000 cGy) can result in injury to the mucosa and cartilaginous framework of the larynx if it is included in the radiation field. These injuries are an expected outcome of radiation therapy and can include mucosal drying, soft tissue edema, and laryngeal radionecrosis. The treatment of mucosal drying is symptomatic, encouraging frequent water ingestion. Several preparations are available to minimize xerostomia in patients receiving radiation therapy to the head and neck. These work with variable success. Laryngeal edema from radiation can become problematic, resulting in narrowing of the airway. In some patients, this can be treated effectively with intermittent steroid use. In others, tracheotomy is necessary to help maintain an adequate airway.[69]

The incidence of radionecrosis of the larynx is approximately 1% of patients who receive doses in the range of 6000 cGy to 7000 cGy and increases with larger daily fractions.[70] Patients who continue to smoke or drink alcohol during and after radiation therapy are at increased risk. The presence of laryngopharyngeal reflux may contribute to the development and exacerbation of radionecrosis. Radionecrosis can pose a diagnostic dilemma to the clinician, because the symptoms are similar to the symptoms of recurrent cancer; and there is often associated edema and/or ulceration overlying the devitalized tissue. It is often difficult to distinguish between recurrent or persistent tumor and radionecrosis. These patients should undergo direct laryngoscopy and biopsy. Biopsy of radiation-damaged tissue often shows necrotic debris. However, in an inadequately biopsied area, a similar specimen can be obtained in the face of recurrent tumor. Although deep biopsies may exacerbate necrosis, tumor recurrence must be ruled out.[65] Hyperbaric oxygen treatments can be offered to patients with radionecrosis of the larynx, as the increased tissue oxygenation induced by such treatments may promote healing and prevent further damage to the laryngeal framework.[66,67] If the signs and symptoms worsen or are not improved with conservative treatment, partial or total laryngectomy should be considered because of the risk of a life-threatening infection with a retained necrotic larynx and because of the high risk of malignancy in this scenario.[65-67]

The most common iatrogenic injury to the larynx results from intubation trauma.[68] Because children are more often subjected to prolonged intubation as premature infants and neonates in the intensive care unit, they are more likely to experience complications as a result of being intubated.[69] The reported incidence of intubation injury in adults and children has decreased in the last 20 years from 18% to 3% due to improved equipment and methods of intubation.[21] The advent of low-pressure cuffed endotracheal tubes of uniform diameter has significantly decreased the incidence of subglottic stenosis in adults. In addition, the development of ventilator adapters to prevent excessive movement of the endotracheal tube has also contributed to a decrease in the incidence of intubation trauma.[21,68]

In neonates, prolonged intubation often leads to circumferential granulation tissue, scarring, and eventual stenosis of the subglottis. This region is most often affected because the cricoid is the narrowest portion of the airway in the neonate and is, thus, most traumatized by the endotracheal tube. The posterior tilt of the cricoid cartilage in neonates likely helps to prevent damage to the interarytenoid region, which is the most common site of injury in the adult.

Subglottic stenosis from intubation injury in the infant can be managed similarly to congenital subglottic stenosis. For stenoses that are less than 50% obstructing, management can consist of observation, dilatation, or CO_2 laser excision. If CO_2 laser is used for a circumferential stenosis, it is done serially with no more than 30% of the circumference resected during any one procedure to prevent restenosis. If the stenosis is

50 to 70% obstructing, one may consider either endoscopic procedures or open procedures, depending on the location and potential ease of an endoscopic procedure. Stenotic regions that are more than 70% obstructing are managed best using open techniques. Lesions isolated to the subglottic region may be treated with an anterior cricoid split procedure. Longer stenotic regions may be treated with either cartilage grafting or resection with end-to-end anastomosis. Completely stenotic regions require resection and reanastomosis.[70]

In the adult, the glottis is the narrowest portion of the airway, and the posterior glottis often supports the endotracheal tube in the adult. Movement of the arytenoids against the endotracheal tube with respiration often contributes to ischemic necrosis of the thin mucosa overlying the vocal process. This can be followed by ulceration, chondritis, granulation, granuloma formation, and scarring. Often, removal of the endotracheal tube will allow for normal healing in the absence of gastroesophageal reflux, which should be treated presumptively during the healing process.

Scarring of the posterior glottis uncommonly causes problems with airway compromise. Attempts to release posterior glottic scar bands usually should be avoided to prevent worsening stenosis unless substantial symptoms justify the risks. In cases of significant airway compromise and minimal posterior

scarring, treatment with microscopic direct laryngoscopy and carbon dioxide laser division of the scar band is usually successful.[71] Care should be taken during these divisions to protect the normal mucosa of the interarytenoid region.[72] Occasionally, repeat microscopic direct laryngoscopy with repeat laser division is needed. In cases with moderate to severe interarytenoid scarring, a laryngofissure with a mucosal advancement flap from the interarytenoid notch or from an aryepiglottic fold or a similar endoscopic procedure can be performed (Fig 20–22).[73] The value of adjunctive treatment with topical mitomycin-C to prevent restenosis is being studied currently, but preliminary results are encouraging.[74]

Conclusion

Injury to the laryngotracheal complex can result from blunt, penetrating, caustic, thermal, and iatrogenic insults. The primary concern in the initial management of these injuries is the establishment and maintenance of an adequate airway. Treatment can then address the reconstruction of the normal anatomical relationships of the larynx and trachea in an attempt to restore the normal phonatory, respiratory, and protective functions of the larynx.

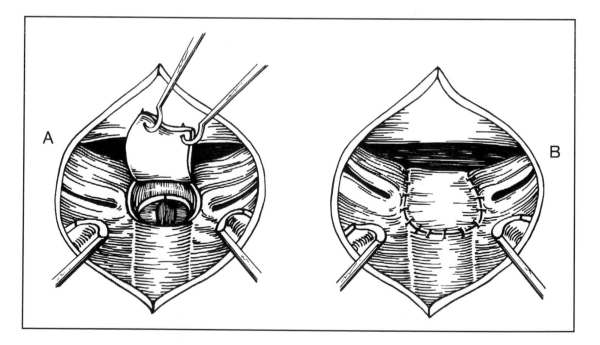

Fig 20–22. A. After resection of posterior glottic stenosis, a superiorly based mucosal flap is elevated. **B.** The mucosal flap is advanced into the defect and fixed with fine, absorbable sutures.

References

1. Bent JP III, Silver JR, Porubsky ES. Acute laryngeal trauma: a review of 77 patients. *Otolaryngol Head Neck Surg.* 1993;109:441–449.

2. Schaefer SD. The treatment of acute external laryngeal injuries. *Arch Otolaryngol Head Neck Surg.* 1991;117:35–39.

3. Jewett BS, Shockley WW, Rutledge R. External laryngeal trauma analysis of 392 patients. *Arch Otolaryngol Head Neck Surg.* 1999;125:877–880.

4. Gussack GS, Jurkovich GJ, Luterman A. Laryngotracheal trauma: a protocol approach to a rare injury. *Laryngoscope.* 1986;96:660–665.

5. Minard G, Kudsk KA, Croce MA, Butts JA, et al. Laryngotracheal trauma. *Am Surg.* 1992;58:181–187.

6. Angood PB, Attia EL, Brown RA, Mudder DS. Extrinsic civilian trauma to the larynx and cervical trachea—important predictors of long-term morbidity. *J Trauma.* 1986;26:869–873.

7. Schaefer SD, Close LG. Acute management of laryngeal trauma. *Ann Otol Rhinol Laryngol.* 1989;98:98–104.

8. Komisar A, Blaugrund SM, Camins M. Head and neck trauma in taxicabs. *Arch Otolaryngol Head Neck Surg.* 1991;117:442–445.

9. Blanc VF, Tremblay NA. The complications of tracheal intubation: a new classification with a review of the literature. *Anesth Analg.* 1974;53:202–213.

10. Whited RE. A prospective of laryngotracheal sequelae in long-term intubation. *Laryngoscope.* 1984;94:367–377.

11. Leopold DA. Laryngeal trauma: a historical comparison of treatment methods. *Arch Otolaryngol.* 1983;109:106–112.

12. Cohn AM, Larson DL. Laryngeal injury: a critical review. *Arch Otolaryngol.* 1976;102:166–170.

13. Olson NR. Surgical treatment of acute blunt laryngeal injuries. *Ann Otol Rhinol Laryngol.* 1978;87:716–721.

14. Potter LR, Sessions DG, Ogura JH. Blunt laryngotracheal trauma. *Otolaryngology.* 1978;86:909–923.

15. Trone TH, Schaefer SD, Carder HM. Blunt and penetrating laryngeal trauma: a 13-year review. *Otolaryngol Head Neck Surg.* 1980;88:257–261.

16. Holinger PH, Schild JA. Pharyngeal, laryngeal, and tracheal injuries in the pediatric age group. *Ann Otol Rhinol Laryngol.* 1972;81:538–545.

17. Pennington CL. External trauma of the larynx and trachea: immediate treatment and management. *Ann Otol Rhinol Laryngol.* 1972;81:546–554.

18. Travis LW, Olson NR, Melvin JW, Snyder RG. Static and dynamic impact trauma of the human larynx. *Am Acad Ophthamol Otolaryngol.* 1975;80:382–390.

19. Ashbaugh DG, Gordon JH. Traumatic avulsion of the trachea associated with cricoid fracture. *J Thorac Cardiovasc Surg.* 1975;69:800–803.

20. Gold SM, Gerber ME, Shott SR, Myer CM III. Blunt laryngotracheal trauma in children. *Arch Otolaryngol Head Neck Surg.* 1997;123:83–87.

21. Bryce DP. Current management of laryngotracheal injury. *Adv Otorhinolaryngol.* 1983;29:27–38.

22. Ford HR, Gardner MJ, Lynch JM. Laryngotracheal disruption from blunt pediatric neck injuries: impact of early recognition and intervention on outcome. *J Pediatr Surg.* 1995;30:331–334.

23. Myer CM III, Orobello P, Cotton RT, Bratcher GO. Blunt laryngeal trauma in children. *Laryngoscope.* 1987;97:1043–1048.

24. Offiah CJ, Endres D. Isolated laryngotracheal separation following blunt trauma to the neck. *J Laryngol Otol.* 1997;111:1079–1081.

25. Alonso WA, Caruso VG, Roncace EA. Minibikes, a new factor in laryngotracheal trauma. *Ann Otol Rhinol Laryngol.* 1973;82:800–804.

26. Schild JA, Denneny EC. Evaluation and treatment of acute laryngeal fractures. *Head Neck.* 1989;11:491–496.

27. Hirano M, Kurita S, Terasawa R. Difficulty in high-pitched phonation by laryngeal trauma. *Arch Otolaryngol.* 1985;111:59–61.

28. Stanley RB Jr, Cooper DS, Florman SH. Phonatory effects of thyroid cartilage fractures. *Ann Otol Rhinol Laryngol.* 1987;96:493–496.

29. Hoffman HT, Brunberg JA, Winter P, et al. Arytenoid subluxation: diagnosis and treatment. *Ann Otol Rhinol Laryngol.* 1991;100:1–9.

30. Sataloff RT, Feldman M, Darby KS, et al. Arytenoid dislocation. *J Voice.* 1988;1:368–377.

31. Sataloff RT, Spiegel JR, Hawkshaw MJ, Rosen DC. Vocal fold hemorrhage: diagnosis and treatment. *NATS J.* 1995;51(5):45–48.

32. Reece CP, Shatney CH. Blunt injuries to the cervical trachea: review of 51 patients. *South Med J.* 1988;81:1542–1547.

33. Chodosh PL. Cricoid fracture with tracheal avulsion. *Arch Otolaryngol.* 1968;87:461–467.

34. Harris HH. Management of injuries to the larynx and trachea. *Laryngoscope.* 1972;82:1924–1929.

35. Ogura J. Management of traumatic injuries of the larynx and trachea including stenosis. *J Laryngol Otol.* 1971;85:1259–1261.

36. Fuhrman GM, Stieg FH, Buerk CA III. Blunt laryngeal trauma: classification and management protocol. *J Trauma.* 1990;30:87–92.

37. Sataloff RT, Bough ID, Spiegel JR. Arytenoid dislocation: diagnosis and treatment. *Laryngoscope.* 1994;104:1353–1361.

38. Olson NR. Laryngeal suspension and epiglottic flap in laryngopharyngeal trauma. *Ann Otol Rhinol Laryngol.* 1976;85:533–537.

39. Thomas GK, Stevens MH. Stenting in experimental laryngeal injuries. *Arch Otolaryngol.* 1975;101:217–221.

40. Dedo HH. Endoscopic Teflon keel for anterior glottic web. *Ann Otol Rhinol Laryngol.* 1979;88:467–473.

41. McNaught RC. Surgical correction of anterior web of the larynx. *Trans Am Laryngol Rhinol Otol Soc.* 1950:232–242.

42. Woo P, Kellman R. Laryngeal framework reconstruction with miniplates: indications and extended indications in 27 cases. *Oper Techn Otolaryngol Head Neck Surg.* 1972;3:159–164.

43. Woo P. Laryngeal framework reconstruction with mini-plates. *Ann Otol Rhinol Laryngol.* 1990;99:772–777.

44. Pou AM, Shoemaker DL, Carrau RL, et al. Repair of laryngeal fractures using adaptation plates. *Head Neck.* 1998;20:707–713.

45. Grillo HC, Donahue DM, Mathisen DJ, et al. Postintubation tracheal stenosis: treatment and results. *J Thorac Cardiovasc Surg.* 1995;109:486–492.

46. Crumley RL. Teflon versus thyroplasty versus nerve transfer: a comparison. *Ann Otol Rhinol Laryngol.* 1990; 99:759–763.

47. Crumley RL. Update: ansa cervicalis to recurrent laryngeal nerve anastomosis for unilateral recurrent laryngeal nerve paralysis. *Laryngoscope.* 1991;100:384–387.

48. Harrison DF. Bullet wounds of the larynx and trachea. *Arch Otolaryngol.* 1984;110:203–205.

49. Grewal H, Rao PM, Mukerji S, Ivatury RR. Management of penetrating laryngotracheal injuries. *Head Neck.* 1995;17:494–502.

50. Feliciano DV, Bitondo CG, Mattox KL, et al. Combined tracheoesophageal injuries. *Am J Surg.* 1985;150:710–715.

51. Defore WW Jr, Mattox KL, Hansen HA, et al. Surgical management of penetrating injuries to the esophagus. *Am J Surg.* 1977;134:734–738.

52. Glatterer MS Jr, Toon RS, Ellestad C, et al. Management of blunt and penetrating external esophageal trauma. *J Trauma.* 1985;25:784–792.

53. Hawkins DB, Demeter MJ, Barnett TE. Caustic ingestion: controversies in management. A review of 214 cases. *Laryngoscope.* 1980;90:98–109.

54. Schild JA. Caustic ingestion in adult patients. *Laryngoscope.* 1985;95:1199–1201.

55. Einhorn A, Horton L, Altieri M, et al. Serious respiratory consequences of detergent ingestions in children. *Pediatrics.* 1989;84:472–474.

56. Holinger LD. Caustic ingestion, esophageal injury and stricture. In: Holinger LD, Lusk RP, Green CG, eds. *Pediatric Laryngology and Bronchoesophagology.* Philadelphia, Pa: Lippincott Williams and Wilkins; 1996:295–304.

57. Wijburg FA, Beukers MM, Heymans HS, et al. Nasogastric intubation as sole treatment of caustic esophageal lesions. *Ann Otol Rhinol Laryngol.* 1985;94:337–341.

58. Jones JE, Rosenberg D. Management of laryngotracheal thermal trauma in children. *Laryngoscope.* 1995;105:540–542.

59. Moylan JA. Smoke inhalation and burn injury. *Surg Clin North Am.* 1980;60:1533–1540.

60. Miller RP, Gray SD, Cotton RT, Myer CM III. Airway reconstruction following laryngotracheal thermal trauma. *Laryngoscope.* 1988;98:826–829.

61. Lund T, Goodwin CW, McManus WF, et al. Upper airway sequelae in burn patient requiring endotracheal intubation or tracheostomy. *Ann Surg.* 1985;201:374–382.

62. Eckhauser FE, Billote J, Burke JF, Quinby WC. Tracheotomy complicating massive burn injury. *Am J Surg.* 1974;127:418–423.

63. Calhoun KH, Deskin RW, Garza C, et al. Long-term airway sequelae in a pediatric burn population. *Laryngoscope.* 1988;98:721–725.

64. Calcaterra TC, Stern F, Ward PH. Dilemma of delayed radiation injury of the larynx. *Ann Otol Rhinol Laryngol.* 1972;81:501–507.

65. Parsons JT. The effect of radiation on normal tissues of the head and neck. In: Million RR, Cassisi NJ, eds. *Management of Head and Neck Cancer: A Multidisciplinary Approach.* Philadelphia, Pa: JB Lippincott; 1984:183–184.

66. Feldmeier JJ, Heimbach RD, Davolt DA, Brakora MJ. Hyperbaric oxygen as an adjunctive treatment for severe laryngeal necrosis: a report of nine consecutive cases. *Undersea Hyperb Med.* 1993;20:329–335.

67. Ferguson BJ, Hudson WR, Farmer JC Jr. Hyperbaric oxygen therapy for laryngeal radionecrosis. *Ann Otol Rhinol Laryngol.* 1987;69:1–6.

68. Richardson MA. Laryngeal anatomy and mechanisms of trauma. *Ear Nose Throat J.* 1981;60:346–351.

69. Cotton RT, Seid AB. Management of the extubation problem in the premature child: anterior cricoid split as an alternative to tracheotomy. *Ann Otol Rhinol Laryngol.* 1980;89:508–511.

70. Lusk RP, Wooley AL, Holinger LD. Laryngotracheal stenosis. In: Holinger LD, Lusk RP, Green CG, eds. *Pediatric Laryngology and Bronchoesophagology.* Philadelphia, Pa: Lippincott Williams & Wilkins; 1996:172–184.

71. Dedo HH, Rowe LD. Laryngeal reconstruction in acute and chronic injuries. *Otolaryngol Clin North Am.* 1983; 16:373–389.

72. Dedo HH, Sooy FA. Endoscopic laser repair of posterior glottic, subglottic, and tracheal stenosis by division or micro-trapdoor flap. *Laryngoscope.* 1984;94:445–450.

73. Dedo HH, Sooy FA. Surgical repair of late glottic stenosis. *Ann Otol Rhinol Laryngol.* 1968;77:435–441.

74. Correa AJ, Reinisch L, Sanders DL, et al. Inhibition of subglottic stenosis with mitomycin-C in the canine model. *Ann Otol Rhinol Laryngol.* 1999;108:1053–1060.

21

Cricoarytenoid and Cricothyroid Joint Injury: Evaluation and Treatment

Robert Thayer Sataloff

Cricoarytenoid Joint Injury

Vocal fold hypomobility immobility may occur following internal or external neck trauma. The impaired mobility may be due to vocal fold paresis or paralysis, cricoarytenoid joint fixation, or arytenoid dislocation or subluxation. Dislocation is the displacement of a structure, particularly a disarrangement of the normal relation of bones or cartilages entering into the formation of a joint. Dislocation and luxation are synonymous. Subluxation is an incomplete dislocation, such that there is still contact between joint surfaces, although the relationship is altered. Subluxation is synonymous with semiluxation, and it constitutes a specific form of dislocation. Most arytenoid dislocations are actually subluxations; but the term dislocation encompasses partial and complete malposition and will be used throughout this chapter. Arytenoid dislocation is misdiagnosed commonly as vocal fold paralysis. When accurate diagnosis is delayed, surgical repair becomes more difficult, although not impossible as previously thought.[1,2] Many laryngologists were taught that arytenoid reduction was impossible or inappropriate beyond the first or second week following injury. Our experience suggests that reasonably good results are common so long as the arytenoid is reduced within about 10 weeks.[2] Although reduction can be performed even many years following arytenoid dislocation, late reductions usually result in correction of the vertical height disparity without restoration of joint motion.

Embryology and Anatomy

Understanding the complicated embryology and anatomy of the arytenoid cartilages is helpful in clarifying surgical principles and avoiding complications. The primordium of the larynx, trachea, bronchi, and lungs arises as an outgrowth of the pharynx during the third week of embryonic life, forming a laryngotracheal groove.[3] This anterior groove lies immediately posterior to the hypobranchial eminence and becomes the primitive laryngeal aditus. The aditus lies between the sixth branchial arches. The laryngotracheal groove fuses in a caudocranial direction at about the fourth week. The ventral ends of the sixth branchial arches grow and form the arytenoid eminences. During the seventh week, a fissure appears on each arytenoid eminence extending into the primitive vestibule. This is the laryngeal ventricle. The last portion of laryngotracheal groove to be obliterated is the intra-arytenoid sulcus at about 11 weeks.

Laryngeal hyaline cartilages develop from branchial arch mesoderm, and elastic cartilages are derived from mesoderm of the floor of the pharynx.[4] Most of the arytenoid is composed of hyaline cartilage. However, the vocal processes are developed separately in association with the vocal folds and consist of elastic cartilage. "Arytenoid" comes from the Greek word *arytainoeides*, meaning ladle-shaped. The cartilages are pyramidal, consisting of an apex, base, and two processes. The base articulates with the cricoid cartilage. The apex attaches to the corniculate cartilage of Santorini and to the aryepiglottic fold. The vocal process projects anteriorly to connect with the vocal ligament, and the muscular process is the point of insertion for most of the muscles that move the arytenoid.[5] The cricoarytenoid facets are well-defined, smooth, and symmetrical. Each arytenoid articulates with an elliptical facet on the posterior superior margin of the cricoid ring. The cricoid facet is about 6 mm long and is cylindrical.[6] Traditional teaching holds that the cricoarytenoid joint motion includes rotating, gliding, and rocking. Most of the cricoarytenoid motion is rocking. However, along the long axis of the cricoid facet, gliding also occurs.[7] Limited rotary pivoting is permitted as well. More recent studies suggest that these traditional descriptions are not fully accurate and that complex revolution may more succinctly describe arytenoid behavior.[8] The arytenoid cartilages and the cricoarytenoid facets are extremely symmetric and consistent.[9] The cricoarytenoid joint is an arthrodial join, supported by a capsule lined with synovium. The capsule is strengthened posteriorly by the cricoarytenoid ligament.[9] This ligament is strong and ordinarily prevents anterior subluxation. The axis of the joint is at an angle of about 45 degrees from the sagittal plane and 40 degrees from the horizontal plane. The cricoarytenoid joint controls abduction and adduction of the true vocal folds, thereby facilitating respiration, protection of the airway, and phonation.

Arytenoid motion is controlled directly by intrinsic laryngeal muscles, including the posterior cricoarytenoid, lateral cricoarytenoid, interarytenoid, and thyroarytenoid. It is also affected by the cricothyroid muscle, which increases longitudinal tension of the vocal fold (which attaches to the vocal process of the arytenoid), and to a lesser degree by the thyroepiglottic muscle, which tenses the aryepiglottic fold.

Arytenoid Dislocation: Diagnosis

Traditionally, arytenoid dislocation has been suspected on the basis of history and absence of the jostle phenomenon present in many cases of unilateral vocal fold paralysis.[10] Often it is not diagnosed until direct laryngoscopy reveals impaired passive mobility of the vocal fold. Preoperative differentiation between vocal fold paralysis and arytenoid dislocation should be possible in virtually all cases. However, if not considered specifically, it will often be missed. Disparity in height between the vocal fold processes is much easier to see in slow motion under stroboscopic light at various pitches than with continuous light. In posterior dislocations, the vocal process and vocal fold are usually higher on the dislocated side[11] (Fig 21–1). In anterior dislocations, generally they are lower on the abnormal side[12] (Fig 21–2). In either case, the injured vocal fold may move sluggishly or be immobile. Rarely, abduction and adduction may appear almost normal under continuous light. Video documentation

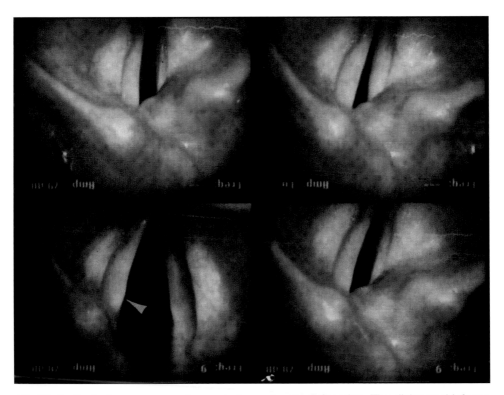

Fig 21–1. Typical appearance of a posterior arytenoid dislocation. The dislocated left arytenoid lifts the vocal process (*arrowhead*) so the abnormal side overlaps the mobile vocal fold.

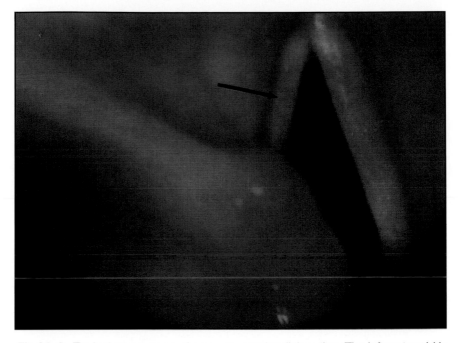

Fig 21–2. Typical appearance of a severe anterior dislocation. The left arytenoid is tilted forward, and the vocal process pulls the vocal fold to a lower level (*arrow*), so the mobile right vocal fold overlaps the abnormal side during adduction.

of the pre- and postoperative appearance can prove particularly helpful in cases of arytenoid dislocation not only diagnostically, but also because many of these patients are involved in litigation related to their injuries.

The most valuable tests are the stroboscopic examination to visualize differences in vocal process height; CT scan of the larynx, which should image the arytenoid dislocation and reveal clouding or obliteration of the cricoarytenoid joint space; and laryngeal electromyography to differentiate an immobile dislocated arytenoid joint from vocal fold paralysis. Airflow analysis is also helpful in documenting changes before and after therapy. Strobovideolaryngoscopy is also important to assess other vocal fold injuries. Stiffness and scar of the musculomembranous portion of the vocal folds are found commonly in association with arytenoid dislocation. The trauma causing dislocation frequently involves considerable force that results in vocal fold hemorrhage. It is important to recognize the presence of vocal fold scar prior to reducing an arytenoid dislocation so that the patient can be informed about reasonable expectations for surgical outcome.

When the author reported his series of 26 cases in 1994, only 31 additional cases had been reported in the literature.[2] Since that time, additional cases have been documented.[10-22] Although anterior and posterior dislocations are described most commonly, the arytenoid can be dislocated in any direction.[2] Complex disloca-

tions have been observed in some of the more than two dozen cases cared for by the author since our last report.[2]

Posterior dislocation is commonly an extubation injury. The arytenoid is displaced posterolaterally, and the vocal process is high and laterally positioned. Anterior dislocation is commonly most caused by intubation. The laryngoscope engages the posterior lip of the arytenoid, tearing the posterior cricoarytenoid ligament and tipping the arytenoid anteromedially (Fig 21–3). The vocal process ordinarily is lower than normal in such cases. Complex arytenoid dislocations also occur and can be particularly challenging. In our more recent (unreported) cases, direct anterior dislocation was seen in two patients. In these cases, the arytenoid was displaced anteriorly, but the vocal process was high. This injury requires considerable trauma, with disruption of cartilage. Both cases followed intubation. With injury of this severity, endoscopic reduction has been less satisfactory than with more typical anterior or posterior dislocations. In rare instances, even more complicated situations can be encountered, including bilateral arytenoid dislocation (Fig 21–4).

Techniques for Surgical Reduction of Arytenoid Dislocation

Although early spontaneous reduction of arytenoid dislocation has been reported,[2] surgical reduction

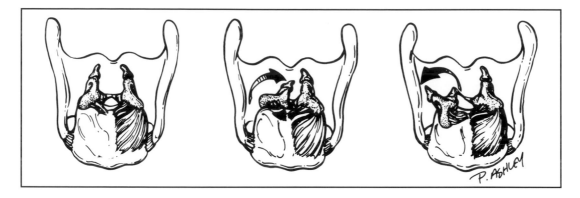

Fig 21–3 On the left, a normal larynx can be visualized from the back. The cricoarytenoid ligament is seen on both sides. The interarytenoid muscle has been removed. The posterior cricoarytenoid muscle is preserved on the right. In posterior arytenoid dislocation (*center image*), the posterior cricoarytenoid ligament is generally made more lax, and it is not torn. In an anterior dislocation (*right image*), the posterior cricoarytenoid ligament is generally torn (as illustrated) or avulsed from its insertion into the cricoid or arytenoid cartilage.

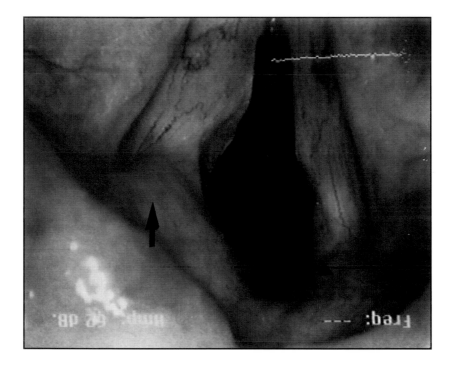

Fig 21–4. This 62-year-old artist and teacher awoke from abdominal surgery with severe hoarseness, breathiness, and sore throat 10 months prior to our evaluation. Both vocal folds were immobile, and laryngeal electromyography was normal. Note the very unusual position of the arytenoids. They are at different heights. The right arytenoids (*curved arrow*) is dislocated posteriorly. The left arytenoid has suffered a complex anterior arytenoid dislocation (*straight arrow*) with the vocal process displaced straight forward and high. Note the bowing and laxity of the left vocal fold.

generally is required. Voice therapy for at least a brief period may be helpful in some cases, and preoperative evaluation by a speech-language pathologist is generally recommended. Surgeons also should be aware that nonsurgical approaches have been suggested. For example, Rontal and Rontal have introduced the concept of chemical tenotomy using Botulinum toxin to enhance spontaneous reductions.[23] In some cases, adjunct procedures performed at the time of arytenoid reduction may also be advisable, as discussed below.

Closed Reduction for Posterior Arytenoid Dislocation

The author has found the anesthesiologist's old-fashioned, straight, Miller-3 laryngoscope blade to be the most useful instrument for posterior arytenoid dislocation (Fig 21–5). Newer models do not have the distal rolled lip. The instrument is placed in the piriform sinus with the rolled tip of the laryngoscope against the infralateral edge of the dislocated cartilage (Fig 21–6). The surgeon's other hand is placed on the opposite side of the larynx externally to apply counterpressure. The arytenoid is distracted cranially, then manipulated anteromedially to pop the arytenoid back into position. Substantial force is often necessary, sometimes the full strength of the author's right arm.

A Holinger laryngoscope usually is used to reduce anterior dislocations. More delicate instruments such as cupped forceps are not strong enough and are more likely to lacerate the mucosa and expose cartilage to the risk of infection. No instrument should be placed under the vocal process because of the risk of fracture at the embryologic fusion plane between the vocal process and body of the arytenoid. The Holinger laryngoscope is rotated so that its supralateral surface makes broad contact with the anteromedial face of the arytenoid. The surgeon's other hand is placed against the larynx externally and posteriorly for manipulation and counterpressure (Fig 21–7).

For complex dislocations, a combination of these techniques is used. It may be necessary to refracture the cartilage and/or separate the joint in order to manipulate the arytenoid. For example, in lateral and anterolateral dislocations, it has been helpful to use the Holinger laryngoscope to disrupt the cartilage and fibrosis, bringing the arytenoid posteriorly. Then, a combination of the Holinger laryngoscope and Miller-3 laryngoscope is used to return the arytenoid to optimal position.

When endoscopic closed reduction is not successful or is so unstable that dislocation recurs, open reduc-

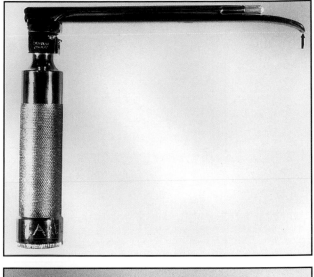

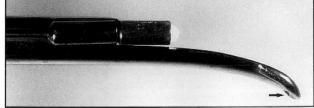

Fig 21–5. Straight Miller-3 laryngoscope blade (*top*) used by anesthesiologists. Below, the curved tip with a slight lip (*arrow*) has proven ideal for the reduction of posterior arytenoid dislocation.

tion and fixation should be considered. The procedure is performed using a standard arytenoid adduction/rotation approach. Usually, the joint is entered. If the joint has been obliterated by scar, a "joint" is created sharply, usually using an iris scissors. The arytenoid is moved to optimize vocal process position. The surgery is performed with the patient awake, and it is important to adjust vocal process position while the patient is phonating at his or her habitual frequency, rather than using a high-pitch /i/. If the arytenoid is unstable or hypermobile, it is sometimes possible to stabilize it with three to six fine sutures placed through the soft tissue attached to the cricoid and arytenoid cartilages. This approach has not been discussed prior to this publication; but the author has found it useful to stabilize a hypermobile cartilage in selected cases, particularly if the arytenoid is tending to fall anteriorly. Essentially, the sutures replace the posterior cricoarytenoid ligament.

Special situations and challenging clinical conditions sometimes demand other solutions to the problems of arytenoid dislocation. On three occasions, the

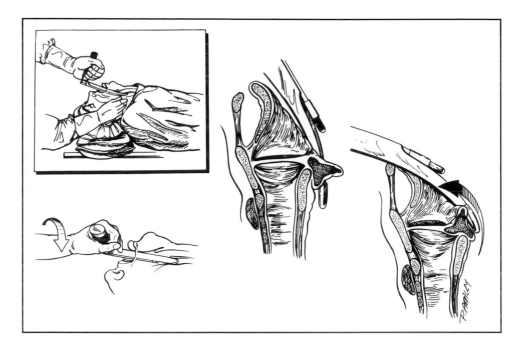

Fig 21–6. To reduce a posterior arytenoid dislocation, the tip of a Miller-3 blade is placed in the piriform sinus (*upper left*). To reduce a left posterior dislocation, the laryngoscope is rotated medially (*lower left*) so that the lip on the laryngoscope engages the dislocated arytenoids as the laryngoscope is drawn superiorly out of the piriform sinus. Digital external counterpressure (*upper left*) is required; and the right hand ordinarily needs to be placed more anteriorly than illustrated in this figure. If illustrated in proper position, the hand would block visualization of the tip of the laryngoscope. Once the arytenoid has been hooked by the lip of the laryngoscope (*center*), considerable force is necessary to distract the arytenoid in a cephalad direction and then to rotate it anteromedially, reducing it (*right*).

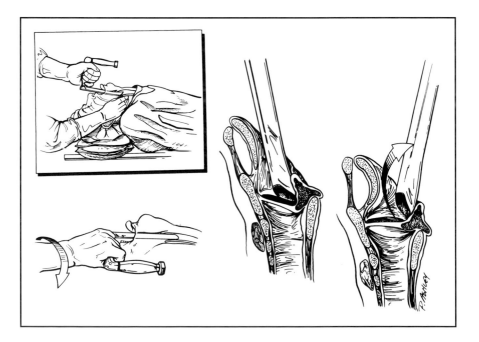

Fig 21–7. To reduce an anterior dislocation, a Holinger laryngoscope is positioned (*upper left*). To reduce a right arytenoid dislocation, the laryngoscope is rotated about 130° (*lower left*) so that the upper surface of the laryngoscope makes broad contact with the medial surface of the dislocated arytenoid (*center*). The surgeon's contralateral hand is placed externally, posteriorly on the larynx (*upper left*), so that the arytenoid is manipulated between the laryngoscope tip and the fingers of the surgeon's right hand, to reduce this right arytenoid anterior dislocation. Considerable force is required to reduce the arytenoid (*right*); and care must be taken not to injure or avulse the vocal process.

author has used digital reduction (Fig 21–8). The first was on an edentulous patient in an intensive care unit who had extubated herself repeatedly. Her physicians were concerned about even the risk of transporting her to the operating room, let alone sedating her. Yet, she had respiratory problems, and it was important to restore the efficiency of her cough. Her tongue was held with gauze in the manner of indirect laryngoscopy, at the bedside. An assistant helped stabilize her larynx externally. A finger was placed in her piriform sinus, and her posterior arytenoid dislocation was manually reduced. It maintained good position and mobility returned. This technique has been used on two other patients whose arytenoids redislocated within 48 hours following surgical reduction.

Most recently, another new technique was utilized. The author was called to see a patient who had awakened with a hoarse, weak, breathy voice and ineffective cough following anterior cervical fusion. Posterior arytenoid dislocation was diagnosed easily, and good vocal fold innervation was confirmed by electromyography. However, the patient had a short, thick neck and was flexed in a halo, and on full-dose coumadin. In the operating room, the arytenoid was re-

duced indirectly under nasal fiberoptic laryngoscopic control. A right-angle bayonet forceps was used. This is the instrument that used to be utilized routinely for holding cocainized cotton in the piriform sinuses to provide local anesthesia to the larynx. The tip of the forceps was covered with a red rubber catheter. The instrument was placed in the piriform sinus, and the arytenoid was lifted cranially, anteriorly and medially; and it popped back into position easily (Fig 21–9).

It is worthwhile attempting endoscopic reduction even long after the injury.[1,2,22] In 1998 (not yet reported in detail), the author successfully reduced an anterior arytenoid dislocation that had occurred 38 years previously, restoring vertical symmetry of the vocal process and fold, although thyroplasty was necessary to provide adequate medialization.

Adjunctive Measures

Several adjunctive measures should be considered when performing arytenoid reduction. For a long-standing posterior dislocation, especially when the reduction seems unstable, simultaneous medialization should be considered. Thyroplasty or injection of autol-

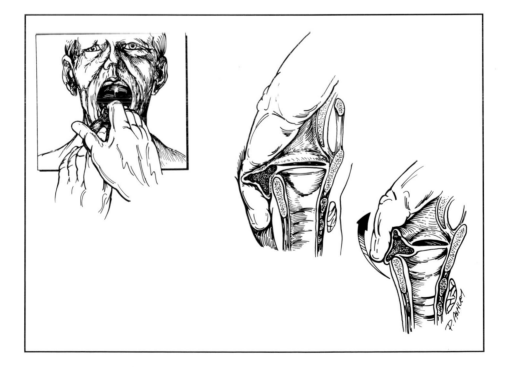

Fig 21–8. Digital reduction can be accomplished occasionally, especially for patients who are edentulous and who have had recent posterior dislocation or redislocation following recent arytenoid reduction. The patient's tongue is retracted by the patient or an assistant, leaving the surgeon's other hand free for external counterpressure (*left*). The surgeon's index or middle finger is placed in the piriform sinus, engaging the dislocated arytenoid (*center*). The surgeon's other hand applies external counterpressure, and the arytenoid is reduced digitally (*right*).

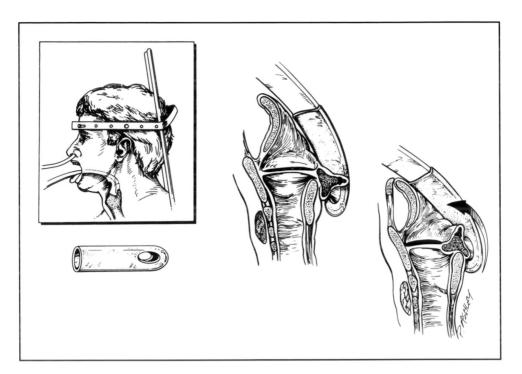

Fig 21–9. This previously undescribed procedure can be used for patients with posterior arytenoid dislocation and difficult anatomical constraints, such as this patient in a halo. A flexible laryngoscope is placed in the nostril to observe the larynx. A right-angle instrument such as a laryngeal bayonet forceps is covered with a shortened red rubber cathe- ter. The hole in the red rubber catheter (*lower left*) assists in making stable contact with the dislocated arytenoid. The posterior aspect of the dislocated arytenoid is engaged (*center*) and then drawn superiorly, and anteromedially, to reduce the dislocated cartilage (*right*).

ogous fat or collagen not only helps medialize the vocal fold, but also tends to pull the vocal process forward. This helps maintain the desired arytenoid position.

Following anterior dislocation, Rontal and Rontal have suggested Botulinum toxin injection into adductor muscles that tend to pull the arytenoid forward.[23] In fact, they have suggested that Botulinum toxin alone may result in "spontaneous" reduction without the need for surgical intervention. In this author's opinion, although this may be true in rare cases, it is not likely to occur once the joint has been fibrosed. More investigation of this novel concept is certainly warranted. However, the author (RTS) has used Botulinum toxin intraoperatively on several occasions when arytenoid reductions have appeared somewhat unstable. If a posterior dislocation can be reduced but tends to redislocate posteriorly when the patient is asked to cough in the operating room, Botulinum toxin can be injected into the posterior cricoarytenoid muscle. This permits unopposed pull from the adductor muscle, which tends to move the arytenoid in the desired direction. When combined with autologous fat injection, this technique has proven very effective.

Cricothyroid Joint Injury

Although injuries to the cricoarytenoid joint have been discussed in considerable detail, as noted above, dysphonia related to injury of the cricothyroid joint has been reported only rarely. [24,25] Otolaryngologists should be aware that injury to this structure can occur and cause severe voice dysfunction. The cricothyroid joint is a synovial articulation between the inferior cornu of the thyroid cartilage and the side of the cricoid cartilage, as described previously in chapter 6. In 1978, Schultz-Coulon described a 44-year-old professional singer who suffered a severe laryngeal contusion following a sports accident.[24] He recovered from the acute injury but complained of persistent loss of his falsetto voice. Left unilateral subluxation of the cricothyroid joint was diagnosed by xero-radiography. At lower pitches, his voice reportedly returned to normal, but he failed to recover his falsetto despite more than 12 months of intensive voice therapy. The authors attributed this permanent impairment to disturbance of the tilting mechanism between the cricoid and thyroid cartilages.

In 1998, Sataloff et al reported two patients with cricothyroid joint dysfunction.[25] Case 1 was a 38-year-old retired professional basketball player. He had been struck in the anterior neck 12 times during his ca-

reer. The last injury resulted in immediate and persistent breathiness, decreased volume, hoarseness, very low pitch, and inability to project his voice. His cricothyroid joint was fused and ossified (Fig 21–10);

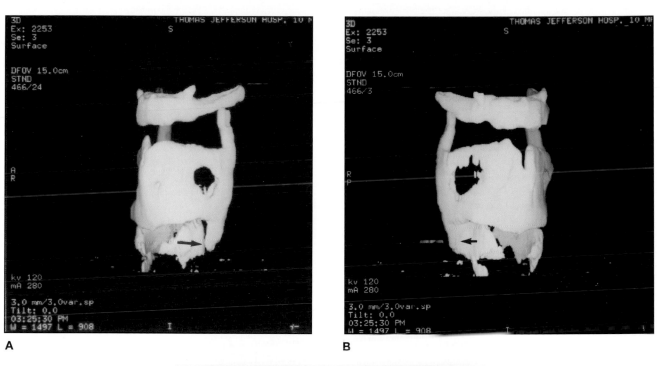

A

B

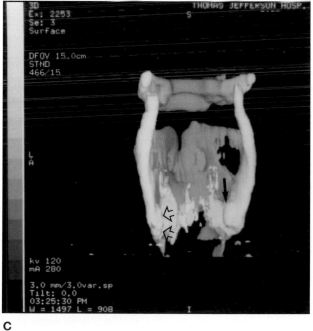

C

Fig 21–10. A. Anterior oblique CT scan of larynx showing normal left cricothyroid joint (*arrow*). **B.** Anterior oblique 3-D CT scan showing fusion of cricoid and thyroid in region of obliterated cricothyroid joint (*arrow*). **C.** Posterior-anterior 3-

D CT scan showing the left cricothyroid joint intact *(open arrows)* and fusion with new cartilage formation in the right cricothyroid joint region (*straight arrow*).

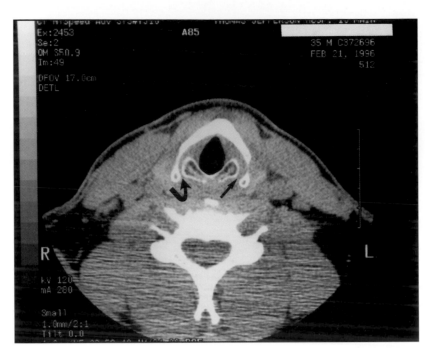

Fig 21–11. Axial CT scan showing normal right cricothyroid joint (*curved arrow*) and separated left cricothyroid joint (*straight arrow*). This appearance was consistent throughout the CT scans and is not due to rotation.

and his cricothyroid space was widened, fixing his voice in vocal fry. Case 2 was a 36-year-old male who had been involved in an altercation. He complained of dysphagia, mild vocal weakness, and laryngeal pain that was most pronounced during sneezing and coughing. His left cricothyroid joint was separated (Fig 21–11). Both patients had significant dysphonia due to impairment of the tilting mechanism between the cricoid and thyroid cartilages. In Case 1, motion between the cricoid and thyroid cartilages was eradicated completely. Voice therapy alone was not adequate, and surgery was necessary to restore mobility. In Case 2, motion was impaired but still present. Voice therapy permitted restoration of vocal quality and endurance adequate for the patient's purposes. If the patient had greater professional voice demands, surgery to realign the cricoid and thyroid cartilages (reduction of the joint separation) would have been offered.

Conclusion

Arytenoid dislocation is not rare, although it often is misdiagnosed as vocal fold paralysis. Although the goal of treatment is restoration of normal position and function, this cannot always be achieved. However, even correcting the vertical height abnormality is worthwhile. Essentially, this simplifies the problem,

converting it to one that can be managed easily by standard medialization surgery. It is essential for the surgeon to understand the anatomy and surgical principles involved, because visualization during surgical manipulation is extremely limited and considerable force is required. In virtually all cases, the patient's voice can be improved; and airway problems and other significant complications have not been encountered thus far.

Injury to the cricothyroid joint has been reported rarely, although it is certain that it has occurred more frequently but not been recognized. Laryngologists should be familiar with the nature and the importance of the cricothyroid joint and the potential for symptomatic injury of this structure. Additional experience is needed to determine optimal treatment.

References

1. Sataloff RT, Feldman M, Darby KS, et al. Arytenoid dislocation. *J Voice.* 1987;1(4):368–377.
2. Sataloff RT, Bough ID Jr, Spiegel JR. Arytenoid dislocation: diagnosis and treatment. *Laryngoscope.* 1994;104(10): 1353–1361.
3. Lee GJ. *Essential Otolaryngology.* 3rd ed. New York, NY: Medical Examination Publishing; 1983:306–310.
4. Langman J. *Medical Embryology.* 3rd ed. Baltimore, Md: Williams and Wilkins; 1975:269, 272.
5. Hollinshead WH. *Anatomy for Surgeons.* Vol 1. 3rd ed. New York, NY: Harper and Row; 1982:423–427.

6. Maue W, Dickson DR. Cartilages and ligaments of the adult human larynx. *Arch Otolaryngol.* 1971;94:432–439.

7. von Leden H, Moore P. The mechanics of the cricoarytenoid joint. *Arch Otolaryngol.* 1961;73:541–550.

8. Letson JA, Jr, Tatchell R. Arytenoid joint. In Sataloff RT. *Professional Voice: Science and Art of Clinical Care.* 2nd ed. San Diego, Calif: Singular Publishing Group, Inc; 1997: 131–146.

9. Pennington CL. External trauma of the larynx and trachea. Immediate treatment and management. *Ann Otol Rhinol Laryngol.* 1972;81:546–554.

10. Jackson C, Jackson CL. *Disease and Injuries of the Larynx.* New York, NY: Macmilian; 1942:321.

11. Sataloff RT, McCarter AA, Hawkshaw M. Posterior arytenoid dislocation. *Ear Nose Throat J.* 1998;77(1):12.

12. Sataloff RT, Spiegel JR, Heuer RJ, Hawkshaw M. Pediatric anterior arytenoid dislocation. *Ear Nose Throat J.* 1995;74(7):454–456.

13. Szigeti CL, Baeuerle JJ, Mongan PD. Arytenoid dislocation with lighted stylet intubation: case report and retrospective review. *Anesth Analg.* 1994;78(1):185–186.

14. Alexander AE, Jr, Lyons GD, Fazekas-May MA, et al. Utility of helical computed tomography in the study of arytenoid dislocation and arytenoid subluxation. *Ann Otol Rhinol Laryngol.* 1997;160(12):1020–1023.

15. Gauss A, Treiber HS, Haehnel J, Johannsen HS. Spontaneous reposition of a dislocated arytenoid cartilage. *Br J Anaesth.* 1993;70(5):591–592.

16. Hsu CS, Huang CT, So EC, et al. [Arytenoid subluxation following endotracheal intubation—a case report.] *Acta Anaesthesiol Sin.* 1995;33(1):45–52.

17. Rieger A. Hass I, Gross M, et al. [Intubation trauma of the larynx—a literature review with special reference to arytenoid cartilage dislocation.] *Anasthesiol Intensivmed Notfallmed Schmerzther.* 1996;31(5):281–287.

18. Friedberg J, Giberson W. Failed tracheotomy decannulation in children. *J Otolaryngol.* 1992;21(6):404–408.

19. Talmi YP, Wolf M, Bar-Ziv J, et al. Postintubation arytenoid subluxation. *Ann Otol Rhinol Laryngol.* 1996;105(5): 384–390.

20. Stack BC Jr, Ridley MB. Arytenoid subluxation from blunt laryngeal trauma. *Am J Otolaryngol.* 1994;15(1):68–73.

21. Hiong YT, Fung CF, Sudhaman DA. Arytenoid subluxation: implications for the anaesthetist. *Anaesth Intensive Care.* 1996;24(5):609–610.

22. Sataloff RT. Arytenoid dislocation. *Oper Techn Otolaryngol Head Neck Surg.* 1998;9(4):196–202.

23. Rontal E, Rontal M. Laryngeal rebalancing in the treatment of anteromedial dislocation of the arytenoids. *J Voice.* 1998;12(3):383–388.

24. Schultz-Coulon J, Brase A. [Clinical and roentgenological manifestations of unilateral subluxation of the cricothyroid joint.] *HNO.* 1978;26(2):68–72.

25. Sataloff RT, Rao VM, Hawkshaw M, et al. Cricothyroid joint injury. *J Voice.* 1998;12(1):112–116.

22

Management of Gender Reassignment (Sex Change) Patients

Reinhardt J. Heuer, Margaret M. Baroody, and Robert Thayer Sataloff

Transsexualism is a gender dysphoric disorder characterized by persistent feelings of inappropriateness of biologic sex and preoccupation with eliminating primary and secondary sexual characteristics. Male-to-female transsexualism is encountered more commonly than female-to-male transsexualism and demonstrates more difficult communication problems. In most cases, these patients benefit from communication therapy. Female-to-male transsexuals, due to the influence of hormonal treatment on the larynx and related structures, are less likely to have vocal problems. Male-to-female transsexualism occurs in approximately 1 out of 37,000 births.[1,2] Other related groups of individuals require similar communication assistance. Transgenderists are men who wish to live full time as women but are not so concerned with body issues. Interestingly, in the American culture, it is easier for women to live full time in a masculine role. Cross-dressers are men who enjoy part-time dressing and behaving as women. However, individuals frequently will vacillate from one classification to another over a lifetime. Persons who are primarily cross-dressers will move toward transsexualism or will abandon (purge) their feminine accoutrements. Most males falling into these categories report periods of rejection of the entire issue and work toward becoming hypermasculine, usually early in their lives. Most are married, and many have children. The authors believe that therapy for voice and communication issues is most appropriate when the patient has been diagnosed with gender dysphoria and is living 90 to 100% of the time as a woman. When working with cross-dressers, treatment should be behaviorally based and focus on developing "stage" accent and scripts for use during social events. Other subgroups, such as transvestites and female impersonators, are less likely to look to voice and communication specialists for assistance; but they can be helped similarly when they do.

When developing a program of therapy for the male-to-female transsexual (M/FT), it is important to keep in mind which aspects of communication are based in biology/genetic structure (male/female) and which aspects are based in learned/social behavior (masculine/feminine). Biologic and genetic aspects include, of course, primary and secondary sexual characteristics. Specifically related to communication are lung size and capacity, laryngeal size and configuration, vocal fold mass, resonating cavity sizes, muscle mass of the tongue, and oral orifice size and thickness. These differences affect the pitch, loudness, quality, and resonance of the voice and some aspects of articulation. Learned or social aspects of communication include melody/intonation in voicing, patterns of syllabic emphasis/stress, word choice, sentence structure, semantic structure, gestural communication, and dress.

The major goal for most M/FTs is sexual reassignment surgery with modification of the primary sexual characteristics. This surgery is expensive ($20,000) and is considered elective by many insurance companies. Most responsible sexual reassignment surgeons require psychiatric proof of gender dysphoria and practical evidence of the patient's ability to live successfully in a feminine role prior to consenting to do the surgery.

There are no really good surgical procedures to lower the voice in female-to-male transsexuals. The mass of the vocal folds can be increased by injection of substances, and the vocal folds can be shortened by type III thyroplasty; but neither technique results consistently in both substantial decrease in habitual pitch and retention of good vocal quality. Procedures to feminize the biologically male voice are more successful.

Nonsurgical Therapy for Pitch Modification

Ninety-five percent of the more than 400 M/FTs the author (RJH) has seen had a primary complaint of excessively low pitch. Although this is a male/female trait, the patient frequently elects to work on pitch behaviorally. Surgical considerations for pitch change are discussed later in this chapter.

Gelfer and Schofield[3] report that speech fundamental frequencies above 155 Hz (D3) are more likely to be perceived as feminine. Oates and Dacakis[4] are more generous in reporting a gender ambiguous range between 128 and 260 Hz. The goal of pitch modification in M/FTs is to develop a speaking fundamental frequency high enough to allow down-glides that remain above the masculine/feminine cutoff. Initial evaluation of the M/FT involves determining current speech fundamental frequency and the patient's frequency comfortable range. It would be difficult to modify the pitch range upward for an individual who has little flexibility in the upper voice ranges. Behavioral modification of habitual pitch is not easy. It involves development of vocal flexibility, breath support, relaxation, and practice. General breath support and relaxation exercises can be found in chapters 4 and 9. Several approaches have been successful in raising speech fundamental frequency, hopefully allowing the patient to continue using modal voice. Again, this is possible only if the patient has an adequate range. A series of up, down, and up-and-down glide exercises is helpful in extending the patient's range and flexibility. Exercises may include glides on the vowels /ɑ/, /i/, and /u/. One would like to establish a pitch range of at least four semitones above 155 Hz. Drills on words and phrases following upglides are very helpful. Visual feedback using the Kay Visi-Pitch or Kay Real-Time Pitch programs is also very helpful. The majority of patients who seek help do so because they are unable to modify or monitor their own voices acoustically. A program of practice with and upglide + phrase with visual cues, upglide + phrase without visual cues, followed by fading of the upglide and visual cues has been effective in our clinic.

Patients with limited upper ranges are not good candidates for behavioral modification of modal voice or for surgical modification of voice. A voice modification program called "Melanie Speaks" advocated the use of low falsetto voice.[5] The author describes exercises gliding down from natural falsetto to lower falsetto pitches and modifying pharyngeal tension. This is similar to a classical bel canto exercise used for centuries by singers to integrate registers into a "mixed" voice.

Surgery for Pitch Modification

Once the diagnosis has been established, the patient is living as a female, psychiatry clearance has been obtained, and voice therapy has been completed, pitch modification surgery may be reasonable. Transsexuals often request this surgery even if they have been extremely successful at modifying voice gender recognition through voice therapy. If such patients are awakened suddenly, talk in their sleep, or are startled, they are often "revealed" through unthinking, sudden bursts of masculine phonation. This can be extremely embarrassing; and surgical correction in such patients is appropriate.

Many techniques have been proposed, and none is ideal for all cases. Isshiki's type IV thyroplasty, which is described in chapter 18, has been used for this indication. Unfortunately, even with overcorrection, vocal pitch tends to drop over time. The author's (RTS) cricothyroid fusion procedure (also described in the thyroplasty section of chapter 18) produces better long-term results. However, it is only suitable for use in young transsexuals. The cricoid cartilage must be sufficiently flexible to permit its placement just inside the lower border of the thyroid cartilage. When pulling the cricoid toward the thyroid cartilage, it is extremely important to exert all forces under the cricoid arch laterally. The cricoid arch is thin in the midline. If attempts are made to pull the cricoid superiorly with hooks placed in or near the midline, midline fracture is likely to occur. In patients under 40, this operation tends to work well. In patients over 60, ossification is usually too advanced to permit subluxation of the cricoid arch behind the thyroid cartilage. In those between 40 and 60 years old, success depends on the degree of ossification. In such patients, Isshiki's technique can be used as described originally or with suture placement as modified by Lee et al.[6] Anterior commissure advancement was described by LeJeune and coworkers in 1983.[7] LeJeune created a cartilage window that was pulled forward, along with the vocal folds. The space between the advanced cartilage and the rest of the thyroid cartilage was maintained with a titanium splint. Tucker modified the procedure by placing the cartilage window in a more cranial position.[8] However, both of these procedures result in increased prominence of the thyroid cartilage. Because many transsexual patients have already undergone laryngeal shave to reduce the thyroid prominence, this cosmetic disadvantage may be unacceptable to the patient.

A few authors have used scarring obtained by parallel cuts near the vibratory margin[9] or vocal fold stripping[10] to elevate pitch. Although increased stiffness does elevate pitch, it is also associated with decreased volume and substantial hoarseness. This author (RTS) does not advocate these procedures. Abitbol has utilized endoscopic thyroarytenoid myomectomy successfully (Jean Abitbol, MD, Paris, France, personal communication, 2001). In this operation, a large ellipse of thyroarytenoid muscle is removed using a CO_2 laser through an incision placed laterally on the superior surface of the vocal fold. The vibratory margin is not disturbed. This procedure results in decreased mass and, consequently, elevated pitch. The voices are slightly breathy but clear. This procedure can be done unilaterally or bilaterally and has a place in the management of these patients.

Another approach to pitch elevation involves shortening of the vocal folds. Initially, Donald proposed performing such surgery through an external approach.[11] The anterior commissure was divided, the anterior portion of the vocal folds was de-epithelialized, and the vocal folds were sutured together. This procedure was modified by Wendler[12] and Gross[13,14] and more recently by the author (RTS, unpublished data). The procedure described by Wendler and by Gross essentially creates a web, as did Donald; but it is created endoscopically. The anterior portion of the vocal fold is de-epithelialized, and the vocal fold are sutured together firmly through the laryngoscope, creating a V-shaped anterior commissure but a shorter vibrating vocal fold. As in patients who have vocal fold webs for other reasons, this usually results in a clear voice of higher pitch; because the remaining vibrating segment is short, but the vibratory margin has not been disturbed. This author (RTS) has modified the procedure slightly, preserving approximately 2 mm of mucosa adjacent to the anterior commissure. This small area does not interfere with the result. However, although it is unlikely that anyone would elect to have this procedure reversed, should it ever be necessary to try to correct the surgically created web, retaining the anterior commissure will probably prove helpful. To elevate pitch substantially, it has been necessary to de-epithelialize at least one-third to one-half of the musculomembranous vocal fold. This author prefers to accomplish this procedure by marking the anterior and posterior limits of the intended resection with a CO_2 laser. Submucosal infusion is then performed. Flaps of mucosa can be elevated bilaterally using cold instruments or the CO_2 laser. However, because the intention is to scar the vocal fold together, there is no disadvantage to using the laser during this procedure. The vocal folds are approximated using one or two Vicryl sutures. The procedure can be performed under local or general anesthesia. This operation has proven useful both as a primary procedure and as a secondary procedure when cricothyroid approximation has proven insufficient for the patient's needs. Following successful pitch modification surgery, it is reasonable to expect an increase in pitch of about 5 to 9 semitones (about one-fourth to one-sixth of an octave). Pitch elevations as low as 3 or 4 semitones and as high as about 12 semitones occur occasionally. With the increase in pitch, there usually is some decrease in pitch range, particularly loss of a one-fourth or one-fifth of an octave on the lower end of the pitch range. The highest notes that can be produced do not tend to change much as a result of the surgery.

Therapy for Other Aspects of Voice Gender Identification

Speech fundamental frequency is not the sole answer to a more feminine voice, even following surgical modification. As noted above, Oates and Dacakis[4] reported the gender ambiguous frequency range as quite large. Probably of more importance to gender identification is the inclusion of increased melody within the spoken syllable. This voice attribute appears to be learned and is an aspect of the masculine/feminine continuum not the male/female continuum. The more feminine individual tends to utilize increased intrasyllabic melody on vowels within the syllable. The more masculine individual tends to utilize a flatter, less melodic pattern. Listen to the way masculine individuals say "Hello" or "Good morning," and this difference is obvious immediately. Pitch modification does not change this voicing attribute and may only create the impression of a masculine individual with a high-pitched voice.

Practice in melodic intonation should include visual feedback using a device such as the Kay Visi-Pitch overwrite feature for short phrases and sentences. Initially, vowels may need to be elongated, and consonants may have to be shortened and made more precise to allow time to shift pitch on each vowel. Extensive drill is necessary. Practice on varying intonation patterns (particularly upglides) within phrases is also helpful. Over time, visual feedback should be faded, speaking rate increased, and carryover procedures should be initiated. Matching melody to emotional content should be encouraged once the patient is able to free herself from the more monotone masculine pattern. Phrases and sentences taken from the patient's own corpus of frequently said sentences should be used for practice purposes. Melanie Phillips[5] suggests pharyngeal constrictions similar to that obtained when mimicking "the wicked witch of the west" voice and then relaxing the throat to the point of resonance desired. Moya Andrews[15] discusses elevation of the larynx and pharyngeal constriction as another possibility. Currently, there is no evidence of safety from vocal discomfort or disorders in developing these vocal misuse patterns.

Using a relaxed jaw and gentle smile is very effective in reducing the strength of the lower partials in the voice. More feminine individuals are found to smile more frequently during speech in any case. Better oral resonance and a relaxed open jaw can be facilitated by an exercise that involves clenching the jaw while monitoring the masseter muscles with the fingertips and then relaxing the jaw until the muscle bulk has diminished but the muscle is not stretched. Mirrors and videotapes are helpful feedback devices for practicing smiling speech. Over-rounding of the lips or a chimneylike anterior resonance chamber should be avoided.

The female oral cavity is somewhat smaller in most cases than the male oral cavity. Tongue bulk is also less. More feminine articulation is characterized by lighter contacts and shorter articulatory gesture distances that result in less impact on contact. The patient should practice reducing the vowel triangle both posteriorly/anteriorly and inferiorly/superiorly; moving the posteriorly articulated consonants /k/ and /g/ and /ŋ/ forward may create a more feminine articulatory production. Utilizing a modified paired-stimuli approach is helpful. The target consonant-vowel (CV) syllable /ki/ can be contrasted with /ku/ and other back vowels, striving to keep the place of articulation of /k/ and the vowel in the forward position. These modifications in articulation tend to change the positioning of formant II, which is correlated with more feminine speech. Extensive practice at home is necessary to modify these basic speech patterns. Drilling on words from the Thorndike/Lorge Lists of the 1000 Most Frequently Used Words[16] may be helpful.

In addition to working on anteriorizing vowels and consonants, narrowing the productions of sibilants may also improve femininity of speech. More masculine sibilants tend to be more dull and strong. All of these aspects of voicing, resonance, and articulation benefit from singing as well as speech practice.

Carol Gilligan, in her book *In a Different Voice* discusses the differences in the developmental patterns of boys and girls and how differences affect a person's worldview, what he or she talks about, and how he or she phrases speech.[17] Women develop other-orientation, oligarchical superiority, and relationship maintenance preferences. Apparently differences between boys' and girls' attitudes begin very early in life and are probably related, at least in part, to differential parental patterns. Gilligan demonstrates these differences even in the play patterns of young children. More feminine individuals tend to soften the harshness of their speaking patterns by including more tag question sentences such as, "It's time to go, isn't it?" They tend to use more psychological verbs, such as "I feel, I think," and so on. These kinds of changes are difficult to train later in life when we work with gender dysphoria, because they are related directly to the person's mindset. However, the patient should be aware of these kinds of differences, as well.

Gesture and body language also may need to be modified. More masculine individuals tend to take up all of the available space with their bodies; whereas more feminine individuals tend to compact themselves with more upright posture, crossed legs or ankles, and arms held close to the body. More masculine individuals tend to walk with a broad-based gait and the palms of the hands facing backwards; more feminine individuals walk with the feet placed in front of each other and the palms of the hands facing toward the thighs. Feminine arm gestures tend to be more lateral and less often in front of the gesturer. Arm gestures focus on the wrists and fingers of more feminine gesturers.

The major goal in behavioral therapy with male-to-female transsexuals is the development of comfort and a feeling of confidence in the patient's femininity. If a true relationship exists between communicating partners, after about 5 minutes of conversation, the voice and speech patterns of the individual become irrelevant and/or are simply part of that person's persona. A conundrum always exists within the male-to-female transsexual because of the feeling of being "female" trapped in a "male" body. "If I already feel as though I am a woman, why do I have to change my behavior?" Yet, there is an anxiety about "passing" and "being ready" as the opposite sex. The development of confidence and the ability to recognize what constitutes more feminine behavior assist patients in developing comfort and ease with whatever level of feminine voice and speech they are capable of reaching.

References

1. Brown GR. A review of clinical approaches to gender dysphoria. *J Clin Psychiatry*. 1990;51(2):57–69.

2. Landen M, Walinder J, Lundstrom B. Prevalence, incidence and sex ratio of transsexualism. *Acta Psychiatr Scand.* 1996;93:221–223.

3. Gelfer MP, Schofield KJ. Comparison of acoustic and perceptual measures of voice in male-to-female transsexuals perceived as female versus those perceived as male. *J Voice.* 2000:14(1) 22–33.

4. Oates JM, Dacakis G. Speech pathology considerations in the management of transsexualism–a review. *Br J Disord Commun.* 1983:18(3) 139–151.

5. Phillips M. *Melanie Speaks!* Burbank, Calif: Heart Corp (PO Box 295, Burbank, CA 91503). [Video.]

6. Lee SY, Liao TT, Hsieh T. Extralaryngeal approach in functional phonosurgery. In: *Proceedings of the 20th Congress of the IALP*. Tokyo, Japan: The Organizing Committee of the XXth Congress of the International Association of Logopedics and Phoniatrics; 1986:482–483.

7. LeJeune FE, Guice CE, Samuels PM. Early experiences with vocal ligament tightening. *Ann Otol Rhinol Laryngol.* 1983;92:475–477.

8. Tucker HM. Anterior laryngoplasty for adjustment of vocal fold tension. *Ann Otol Rhinol Laryngol.* 1985;94:547–549.

9. Tanabe M, Haji T, Isshiki N. Surgical treatment for androphonia. An experimental study. *Folia Phoniatr (Basel).* 1985;37:15–21.

10. Hirano M, Ohala J, Vennard W. The function of laryngeal muscles in regulating fundamental frequency and intensity of phonation. *J Speech Hear Res.* 1969;12:616–628.

11. Donald PJ, Voice change in the transsexual. *Head Neck Surg.* 1982;4:433–437.

12. Wendler J. Pitch elevation after transsexualism male to female. Presented at the XVI UEP Congress; October 10–14, 1990; Salsomaggiore, Italy.

13. Gross M, Fehland P. Ergebnisse nach operativer Anhebung der mittleren Sprechstimmlage bie Transsexuellen durch Verkurzung des schwingenden Stimmkippenanteils. In: Gross M, ed. *Aktuelle phoniatrisch-padaudiologische Aspekte 1995*. Berlin: Germany: RGV; 1996:88–89.

14. Gross M. Pitch-raising surgery in male-to-female transsexuals. *J Voice.* 1999;13(2):246–250.

15. Andrews ML. *Manual of Voice Treatment: Pediatrics through Geriatrics*. San Diego, Calif: Singular Publishing Group, Inc; 1995:391–404.

16. Thorndike E L, Lorge I. *The Teacher's Wordbook of 30,000 Words*. New York, NY: Teacher's College, Columbia University; 1944.

17. Gilligan C. *In A Different Voice: Psychological Theory and Women's Development*. Cambridge, Mass: Harvard University Press; 1982.

23

Laryngeal Cancer

Timothy D. Anderson and Robert Thayer Sataloff

Carcinoma of the larynx represents approximately 1.3% of all new cancer diagnoses, and approximately 20% of all head and neck cancers. In 2001, the American Cancer Society estimated that in the coming year there would be approximately 10,000 new cases of laryngeal cancer with a 4:1 male to female ratio and that there would be 4,000 deaths due to laryngeal cancer.[1] Thirty-five years ago the male to female ratio was between 10:1 and 50:1, the change is probably due to increasing use of tobacco and alcohol among women.[2] Although laryngeal cancer is primarily a disease of older age with peak incidence in the sixth and seventh decades, it does occur in younger patients, including children.[3] Younger patients who present with laryngeal carcinoma most often are nonsmokers who do not have other identifiable risk factors for laryngeal cancer, suggesting a genetic predisposition.[3] Overall, the major etiologic factor in laryngeal cancer is exposure to tobacco. Studies have shown an increased incidence of both premalignant and malignant lesions in smokers and a dose-dependent relationship between cigarette use and the development of cancer.[4-6] Laryngeal cancer in nonsmokers is rare. Heavy alcohol use is also a factor in the development of laryngeal cancer, and there appears to be a synergistic effect with tobacco, especially in the development of supraglottic tumors.[7] Radiation exposure and exposure to occupational pollutants such as nickel, mustard gas, wood products, and pesticides also have been implicated as etiologic factors.[4,8,9] The etiologic effect of asbestos on laryngeal cancer is not yet well documented, but it appears to be limited to active smokers.[10,11] Laryngopharyngeal reflux and laryngeal papillomatosis may be causally related to cancer, as discussed elsewhere in this book.

Because of the larynx's unique functions of speech, swallowing, and airway protection, treatment of laryngeal cancer has always been complex and controversial. Carcinoma of the larynx is a potentially curable disease with a 5-year survival rate of over 67%. However, early detection of smaller lesions offers a much better opportunity for both survival and preservation of laryngeal function. Thus, aggressive clinical evaluation of laryngeal lesions is critical. In early lesions, treatment usually consists of either surgery or radiation therapy, with the choice based on the individual history and tumor characteristics, as well as the potential effects on laryngeal function. In advanced lesions, usually both surgery and radiation therapy are necessary to optimize long-term survival. New protocols utilizing neo-adjuvant or concomitant chemotherapy have offered some patients with advanced lesions the opportunity to be cured without the need for total laryngectomy.[12]

Supraglottic Tumors

The supraglottic larynx extends from the tip of the epiglottis to the ventricles. It includes the laryngeal surface of the epiglottis, the aryepiglottic folds, the false vocal folds, the laryngeal surface of the arytenoids, and the ventricles (Fig 23–1). The mucosa of

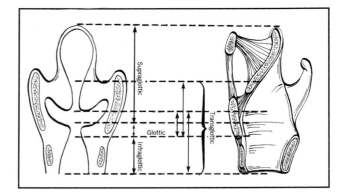

Fig 23–1. Regions of the larynx.

the lingual surface of the epiglottis is in the supraglottic larynx, but the mucosa of the vallecula is oropharyngeal. The lymphatic drainage of the supraglottis is extensive. It traverses the thyrohyoid membrane and travels with the superior laryngeal vessels to the deep jugular nodes. This lymphatic pathway is separate from the inferior drainage of glottic and subglottic tumors owing to a difference in embryologic development. Thus, surgical management of supraglottic tumors is a distinct entity.

Supraglottic cancer spreads in patterns dependent on its site of origin. It can spread over mucosal surfaces to adjacent structures, or it can traverse cartilaginous or fibrous barriers into deeper spaces. The pre-epiglottic space anteriorly is a common site for spread of the epiglottic tumors. This area is supplied richly with lymphatics and invasion of the pre-epiglottic space predisposes to neck metastases and allows unobstructed cancer extension inferiorly to the anterior commissure and subglottis. The paraglottic space, lateral to the endolarynx, is an early site of spread of false vocal fold and ventricular tumors (Fig 23–2). Paraglottic space involvement provides for rapid transglottic and subglottic extension.[13]

Most clinicians utilize the staging system based on the American Joint Committee (AJC) for Cancer Staging and End Result Reporting. Its most recent revision (1988) is seen in Table 23–1.[14] There is little emphasis on tumor size, with extent of mucosal spread determining the tumor's class. Progression to T_3 status is determined by fixation of the hemilarynx, involvement of postcricoid and piriform mucosa, or pre-epiglottic extension. Lymph node staging is standard for all head and neck cancer (Table 23–2).

Patients with supraglottic cancer can present with sore throat, voice change such as hoarseness and dysphagia, otalgia, halitosis, weight loss, or neck mass. The voice is usually muffled, but true hoarseness is usually a sign of a transglottic tumor, vocal fold fixation, or a low false vocal fold lesion. Symptoms are often subtle and insidious, and many tumors are quite extensive at presentation. The clinician must be especially suspicious of supraglottic cancer in patients with persistent complaints of sore throat and otalgia.

Lymph node metastases occur in 25 to 50% of patients with supraglottic cancer; 30 to 50% are palpable at presentation; and 20 to 40% are occult in necks with clinically negative findings.[15-19] Contralateral disease is common. The rate of metastasis increases with tumor size but ranges from 15 to 40% even in T_1 tumors.[15-18]

Treatment Considerations

Accurate assessment and staging are critical in determining treatment. Computed tomography scanning

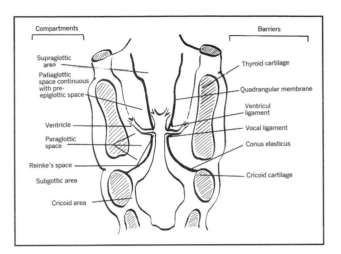

Fig 23–2. Compartments and barriers in the larynx.

Table 23–1. Staging of Primary Tumor in Laryngeal Cancer.

Supraglottis

T_1—Tumor limited to one subsite of the supraglottis with normal vocal fold mobility

T_2—Tumor invades more than one subsite of supraglottis or glottis with normal vocal fold mobility

T_3—Tumor limited to the larynx with vocal fold fixation and/or invades postcricoid area, medial wall of piriform sinus, or pre-epiglottic tissues

T_4—Tumor invades through thyroid cartilage and/or extends to other tissues beyond the larynx

with contrast infusion can help in judging the size and location of the primary tumor and the extent of lymph node involvement.[19] Magnetic resonance imaging may be useful, but in most cases CT imaging of the larynx is sufficient. All patients should undergo operative laryngoscopy to visualize and palpate the extent of the cancer. However, fiberoptic laryngoscopy, especially with stroboscopy and video documentation, can provide an excellent overall assessment and allow operative endoscopy to be reserved for the time of definitive treatment. This is especially helpful in patients with airway compromise or other significant medical conditions. A thorough search for a metachronous primary must be completed, because the incidence has been reported to be as high as 20 to 30% with aerodigestive tract tumors.[20]

In stage I lesions, cure rates with surgery and radiation therapy are equivalent (75-80%).[21,22] Radiation therapy, at least within the first year, results in less

Table 23–2. Staging of Lymphatic Metastasis in Laryngeal Cancer.

N_x— Regional lymph nodes cannot be assessed.

N_0— No regional lymph node metastasis.

N_1— Metastasis in a single ipsilateral lymph node, 3 cm or less in greatest dimension.

N_2— Metastasis in a single ipsilateral lymph node, more than 3 cm, but not more than 6 cm in greatest dimension, or multiple ipsilateral lymph nodes, none more than 6 cm in greatest dimension, or bilateral or contralateral lymph nodes none more than 6 cm in greatest dimension.

N_{2a}— Metastasis in a single ipsilateral lymph node more than 3 cm but no more than 6 cm in greatest dimension.

N_{2b}— Metastasis in multiple ipsilateral lymph nodes, none more than 6 cm in greatest dimension.

N_{2c}— Metastasis in bilateral or contralateral lymph nodes, none more than 6 cm in greatest dimension.

N_3— Metastasis in a lymph node more than 6 cm in greatest dimension.

---

speech and swallowing morbidity than laryngeal surgery and generally is well tolerated. Voice results following treatment (radiation vs surgery) have not been studied convincingly, and there is at least a possibility that voice results 5 and 10 years after treatment may prove superior after limited surgery than after irradiation. Surgery is advantageous in patients with limited primary lesions and in younger patients (thus reserving radiation for those who may develop another primary tumor later in life).[21,22] In stage II and III lesions, treatment options are varied. For treatment of the primary site, neither surgery nor radiation with surgical salvage has shown a superior cure rate; and the use of combined therapy is not supported clearly.[23-25] Using primary radiation therapy is an attractive alternative to surgery.[26,27] However, the cervical nodes cannot be assessed, and the morbidity of salvage surgery must be considered. Most patients undergoing salvage surgery will require total laryngectomy, although partial laryngectomies can be performed safely in selected post-irradiation patients. Primary supraglottic laryngectomy can yield local control rates as high as 90% with low morbidity.[27,28] Stage IV lesions can be treated either with combined surgery (usually a total laryngectomy) in combination with radiation therapy or with combined chemotherapy and radiation therapy in selected patients. Proto-cols combining chemotherapy and radiation have the advantage of laryngeal preservation in up to two-thirds of patients with equivalent survival.[12]

Treatment of metastatic neck disease is another controversial area in the care of supraglottic cancer. Patients with primary lesion T_2 or larger and N_0 neck are at risk for bilateral occult neck metastasis and should be treated. Radiation therapy and modified neck dissection are equally effective.[17] In smaller tumors that are treated with primary radiotherapy, both sides of the neck should also be radiated. Patients who are going to undergo planned postoperative radiotherapy can also be spared bilateral neck dissections through irradiation of one or both N_0 necks. However, there are significant advantages to treating the primary lesion surgically and performing simultaneous, bilateral, modified neck dissections.[27,29-32] If there are no metastases, postoperative radiation may not be warranted. The discovery of occult nodes can guide the use of postoperative radiation. Ultimately, the decision will be influenced by the patient's history and condition, the quality of radiation treatment available, and the surgeon's experience in performing conservation modified neck dissection. Recognized indications for postoperative radiotherapy include large tumors, bulky neck disease, extracapsular spread of nodal disease, and perineural or angio-lymphatic invasion.

Few data support the need for neck dissection following chemoradiation therapy for supraglottic tumors. Certainly, most residual neck masses should be treated by a neck dissection. In addition, patients who had neck disease larger than 2 to 3 cm in size prior to chemoradiation probably should undergo neck dissection following chemoradiation therapy; because there is a higher incidence of residual disease in these patients.[33,34] Local and regional recurrence rates are higher after primary chemoradiation when compared to surgery and radiation, which underscores the importance of aggressive surveillance of the primary site and the need for neck dissections in patients with poor prognostic features.[12]

Surgical Procedures

Small T_1 cancers limited to the epiglottis can be treated by transoral, subtotal supraglottic laryngectomy. Relative contraindications to this approach are involvement of the pre-epiglottic space, the petiole of the epiglottis, the free margin of the false vocal fold, or the presence of palpable neck disease. Additionally, endoscopic visualization is difficult without a large or bivalved laryngoscope designed to provide a wide field of view in the supraglottis.[35] The procedure is performed under general anesthesia usually with the carbon dioxide (CO_2) laser. A laser-safe endotracheal tube is used, and a tracheotomy is not necessary. The pre-epiglottic space is evaluated during the dissection. If pre-epiglottic space invasion is noted, the procedure is converted to an open, supraglottic laryngectomy. When endoscopic visualization is difficult, external access to the supraglottic larynx can be obtained through a transverse, suprahyoid pharyngotomy, or a lateral pharyngotomy in the piriform sinus.

Although not yet widely used, endoscopic transoral CO_2 laser resection of larger supraglottic tumors has been reported in the literature.[36-39] This technique is also performed under general anesthesia with a laser-protected endotracheal tube and wide exposure using a bivalved laryngoscope. Although various techniques have been described,[37-39] most begin with dividing the epiglottis in half and dissecting the midline pre-epiglottic space until the superior surface of the thyroid cartilage is identified. Dissection is then carried along the edge of the superior portion of the thyroid cartilage from anterior to posterior, exposing the entire top of the thyroid cartilage. The laser is then used to dissect along the inner surface of the thyroid cartilage preferably leaving the perichondrium in situ unless it is needed as a tumor margin. Dissection is carried down to the level of the vallecula. Posterior cuts are made through the false vocal folds into the ventricle distant from the tumor. The tumor is then removed through the mouth. In addition to the bivalved laryngoscope, especially designed bipolar cautery forceps and unipolar cautery instruments are needed for control of larger blood vessels. Specialized grasping instruments are desirable to provide exposure and retraction of the area to be dissected. Healing occurs over the next several weeks, and most reports indicate that swallowing function and sensation of the remucosalized larynx are excellent. Neck dissections are performed several days to weeks after the primary operation. Oncologic results have been reported to be equal or superior to open supraglottic laryngectomy.[36-39] Recurrences often can be treated adequately with repeat transoral laser excision.[40]

The standard surgical procedure for cancer isolated above the vocal folds is the horizontal supraglottic laryngectomy. It can be used for any laryngeal tumor superior to the ventricles including tumors that involve the laryngeal surface of the epiglottis, the medial wall of the piriform sinus above the apex, and the aryepiglottic folds. It is contraindicated in patients with vocal fold fixation, thyroid cartilage invasion, or if there is involvement of the arytenoid cartilage, ventricle, apex of the piriform sinus, anterior commissure,

intra-arytenoid area, base of tongue, paraglottic space, or soft tissues of the neck. Additionally, patients must be in good general health. A horizontal hemilaryngectomy allows for normal or near-normal deglutition postoperatively due to the sparing of the vocal folds, which will continue to perform their role in airway protection. However, the patient must be able to learn a new swallowing technique and must be able to sense and cough out any aspirated material. The patient must be cooperative, motivated, and strong enough to tolerate prolonged postoperative rehabilitation. Patients with inadequate pulmonary function or poor compliance may suffer life-threatening aspiration postoperatively, and total laryngectomy is indicated in this patient population.

The supraglottic laryngectomy is performed under general anesthesia with a tracheotomy in place. A separate horizontal skin incision is performed and subplatysmal flaps are raised (Fig 23–3). The strap muscles are divided in the midline, and the thyroid cartilage is exposed. The perichondrium is incised along the superior edge of the cartilage and dissected inferiorly (Fig 23–4). This dissection must be performed with care using fine elevators. The perichondrial layer is dissected halfway between the superior and inferior edges of the thyroid cartilage in males and one third of the distance from the superior edge in females. The cartilage incision is carried superiorly, medial to the

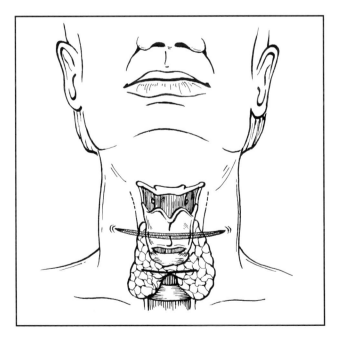

Fig 23–3. A separate transverse incision, superior to the tracheotomy site, is suitable for most partial laryngectomies, and yields the best cosmetic result.

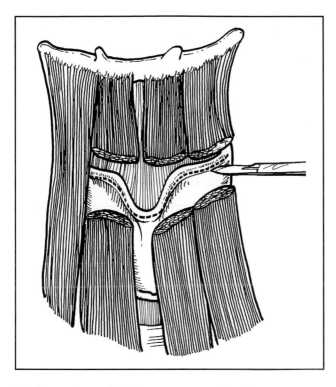

Fig 23–4. Supraglottic laryngectomy. After the strap muscles are divided, the perichondrium is incised along the superior margin of the thyroid cartilage.

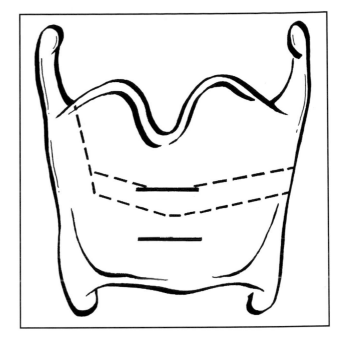

Fig 23–5. Supraglottic laryngectomy. The transverse cartilage cut is made at the presumed level of the glottis (the superior line is used for females) and angled superiorly on the unaffected side.

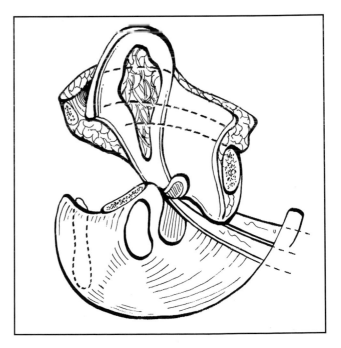

Fig 23–6. Supraglottic laryngectomy. The scissors are placed in the ventricle internally and the cartilage is cut externally in the final maneuver to remove the supraglottic larynx.

superior cornua on the nondominant side (Fig 23–5). The suprahyoid muscles are then transected, and the entire hyoid bone is dissected free. The superior laryngeal vessels are identified and controlled between the greater cornu of the hyoid and superior cornu of the thyroid cartilage on each side. The pharyngeal mucosa is identified superior to the hyoid bone, and the pharynx is entered through the vallecula. The epiglottis is grasped and retracted anteriorly, and incisions are extended with scissors along the lateral borders of the epiglottis. In tumors involving the tip of the epiglottis or vallecula, the larynx is entered laterally through the piriform mucosa on the side opposite the tumor. When the epiglottis is retracted anteriorly, the glottis is visualized directly and the extent of the tumor is identified. With the medial blade of the scissors in the ventricle and the lateral blade in the cartilage incision, the supraglottic larynx is excised (Fig 23–6). The perichondrium is closed to the base of the tongue using 3-0 or 4-0 absorbable sutures. Before tying the first layer of closure, the neck is flexed and the remaining larynx is suspended superiorly. The most secure suspension is accomplished by passing heavy permanent suture (prolene or stainless steel) through drilled holes in the thyroid cartilage and through the mandibular symph-

ysis (Fig 23–7). The sutures can also be fixed to the mandibular periosteum or the digastric tendons bilat-

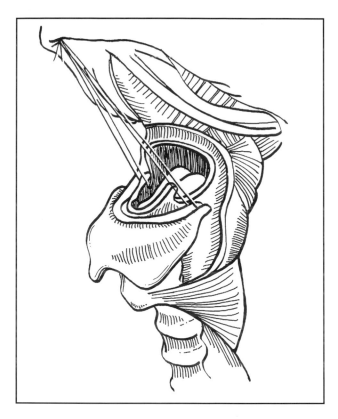

Fig 23–7. Supraglottic laryngectomy. The larynx is suspended superiorly and anteriorly by wiring to the mandibular symphysis.

erally. The larynx must be suspended as far anteriorly and superiorly as possible in order to allow it to remain under the tongue base during the oropharyngeal phase of swallowing. A cricopharyngeal myotomy should be performed before closure as well. The laryngeal closure sutures are tied and a second layer of suture is placed. The skin is closed over a small drain.

The basic supraglottic laryngectomy can be extended to include additional involved structures. When the mucosa over the arytenoid cartilages is involved, the entire cartilage can be removed. However, any extension of the resection that affects vocal fold mobility adversely increases the risk of aspiration; and the removal of additional cartilage may result in glottic stenosis.

The two most important factors in the postoperative care of a supraglottic laryngectomy patient are the healing of the laryngeal closure and mastering of the supraglottic swallowing technique. As in most partial laryngectomies, mucosal closure is not possible; thus initial healing is by secondary intention. Patients with conditions that would affect wound healing adversely, such as malnutrition, diabetes mellitus, chronic alcoholism, uncontrolled reflux laryngitis, and prior

radiation therapy, are poorer candidates for this procedure than patients who do not have such conditions. Successful supraglottic laryngectomy can be performed in previously irradiated patients, but other factors must be optimal; and there is an increased rate of complications.[41] Initial swallowing trials are accomplished best after the nasogastric tube has been removed and, if at all possible, after the tracheotomy has been removed. Patients are taught to swallow slowly, stopping to cough before each inhalation. Most nonirradiated patients can maintain adequate nutrition by an oral diet within 10 to 14 days after surgery. Irradiated patients frequently remain partially dependent on tube feedings for weeks or months following surgery.

Glottic Tumors

Glottic tumors include neoplasms involving the true vocal folds, the anterior commissure, and the posterior larynx at the level of the true vocal folds. The superior limit of the glottis is the lateral recess of the ventricles. The inferior limit extends 10 mm below the free margin of the vocal folds at the anterior commissure, decreasing to 5 mm below the free margin posteriorly (see Fig 23–1). The lymphatic channels of the glottis are quite sparse and lie in the submucosal space. Glottic tumors usually spread along the mucosa, and small lesions rarely invade deeper structures. When deep invasion occurs, violation of the inner perichondrium of the thyroid cartilage or the conus elasticus into the paralaryngeal space is the most important consideration in treatment decisions[42] (see Fig 23–2).

By far, the most common presenting symptom of glottic carcinoma is hoarseness. Sore throat, dysphagia, hemoptysis, and airway obstruction usually are present in patients with advanced tumors. Otalgia or dry cough occasionally can accompany hoarseness as early symptoms. Almost all patients with glottic cancer have a history of cigarette smoking. There is a 4:1 male predominance with a peak incidence in the sixth and seventh decades.

In early glottic carcinoma, accurate diagnosis and staging are critical. The most important factor in staging is the presence of vocal fold fixation, which makes the tumor at least T_3 (Table 23–3). The first step in evaluation is adequate laryngeal visualization to determine the indications and plan for endoscopic biopsy. With fiberoptic laryngoscopy, it should be possible to visualize most patients. The addition of video improves documentation and the patient's understanding and acceptance of future treatment. Stroboscopy can be invaluable in determining the need for biopsy

Table 23–3. Staging of Primary Tumor in Laryngeal Cancer.

Glottis

T_1— Tumor limited to vocal fold(s) (may involve anterior commissure or posterior larynx) with normal mobility.

T_{1a}—Tumor limited to one vocal fold.

T_{1b}—Tumor involves both vocal folds.

T_2— Tumor extends to supraglottis and/or subglottis and/or with impaired vocal fold mobility.

T_3— Tumor limited to larynx with vocal fold fixation.

T_4— Tumor invades through the thyroid cartilage and/or extends to other tissues beyond the larynx.

and the depth of tumor spread, especially in a professional voice user. The absence of mucosal vibration in the region of a suspicious lesion is not diagnostic for an invasive process, but it generally increases the clinical suspicion of cancer. Patients suspected of having carcinoma should undergo operative endoscopy and biopsy. Panendoscopy is recommended because, even with small glottic tumors, the risk of a metachronous primary is 15%.[20]

The differential diagnosis of a small glottic lesion includes hyperkeratosis, dysplasia, carcinoma *in situ*, and invasive carcinoma. Accuracy in pathologic diagnosis is critical. All lesions except invasive carcinoma are treated by simple excision without large margins and with close observation.[43] Invasive cancer requires either total surgical excision with free margins or radiation therapy.

For most T_1 and T_2 glottic tumors, long-term cure rates are equal after surgery or radiation.[44] The treatment decision is made by comparing the time, expense, and morbidity of radiation therapy to the operative risk and morbidity associated with surgery. It has always been assumed that radiation therapy will not alter vocal quality as much as surgical procedures. However, no study to evaluate this finding objectively has been completed. Anecdotally, in most cases, voice quality appears to be better during the first year following radiation therapy than during the first year after surgery. However, it is not certain that postradiation voice quality is better than postoperative voice quality after longer periods, because the late effects of radiotherapy become more evident. When voice is a primary concern, the location of the tumor and potential depth of the surgery must be taken into account along with other factors. The patient must be informed fully about the advantages, disadvantages, and uncertainties associated with each treatment modality

before the patient selects a therapeutic plan. Radiation failures can be salvaged by partial laryngectomy. Operative morbidity is higher than in nonirradiated patients and the need for eventual salvage with total laryngectomy may be as high as 25%.[45-47]

Surgical Treatment

Excisional Biopsy

A retrospective study of patients who had partial laryngectomy for small glottic cancers revealed no tumor in the resected specimen in as many as 20%.[48] This means that at least this percentage of tumors can be adequately removed with a generous excisional biopsy. When preoperative suspicion of cancer is high, and the patient's larynx can be visualized well by suspension laryngoscopy, excisional biopsy can be planned and accomplished safely.

Endoscopic Surgery

The indications for endoscopic excision of a vocal fold carcinoma include lesions isolated to the membranous portion of one or both vocal folds, no impairment of vocal fold mobility, and the ability to obtain adequate visualization by suspension laryngoscopy. Difficulty in obtaining adequate visualization can be expected in patients who are obese; have short necks, short mandibles, or large tongues; have a narrow dental arch with full dentition; or cervical spine disease. Tracheotomy is almost never necessary. General anesthesia is utilized with a laser-safe endotracheal tube. A Dedo, Fragen, or Sataloff suspension laryngoscope is preferred by the authors, but any large laryngoscope that provides good visibility is satisfactory. Toluidine blue may be painted on the vocal fold to reveal areas of increased DNA activity, and rigid endoscopes are helpful in visualizing the full extent of the lesion. The lesion(s) can be excised using either cold microscopic technique or a carbon dioxide laser. The laser is advantageous because of its accuracy and ability to provide ongoing hemostasis. However, when treating superficial lesions with the laser, damage to the underlying lamina propria or muscle is possible. Noninvasive lesions are removed including the full thickness of mucosa, but the vocalis muscle is not exposed. Invasive lesions are outlined with a 1-millimeter margin and are resected with underlying muscle (Fig 23–8). Contact endoscopy may be helpful in mapping the margin. With fine microscopic technique, a separate margin can be obtained to ensure adequate resection. Studies have shown endoscopic techniques to be equal to open surgery in obtaining long-term, disease-free survival in selected patients with small cancers.[48,49]

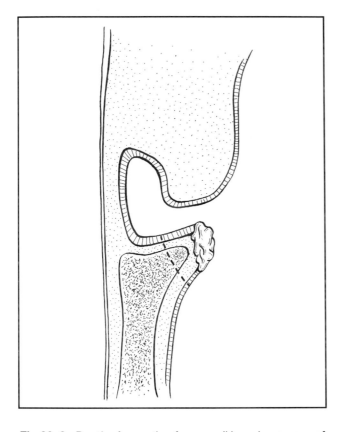

Fig 23–8. Depth of resection for a small invasive cancer of the vocal fold.

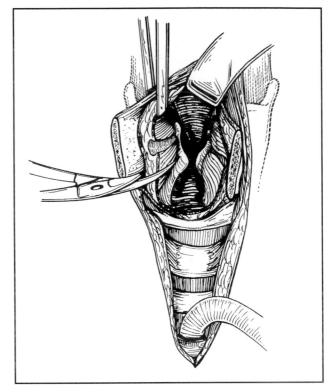

Fig 23–9. Cordectomy performed through a laryngofissure.

Photofrin-radiated photodynamic therapy has shown some promise in treating early lesions with preservation of the mucosal wave.[50] After administering a photosensitizer, intraoperative laser light activation causes irreversible cellular change to cells that concentrate the photosensitizing agent. As cancer cells concentrate porfimer sodium, they are preferentially destroyed. Small studies have had good results,[50] but larger, randomized, controlled studies have not been done.

Cordectomy

Cordectomy remains the standard by which all other surgical treatments of small glottic cancers are measured.[51] Cordectomy involves removal of the entire musculomembranous vocal fold with the vocalis muscle (Fig 23–9). The inner perichondrium of the thyroid cartilage also can be removed, either partially or completely. Cordectomy is contraindicated when vocal fold mobility is impaired, when the thyroid cartilage is invaded by the tumor, or when there is supraglottic or subglottic extension. Cordectomy can be accomplished endoscopically with a carbon dioxide laser. However,

it may be difficult to assess lateral tumor extension in many cases; and the patient should be prepared for conversion to an open procedure. Traditionally, cordectomy is performed through a laryngofissure. A tracheotomy is performed, and general anesthesia is utilized. A separate, superior transverse incision is adequate for exposure and provides a good cosmetic result, but a single vertical incision can be used. A vertical midline thyrotomy is performed in most cases; but if endoscopic examination reveals involvement of the anterior commissure, the vertical thyrotomy can be made off-center on the uninvolved side. Once the larynx is opened, the tumor's margins are defined and the involved vocal fold is resected with a 1- to 2-mm mucosal margin. Resection of the underlying vocalis muscle must be generous due to the inability to obtain reliable margins in muscle fascicles. Thus, even in cases in which some mucosa can be spared, a large bulk of the vocal fold usually is resected. Tumors that involve the inner thyroid perichondrium or abut the thyroid cartilage require vertical hemilaryngectomy in most cases. However, even with bulky disease, the cartilage can be spared in many patients with early glottic carcinoma. Most cases should be approached with the hope of performing a soft tissue resection alone. In rare cases, small lesions on both vocal folds can be resected simultaneously by this technique.[52] CT and MRI scanning may be helpful preoperatively, but examination and biopsy at the time of open surgery provide the most definitive indications for cartilage resection.

Endoscopic Laser-Assisted Vertical Hemilaryngectomy

Glottic carcinoma can be resected using a transoral CO_2 laser-assisted approach in patients in whom adequate exposure can be obtained.[36-39] Contraindications to this approach include T_4 lesions, especially in patients with invasion of thyroid cartilage, extension into the subglottis, or extensive supraglottic extension, as well as tumors with fixed vocal folds (which implies invasion of the cricoarytenoid joint). Patients in whom adequate exposure cannot be obtained are not candidates for this technique.

After obtaining adequate exposure with the bivalved laryngoscope, the false vocal fold is excised as a separate specimen in order to expose fully the lateral tumor extent. Tumors involving the anterior commissure can be exposed through excision of the petiole of the epiglottis. If the full extent of the tumor cannot be visualized easily after these maneuvers, endoscopic excision is likely to result in positive margins and generally should not be performed. Once the tumor is visualized completely, superficial marking incisions are made to outline the extent of resection. The success of this procedure requires meticulous dissection and hemostasis usually with the CO_2 laser and, occasionally, monopolar or bipolar electrocautery. Forceps are used to retract the vocal fold and tumor medially, providing counter traction, while the laser is used as a cutting instrument. The area undergoing dissection should always be under tension to aid cutting and allow identification of tissue planes and deep cancer extension. Cancer up to and including the anterior commissure can be resected using this technique, although adequate removal of the anterior commissure is technically difficult and the defect resulting from this procedure creates an extremely breathy voice that requires further surgery to improve voice quality. With this technique, intraoperative frozen sections and control of margins are essential to verify complete extirpation of the tumor.

No primary reconstruction is undertaken during this procedure. The resected areas generally mucosalize over the next few weeks. Resection of the false vocal fold and infrapetiole region has the added advantage of aiding postoperative surveillance for recurrence.

Frequent postoperative surveillance is important, because early recurrences often can be cured with a second transoral laser excision.[40] Most patients will form a scar band opposing the contralateral normal vocal fold, allowing phonation. Patients with breathy voices after this procedure can be helped by a variety of procedures to increase the bulk and size of the scar band on the operated side.

Vertical Hemilaryngectomy

When glottic carcinoma invades deeply to involve the perichondrium, removal of the thyroid cartilage is necessary. If the cartilage itself is invaded, which means a stage IV tumor, most authors recommend total laryngectomy.[53] However, when the area of cartilage involvement is small and the vocal fold is mobile, a partial laryngectomy with postoperative radiation therapy may be considered.[53]

A standard hemilaryngectomy is approached in the same way as a cordectomy (Fig 23–10). A second cartilage cut is made laterally on the involved side leaving a 3- to 4-mm strip of the posterior thyroid ala, including the superior and inferior cornua (Fig 23–11). The cartilage cuts can be tailored based on the preoperative examination and intraoperative assessments. The anterior incision can be moved off the midline to

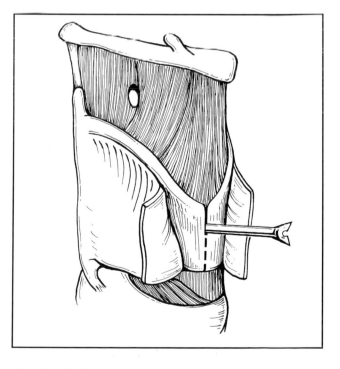

Fig 23–10. Standard midline thyrotomy approach for cordectomy or vertical hemilaryngectomy.

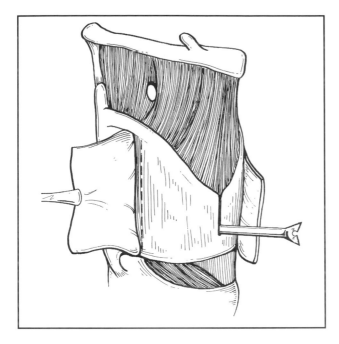

Fig 23–11. For vertical hemilaryngectomy, the second cartilage cut (*dashed line*) is made leaving a 4- to 5-mm strip of posterior thyroid ala.

include the anterior commissure, or to remove up to two thirds of the contralateral ala. The cartilage resection can also be quite narrow, involving a strip 8- to 10-mm wide, in select cases. The outer perichondrium is dissected off the cartilage to be resected and is utilized for closure. A standard hemilaryngectomy must be extended to include the anterior commissure if it is found to be involved (anterolateral laryngectomy) and can be performed to remove only the anterior commissure (anterior vertical laryngectomy).[54,55] It also can be extended to include part or all of the arytenoid cartilage. Additionally, a vertical laryngectomy can be performed with a supraglottic laryngectomy (suprahemilaryngectomy) or even in an extended fashion as a near-total laryngectomy. However, extension of the procedure increases the risks of postoperative glottic stenosis and aspiration, and decreases local control rates.[56]

Patients should be treated with perioperative prophylactic antibiotics and remain *non per os* (NPO) for 5 to 10 days postoperatively. Usually, the tracheotomy can be removed 1 to 2 weeks after surgery, but it may need to be left in place longer in patients who have extended resections, delayed healing (due to previous radiation therapy, diabetes, malnutrition, and so on) or aspiration. However, most patients swallow much more effectively after decannulation. Thus, early removal of the tracheotomy tube is encouraged.

Reconstruction After Partial Laryngectomy

Primary mucosal closure cannot be obtained after almost all forms of partial laryngectomy. In most cases, the thyroid perichondrium is used to close the operative site. In others, the area of mucosal resection is left open. In either situation, healing proceeds by granulation and epithelialization from the remaining mucosa. For this reason, most surgeons have suggested that a history of prior radiation therapy or the presence of systemic conditions that slow healing (diabetes mellitus, malnutrition, alcoholism, or renal failure) are contraindications to laryngeal conservation with a partial laryngectomy. However, with meticulous technique, a cooperative patient, and mucosal and cartilaginous reconstruction, partial laryngectomy can be considered in most cases. The simplest forms of reconstruction utilize advancement and rotation flaps of local mucosa to cover exposed areas. A posterior mucosal defect can be closed by advancing postcricoid mucosa and rotating tissue from the aryepiglottic fold or medial wall of the piriform sinus. More generous portions of piriform or posterior pharyngeal wall mucosa can be rotated to cover almost an entire hemilarynx, but this narrows or closes the piriform sinus and may increase the risk of aspiration. Amin and Koufman have described a reconstructive technique for cases in which an arytenoid is sacrificed in which the ipsilateral cricoid cartilage is resected and reconstructed with a local muscle flap and stent.[57]

Many methods have been used successfully to provide bulk to the operated side and thus improve the postoperative voice. Probably the most reliable is a bipedicled, strap muscle flap that is developed from the anterior half of the muscle and interposed deep to the perichondrium of the operated side[58] (Fig 23–12). An inferiorly based sternohyoid flap can be interposed to cover the arytenoid cartilage and provide bulk for a neo-vocal fold[59] (Fig 23–13). Portions of thyroid cartilage, especially the superior cornua, can be rotated into the defect and then covered with muscle or mucosa to provide a ridge apposing the remaining mobile vocal fold.[60]

When cartilage support and mucosal coverage are necessary, an epiglottic flap is usually the first choice for reconstruction after hemilaryngectomy or extended partial laryngectomy procedures.[61,62] The petiole must be uninvolved by tumor. The epiglottis is grasped at the petiole, and dissection is carried out superiorly along the lateral margins as the cartilage is retracted inferiorly. The mucosa over the laryngeal surface is usually left intact, and the cartilage can be released enough to suture to the cricoid cartilage inferiorly. There is no evidence of an increased risk of aspiration

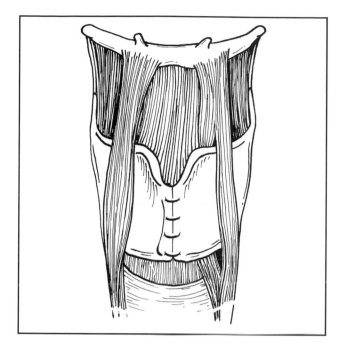

Fig 23–12. Bipedicled sternohyoid muscle flap interposed deep to the perichondrium.

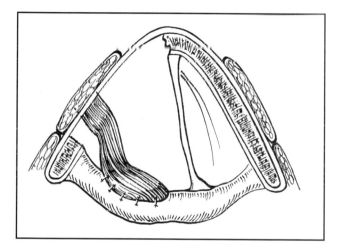

Fig 23–13. An inferiorly based sternohyoid muscle flap used to reconstruct the arytenoid bed.

after use of an epiglottic flap, and results in radiated patients are excellent.[63] Composite grafts of nasal septum or auricular cartilage and skin also can be used, but healing of these free grafts in radiated tissue is unpredictable.

Supracricoid Hemilaryngectomy

Select T_2 and T_3 glottic and supraglottic carcinomas can be treated using supracricoid hemilaryngectomy

with either cricohyoidopexy (CHP) or cricohyoepiglottopexy (CHEP) for reconstruction.[64-67] Supracricoid hemilaryngectomy provides equivalent local control to total laryngectomy in carefully selected T_3 tumors, and better local control than vertical partial laryngectomy in most T_2 carcinomas.[64-67] The technique involves removal of the entire thyroid cartilage, both vocal folds, and resection of up to one arytenoid cartilage. Voice and swallowing results are better when both arytenoid cartilages can be preserved. Contraindications to this procedure include lesions originating in the ventricle or the anterior commissure with pre-epiglottic space invasion, arytenoid cartilage fixation (indicating invasion of the cricoarytenoid joint), and subglottic extension of more than 10 mm anteriorly or 5 mm posteriorly. Patients with poor preoperative pulmonary function are not candidates as micro-aspiration is an expected consequence despite swallowing rehabilitation. The swallowing rehabilitation process after supracricoid hemilaryngectomy is very involved and patients must be able to participate actively in the rehabilitation process.

Supracricoid hemilaryngectomy is performed under general anesthesia with orotracheal intubation. A standard apron flap incision is made with elevation of the skin flap to at least 1 centimeter above the hyoid bone and down to the clavicles. Neck dissections are performed if indicated. The sternohyoid and thyrohyoid muscles are transected along the superior part of the thyroid cartilage; these muscles are then mobilized inferiorly to expose the sternothyroid muscle. The sternothyroid muscle is transected at the inferior border of the thyroid cartilage, and the pharyngeal constrictor muscles are incised along the lateral alae of the thyroid cartilage. The thyroid perichondrium is incised along the lateral border, and the piriform sinuses are dissected free of the thyroid cartilage. The cricothyroid joints are disarticulated carefully to avoid damaging the recurrent laryngeal nerves. A cricothyroidotomy is performed, and the endotracheal tube is removed from the mouth and placed through the cricothyroid membrane. For glottic tumors, the thyrohyoid membrane is incised just above the thyroid cartilage, entering the pharynx. In supraglottic cancer, the hyoid bone periosteum is incised and stripped from the deep surface of the bone. A tunnel is used to traverse the pre-epiglottic space and enter the pharynx just above the epiglottis. In either case, the tumor is visualized through the pharyngotomy; and the pharyngotomy is connected to the cricothyroidotomy on the less involved side using heavy Mayo scissors, sparing as much mucosa as is possible. This maneuver provides adequate visualization for mucosal cuts on the tumor-bearing side. If it is necessary for adequate margins, excision of the ipsilateral arytenoid cartilage may be performed. If the arytenoid is to be spared, the incision should be performed just anterior to or through the vocal process of the arytenoid. More posterior cuts are likely to violate the joint capsule and result in an immobile arytenoid. Once the tumor is released and removed, the mucosa of the upper part of the arytenoid cartilage is closed over the exposed arytenoid cartilage. No sutures are placed near the inferior portion of the arytenoid to preserve mobility. A suture is then used to pull the arytenoid cartilage anteriorly and attach it to the cricoid cartilage to prevent posterior rotation of the arytenoids due to unopposed posterior cricoarytenoid muscle pull. The primary closure of the surgical defect is then performed using three submucosal 0-Vicryl sutures that are looped around the cricoid cartilage and passed through either the remaining epiglottic cartilage and around the hyoid bone in a CHEP, or around just the hyoid bone in CHP. A large portion of the tongue base should be included in each of these sutures. The sutures are then pulled together and tied to impact the cricoid cartilage into the hyoid bone. Prior to tying these sutures, a tracheotomy is performed with the cricoid cartilage and trachea pulled up to their eventual locations.

Postoperative care includes aggressive speech and swallowing therapy. Nutrition is maintained through a feeding tube until the patient is able to tolerate a full diet. In the immediate postoperative period, the patient is instructed to expectorate all secretions forcefully in order to improve tongue mobility and future swallowing ability. As the patient is able to tolerate his or her own secretions, the diet is advanced slowly under the close supervision of the speech and swallowing therapists. Tracheotomy decannulation and full oral diet are possible in 95% of patients.[64,66]

Total Laryngectomy

In the opinion of most laryngologists, advanced tumors that impair vocal fold motion, exhibit transglottic extension, or deeply invade adjacent tissues are treated best by total laryngectomy, usually combined with postoperative radiation therapy. However, Harwood et al[68] have shown the efficacy of primary radical radiotherapy with surgical salvage. The addition of chemotherapy will allow 30 to 50% of patients who are cured to retain their larynges.[12] Patients whose tumors recur after nonsurgical treatment are most often salvaged with total laryngectomy. Standard wide-field laryngectomy includes resection of the entire larynx, the hyoid bone, overlying strap muscles, and the upper trachea. The thyroid lobe on the dominant side of the tumor is usually removed, as well. The

surgery can be extended to include part or all of the hypopharyngeal mucosa, the entire esophagus, and the entire cervical trachea. Unilateral or bilateral modified or radical neck dissections are performed in combination with total laryngectomy, if indicated. Patients presenting with advanced, obstructing tumors often need airway protection prior to definitive surgery. Although tracheotomy provides a definitively safe airway, there has been some concern that performing tracheotomy before total laryngectomy increases the risk of stomal recurrence. An alternative, temporizing measure to re-establish an adequate airway is to debulk the obstructing portion of tumor, often at the time of biopsy, for definitive diagnosis. Debulking can be accomplished through the use of the CO_2 laser or with the use of powered instrumentation with specially designed laryngeal attachments.

Prior to total laryngectomy, patients should be treated with prophylactic antibiotics and are prepared for possible intraoperative transfusion. Many patients require tracheotomy under local anesthesia for airway support prior to the induction of general anesthesia. If orotracheal intubation is accomplished, the tube can be left in place until the trachea is incised.

The incision is determined by the extent of the resection. A wide, superiorly based apron flap, including a tracheal stoma, is performed for simple laryngectomies (Fig 23–14). This can be extended laterally, and an inferior limb can be added when a neck dissection is performed (Fig 23–15). A full or half "h" incision with its modifications also can provide excellent exposure. The skin flaps are elevated deep to the platysma

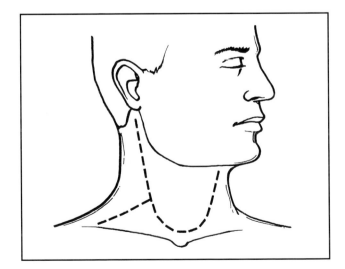

Fig 23–14. An apron flap incision as utilized for total laryngectomy. The lateral extension can be added for simultaneous radical dissection.

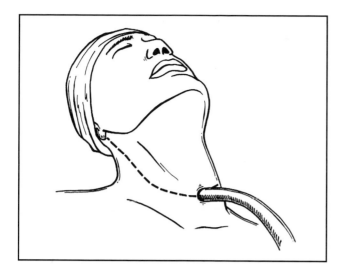

Fig 23–15. A utility incision is preferred when laryngectomy is combined with a neck dissection.

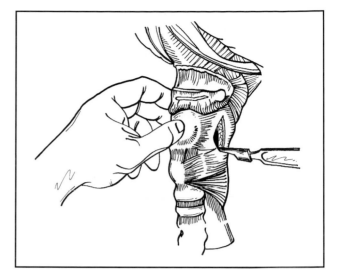

Fig 23–16. Total laryngectomy. The inferior constrictor muscle is divided form the lateral margin of the thyroid ala.

muscle. They must be handled gently, especially in radiated patients. The strap muscles are divided inferiorly, and the thyroid gland is exposed. The carotid sheath structures are identified, isolated from the larynx, and retracted laterally with the sternocleidomastoid muscle. The thyroid isthmus is divided, and the lobe on the uninvolved side is dissected sharply from the trachea. On the involved side, dissection proceeds lateral to the thyroid lobe, isolating and controlling the inferior and superior vascular pedicles. The larynx is rotated, and the inferior constrictor muscles are dissected sharply from the lateral margins of the thyroid ala on each side (Fig 23–16). The suprahyoid muscles are dissected from the hyoid bone, and the greater cornua are freed. Care must be taken to dissect close to the bone to prevent hypoglossal nerve injury. Control and ligation of the superior vascular pedicles of the larynx are the last steps in separating the larynx from external muscular structures (Fig 23–17).

The larynx is removed by separating its mucosal attachments. The trachea is divided below the second ring or one ring below a pre-existing tracheotomy. The incision in the tracheal mucosa is carried superiorly on the posterior wall to provide extra length for the stoma. Once the trachea is divided, it must be sutured to the inferior skin margin to prevent retraction into the mediastinum. Scalpel dissection proceeds through the posterior wall incision until the "gray line" between the trachea and esophagus is identified. This reveals a plane that can be opened bluntly to the level of the arytenoid cartilages. The lateral attachments along this plane are divided. The pharynx is entered superior to the hyoid bone, through the mucosa of the vallecula. If there is tumor extension into the epiglottis

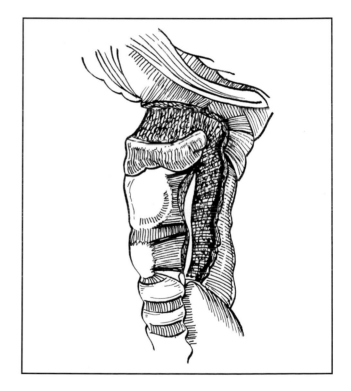

Fig 23–17. Total laryngectomy. After division of the strap muscles and the inferior constrictors, the larynx is freed from all muscular attachments.

or vallecula, the pharynx is opened through the contralateral piriform sinus (Fig 23–18). The epiglottis is grasped and mucosal incisions are carried inferiorly to allow the larynx to be opened on the contralateral side to visualize the tumor directly (Fig 23–19). Mucosal

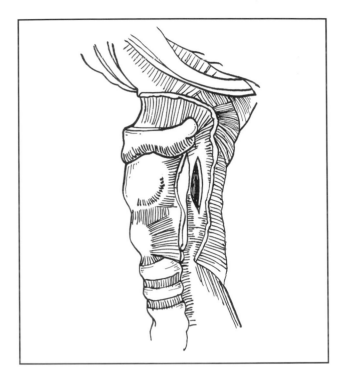

Fig 23–18. Total laryngectomy. When the pre-epiglottic space is involved, the larynx is entered through the contralateral piriform sinus, and the larynx is rotated to expose the tumor.

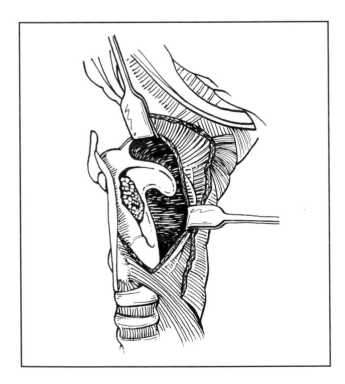

Fig. 23–19. Total laryngectomy. The final mucosal incisions are made with the tumor visualized directly to allow adequate surgical margins.

incisions proceed as medially as possible along the piriform sinus mucosa leaving at least a 2-cm mucosal margin. The incisions are connected inferiorly, and the larynx is removed. Mucosal closure of the pharynx is usually performed in a "T" fashion (Fig 23–20). When extensive pharyngectomy is required, a straight-line closure may be appropriate. The closure is in two layers: a running, inverting Connell (inverting horizontal mattress) suture in the mucosa and interrupted imbricating sutures in the muscularis. Absorbable suture is used. A nasogastric tube is placed under direct visualization prior to closure.

Creation of a stoma begins by resecting a circular ellipse of skin slightly larger than the tracheal diameter and removing subcutaneous fat from the margin. The stoma is secured with interrupted vertical mattress sutures around the distal tracheal cartilage ring. A continuous 4-0 or 5-0 absorbable suture may be placed circumferentially to closely appose the mucosa and the skin. Large suction drains are placed and the skin flaps are closed in layers.

Voice and Swallowing Rehabilitation After Total Laryngectomy

Voice rehabilitation can be accomplished with an electrolarynx (oral or neck placement), esophageal speech,

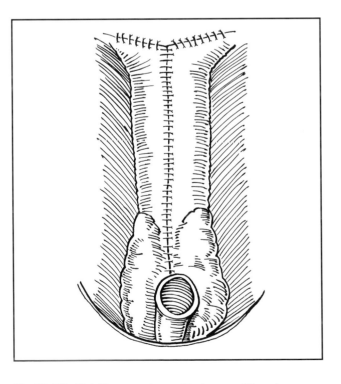

Fig 23–20. Total laryngectomy. T-closure of the pharynx.

or by means of a valve prosthesis placed in a tracheoesophageal conduit. Historically, multiple attempts have been made to create a vocal tract surgically using pharyngeal mucosal flaps placed over the tracheal air column. However, most of these methods have been abandoned due to the risk of aspiration. Almost all patients use an electrolarynx at some point during their rehabilitation, and approximately one third of laryngectomy patients can obtain good results with esophageal speech.

The valve voice prosthesis can provide a controllable, nonmechanical voice for over 90% of total laryngectomy patients.[69,70] It can be considered even after hypopharyngeal or esophageal reconstruction.[71,72] However, the prosthesis requires frequent maintenance and sometimes considerable speech training. Patient selection is based on intelligence, compliance, and manual dexterity. The fistula can be formed at the time of total laryngectomy or anytime after primary healing is completed. When prosthesis fistula creation is considered as a delayed procedure, the patient is first evaluated with a barium swallow, to rule out pharyngeal stenosis; and an air insufflation test is used to prove the patient can produce voice. Usually, the operation is performed under general anesthesia. A rigid esophagoscope is placed at the level of the superior margin of the tracheal stoma. A needle is placed 2 to 3 mm proximal to the mucocutaneous junction and visualized in the esophageal lumen. A silk suture is pulled through the esophagoscope (Fig 23–21). The suture is attached to progressively enlarging dilators (usually filiform and followers) until a 16-gauge French red rubber catheter is pulled through. The internal portion of the catheter is pushed into the distal esophagus, and the external portion is sutured to the skin superior to the stoma. Three to five days later, the catheter is removed, and the patient is fitted with a prosthesis. Kits are available with some prostheses that allow placement of the valve at the time of tracheoesophageal puncture, although surgical edema usually prevents adequate voicing for several days after placement.

The fistula also can be formed at the time of total laryngectomy. The common tracheal and esophageal walls are grasped with ring forceps, and the incision is made high on the posterior tracheal wall. A 16-gauge French red rubber catheter is placed through the incision into the esophagus directly. The distal catheter is pushed into the esophagus and used as a feeding tube postoperatively. Placement of the prosthesis within a week of laryngectomy has the advantages of providing early, excellent voice rehabilitation. Patients become more involved in their postoperative care and return to work sooner. However, the fistula can be difficult to manage during radiation therapy; and the patient may not have useful voice during that time. Additionally, the incidence of stomal stenosis is somewhat increased; and stenting with laryngectomy tubes may be necessary.[73]

Swallowing rehabilitation is easier after total laryngectomy than after partial laryngectomy due to the total separation of the digestive and respiratory passages by total laryngectomy. Most patients who do not develop pharyngocutaneous fistulae can begin oral feedings 5 to 10 days after surgery. Oral feeding is generally delayed by several weeks in previously irradiated patients due to the relatively high incidence of delayed fistulas in this patient population. A recent article demonstrated the safety of oral feedings in selected patients 48 hours after total laryngectomy.[74]

Subglottic Cancer

The cricothyroid membrane is found about 10 mm inferior to the anterior commissure and 5 mm inferior to the posterior margin of the vocal fold. Tumor extension to this membrane allows lymphatic spread to the paratracheal lymph nodes and the thyroid gland. Inferiorly, tumor may extend submucosally to involve the cricoid cartilage. Circumferential involvement and extensive posterior growth into the hypopharynx are not uncommon.[75]

Most subglottic tumors are extensions from glottic primary lesions. Primary subglottic carcinoma is rare. Patients usually present with airway obstruction, and hoarseness is common secondary to a greater than 75% incidence of vocal fold fixation.[76] Accurate diagnosis and staging are important (Table 23–4).

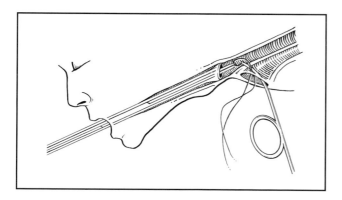

Fig 23–21. A silk suture is placed through the tracheoesophageal puncture and brought through the esophagoscope into the oral cavity. The suture is attached to dilators; and after adequate dilatation, a 16-gauge red rubber catheter is introduced in the distal esophagus and fixed to the skin.

Table 23–4. Staging of Primary Tumor in Laryngeal Cancer.

Subglottis

T_1— Tumor limited to subglottis.

T_2— Tumor extends to vocal folds with normal or impaired mobility.

T_3— Tumor limited to larynx with vocal fold fixation.

T_4— Tumor invades the cricoid or thyroid cartilage and/or extends to other tissues beyond the larynx.

Surgical excision of primary subglottic tumors always requires a total laryngectomy, because resection of the cricoid cartilage destroys the protective function of the larynx during swallowing. However, some tumors extending from glottic cancers can be resected by vertical hemilaryngectomy with partial cricoid resection.[77] Biller and Som have described a technique of rotating the remaining posterior margin of the thyroid lamina into the cricoid defect with mucosal flap coverage.[78] Contraindicatons to vertical hemilaryngectomy with partial cricoid resection include prior radiation therapy, vocal fold fixation, and extensive invasion of the cricoid cartilage. The incidence of occult lymph node metastasis in subglottic tumors is less than 10%, so elective neck dissection is not indicated.[63]

Conclusion

Laryngeal carcinoma remains a complex clinical challenge. Intimate knowledge of anatomy, patterns of malignant spread, and diverse treatment options is essential. Treatment decisions often are difficult when attempting to balance adequate tumor control and maintenance of voice and swallowing function. The curability of laryngeal cancer has improved only minimally over the past few decades. However, functional treatment results have improved substantially thanks to adjuvant chemotherapy, radical radiotherapy, and innovative conservation and reconstructive surgical techniques.

References

1. American Cancer Society. *Cancer Facts and Figures.* Atlanta, Ga: Author; 2001:7.
2. Silverberg E. Cancer statistics, 1984. *CA.* 1984;34:7–23.
3. Albright JT, Karpti R, Topham A, et al. Second malignant neoplasms in patients under 40 years of age with laryngeal cancer. *Laryngoscope.* 2001;111:563–567.
4. Burch JD, Howe GR, Miller AB, Semenciw R. Tobacco, alcohol, asbestos, and nickel in the etiology of cancer of

the larynx: a case-control study. *J Natl Cancer Inst.* 1981; 67:1219–1224.
5. Wynder EL, Bross IJ, Day E. Epidemiological approach to the etiology of cancer of the larynx. *JAMA.* 1956;160: 1384–1391.
6. Auerbach O, Hammond EC, Garfinkel L. Historic changes in the larynx in relation to smoking habits. *Cancer.* 1970;25:92–104.
7. Flanders WD, Rothman KJ. Interaction of alcohol and tobacco in laryngeal cancer. *Am J Epidemiol.* 1982;115: 371–379.
8. Wynder EL, Cover LS, Marbuchi K, Mushinski M. Environmental factors in cancer of the larynx: a second look. *Cancer.* 1976;38:1591–1601.
9. Pedersen E, Hogetveit AC, Andersen A. Cancer of respiratory organs among workers at a nickel refinery in Norway. *Int J Cancer.* 1973;12:32–41.
10. Stell PM, McGill T. Asbestos and laryngeal carcinoma. *Lancet.* 1973;2:416–417.
11. Parnes SM. Asbestos and cancer of the larynx: is there a relationship? *Laryngoscope.* 1990;100:254–261.
12. Wolf GT, Hong WK, Fisher S, et al. Induction chemotherapy plus radiation compared with surgery plus radiation in patients with advanced laryngeal cancer. *New Eng J Med.* 1991;324:1685–1690.
13. McDonald TJ, DeSanto LW, Weiland LH. Supraglottic larynx and its pathology as studied by whole laryngeal sections. *Laryngoscope.* 1976;86:635–648.
14. American Joint Committee on Cancer. *Manual for Staging Cancer.* 3rd ed. Philadelphia, Pa: JB Lippincott; 1988.
15. Coates HL, DeSanto LW, Devine KD, Elveback LR. Carcinoma of the supraglottic larynx: a review of 221 cases. *Arch Otolaryngol.* 1976;102:686–689.
16. Bocca E. Supraglottic cancer. *Laryngoscope.* 1975:85:1318–1326.
17. Shah JP, Tollefsen HR. Epidermoid carcinoma of the supraglottic larynx: role of neck dissection in initial surgical treatment. *Am J Surg.* 1974;128:494–499.
18. Som ML. Conservation surgery for carcinoma of the supraglottis. *J Laryngol Otol.* 1970;84:656–678.
19. Archer CR, Yeager VL. Computed tomography of laryngeal cancer with histopathological correlation. *Laryngoscope.* 1982;92:1173–1180.
20. Larson JT, Adams GL, Fattah HA. Survival statistics for multiple primaries in head and neck cancer. *Otolaryngol Head Neck Surg.* 1990;103:14–24.
21. Fayos JV. Carcinoma of the endolarynx: results of irradiation. *Cancer.* 1975;35:1525–1532.
22. DeSanto LW: Early supraglottic cancer. *Ann Otol Rhinol Laryngol.* 1990;99:593–597.
23. Goepfert H, Jessie RH, Fletcher GH, Hamberger A. Optimal treatment for the technically resectable squamous cell carcinoma of the supraglottic larynx. *Laryngoscope.* 1975;85:14–32.
24. Snow JB Jr, Gelber RD, Kramer S, et al. Evaluation of randomized preoperative and postoperative radiation therapy for supraglottic carcinoma. *Ann Otol Rhinol Laryngol.* 1978;87:686–691.
25. Schuller DE, McGuirt WF, Krause CJ, et al. Symposium: adjuvant cancer therapy of head neck tumors. Increased

survival with surgery alone vs. combined therapy. *Laryngoscope*. 1979;89:582–594.

26. Harwood AR. Cancer of the larynx: the Toronto experience. *J Otolaryngol*. 1982;11(suppl 11):S10–S13.

27. DeSanto LW. Cancer of the supraglottic larynx: a review of 260 patients. *Otolaryngol Head Neck Surg*. 1985;93:705–711.

28. Burstein FD, Calcaterra TC. Supraglottic laryngectomy: series report and analysis of results. *Laryngoscope*. 1985; 95:833–836.

29. Mendenhall WM, Parsons JT, Stringer SP, et al. Carcinoma of the supraglottic larynx: a basis for comparing the results of radiotherapy and surgery. *Head Neck*. 1990;12: 204–209.

30. Lutz CK, Jahnson JT, Wagner RL, Myers EN. Supraglottic carcinoma: patterns of recurrence. *Ann Otol Rhinol Laryngol*. 1990;99:12–17.

31. DeSanto LW, Magrina C, O'Fallon WM. The "second" side of the neck in supraglottic cancer. *Otolaryngol Head Neck Surg*. 1990;102:351–361.

32. Bocca E. Surgical management of supraglottic cancer and its lymph node metastases in a conservative perspective. Sixteenth Daniel C. Baker Jr Memorial Lecture. *Ann Otol Rhinol Laryngol*. 1991;100:261–267.

33. Boyd TS, Harari PM, Tannehill SP, et al. Planned postradiotherapy neck dissection in patients with advanced head and neck cancer. *Head Neck*. 1998;20(2):132–137.

34. Chan AW, Ancukiewicz M, Carballo N, et al. The role of postradiotherapy neck dissection in supraglottic carcinoma. *Int J Radiat Oncol Biol Phys*. 2001;50(2):367–375.

35. Zeitels SM, Vaughan CW, Domanowski GF. Endoscopic management of early supraglottic cancer. *Ann Otol Rhinol Laryngol*. 1990;99:951–956.

36. Iro H, Waldfahrer F, Altendorf-Hofmann A, et al. Transoral laser surgery of supraglottic cancer: follow-up of 141 patient. *Arch Otolaryngol Head Neck Surg*. 1998;124(11): 1245–1250.

37. Rudert I II I, Werner JA, Hoft S. Transoral carbon dioxide laser resection of supraglottic carcinoma. *Ann Otol Rhinol Laryngol*. 1999;108(9):819–827.

38. Quer M, Leon X, Orus C, et al. Endoscopic laser surgery in the treatment of radiation failure of early laryngeal carcinoma. *Head Neck*. 2000;22(5):520–523.

39. Eckel HE, Thumfart W, Jungehulsing M, et al. Transoral laser surgery for early glottic carcinoma. *Eur Arch Otorhinolaryngol*. 2000;257(4):221–226.

40. Eckel HE. Local recurrences following transoral laser surgery for early glottic carcinoma: frequency, management, and outcome. *Ann Otol Rhinol Laryngol*. 2001;110(1): 7–15.

41. DeSanto LW, Lillie JC, Devine KD. Surgical salvage after radiation for laryngeal cancer. *Laryngoscope*. 1976;86:649–657.

42. Kirchner JD. Two hundred laryngeal cancers: patterns of growth and spread as seen in serial section. *Laryngoscope*. 1977;87:474–482.

43. Maran AG, Mackenzie IJ, Stanley RE. Carcinoma in situ of the larynx. *Head Neck Surg*. 1984;7:28–31.

44. Kaplan MJ, Johns ME, Clark DA, Cantrell RW. Glottic carcinoma: the roles of surgery and irradiation. *Cancer*. 1984;53:2641–2648.

45. Nichols RD, Mickelson SA. Partial laryngectomy after irradiation failure. *Ann Otol Rhinol Laryngol*. 1991;100: 176–180.

46. Shaw HJ. Role of partial laryngectomy after irradiation in the treatment of laryngeal cancer: a view from the United Kingdom. *Ann Otol Rhinol Laryngol*. 1991;100:268–273.

47. Shah JP, Loree TR, Kowalski L. Conservation surgery for radiation-failure carcinoma of the glottic larynx. *Head Neck*. 1990;12:326–331.

48. Shapshay SM, Hybels RL, Bohigan RK. Laser excision of early vocal cord carcinoma: indications, limitations, and precautions. *Ann Otol Rhinol Laryngol*. 1990;99:46–50.

49. Ossoff RH, Sisson GA, Shapshay SM. Endoscopic management of selected early vocal cord carinoma. *Ann Otol Rhinol Laryngol*. 1985;94:560–564.

50. Schweitzer VG. Photofrin-mediated photodynamic therapy for treatment of early stage oral cavity and laryngeal malignancies. *Lasers Surg Med*. 2001;29:305–313.

51. Sessions DG, Maness GM, McSwain B. Laryngofissure in the treatment of carcinoma of the vocal cord: a report of forty cases and a review of the literature. *Laryngoscope*. 1965;75:490–502.

52. Biller HF, Lawson W. Bilateral vertical partial laryngectomy for bilateral vocal cord carcinoma. *Ann Otol Rhinol Laryngol*. 1981;90:489–491.

53. Biller HF, Ogura JH, Pratt LL. Hemilaryngectomy for T2 glottic cancer. *Arch Otolaryngol*. 1971;93:238–243.

54. Kirchner JA, Som ML. The anterior commissure technique of partial laryngectomy: clinical and laboratory observations. *Laryngoscope*. 1975;85:1308–1317.

55. Sessions DG, Ogura JH, Fried MP. The anterior commissure in glottic carcinoma. *Laryngoscope*. 1975;85:1624–1632.

56. Biller HF, Lawson W. Partial laryngectomy for vocal cord cancer with marked limitation or fixation of the vocal cord. *Laryngoscope*. 1986;96:61–64.

57. Amin MR, Koufman JA. Hemicricoidectomy for voice rehabilitation following hemilaryngectomy with ipsilateral arytenoid removal. *Ann Otol Rhinol Laryngol*. 2001; 110(6):514–518.

58. Bailey BJ. Partial laryngectomy and laryngoplasty: a technique and review. *Trans Am Acad Ophthalmol Otolaryngol*. 1966;70(4):559–574.

59. Biller HF, Lucente FE. Reconstruction of the larynx following vertical partial laryngectomy. *Otolaryngol Clin North Am*. 1979;12:761–766.

60. Biller HF, Lawson W. Partial laryngectomy for transglottic cancers. *Ann Otol Rhinol Laryngol*. 1984;93:297–300.

61. Schechter GL. Epiglottic reconstruction and subtotal laryngectomy. *Laryngoscope*. 1983;93:729–734.

62. Nong HU, Mo W, Huang GW, et al. Epiglottic laryngoplasty after hemilaryngectomy for glottic cancer. *Otolaryngol Head Neck Surg*. 1991;104:809–813.

63. Tucker HM, Benninger MS, Roberts JK, et al. Near-total laryngectomy with epiglottic reconstruction. *Arch Otolaryngol Head Neck Surg*. 1989;115:1314–1344.

64. Laccourreye L, Salzer SJ, Brasnu D, et al. Glottic carcinoma with a fixed true vocal cord: outcomes after neoadjuvant chemotherapy and supracricoid partial laryngectomy with cricohyoidoepiglottopexy. *Otolaryngol Head Neck Surg.* 1996;114:400–406.

65. Laccourreye O, Weinstein G, Brasnu D, et al. A clinical trial of continuous cisplatin-flurouracil induction chemotherapy and supracricoid partial laryngectomy for glottic carcinoma classified as T2. *Cancer.* 1994;74(10): 2781–2790.

66. Laccourreye O, Weinstein G, Naudo P, et al. Supracricoid partial laryngectomy after failed laryngeal radiation therapy. *Laryngoscope.* 1996;106:495–498.

67. Laccourreye O, Weinstein G, Brasnu D, et al. Vertical partial laryngectomy: a critical analysis of local recurrence. *Ann Otol Rhino Laryngol.* 1991;110:68–71.

68. Harwood AR, Bryce DP, Rider WD. Management of T3 glottic cancer. *Arch Otolaryngol.* 1980;106:697–699.

69. Wood BG, Rusnove MG, Tucker HM, et al. Tracheoesophageal puncture for alaryngeal voice restoration. *Ann Otol Rhinol Laryngol.* 1981;90:492–494.

70. Singer MI. Tracheoesophageal speech: vocal rehabilitation after total laryngectomy. *Laryngoscope.* 1983;93:1454–1465.

71. Bleach N, Perry A, Cheesman A. Surgical voice restoration with the Blom-Singer prosthesis following laryngopharyngoesophagectomy and pharyngogastric anastomosis. *Ann Otol Rhinol Laryngol.* 1991;100:142–147.

72. Kinishi M, Amatsu M, Tahara S, Makino K. Primary tracheojejunal shunt operation for voice restoration following pharyngolaryngoesophagectomy. *Ann Otol Rhinol Laryngol.* 1991;100:435–438.

73. Ho CM, Wei WI, Lau WF, Lam KH. Tracheostomal stenosis after immediate tracheoesophageal puncture. *Arch Otolaryngol Head Neck Surg.* 1991;117:662–665.

74. Medina JE, Khafif A. Early oral feeding following total laryngectomy. *Laryngoscope.* 2001;111(3):368–372.

75. Micheau C, Luboinski B, Sancho H, Cachin Y. Modes of invasion of cancer of the larynx: a statistical, histological, and radioclinical analysis of 120 cases. *Cancer.* 1976;38: 346–360.

76. Stell MP. The subglottic space. In: Alberti PW, Bryce DP, eds. *Workshops from the Centennial Conference on Laryngeal Cancer.* New York, NY: Appleton-Century-Crofts; 1976: 620.

77. Sessions DG, Ogura JH, Fried MP. Carcinoma of the subglottic area. *Laryngoscope.* 1975;85:1417–1423.

78. Biller HF, Som ML. Vertical partial laryngectomy for glottic carcinoma with posterior subglottic extension. *Ann Otol Rhinol Laryngol.* 1977;86:715–718.

24

Nursing Considerations in the Care of Professional Voice Users

Mary J. Hawkshaw and Robert Thayer Sataloff

The profession of nursing has long been in a state of transition, and nursing literature is replete with contributions that attempt to keep its practitioners abreast of the changing status and role of the professional registered nurse. Clearly, all professionals are affected by external and internal forces, including an expanding base of scientific knowledge, the changing scope of practice, and social and financial factors. These make it clear that the profession of nursing will continue to undergo redefinition. Nurses have gained an increasingly independent function in the primary care of patients in many settings, for example, the nurse practitioner's role, which is now commonplace and widely accepted. Nonetheless, the basic definition of nursing and the core of nursing care is unchanged from nursing's earliest history; nursing is a profession devoted to the prevention and relief of physical and emotional suffering. Inherent in that practice is the "control of disease, the care and rehabilitation of the sick and the promotion of health through teaching and counseling."[1,2(p3)] Nurses apply interventions with a scientific, research-based understanding of pathophysiology, clinical experience, and competence with physical procedures. Through contributions of insight and empathy, they also assist in the management of psychological distress.

It is incumbent on the nurse specialist in the field of otolaryngology to thoroughly understand the anatomy and physiology of the head and neck.[3] Pathophysiologic conditions unique to otorhinolaryngology may be present in the professional voice user, in addition to the chief presenting voice complaint. Additionally, a comprehensive knowledge of the pharmacology of the medications used in the treatment of illnesses specific to the head and neck, as well as those used in the management of generalized medical conditions, must be acquired and frequently updated by the nurse practicing in this field.

One source of ongoing continuing education for nurses practicing in the medical-surgical subspecialty of otorhinolaryngology is the Society of Otorhinolaryngology and Head-Neck Nursing (SOHN). This society, which promotes excellence in care and nursing research, also provides certification for its practitioners.

As a member of a voice care team, the otolaryngologic nurse-clinician must develop an extensive recognition and understanding of the special problems of professional voice users. In addition to knowledge of the most common medical diagnoses, etiologies, and treatments for voice disorders, she or he must acquire extra training in technical aspects of voice production in speech and singing and work collaboratively with specialists in these disciplines as a member of a voice care team. It is especially helpful if the professional nurse functioning in this role has personal experience as a vocal performer. Not only does this permit him or her to assess the potential role demands in the patient's repertoire, it allows for greater empathy derived from experiential understanding of the professional and emotional impact of possible damage to the performer's vocal mechanism.

Functions of the Otolaryngologic Nurse-Clinician

Although many clinical voice centers function without the expertise of an otolaryngologic nurse-clinician, the role is essential in our practice model. The nurse, as a member of our multidisciplinary team, provides care for patients both directly and indirectly. Direct responsibilities involve patient care and the coordination of care provided by all members of the voice team. Indirect care includes providing and maintaining a safe physical environment in which the patient receives care and treatment from all members of the team. Additionally, our nurses devote a large percentage of their time to educating patients and their families, colleagues, and the profession as a whole.

Care of the professional voice user generally begins with triage based on telephone contact. When a patient contacts the voice center by telephone, his or her call is first taken by one of the secretarial staff who have been trained by the laryngologist (RTS) and nurse-clinician (MJH) to ask specific questions designed to elicit the information essential in deciding how urgently the patient needs evaluation. If the situation is equivocal or emergent, the secretaries are instructed to contact one of the nurse-clinicians or physicians. During clinical questioning, the nurse-clinician listens critically to the quality of the patient's voice on the telephone, as well as the description of the onset of the voice complaint and imminent performances. This allows the nurse to assess for vocal problems that require immediate, absolute voice rest, and/or an emergency evaluation. Of course, all nursing decisions involve collaboration with the laryngologist when necessary. Immediate performance demands in a professional performer with voice complaints necessitate that the patient be seen emergently. Thus, caring for professional voice users, singers, and actors is a 24-hour, 7 days a week commitment of access to laryngological care. Voice patients who seek care at our voice center for the first time are provided with our specialized questionnaire, which is included in Appendix Ib. When there is sufficient time prior to the evaluation, this form is mailed to the patient so that she or he may consider the questions carefully and answer them fully. When the patient is scheduled for an urgent evaluation, the form is completed in the waiting room once the patient arrives at the center.

Using the printed history form as a guide, the nurse will perform a complete medical and nursing history. The medical history follows the routine format: identifying data; chief complaint; history of the presenting illness; past medical and surgical history, including current medications and medication allergies; family history; social history (which includes current performance commitments in professional voice users); smoking, alcohol, and recreational drug use; and toxic exposure. The nurse should also assess the ways in which the patient's voice problem interferes with activities of daily living and how it affects emotional responses and other health problems. Once the nurse

has obtained a patient's medical and surgical history, she or he then takes a "voice" history. Questions asked include (but are not limited to): When did your voice problem begin? Is it getting better or worse? Have you had similar or any other history of voice problems? and many other questions. A more complete discussion on taking the history can be found in *Clinical Assessment of Voice*.[4] The otolaryngologic nurse-clinician then presents the history to the laryngologist before the patient enters the room to be examined. The laryngologist reviews this information, as well as the patient's written responses. He or she will then expand the history and pursue areas relevant to the differential diagnoses.

In our center, nurses assist the physician in performing a complete head and neck physical examination. However, the nurse's role involves not only physical assistance to the physician, but also emotional support and education of the patient throughout the examination. The nurse is also responsible for thoroughly documenting the physician's physical findings on the medical record. After completion of the examination, the laryngologist may order additional laboratory tests, imaging studies, and referrals to consultants as part of the comprehensive voice evaluation. In our center, the initial evaluation of a patient with a voice disorder generally includes a strobovideo-olaryngoscopic evaluation of laryngeal function. This, slow-motion visual analysis of laryngeal function is the current standard of care in evaluating patients with voice disorders. Nurses interested in learning more about this procedure are encouraged to read *Clinical Assessment of Voice*[4,5]. Prior to the strobovideo-laryngoscopy, the laryngologist (or the nurse-specialist on the laryngologist's order) will administer topical anesthesia to facilitate patients' comfort and a thorough endoscopic examination with optimal visualization. Among the nurse's roles is explaining to the patient the sensations associated with anesthesia in the nasopharynx, oropharynx, and hypopharynx. The patient receives both oral and written instructions for the prevention of aspiration and other problems that could occur before the anesthesia effect wears off. In our hands, the amount of topical anesthesia administered generally lasts no more than 30 to 40 minutes. The nurse then begins the first part of the videostroboscopic examination by placing a microphone and EGG (electroglottograph) leads on the patient and then records a baseline EGG and a conversational voice sample on videotape.[6] The patient receives instruction and demonstration of techniques that are useful in suppressing the gag reflex (common during endoscopy); one of the nurse's responsibilities during the examination is to support and coach the patient in the use of these techniques.

The strobovideolaryngoscopic examination is performed by the laryngologist in the author's practice. Occasionally, in other voice centers, speech-language pathologists may perform and record a rigid endoscopic examination for later review by the laryngologist. In Pennsylvania (where the authors practice), registered nurses who have been specially trained are permitted to intubate and may use both flexible and rigid endoscopes under the supervision of a physician. Occasionally, it may be appropriate for the otolaryngologic nurse-clinician to perform a strobovideolaryngoscopic examination during a follow-up visit. The laryngologist subsequently reviews all of the examinations, and diagnoses are made only by the laryngologist. During the examination, the nurse will operate the computer and video equipment and document the physical findings on a standard report form. These are reviewed, amended, and expanded by the laryngologist, who prepares an operative report for the patient's medical record. At the conclusion of the examination, the nurse provides the patient with additional explanation of the diagnoses rendered by the laryngologist following his or her examination, the treatment prescribed, and explanations or instructions for additional studies the laryngologist has ordered for further assessment. Both short- and long-term plans of care are defined.

The professional nurse is responsible for supervising the implementation of the plan of care and for communication with the laryngologist and other voice team members (speech-language pathologists, singing voice specialists, and others) regarding its implementation and time frame.

We have found that patients frequently do not retain all of the information they receive during their first visit. Psychological research indicates that emotional distress radically diminishes recall of information provided during a crisis. For that reason, professional voice patients often require repetition, amplification, expansion, and documentation of information regarding their diagnoses and treatment plan. They also need the opportunity to discuss their emotional responses and the social impact they are experiencing. When the patient's emotional responses seem extreme, complex, and/or dangerous, the patient is referred to the clinical psychologist or psychiatrist for further assessment and possible treatment. The vocal rehabilitation of a professional voice user is an exquisitely slow, carefully monitored process whether or not surgery is required. For some patients, this becomes difficult to manage emotionally; and it is especially stressful for professional voice users, because their voice (treatment and outcome) and their sense of self are so closely intertwined, as discussed previously. In our setting, patients always have access to a nurse, either by tele-

phone or in person. Supporting patients in this manner has proven to be very beneficial in allaying fears and anxiety, which, in turn, enhances voice rehabilitation. When absolute voice rest is ordered, the nurse will instruct the patient on ways to maintain communication, such as the use of writing pads, magic slates, and laptop computers. Certain types of voice surgery may require a period of absolute voice rest for 1 week following surgery. One of our patients devised a means for helping herself during this situation. A badge was suggested by this patient, and the authors' gratefully share her creativity! The badge contains the patient 's name and also the phrase, "I've had voice surgery. I can't speak but I can hear and write. Please don't shout."

Another indirect function of the nurse in an outpatient setting is the establishment of and adherence to the Occupational Safety and Health Administration (OSHA) mandated infection control policies and procedures. The nurse is responsible for ensuring that Universal Precautions are employed during the examination of any patient when contact with body fluids might be anticipated. In addition, instruments, endoscopes, and equipment are disinfected according to current OSHA guidelines. Supervision of proper disposal of medical waste also falls under the nursing purview. In-service education of other professionals on the voice team and office staff members who have a potential risk of exposure is conducted when they are newly hired and on a yearly basis. Appropriate records are maintained.

Patients cannot be examined properly without adequate lighting, instrumentation, and functioning electronic and suction equipment. The nurse is responsible for the purchasing and maintenance of equipment, as well as assisting the laryngologist in evaluating new products that might enhance the quality of patient assessment and care. In the authors' practice, the nurse-clinician is also responsible for the orientation and education of other voice team colleagues on the proper use of the equipment in the examination of the professional voice patient.

A clinical practice with quality and breadth will emphasize the need for education. This always includes education of the patient. Current nursing practice views the patient as the central participant in his or her own therapy. Nurses help direct a patient by focusing his or her energy on the goals of therapy, as designed by the laryngologist, other voice team members, and the patient. In order for this to happen, the patient must be informed of the therapeutic goals of the entire team and his or her cooperation and consent must be obtained. It is a matter of professional nursing judgment, as well as the policy of each individual medical practice, regarding which facts to impart, when, and by whom. The nurse will need to assess the patient's physical and psychological readiness to learn, and all of the factors affecting the patient's learning ability, such as educational experience, occupation, or affect. Special adaptations relating to any potential intellectual, physical, or sensory impairment must be considered. Teaching aids including written reiteration of the verbal instructions and visual aids are provided whenever possible.[3] Although voice care, as a subspeciality of laryngology, has advanced dramatically over the past two decades, new information about the voice and how it works is still being discovered. It is incumbent on all nurses involved in caring for patients with voice disorders to remain current in their knowledge of the advancements made in the diagnosis and treatment of these most interesting and challenging patients.

Continuing education for the professional staff should also be an ongoing component in any voice center. In the authors' practice, regular meetings with all members of the voice team are held to discuss the care of all voice patients. Interdisciplinary collaboration provides additional clinical insight and direction in the therapeutic goals.

Finally, the nurses in our practice devote time and energy to the growth of their professional nursing organizations, such as the Society of Otorhinolaryngology and Head-Neck Nursing. There are no graduate nursing programs that provide in-depth, additional education for the professional nurse who chooses to practice in the specialized care of voice patients. Most undergraduate nursing programs (diploma, associate nursing degrees, or baccalaureate nursing degrees) offer only minimal exposure to the anatomy and physiology, pathophysiology, medical and surgical treatment, pharmacology, and psychosocial needs in this unique patient population. Most professional nurses practicing in the field have developed their skills through on-the-job training, continuing education through the literature and seminar attendance, and networking. SOHN, with its regional education offerings and its annual Congress, provides the nurses with the most current information in otorhinolaryngology—head and neck nursing offered by colleagues who are actively working at the forefront of research, in clinical practice, and in education. The authors strongly encourage membership and attendance at SOHN educational meetings. In addition, a number of symposia dedicated to care of the professional voice offer additional training by practitioners in all disciplines in this field. The Voice Foundation offers the most extensive annual symposium, which is held yearly in June. Information may be obtained by writing to The Voice Foundation at 1721 Pine Street, Philadelphia, Pennsylvania 19103 or by calling them directly at (215) 735-7999. An internship in our voice center and others provides a unique opportunity for intense observation of all aspects of voice care and, in some centers, may also include supervised nursing intervention with these patients.

Conclusion

The face of nursing has changed since its emergence and continues to evolve rapidly. Ongoing changes in health care delivery undoubtedly will be accompanied by changes in the roles of professional nurses, particularly in the care of professional voice users. Nursing intervention is critical to the healing process in any patient as are all of the other dimensions of treatment. In professional voice users, the sense of being known, understood, and respected as an individual is critical. The laryngologist shares responsibility with the otolaryngologic nurse-clinician, for the ongoing coordination of care for professional voice patients.

References

1. Fuerst EV, Wolff L. Fundamentals of nursing. *The Humanities and Sciences in Nursing.* 4th ed. Philadelphia, Pa: JB Lippincott Co; 1969:3–8.
2. Bruner LS, Emerson CP, Ferguson LK, Suddarth DS. *Textbook of Medical Surgical Nursing.* 2nd ed. Philadelphia, Pa: JB Lippincott Co; 1970:3.
3. Sigler BA, Schuring LT. *Ear, Nose, and Throat Disorders.* Mosby's Clinical Nursing Series. St Louis, Mo: CV Mosby; 1993:18:182–186.
4. Sataloff RT, Anticaglia J, Hawkshaw MJ. Patient history. In: Sataloff RT. *Clinical Assessment of Voice.* San Diego, Calif: Plural Publishing Inc; 2005:1–16.
5. Heuer RT, Hawkshaw MJ, Sataloff RT. The clinical voice laboratory. In: Sataloff RT. *Clinical Assessment of Voice.* San Diego, Calif: Plural Publishing Inc; 2005:33–81.
6. Sataloff RT, Spiegel JR, Carroll LM, et al. The clinical voice laboratory: practical design and clinical application. *J Voice.* 1990;4(3):264–279.

25

Controversy in the Care of the Singer and Professional Voice Users

Clark A. Rosen and Kimberly M. Steinhauer

A multitude of controversial subjects surrounds the medical care of singers and professional voice users. These controversies typically arise from a paucity of definitive, scientific information regarding the use of the vocal mechanism during a variety of situations. The scarcity of rigorous, experimental testing of the professional voice has relegated voice care to an art form equally as complex and mysterious as that of performing an art song. The purpose of this chapter is to highlight the controversies in order to provide a dialogue for future research and to heighten the awareness of voice care professionals who deal daily with these issues; however, as is the nature of controversy, identifying the issues is the easy first step in a long complicated process of resolution.

Choral Versus Solo Singing

Choral singing is viewed in a negative light frequently within the area of medical care of the singer. Often, the voice care professional recommends that the patient limit or withdraw from choral singing, regardless of the diagnosis and treatment plan. This overtly disapproving approach regarding choral singing stems mostly from anecdotal incidents whereby choral singers report an increase in dysphonia during or after rehearsal. Another source is the laryngologist's past patient experience of caring for singers who have developed a voice problem related to choral singing. It is important to note that a significant selection bias exists in this type of approach, because the laryngologist cannot possibly know the number of countless choral singers who never developed a voice problem. Similarly, when a singer develops a vocal injury from solo singing, the negative connotation that is applied to choral singers is not applied to solo singers.

There are multiple reasons for voice complaints associated with choral singing, including competition with the neighboring choral singer by trying to match intensity and voice quality and oversinging as a result of the decreasing ability to monitor one's voice in the large group (Lombard effect). However, the most serious risk factor in developing vocal injury occurs when the choir member follows a choral conductor who does not fully understand the intricate details, demands, and needs of a singer. All too frequently, choral conductors have an instrumental background and may not fully understand the technical aspects of singing.[1] Inexperienced choral conductors will place inappropriate expectations and demands on the choral singer to achieve a specific vocal quality or "color," which can be potentially damaging to the singer. Therefore, the tendency for choral singers to oversing, compete, or develop injurious singing techniques or habits frequently has led voice care professionals to view choral singing negatively.

A variety of potential difficulties associated with choral singing must be considered carefully when advising singers; however, there are significant advantages to choral singing that must not be dismissed. The advantages include the development of musicianship, ear training, and an esprit de corps that one misses as a soloist. An additional benefit is the positive professional development associated with choral singing (ie, exposure and financial reward). When addressing the appropriateness of a singer's participation or continuation in choral singing activities, the pros and cons need to be balanced. This decision-making process must incorporate the vocal experience of the conductor, maturity of the singer, and a healthy collaboration between the choral director and private singing teacher.[2]

Surgery for Singers and Professional Voice Users

A widespread misconception among singers and singing teachers concludes that a singer will never return to full vocal function following vocal fold surgery. This grave error has led many vocalists to end their careers prematurely, fearing that surgery will not improve their singing voices. Furthermore, significant morbidity and loss of professional development have occurred from this fallacy; because many singers delay surgery and, as a result, lose income.

Singers, singing teachers, speech-language pathologists, and otolaryngologists must be informed that the appropriate use of surgery to improve the voice (specifically phonomicrosurgery for benign vocal fold lesions) usually can restore a singer's voice to its premorbid condition; however, complete recovery of the singing voice depends on a multitude of factors, including compliance of the patient and expertise of the voice care team. Surgery must be reserved until all nonsurgical rehabilitative treatment options have been exhausted. It is reasonable to state that a "specialist of specialists" should perform surgery on the singer and professional voice user. These surgeons have a great deal of training and expertise in this type of highly specialized voice surgery. In addition to finding the right surgeon, the best results typically are achieved by working closely with a voice team that should, at a minimum, be comprised of an otolaryngologist specializing in voice care (laryngologist), a speech-language pathologist specializing in voice care, and a singing voice specialist.

Laser Versus Cold Steel Phonomicrosurgery

The debate between laser surgery versus "cold steel" surgery of the vocal fold has continued for over a decade. The crux of the debate rests on which surgical technique is best to achieve optimal voice results. Several key concepts need to be understood to assist in the framing of this controversy.

Laser and cold steel surgery are methods used to cut tissue but are not actual operative philosophies or surgical techniques. Most importantly, it is essential to recognize that the surgeon behind the instrument (laser or cold steel) is usually the essential component to surgi-

cal success. Thus, excellent results can most often be obtained with either laser or cold steel if the surgeon understands the appropriate use of the technique, uses good judgment, and has a high degree of skill.[3]

The history behind this controversy arose when the laser was developed and was touted as a panacea for laryngeal surgeons. The enthusiasm for the laser was driven, in part, by the "if it is new and high-tech, it must be better" concept and by the companies selling the laser. Another attractive aspect of the laser was the "no instrument in the laryngoscope" aspect to the laser surgery. If one performs laryngeal surgery through a small laryngoscope, the laser affords the surgeon the ability to make incisions in the vocal fold without having to have an instrument within the already crowded and narrow laryngoscope operating space. Similarly, if a surgeon has difficulty controlling his nondominant hand during bimanual surgery, the laser could be an advantage from a precision and control aspect.

The risks of laser surgery of the vocal fold arise from the fact that the laser works by vaporizing tissue using extreme heat. The heat associated with laser use can cause significant thermal injury to adjacent areas of the vocal fold. This injury results in scar formation within the vocal fold. The other disadvantages of laser surgery include cost and airway fire risk. The laser used most frequently for surgery of the vocal fold is the carbon dioxide (CO_2) laser. This laser has been through several generations of development of laser delivery methods (micromanipulator) and requires routine maintenance. An essential aspect to this controversy is the availability of the most recent micromanipulator that delivers a laser spot size of about 0.3 mm. No laser surgery of the vocal fold for benign disease should be performed that does not have this level of micromanipulator and is not regularly maintained. Many hospitals in the United States of America purchased a CO_2 laser a decade or more ago and have not continued proper maintenance. Therefore, many CO_2 lasers are dated in their technology and not properly maintained. Furthermore, laser surgery of the vocal folds requires special skill, knowledge, and maintenance of these skills by the surgeon. If the surgeon does not regularly use the laser, the outcome can be disastrous.

For the majority of phonomicrosurgerical procedures, the present principles and techniques negate the advantages of the laser. This includes the use of large-bore laryngoscopes, miniaturized cold steel instruments, and specialized training for the nondominant hand. Thus, cold steel phonomicrosurgery is usually the preferred technique for precise, accurate microsurgery of the vocal fold.[4] There are still indications for laser surgery, but most laryngologists consider them rare and for highly specialized situations.

Voice Rest

Significant debate exists regarding voice rest for singers and professional voice users. Some individuals feel that healthy professional voice users are served best by having regularly scheduled periods of "voice rest." Also, when a minor voice problem does occur in a heavy voice user, there is much controversy regarding the utility of voice rest.

An important issue regarding voice rest involves the use of scheduled breaks to prevent vocal fatigue or injury in the healthy voice professional (eg, a 20-minute silent period for the school teacher, abstaining from singing during the opening hymn for the minister, or preperformance quiet meditation for the singer). The benefits of this practice may be correlated with positive physical and/or psychological effects. Despite the widespread use of this practice and the positive anecdotal results, the mechanism underlying the positive effects of voice rest are unknown.

Another controversy regarding voice rest for the singer and professional voice user concerns the prescription of voice rest during vocal malady. Arguments have been made for the use of voice rest to allow the temporary inflammation of the vocal folds associated with medical illness to subside. In contrast, equally impassioned arguments have been made for appropriate and controlled voice *use* to facilitate healing associated with vocal fold swelling and/or the postoperative condition.[5,6] Specifically, the use of vocal fold high-amplitude, low impact vocal tasks has been likened to rehabilitative stretching and exercises that are used in sports medicine rehabilitation.

Future research will address much of the unknown aspects regarding voice rest controversies. Until then, the art of medicine must invoke the psychological profile, experience level, and physical diagnosis of the professional voice user to determine the appropriate use(s) of voice rest.

Age and Maturational Development of the Voice

The voice care professional is often asked to make a decision or give an opinion regarding the duration and type of singing obligations young singers should assume. This area of great controversy arises most notably when factors such as style of singing, amount of singing, and age of the singer are implicated as causes of a vocal injury. Specifically, this section highlights both the psychological and physical issues young singers may confront as they embark on a performing career.

Unequivocal guidelines for decisions regarding vocal performance are inappropriate due to the different psychological and physical rates of development of young singers. An 8-year-old girl may be able to manage multiple performances per week with very little psychological trauma; however, a 15-year-old boy may experience significant psychological difficulties and negative repercussions from a single, monthly performance.

This area is complicated further by the anecdotally documented but poorly understood physical development of the operatic female singer, who does not fully develop vocally until the third decade of life. It is important to remember that, even though the 22-year-old female singer is physically an adult, vocally she is not. Thus song selection, vocal demands, and training must be adjusted with this in mind.

Young boys endure adolescent voice changes that can have a great impact on both their physical and psychological ability to perform during this time period. This is another example of a time period in a singer's development that may require special consideration. One study found that boys at these time periods did well with vocal training.[7] This study has not been replicated and runs contrary to current opinion and dogma.

Little research has explored the physical impact of singing on the vocal mechanism of the young performer. In addition, the small amount of anecdotal information used in directing singers and their families in the development of young voices is based on Western European classical musical styles (bel canto is acceptable; however, belting is not). The overlying principle guiding development in young performers should involve nurturing the singer, while simultaneously avoiding injury or inhibition of the growth of the singer.

Incidence, Importance, and Impact of Laryngopharyngeal Reflux Disease (LPRD) on Singers and Professional Voice Users

In the last decade, there has been an upsurge in the recognition of the impact of laryngopharyngeal reflux disease on a variety of voice disorders (ie, vocal fold nodules, vocal fold granulomas, etc). This has been especially noted in singers and professional voice users, because a multitude of factors in this group may make them more prone to laryngopharyngeal reflux disease. In addition, any minor changes that occur to the voice from LPRD may affect singers to a greater degree. The controversy within this subject matter involves the unknown true incidence and impact of this disease on singers and professional voice users. The majority of information that we have about the impact of LPRD on the development of voice disorders is anecdotal and descriptive. Thus, the present philosophy of many laryngologists is to treat singers and professional voice users as if they have LPRD even without definitive diagnosis; because the diagnostic process is costly, time-consuming, and can often lead to a quagmire of results. To proceed without definitive diagnosis is simpler, and the negative sequelae of not treating can be significant.

The difficulties and controversies that arise with LPRD in this patient population stem from our limited knowledge base regarding baseline incidence of LPRD, lack of understanding of the pathophysiology of LPRD as related to voice disorders, and lack of definitive diagnostic testing. The impact of laryngopharyngeal reflux disease was previously underrecognized in laryngology and most likely is presently overrecognized and, therefore, overdiagnosed and overtreated.

The direct impact of LPRD on the voice is difficult to assess fully on physical examination or diagnostic testing. We are often left to rely on anecdotal reports of patients' symptoms that can be biased due to a poorly controlled situation, as well as to a possible placebo effect and empiric treatment. Specific questions regarding the impact and incidence of laryngopharyngeal reflux disease in singers and professional voice users include:

1. What is the direct mechanism(s) of LPRD affecting voice production in this population?
2. What is the incidence of LPRD in singers, and is it higher or lower than in nonsingers?
3. How does one accurately identify significant, active LPRD?

The latter will lead to more appropriate treatment recommendations and minimize expensive and possibly complicated treatment for disorders that are not present.

The most common problems in this area have been that it appears that any type of history of having reflux irritation to the larynx results in changes to the posterior aspect of the larynx (posterior laryngitis), and these changes do not resolve quickly or at all. Therefore, when a singer is evaluated for a nonspecific voice problem, and these changes are identified on laryngeal examination, the common assumption is that the

patient's voice problem is due to LPRD when, in fact, these physical examination findings are a holdover from a past experience. This typical patient may have no active laryngopharyngeal reflux disease, and his or her voice problem may be due to a separate matter. This can lead to delayed diagnosis and missed diagnosis, which are not helpful to the patient or to the overall cost of health care.

Instrumental Music and Singing

Often the laryngologist is asked to address the possible detrimental situation of a young singer who also plays a wind instrument. Because most wind instruments do not use the larynx as an articulator, there should generally not be a problem with singers also playing a wind instrument. There are anecdotal experiences of a variety of wind instruments, specifically of flute and French horn, using the larynx as a possible articulator, which in theory could impact the singing voice. More important than the wind instrument's use of the larynx as another level of articulation is the role of the musculature in the instrumental music production and the negative impact of the wind instrumental music playing on the singing voice. Specifically, it is hypothesized that excessive neck tension created or developed during the instrumental music playing could lead to difficulties with the singing voice. This could occur due to the importance of a full range of motion and relaxation in the laryngeal musculature for normal voice production. As with singers, such problems with tension are less likely to occur with highly skilled instruments. When there is a question regarding the negative aspects of instrumental music on the singing voice, one can evaluate the larynx during instrumental music playing with the flexible nasopharyngoscope and see the degree of laryngeal tension and laryngeal articulation during playing. Furthermore, often laryngeal massage, neck muscle relaxation exercises, and vocal warm-up exercises can be used to release any built-up stress and tension in this region following instrumental music playing prior to the onset of singing.

Singing Styles

A universal question surfacing within each voice evaluation addresses the patient's repertoire. The answer the voice care professional prefers to hear most often is "classical." This reply may mislead the voice care professional into a false state of comfort, just as the reply of "popular" music may mislead the same professional into a false state of discontent. The connotations for classical singing are as enigmatic and varied as those for popular singing; thus, the use of the label "legitimate" as synonymous for classical singing should not imply that any other style is "illegitimate."[8] Singing Wagnerian classic operatic arias may be just as stressful on the laryngeal mechanism as singing a Rolling Stones' classic rock ballad.

Research has shown that the production of different voice qualities relies on a dynamically changing vocal mechanism.[9-13] Yet, voice treatment has embraced the techniques biased toward Western European classical singing (ie, that of the early art song). The voice care professional must evaluate and treat the patient according to demands of the specialized repertoire by highlighting the associated burdens and risks, without unduly frightening the patient.

Typically, power singing (true operatic singing and belting) is associated with vocal injury in both the immature and adult singer who, thereafter, feels branded with the negative stigma of being "damaged goods." Yet, in athletics, such as football, physical injury is to be expected and is dealt with respectfully. We, as the comfortable audience, are thrilled by the power singer who takes risks to provide full dramatic impact. We, as voice care professionals, should provide the highest and most sophisticated quality of treatment to ensure that these performers may walk the vocal tightrope for our enjoyment in the many years to come. After all, longevity in a career is not reserved specifically for the bel canto singer. Lasting success crosses the borders of musical style due to smart choices by the performer and by those who provide the advice—from the managers and agents to the voice care professional.

Sports Medicine and Vocal Medicine

Several areas of vocal medicine frequently use the guiding principles of sports medicine as a basis to make decisions. Specifically, management of vocal performance, vocal training and rehabilitation from vocal injury often cite or use a sports medicine/exercise physiology paradigm (see chapter 15). The essential question regarding this area of controversy is: How valid are these various analogies?

The most reasonable and reliable example of this parallel thinking is the psychological approach and care of the singer and professional voice user with respect to performance. Because the mental aspects of performance are the same or similar for singing and pitching, it is reasonable for voice care professionals to use this area of sports medicine as a guide or basis.

The leap of faith between sports medicine and vocal medicine becomes greater when one attempts to apply training techniques of sports medicine to singing. Until research is done to validate these methods for singers, one needs to be very careful when vocal training methods are proposed based on the principles of athletic training. Our knowledge base regarding the muscular system of the vocal tract and how learning in this region is organized is too limited to assume that training techniques that are used to shoot a basketball will be appropriate for vocal training.

Recently, principles of exercise physiology and sports medicine have been applied to the approaches of care of injuries of the vocal mechanism.[14] In particular, recent research in sports medicine has demonstrated an advantage to mobilization of the musculoskeletal region in question following an injury instead of the traditional immobilization approach. Thus, after knee surgery, the knee is promptly (within hours) mobilized instead of being placed in a cast. Is a similar approach to a vocal injury (ie, vocal fold edema following singing, vocal fold hemorrhage, or vocal fold surgery) appropriate? It is important that voice care professionals proceed with a rational, scientific-based approach to voice care and not just accept the transference of philosophy from one field to another without careful consideration and rigorous testing. Great concern exists regarding the use of sports medicine/exercise physiology principles in designing programs for the care of the injured lamina propria of the vocal fold. The lamina propria is a unique area of the body and certainly has great differences in composition and metabolism in comparison with large, striated muscle groups of the body.

Conclusion

A substantial number of controversial areas exist regarding the medical care of singers and professional voice users. Many of these areas of controversy stem from lack of scientific understanding and/or ethical limitations regarding the testing of certain hypotheses. The field of care for the professional voice is moving from antidotal medicine to teleological medicine toward scientific medicine. The first step in this progression is the essential question: Why does this happen, and why is it treated in this fashion? From that stepping-stone, the field will move forward to provide singers and professional voice users with improved care.

References

1. Smith B, Sataloff RT. *Choral Pedagogy*. San Diego, Calif: Singular Publishing Group; 2000:3–12,105–169.

2. Edwin R. The good, the bad, and the ugly: singing teacher-choral director relationships. *J Singing.* 2001; 57(5):53–54.

3. Benninger MS. Micro-dissection or microspot CO2 laser for limited vocal fold benign lesions: a prospective randomized trial. *Laryngoscope.* 2000;110(2 Pt 2):1–17.

4. Zeitels SM. Laser versus cold instruments for microlaryngoscopic surgery. *Laryngoscope.* 1996;106(5 Pt 1):545–552.

5. Verdolini K, Zeitels SM, Maniotis A, Desloge RB, Hillman RE. Role of mechanical stress in tissue recovery subsequent to acute phonotrauma. Paper presented at the Twenty-Eighth Annual Symposium: Care of the Professional Voice; June 1999; Philadelphia, Pa.

6. Spiegel JR, Emerich K, Abaza MM, Sataloff RT. Voice rest after phonosurgery: current concepts of post–operative management. Paper presented at the Twenty-Eighth Annual Symposium: Care of the Professional Voice; June 15, 1999; Philadelphia, Pa.

7. Blatt IM. Training singing children during the phases of voice mutation. *Ann Otol Rhinol Laryngol.* 1983;92(5, Pt 1):462–468.

8. Delp R. From the president: now that the belt voice has become legitimate. *J Singing.* 2001;57 (5):1–2.

9. Colton RH, Estill J. Elements of voice quality: perceptual, acoustic and physiological aspects. In: Lass N, ed. *Speech and Language: Advances in Basic Research and Practice.* New York, NY: Academic Press; 1981.

10. Schutte HK, Miller DG. Belting and pop, nonclassical approaches to the female middle voice: some preliminary considerations. *J Voice.* 1993;7(2):142–150.

11. Sundberg J. *The Science of the Singing Voice.* Dekalb: Northern Illinois University Press; 1987.

12. Titze IR. *Principles of Voice Production.* Englewood Cliffs, NJ: Prentice Hall; 1994.

13. Zemlin WR. *Speech and Hearing Science: Anatomy and Physiology.* 4th ed. Boston, Mass: Allyn & Bacon; 1997.

14. Verdolini K, Ronan D, Saxon K. Mechanisms of wound healing: implications for the exercise hypothesis in voice therapy. Paper presented at the Twenty-Ninth Annual Symposium: Care of the Professional Voice; June 2000; Philadelphia, Pa.

26

Voice Horizons

John S. Rubin and Robert Thayer Sataloff

Communication is central to, and representative of, the human condition. Throughout history the speaking and singing voice have been objects of reverence, joy, and, at times, fear. Even in some societies where physical fitness and prowess were emphasized, for example, Sparta, the singing voice had a major role. Yet, appreciating the voice is not the same as understanding it. Unraveling the mystery of the human voice has been a slow process until the last quarter of the 20th century.

In the modern era of basic science and clinical research, it is hardly surprising that studies of vocal function and vocal health have been interdisciplinary in nature; and this shift in approach has been responsible for great progress. Pioneering researchers have drawn primarily from their own fields of expertise, such as medicine, physics, speech sciences, engineering, and so on. Initially, they brought to the fledgling field of voice a strong basis in physics and mathematics, thereby favoring the areas of acoustical analysis and signal processing, aerodynamics, and computer modeling.

Anatomists have supplied a strong foundation in cross-sectional anatomy and myology of the vocal folds and in the central connections and neural pathways responsible for speech and song. Recently, genetics and the cellular biology underlying laryngeal injury and repair have been emphasized.[1] Understanding aging has also come to the forefront through public demand, including studies on ways to delay the effects of advancing years on all body systems and functions, including the larynx and voice.

Physiologists have investigated the biomechanics of the vocal tract, including the mechano- and chemoreceptors. Much has been gleaned recently on the basic, but complex, function of structures such as the cricoarytenoid joint, for example. Endocrinolo-

gists have advanced the concept that the larynx acts very much as a steroid-receptor organ, with receptors to testosterone and estrogen, as well as with early responses to changes in the thyroid axis. Pedagogists have emphasized research into vocal techniques, not uncommonly fusing the physical (eg, breathing techniques) with the emotional-spiritual components of voice production.

When considering the horizons of laryngology, certain caveats need to be expressed. The authors recognize that there are always resource limitations, (generally inadequate funding) and that voice research in general still lags behind research in many other communications disorders due to a shorter research history. Yet, we also recognize the profound importance of voice for transmitting an individual's ideas and emotions and the potentially devastating effects that a voice disorder can have on patients' quality of life and ability to earn a living. In addition, we recognize the potentially serious systemic medical disorders that may present with laryngeal manifestations but are still often unrecognized by most physicians and lay people.

A useful point of reference, when discussing the future, is the recent past. In 1995, a National Strategic Research Plan[2] for voice research in the United States identified certain specific short-term research priorities. Areas of importance that were identified included: (1) cellular and molecular biology; (2) hormonal effects (mechanisms and sites of action); (3) human development (including embryology, effects of aging on the voice, and genetic transmission of vocal characteristics); (4) neural and vascular factors affecting voice function (and dysfunction); (5) laryngeal biomechanics and respiratory functions and their effects on phonation; (6) the impact of upper digestive tract function and dysfunction on the larynx and pharynx (mechanical and vagal reflex mechanisms); and (7) epidemiology of voice disorders.

Even more recently, throughout the United States and Europe, there has been a move in medicine toward evidence-based outcomes research and a focus on patient satisfaction. To that end, quality of life indicators have been brought to the fore. The concepts of impairment, handicap, and disability, and indices devised to rate them, have had a significant impact on both medical care and the distribution of medical resources. These important issues undoubtedly will play a major role in shaping the next generation of voice research.

The authors believe that this patient-oriented move toward evidence-based outcomes medicine is a very positive step. Together with the research areas identified in the 1995 United States National Strategic Research Plan, and with other areas of research discussed elsewhere in this book and in other literature, these areas represent extremely important pieces of the puzzle that must be completed if we are to understand how the human voice works, why it fails, or how it can be repaired. We believe that the growing appreciation for the societal importance of the voice, the impact of good and expeditious voice care, and the potentially high cost (human and economic) of unsuccessful voice care will lead to the availability of resources sufficient to answer many of the questions posed in this chapter and many more that we do not have space to address.

What then are the horizons of the field? Where is the urgency implicit in clinical need? These questions will determine the next generation of voice research, in concordance with public will and with national and international spending patterns for research.

To answer these questions, and possibly identify others, a thorough review was performed of articles published in the *Journal of Voice* in the 3 years (1998–2000) subsequent to publication of the second edition of this book. The *Journal of Voice* was selected because of its established position as a premier interdisciplinary peer-reviewed journal that involves specialists in virtually all fields related to voice. Of 178 articles reviewed, the major categories of topics included: aerodynamics and acoustics, 44 (25%); clinical voice problems, 35 (20%); surgical issues, 16 (9%); perceptual/profiles, 15 (8%); neurolaryngology, 13 (7%); laryngeal/vocal fold imaging, 12 (7%); biomechanics, 11 (6%); aging, 7 (4%); reflux/upper aerodigestive issues, 6 (3%); psychology, 5 (3%); outcomes measurements 5 (3%); molecular/cellular, 4 (2%); pedagogy, 2 (1%); historical, 2 (1%); and other, 1 (1%). Only a few of these articles will be discussed specifically in this chapter, although all of them, along with the larger world body of voice literature, have influenced our vision of the future of voice care.

Physics and mathematics have dominated the basic science publications in voice research and most likely will continue to do so in the near future. However, there are still significant deficits in our knowledge base and ability to document laryngeal function. The large number of clinically related papers attests to the importance of information designed to improve our abilities to manage the serious, subtle, or overt problems that are inherent to the larynx.

The relative paucity of molecular/cellular research is, perhaps, a matter of concern. The articles are of high quality, however; and the degree of interest throughout the field of voice in the initial results garnered through them suggests that such studies are likely to increase quickly, providing that a secure funding base can be obtained. Such studies have already (and perhaps to a surprising degree) had a profound impact on how surgeons approach the larynx and how scientists think about the larynx. In the authors' opinion, laryngeal molecular and cellular research, now and in the future, should be supported strongly by the voice community.

Let us now review categorically the near-term priorities for laryngeal research identified in the National Strategic Research Plan.[2]

Cellular and Molecular Biology

Interest was stimulated in this area by the works of pioneers in the field, such as Hirano's seminal work on the layered structure of the vocal fold.[3,4] This work has gained significant momentum through the ongoing contributions of Gray and colleagues.[1,5-7] Questions deserving of further investigation are legion. These include, at first examination: the genetic makeup of the laryngeal substrata; distribution of molecular markers throughout the epithelium; expression of proteins necessary for cell-to-cell interactions (eg, the cadherins and other integrins);[8-10] molecular changes leading to disease, both benign and malignant; and immunohistochemical and ultrastructural investigations of the epithelium, basement membrane, and layers of the lamina propria. These have been championed by researchers such as Gray et al[1,11] and Sato.[12]

Hormonal Effects
(Mechanisms and Sites of Action)

There has been extensive interest in the larynx as a hormone target organ. The role of sex hormones has recently been investigated by Abitbol et al[13] and others. The changes in the larynx due to thyroid axis disorders are well recognized.[14] Additional research regarding the nature and location of hormone receptors and of end-organ mechanisms of response to hormonal manipulations (ie, premenstrual and perimenopausal changes and changes in circulating thyroid hormones) may offer ways of blocking adverse effects when hormonal fluctuation or dysfunction is inevitable and possibly produce methods of reversing hormone-related voice changes. It also seems possible that hormonal factors may be operative in vocal fold problems that have gender-specific predilection. For example, it is generally agreed that vocal fold nodules are more common in children and adult females. Reinke's edema appears to occur mainly in adult women. Mechanical reasons have generally been presumed, but these remain unproven; and possible hormone contributions have not been studied adequately.

Human Development (Including Embryology, Effects of Aging on the Voice, and Genetic Transmission of Vocal Characteristics)

The voice changes throughout life. Laryngeal structure and function deteriorate with advancing age, particularly at advanced age, which compromises the cellular, structural, and neural-muscular integrity of the laryngeal system. Control of voice relies not only on the vocal folds, but also on a delicate balance of pulmonary function and laryngeal and articulator activity; and these in turn depend on the functional integrity of the neural, endocrine, and skeletal systems.[15,16]

A review of age-related changes affecting the larynx includes changes in cartilages, articular surfaces, ligaments, and supporting structures, and the true vocal folds. Changes in the laryngeal cartilages include complete ossification by the eighth decade, and often by the sixth decade. This ossification leads to decreased flexibility of cartilages.[17,18] Changes in the articular surfaces include thinning surface and irregularities.[17,19,20]

Changes in the ligaments include loosening of the joint capsules, breakdown in collagen fiber organization, and thinning of elastic fibers.[21-24] Changes in the supporting structures occur in the conus elasticus including waviness, fragmentation, and separation, and changes in connective tissue septae with disorganization.[25-28]

Changes in the true vocal fold include edema of the mucosa, but mainly changes in the lamina propria. Hirano found decrease in density and thinning of the superficial and intermediate layers, collagenous thickening with loss of linearity, and an increase of fibrosis

of the deep layer.[30] The likely effects of these changes on the voice include changes in apposition, pitch, and vocal fold vibration.

Cricoarytenoid articular changes can lead to glottal insufficiency.[17] Stiffer, thinner vocal folds will vibrate more rapidly, perhaps with less amplitude.[17] This is consistent with data that F_0 in men increases after the sixth decade.[16,31] Changes in compliance and elasticity of the lamina propria lead to asynchronous vibrations and incomplete closure thus allowing air to escape during sound production. This leads to aperiodicity.[17]

Changes in the vocal ligament may cause irregularities in vocal fold vibration, which are perceivable as roughness[33-35] and are measured as abnormally high perturbation factors or F_0 variability.[17,32-35] Atrophy of laryngeal muscles could lead to bowing of the vocal folds and weakness. All of the above may lead to increased breathiness and a strained tense voice with changes in voice pitch and resonance, the perceptual correlate of the "elderly" voice.[33]

Published studies on voice changes in elderly versus younger subjects have demonstrated the following findings in the elderly: pitch changes, irregularities in vocal fold vibration, glottal incompetency (air loss and breathiness), voice production changes associated with laryngeal tension, pitch breaks, roughness, hoarseness, harshness, changes in vibrato, development of a tremolo, decreased breath control, and vocal fatigue.[29,31,32,34-36]

It is clear that there is now a substantial body of information in the geriatric literature substantiating physiologic changes that could disrupt the normal process of speech and voice production, and it is not difficult for even inexperienced listeners to reliably categorize speakers as "young" or "old."[37,38] Surprisingly, however, relatively few data are available that correlate the loss of voice with communicative skills of the aging process.[39]

Even less information is available on the potential benefit of speech therapy in vocal rehabilitation of elderly speakers. There is, however, no question but that individual differences in fitness may have a direct impact on the aging voice and that fitness may be improved through vocal rehabilitation with exercise or lifestyle changes.[40-42] In fact, when discussing altered parameters of function, the degree of interindividual variability must be kept in mind.[40]

In a recently published study in the *Journal of Voice*, Decoster and Debruyne examined the voices of radio broadcasters on a longitudinal basis, comparing their voices at 30-year intervals.[43] Recent reviews by Linville and Sataloff have summarized the most current research and clinical management of the effects of age on the voice.[44,45] However, further studies clearly are required to examine prospectively voice-related age changes and to look at the possible communication and psychological benefits obtainable through modification with vocal rehabilitation. Given the continued increase in our society of elderly individuals, such studies should be a research priority.

Neural and Vascular Factors Effects on Voice Function (and Dysfunction)

Investigations into the neural and vascular factors affecting voice production are crucial to advancing our knowledge and understanding of neurolaryngology. Such studies can be considered on a peripheral (laryngeal) and central (supravagal) level. Peripherally, mechanoreceptors and chemoreceptors have been identified throughout the laryngeal mucosa, muscles, the trachea, and the lungs. A body of research is available that focuses on the mucosal receptors.[46-53] Further research is necessary, particularly on the laryngeal and tracheal receptors and their functions and phonatory control. Collapse of transmural pressure receptors in the upper airway has been associated with enhancement of inspiratory activity.[54,55] These receptors may be of particular importance in sudden infant death syndrome.[56] They may also be important in mediating the laryngeal response to systemic and local disease and thus worthy of further research.

Our knowledge of neurolaryngeal feedback controls is rudimentary. Ventilatory inhibition occurs during speech,[57] and there is a clear link between lung pressure and control of inspiration during vocalization.[58] Given the fact that many clinical problems (not the least being dystonia and tremor) appear to be due to defective neural control, any research that sheds light on the anatomy and pathophysiology of the control systems should be of great value to both clinicians and general public. Information on the nature of relevant neurotransmitters, neural interconnections, and controls has the potential to provide us with controllable (and reversible) pharmacological intervention far more sophisticated and specific than agents such as botulinum toxin, our current first-line treatment at the level of the end organ in several of these disorders.

The neural control of voice, in speech or in singing, is still not well understood. As noted by Smith,[59] "while there have been advances in knowledge of neurological control of vocalization, it is readily apparent that there is little information on the laryngeal pathophysiology of many neurological disorders." It has been established that stimulation of the periaqueductal gray region in the midbrain elicits vocalization.[60] This area may be responsible for the integration of laryngeal and respiratory muscle patterns used in vocalizations, as well as for integration of emotional content.[61]

Many neurological disorders affect the voice either early or late in their course. As one example, Parkinson's disease, a nigrostriatal disorder characterized by dopamine deficiency, is common, occurring in 1% of individuals over the age of 60 and 0.1% under that age.[62] At least 89% of the 1.5 million individuals afflicted with Parkinson's disease in the United States have a voice disorder with characteristics of reduced loudness, monotone, hoarseness, and tremor.[62] Hypoadduction of the vocal folds and bowed vocal folds have been observed early in the disorder.[59,63]

It is clear that further research into the entire field of neurolarygology is necessary.

Laryngeal Biomechanics, Respiratory Mechanisms, and Their Effects on Phonation

It has been more than 30 years since Hast published his landmark study on the physiology of the cricothyroid muscle, yet the biomechanics of the larynx are still poorly understood.[64] There has been much more research on laryngeal mucosa than on the laryngeal gesture. Many investigators have linked prolonged mechanical misuse and overuse of the larynx with laryngeal dysfunction and injury. Furthermore, many studies have demonstrated marked improvement through mechanical manipulation utilizing voice therapy (as discussed in preceding chapters) and other techniques.[65] The biomechanics of the laryngeal muscles and skeleton link the inherent properties of the larynx to the gestures that control phonation.[66] Further investigations of laryngeal biomechanics are needed, with emphasis on the development of models to recognize and quantify biomechanical dysfunction and to restore optimal use of laryngeal structures. One such model has been developed by Harris and others.[65,67,68]

Additional work is also needed to clarify the rotational dynamics of the arytenoid cartilage and cricoarytenoid joint and to develop techniques with abilities to measure movements in this region objectively. Such measurements should eventually be applicable to frequency and intensity changes, laryngeal efficiency, and progress in vocal training. In *Professional Voice*, Letson described important new insights into this area, including the vertical component of motion of the arytenoid cartilage that can be overlooked when examining the larynx clinically from the "bird's eye" position that we assume during stroboscopy.

Additionally, research should be encouraged in muscle physiology, in areas such as the metabolic requirements of laryngeal muscles[69] and their fatigue resistance,[66,70] the relationships and functional implications of fast and slow-twitch fibers in laryngeal muscles,[71] and the applicability of sports medicine studies in exercise physiology to laryngeal habilitation and rehabilitation (as discussed by Schneider et al in chapter 15).

In general, computer models created to study laryngeal biomechanics and computer-generated analyses of the effects of various laryngeal configurations on phonation have been beneficial as both research and educational tools.[72] Additional computer research should be encouraged and supported.

It must be remembered that the mass and the expenditure of muscular energy in the larynx are much smaller than those of the muscles supporting respiration. Thus, further biomechanical research is required into the forces generated by the intercostals, diaphragm, abdominal, and back muscles. Bowden, Hixon, Dickson, and others have pioneered this subject, but more research is indicated.[73-75] Research, such as the recent collaboration of Thorpe et al,[76] in which an interdisciplinary team of scientists, speech-language therapists, and singing teachers investigated rib cage position, abdominal motions, and acoustical output of professional opera singers, are seminal to advances in the field, and should be supported.

The Impact of Upper Digestive Tract Dysfunction on the Larynx and Pharynx (Mechanical and Vagal Reflex Mechanisms)

This area continues to generate research interest. The larynx is known to be subject to injury by esophageal reflux, yet our understanding of the interrelationship is still poorly defined. Laryngopharyngeal reflux is clearly a very different disorder than gastroesophageal reflux.[77] To investigate, 24-hour ambulatory pH monitoring has been used increasingly.[77,78] Normative databases for proximal probes in esophageal pH monitoring have been developed recently.[79-81] The concept of a reflux area index has been described to incorporate the number and duration of episodes of reflux.[82] This appears to be a useful indicator of proximal reflux severity. Further investigations on this indicator are needed. More research is also required into the potential role of reflux in such diverse areas as chronic cough, asthma, sudden infant death syndromes, sleep disorders, and common otolaryngologic disorders such as tonsillitis, irritable airway, chronic sinusitis, subglottic stenosis, and others.

Epidemiology of Voice Disorders

The relationships of various potentially carcinogenic factors for laryngeal cancer can require extensive investigation. Cancer of the larynx represents 2.3% of all malignant tumors in males and 0.4% in females, excluding basal and squamous cell carcinomas of the skin.[83] The National Cancer Institute estimates that cancer of the larynx accounts for approximately 1.3% of all new cancer diagnoses and 0.83% of all cancer deaths in the United States,[84] representing approximately 11,000 new cases per year.[83-84] The incidence peaks in the sixth and seventh decades of life.[83] The larynx and hypopharynx are by far the most common sites of head-and-neck squamous cell carcinoma (HNSCC) in the western world.[85]

Known risk factors for laryngeal cancer include tobacco and alcohol use/abuse, industrial exposure to toxins (asbestos, mustard gas, petroleum products, and others), viral agents, radiation exposure, and laryngeal papilloma.[83] There is also some consideration that gastroesophageal reflux may be a significant cofactor.[86] Laryngeal tumors are twice as common in heavily industrialized areas.[85]

Viral agents, especially the human papilloma virus (HPV) and the Epstein-Barr virus (EBV),[83,85,87] have been considered as possible cofactors associated with head-and-neck cancer. Cigarette smoking and alcohol consumption are the two strongest etiological factors for the development of HNSCC and of cancer of the larynx, both independently and synergistically.[83,85]

Occupational exposure to toxic substances is a significant and not satisfactorily researched potential cofactor. For example, in Spain, 4% of cancer deaths are attributed to occupational cancer; over 3 million workers (25.4% of employees) are exposed to potential carcinogens and laryngeal carcinoma incidence is high,[88] yet knowledge of specific problems of occupational cancer in Spain is scarce. Recently, many case control studies have identified a variety of hazardous agents as potentially participating in the development of neoplasia of the larynx or chronic laryngitis.

Maier and Tisch, in their Heidelberg case control study,[89] found that chronic consumption of alcohol and tobacco increased the relative risk of squamous cell carcinoma of the larynx independently in a dose-dependent manner. The majority of cancer patients were found to be blue-collar workers who are exposed to a variety of hazardous working materials such as polycyclic aromatic hydrocarbons, cement dust, metal dusts, asbestos, varnish, lacquer, and others. Environmental exposure to airborne carcinogens like fossil fuel single stove emissions may increase the relative risk of laryngeal cancer. Diesel fumes were associated with laryngeal cancer in one study.[90]

Szeszenia-Dabrowska, in their analysis of malignant neoplasms in Poland from 1971 to 1994, recognized that, in occupational diseases, cancer of the larynx occurred in 25.5% of workers, with asbestos dust, ionizing radiation, chromium and its compounds, and benzidine being the most common causes.[91] Asbestos has been associated with laryngeal carcinoma and hyperplastic laryngitis by several investigators.[92-95] Nickel and chromate dust are principal inorganic chemicals that can cause lesions in the nose, larynx, lung, and paranasal sinuses.[85] Sulfuric acid mist exposure has been associated with an increased risk of development of laryngeal cancer,[96,97] as has fluoride dust.[98]

From the above, it is obvious that further far-reaching epidemiological studies involving the workplace are necessary. Furthermore, as health care providers, we need to be active in continuing to raise public appreciation of the risks of smoking on the larynx and the importance of smoking cessation.

Outcomes Research and Quality of Life

Although not identified specifically in the 1995 review, quality of life issues and outcomes have become seminal in many clinicians' approach to patients with voice problems. The World Health Organization views health to encompass physical, mental, and social states of being.[99] Yet, the study of outcomes is a new area for voice.[100] A patient's perception of the severity of his or her problem can now be assessed using one of several voice-specific outcome measures. The Voice Handicap Index developed by Jacobson and colleagues is one such instrument,[101] and appears to be, perhaps, more specific for our cohort of patients than the previously described medical outcomes instrument study, a short form, 36-item, general health survey otherwise known as the SF-36.[102,103]

Studies of this type are in their infancy and will undoubtedly develop rapidly. These studies emphasize the impact of the voice problem on the affected individual; as such, they are very important. The next step may well be development of new tools, or utilization of present tools on a cross-cultural basis, as the world becomes more and more a global community.

Clinical Practice and Research

Our ability to care for patients presenting with voice problems has changed dramatically in recent years, mainly due to advances in basic research.[104] All of the research discussed above (as well as the many important research considerations not discussed) impact directly on the clinical care of voice patients.

The need to diagnose voice disorders more accurately, and to assess treatment outcomes, has led to the widespread use of clinical voice laboratories. Although advances have been made in our ability to measure voice function objectively, a great deal more research in this area is needed. The authors suspect that advances in voice assessment may be limited by not only current technology, but also our paradigm for voice assessment. Research efforts may develop an entirely new approach to voice assessment, perhaps using different technology such as signal detection methods from the aerospace industry and self-educating neuronets. In the coming years, we anticipate substantial changes and improvements in our ability to analyze acoustic and aerodynamic features of voice and continued improvements in radiological imaging technology, as well.

In addition, our patients' needs have driven clinical research. Considering surgical techniques, examples include the continued interest in implantable and injectable materials (eg, autologous collagen), for vocal fold medialization; the development of animal models (eg,, the use of Lactosorb in a rabbit larynx)[105-107]; continued interest in methods and materials to treat or reduce vocal fold scarring and granulation formation (eg, the agent mitomycin[108]); and many others.

Clinicians are becoming concerned more actively with preventive voice care. We anticipate that this will assume an even greater role in the future. Preventive programs in the near future should include early detection efforts such as vocal evaluations and education in the schools and the workplace. Studies will be necessary to determine the efficacy of such programs and their cost-effectiveness prior to widespread implementation.

Interdisciplinary Collaboration

This text and its first two editions have emphasized the major advances in voice medicine made possible through interdisciplinary collaboration. The importance of voice care teams is now well recognized throughout the world. The value, relevance, and impact on the practice of the laryngologist and speech-language pathologist are clear. Similar benefits exist for singing teachers, acting teachers, and others involved in professional voice use and training. We have witnessed expanded interactions in nonmedical settings in the past decade and anticipate that they will continue. Foundations such as the Voice Foundation in the United States, the British Voice Association in the United Kingdom, the Australian Voice Foundation in Australia, and others appear to act as catalysts for multidisciplinary learning, teaching, and training. Physicians and voice scientists are now serving as faculty and or advisers in more nonmedical organizations, and singing voice teachers and voice therapists are becoming actively involved in medical settings.

A new era is evolving in voice pedagogy and education for singers; voice training for actors and other speakers has begun to follow suit. This should result in additional pedagogical research on the applications of scientific and medical knowledge on voice training and benefit the training of voice educators. The consequent advances undoubtedly will be as exciting for voice teachers as they have been for physicians and speech-language therapists. They should improve substantially the quality and consistency of voice training.

It appears that the evaluation and development of sports medicine and sports science is an appropriate analogy for voice. Advances in sports performance have resulted in large part from the application of scientific information, principles, and technology by far-sighted coaches. Similarly, systematic application of analogous information by skilled voice teachers may lead to the discovery of new performance levels in the healthy voice. This may yet be the most exciting horizon in voice research, as well as in other areas of Arts Medicine.

Conclusion

A review of the recent history of the field of voice care illuminates the importance of inter- and multidisciplinary fellowship. We believe that the level of accomplishments over the past two or three decades will be maintained in the coming years. The field is poised on the brink of a technological explosion, with rapidly improving methodology for investigation, documentation, and treatment.

Clearly, the willingness of specialists from the diverse backgrounds relevant to voice disorders to communicate and collaborate has led to this rapid expansion in the knowledge base. Voice research must continue. It will undoubtedly do so through the combination of scientific curiosity and clinical need.

In this chapter we have identified only a few of the interesting and pressing problems. There are many more that we have not mentioned and more still that have not yet been recognized. We have faith that they will be addressed and supported in clinics and laboratories and that they will lead to a whole new chapter of

pressing issues in time for the following edition of this text.

References

1. Gray SD. Cellular physiology of the vocal folds. *Otolaryngol Clin North Am*. 2000;33(4):679–697.
2. *National Strategic Research Plan*. Bethesda MD: US Dept of Health and Human Services; Publication NIH 95–3711. 1995:261–306.
3. Hirano M. Structure of the vocal fold in normal and disease states. Anatomical and physical study. *ASHA*. 1981; 11:11–30.
4. Hirano M. Phonosurgical anatomy of the larynx. In: Ford CN, Bless DM, eds. *Phonosurgery*. New York, NY: Raven Press; 1991:25–43.
5. Gray SD, Hirano M, Sato K. Molecular and cellular structure of vocal fold tissue. In: Titze IR, ed. *Vocal Fold Physiology: Frontiers in Basic Science*. San Diego, Calif: Singular Publishing Group Inc; 1993:1–23.
6. Gray SD, Pignatari SN, Harding P. Morphologic ultrastructure of anchoring fibers in normal vocal fold basement membrane zone. *J Voice*. 1994;8:48–52.
7. Gray SD, Titze IR, Chan R, et al. Vocal fold proteogylcans and their influences on biomechanics. *Laryngoscope*. 1999;109:845–854.
8. Dorudi S, Hanby AM, Poulsom R, et al. Level of expression of E-cadherin mRNA in colorectal cancer correlates with clinical outcome. *Br J Cancer*. 1995;71:614–616.
9. Dorudi S, Sheffield JP, Poulsom R, et al. E-cadherin expression in colorectal cancer: an immunohistochemical and in situ hybridization study. *Am J Pathol*. 1993:142(4):981–986.
10. Marshall JF, Rutherford DC, McCartney AC, et al. Alpha v beta 1 is a receptor for vitronectin and fibrinogen, and acts with alpha 5 beta 1 to mediate spreading on fibronectin. *J Cell Sci*. 1995;108:1227–1238.
11. Gray SD, Hirano M, Sato K. Molecular and cellular structure of vocal fold tissue. In: Titze IR, ed. *Vocal Fold Physiology: Frontiers in Basic Science*. San Diego, Calif: Singular Publishing Group Inc; 1993:1–23.
12. Sato K. Functional fine structurues of the human vocal fold mucosa. In: Rubin JS, Sataloff RT, Korovin GS, eds. *Diagnosis and Treatment of Voice Disorders*. 2nd ed. Clifton Park, NY: Delmar Thomson Learning; 2003:41–48.
13. Abitbol J, Abitbol P, Abitbol B. Sex hormones and the female voice. *J Voice*. 1999;13:424–426.
14. Simpson CB, Fleming DJ. Medical and vocal history in the evaluation of dysphonia. *Otolaryngol Clin North Am*. 2000;33:719–729.
15. Gould WJ, Rubin JS. Special considerations for the professional voice user. In: Rubin JS, Sataloff RT, Korovin G, Gould WJ, eds. *Diagnosis and Treatment of Voice Disorders*. Tokyo/New York: Igaku-Shoin Medical Publishers; 1995; 424–435.
16. Ringel RL, Chodzko-Zajko WJ. Vocal indices of biological age. *J Voice*. 1987;1(1):31–37.
17. Kahane JC. Connective tissue changes in the larynx and their effects on voice. *J Voice*. 1987;1(1):27–30.

18. Zenker W, Zenker A. Ueber die regelund der stimmilippen-spannung durch von aussen eingreifende menchanismen. *Folia Phoniatr.* 1960;12:1–36.

19. Kahn A, Kahane JC. India ink pinprick assessment of age-related changes in the cricoarytenoid joint (CAJ) articular surfaces. *J Speech Hear Res.* 1986;29:536–543.

20. Kahane JC, Hammons J. Developmental changes in the articular cartilage of the human cricoarytenoid joint. In: Baer T, Harris K, Sasaki C, eds. *Vocal Physiology.* San Diego, Calif: College-Hill Press; 1987:14–18.

21. Segre R. Senescence of the voice. *Eye Ear Nose Throat Mon.* 1971;50:223–233.

22. Hommerich KW. Der alternde larynx: Morphologische aspekt. *Hals Nasen Ohrenaerzte.* 1972;20:115–120.

23. Kofler D. Histopathologische veranderingen an altereskehlkopf. *Monatssche Ohrenkeilk Laryngorhinol* (Wein). 1932;66:1468–1472.

24. Ferreri G. Senescence of the larynx. *Ital Gen Rev Oto-Rhino-Laryngol.* 1959;1:640–709.

25. Kahane JC. Age related changes in the elastic fibers of the adult male ligament. In: Lawrence V, ed. *Transcripts of the 11th Symposium: Care of the Professional Voice.* New York, NY: The Voice Foundation; 1982;116–122.

26. Kahane JC. Postnatal development and aging of the human larynx. *Semin Speech Lang.* 1983;4:189–203.

27. Kahane JC. A survey of age-related changes in the connective tissues of the human adult larynx. In: Bless DM, Abbs JH, eds. *Vocal Fold Physiology. Contemporary Research and Clinical Issues.* San Diego, Calif, College-Hill Press; 1983:44–49

28. Kahane JC, Stadlan EM, Bell JS. A histomorphological study of the aging male larynx. *ASHA.* 1979;20:747.

29. McGlone RE, Hollien H. Vocal pitch characteristics of aged white women. *J Speech Hear Res.* 1963;6:164–170.

30. Hirano M, Kurita S, Nakashima T. Growth, development and aging of human vocal folds. In: Bless DM, Abbs JH, eds. *Vocal Fold Physiology. Contemporary Research and Clinical Issues.* San Diego, Calif: College-Hill Press; 1983:22–43.

31. Hollien H, Shipp T. Speaking fundamental frequency and chronological age in males. *J Speech Hearing Res.* 1972;15:155–159.

32. Wilcox KA, Horii YH. Age and changes in vocal jitter. *J Gerontol.* 1980;35:194–198.

33. Ryan WJ, Burk KW. Perceptual and acoustic correlates of aging in the speech of males. *J Commun Disord.* 1974; 7:181–192.

34. Ryan WJ, Capadano HL. Age perception and evaluative reactions toward adult speakers. *J Gerontol.* 1978;33:98–102.

35. Ptacek PH, Sander EK, Manoley W, et al. Phonatory and related changes with advanced age. *J Speech Hear Res.* 1966;9:353–360.

36. Hartman DE, Danahuer JL. Perceptual features of speech for males in four perceived age decades. *J Acoust Soc Am.* 1976;59:713–715.

37. Shipp T, Hollien H. Perception of the aging male voice. *J Speech Hear Res.* 1969;12:703–710.

38. Linville SE. Acoustic-perceptual studies of aging voice in women. *J Voice.* 1987;1(1):44–48.

39. Morris RJ. Brown WS Jr., Age-related voice measures among adult women. *J Voice.* 1987;1(1):38–43.

40. Finch CE, Schneider EL. *Handbook of the Biology of Aging.* 2nd ed. New York, NY: John Wiley; 1985.

41. Spirduso WW. Physical fitness in relation to motor aging. In: Mortimer JA, Pirizzolo FJ, Maletta GJ, eds. *The Aging Motor System.* New York, NY: Praeger Publishers; 1982:120–151

42. Fries JF, Crapo LM. *Vitality and Aging.* San Francisco, Calif: Freeman; 1981.

43. Decoster W, Debruyne F. Longitudinal voice changes: facts and interpretation. *J Voice.* 2000;14 (2):184–193.

44. Linville SE. Vocal aging. *Curr Opin Otolaryngol Head Neck Surg.* 1995;3:183–187.

45. Sataloff RT, Vocal aging. *Curr Opin Otolaryngol Head Neck Surg.* 1998;421–428.

46. Boggs DF, Bartlett D. Chemical specificity of a laryngeal apneic reflex in puppies. *J Appl Physiol.* 1982;53:455–462.

47. Davis PJ, Bartlett D, Luschei ES. Coordination of the respiratory and laryngeal systems in breathing and vocalization. In: Titze IR, ed. *Vocal Fold Physiology: Frontiers in Basic Science.* San Diego, Calif: Singular Publishing Group Inc; 1993:189–226.

48. Boushey HA, Richardson PS, Widdicombe JG, Wise JCM. The response of laryngeal afferent fibers to mechanical and chemical stimuli. *J Physiol.* 1974;240:153–175.

49. Davis PJ, Nail BS. Quantitative analysis of laryngeal mechanosensitivity in the cat and rabbit. *J Physiol.* 1987; 388:467–485.

50. Mathew OP, Sant'Ambrogio G, Fisher JT, Sant'Ambrogio FB. Laryngeal pressure receptors. *Respir Physiol.* 1984; 54:259–268.

51. Testerman RL. Modulation of laryngeal activity by pulmonary changes during vocalization in cats. *Exp Neurol.* 1970;29:281–297.

52. Sant'Ambrogio G, Mathew OP, Fisher JT, Sant'Ambrogio FB. Laryngeal receptors responding to transmural pressure, airflow, and local muscle activity. *Respir Physiol.* 1983;54:317–330.

53. Sant'Ambrogio G, Brambilla-Sant'Ambrogio F, Mathew OP. Effect of cold air on laryngeal mechanoreceptors in the dog. *Respir Physiol.* 1986;64:45–56.

54. Mathew OP. Upper airway negative-pressure effects on respiratory activities of upper airway muscles. *J Appl Physiol.* 1984;56:500–505.

55. Mathew OP, Farber JP. Effect of upper airway negative pressure on respiratory timing. *Respir Physiol.* 1983;54: 259–268.

56. Benninger MS, Schwimmer C. Functional neurophysiology and vocal fold paresis. In: Rubin JS, Sataloff RT, Korovin GK, Gould WJ, eds. *Diagnosis and Treatment of Voice Disorders.* New York, NY: Igaku-Shoin Medical Publishers; 1995;105–121.

57. Gelfer C, Harris K, Collier R, Baer T. Is declination actively controlled? In: Titze IR, Scherer RC, eds. *Vocal Fold Physiology: Biomechanics, Acoustics and Phonatory Control.* Denver, Colo: The Denver Center for the Performing Arts; 1983:113–116.

58. Garrett JD, Luschei ES. Subglottic pressure modulation during evoked phonation in the anesthetized cat. In: Baer T, Sasaki C, Harris K, eds. *Laryngeal Function in Phonation and Respiration.* Boston, Mass: College-Hill Press; 1987:139–153.

59. Smith ME, Ramig LO. Neurological disorders and voice. In: Rubin JS, Sataloff RT, Korovin G, Gould WJ, eds. *Diagnosis and Treatment of Voice Disorders.* Tokyo/New York: Igako Shoin Medical Publishers; 1995:203–224.

60. Bandler R. Brain mechanisms of aggression as recorded by electrical and chemical stimulation: suggestion of a central role for the midbrain periaqueductal gray region. In: Epstein A, Morrison A, eds. *Progress in Psychobiology and Physiological Psychology.* vol 13. New York, NY: Academic Press; 1988:67–153.

61. Davis P, Zhang SP, Winkworth A, Bandler R. Neural control of vocalization: respiratory and emotional influences. *J Voice.* 1996;10:23–38.

62. Logemann JA, Fisher HB, Boshes B, Blonsky ER. Frequency and occurrence of vocal tract dysfunctions in the speech of a large sample of Parkinson's patients. *J Speech Hear Disord.* 1978;43:47–57.

63. Gracco C, Marek K. Laryngeal manifestations of early Parkinson's disease: data characterizing stage of disease and severity of symptoms. Presented at the Conference of Motor Speech Disorders; March 1994; Sedona, Ariz. .

64. Hast MH. Mechanical properties of the cricothyroid muscle. *Laryngoscope.* 1965;75:537–548.

65. Harris T, Lieberman J. The cricothyroid mechanism, its relation to vocal fatigue and voice dysfunction. *J Voice.* 1993;3:89–96.

66. Cooper DS, Partridge LD, Alipour-Haghighi F. Muscle energetics, vocal efficiency and laryngeal biomechanics. In: Titze IR, ed. *Vocal Fold Physiology: Frontiers in Basic Science.* San Diego, Calif: Singular Publishing Group Inc; 1993:37–92.

67. Rubin JS, Lieberman J, Harris TM. Laryngeal manipulation. *Otolaryngol Clin North Am.* 2000;33(5):1017–1034

68. Harris T. Laryngeal mechanisms in normal function and dysfunction. In: Harris T, Harris S, Rubin JS, Howard DM, eds. *The Voice Clinic Handbook.* London: Taylor and Francis Group/Whurr Publishers; 1998:64–87.

69. Cooper DS, Rice DH. Fatigue resistance of canine vocal fold muscle. *Ann Otol Rhinol Laryngol.* 1990;99:228–233.

70. Cooper DS, Pinczower E, Rice DH. Laryngeal intramuscular pressures. *J Acoust Soc Am.* 1990;88 (suppl 1):S151.

71. Sanders I. The microanatomy of the vocal folds. In: Rubin JS, Sataloff RT, Korovin GS, Gould WJ, eds. *Diagnosis and Treatment of Voice Disorders.* Tokyo/New York: Igaku Shoin Medical Publishers; 1995:70–85.

72. Titze IR, Talkin DT. A theoretical study of the effects of various laryngeal configurations on the acoustics of phonation. *J Acoust Soc Am.* 1979;66:60–74.

73. Bowden REM, Scheuer JL. Weight of abductor and adductor muscles of the human larynx. *J Laryngol Otol.* 1960;74:971–980.

74. Hixon TJ. Kinematics of the chest wall during speech production: volume displacements of the rib cage, abdomen and lung. *J Speech Hear Res.* 1973;16:78.

75. Dickson DR, Maue-Dickson W. *Anatomical and Physiological Bases of Speech.* Boston, Mass: Little, Brown and Co; 1982.

76. Thorpe CW, Cala SJ, Chapman J, Davis PJ. Patterns of breath support in projection of the singing voice. *J Voice.* 2001;15(1):86–104.

77. Sataloff RT, Castell DO, Katz PO, Sataloff DM. *Reflux Laryngitis and Related Disorders.* San Diego, Calif: Singular Publishing Group Inc; 1999;1–112.

78. Koufman JA. The otolaryngologic manifestations of gastroesophageal reflux (GERD): a clinical investigaton of 225 patients using ambulatory 24-hour pH monitoring and an experimental investigation of the role of acid and pepsin in the development of laryngeal injury. *Laryngoscope.* 1991:101(4, suppl 53):1–78.

79. Vincent DA Jr, Garrett JD, Radionoff SL, et al. The proximal probe in esophageal pH monitoring: development of a normative database. *J Voice.* 2000;14(2):247–254.

80. Dublian R, Castell DO. Normal and abnormal proximal esophageal acid exposure: results of ambulatory dual-probe pH monitoring. *Am J Gastroenterol.* 1993:88(1): 25–29.

81. Jacob P, Kahrilas PJ, Herzon G. Proximal esophageal pH-metry in patients with reflux laryngitis. *Gastroenterology.* 1991;100:305–310.

82. Vandeplas Y, Franckx-Goosens A, Pipeleers-Marichal M, et al. Area under pH 4: advantages of a new parameter in the interpretation of esophageal pH monitoring data in infants. *J Pediatr Gastroenterol Nutr.* 1989;9(1): 34–39.

83. Thawley SE, Cysts and tumors of the larynx. In: Paparella MM, Shumrick DA, Gluckman JI, Meyerhoff WL, eds. Otolaryngology. *Vol III. Head and Neck.* Philadelphia, Pa: WB Saunders Co; 1991;2307–2369.

84. Young JL, Asire AJ, Polltell ES. SEER program Cancer incidence and mortality in the United States 1973–1976. BHEW Publication (NIH)78-1837. Washington DC: US Government Printing Office; 1978.

85. Watkinson JC, Gaze MN, Wilson JA, eds. *Stell & Maran's Head and Neck Surgery.* 4th ed. Oxford, England: Butterworth Heineman; 2000:1–9.

86. Koufman J. Gastroesophageal reflux and voice disorders. In: Rubin JS, Sataloff RT, Korovin G, Gould WJ, eds. *Diagnosis and Treatment of Voice Disorders.* Tokyo/New York: Igaku Shoin Medical Publishers; 1995:161–175.

87. Sugar J, Vereczkey I, Toth J. Some etio-pathogenetic factors in laryngeal carcinogenesis. *J Environ Pathol Toxicol Oncol.* 1996;15:195–199.

88. Gonzalez CA, Agudo A. Occupational cancer in Spain. *Environ Health Perspect.* 1999;107(suppl 2):273–277.

89. Maier H, Tisch M. Epidemiology of laryngeal cancer: Results of the Heidelberg case-control study. *Acta Otolaryngol Suppl.* 1997;527:160–164.

90. Muscat JE, Wynder EL. Tobacco, alcohol, asbestos and occupational risk factors for laryngeal cancer. *Cancer.* 1992;69:2244–2251.

91. Szeszenia-Dabrowska N, Strzelecka A, Wilczynska U, Szymczak W. Occupational neoplasms in Poland in the years 1971–1994. *Med-Pr.* 1997;48:1–14.

92. Podol'skaia EV. [Precancerous conditions of the larynx in workers exposed to dust and their prevention.] *Vestn-Oturinolaringol.* 1989;2:67–69.

93. Landrigan PJ, Nicholson WJ, Suzuki Y, Ladou J. The hazards of chrysotile asbestos: a critical review. *Ind Health.* 1999;37:271–280.

94. Vejlupkova J, Lebedova J. Diseases caused by asbestos. *Prakt Lek.* 2000;80:441–446.

95. Gustavsson P, Jakonsson R, Johansson H, et al. Occupational exposures and squamous cell carcinoma of the oral cavity, pharynx, larynx, and oesophagus: a case-control study in Sweden. *Occup Environ Med.* 1998;55:393–400.

96. Soskolne CL, Zeighami EA, Hanis NM, et al. Laryngeal cancer and occupational exposure to sulfuric acid. *Am J Epidemiol.* 1984;120:358–369.

97. Steenland K. Laryngeal cancer incidence among workers exposed to acid mists. *Cancer Causes Control.* 1997;8: 34–38.

98. Grandjean P, Olsen JH, Jensen OM, et al. Cancer incidence and mortality in workers exposed to fluoride. *J Natl Cancer Inst.* 1992;84:1903–1909.

99. World Health Organization. *International Classification of Impairments, Disabilities and Handicaps: A Manual of Classification Relating to the Consequences of Disease.* Geneva, Switzerland: World Health Organization; 1980:25–43.

100. Murry T, Rosen CA. Outcome measurements and quality of life in voice disorders. *Otolaryngol Clin North Am.* 2000;33(4)905–916.

101. Jacobson BH, Johnson A, Grywalsky C, et al. The Voice Handicap Index (VHI): development and validation. *J Voice.* 1998;12:540–550.

102. List MA, Ritter-Sterr C, Lansky SB. A performance status scale for head and neck patients. *Cancer.* 1990;66: 564–569.

103. Ware JE, Sherbourne CD. The MOS 36-item short form health survey (SF-36). Conceptual framework and item selection. *Med Care.* 1992;30:473–483.

104. Sataloff RT. Rational thought: the impact of voice science upon voice care. (G. Paul Moore Lecture). *J Voice.* 1995;9(3):215–234.

105. Dufresne AM, Lafreniere D. Soft tissue response in the rabbit larynx following implantation of LactoSorb (PLA/PGA copolymer) prosthesis for medialization laryngoplasty. *J Voice.* 2000;14(3):387–397.

106. Remacle M, Lawson G, Keghian J, Jamart J. Use of injectable autologous collagen for correcting glottic gaps: initial results. *J Voice.* 2000;14(4):280–288.

107. Ford CN, Staskowski PA, Bless DM. Autologous collagen vocal fold injection: a preliminary clinical study. *Laryngoscope.* 1995;105:944–948.

108. Rahbar R, Valdez TA, Shapshay SM. Preliminary results of intraoperative mitomycin-C in the treatment and prevention of glottic and subglottic stenosis. *J Voice.* 2000;14:282–286.

Glossary

This glossary has been developed from the author's experience and also from a review of glossaries developed by Johan Sundberg (personal communication, June 1995), Ingo Titze (*Principles of Voice Production*, Englewood, NJ: Prentice-Hall, 1994:330–338), and other sources. It is difficult to credit appropriately contributions to glossaries or dictionaries of general terms, as each new glossary builds on prior works. The author is indebted to colleagues whose previous efforts have contributed to the compilation of this glossary.

AAO–HNS: American Academy of Otolaryngology-Head and Neck Surgery

AIDS: Acquired Immune Deficiency Syndrome

abduct: To move apart, separate

abduction quotient: The ratio of the glottal half-width at the vocal processes to the amplitude of vibration of the vocal fold

abscess: Collection of pus

absolute jitter (Jita): A discrete measure of very short term (cycle-to-cycle) variation of the pitch periods expressed in microseconds. This parameter is dependent on the fundamental frequency of the voicing sample. Therefore, normative data differs significantly for men and women. Higher pitch results in lower Jita

absolute voice rest: Total silence of the phonatory system

acceleration: The rate of change of velocity with respect to time (measured in millimeters per square second mm/s^2)

acoustic power: The physical measure of the amount of energy produced and radiated into the air per second (measured in watts)

acoustical zero decibels: 0.0002 microbar

actin: A protein molecule that reacts with myosin to form actinomysin, the contractile part of a myofilament in muscle

acting-voice trainer: (1) *See* **Voice Coach**; (2) A professional with specialized training who may work with injured voices as part of a medical voice team in an effort to optimize speaking voice performance

Adam's apple: Prominence of the thyroid cartilage, primarily in males

adduct: To bring together, approximate

affricate: Combination of plosive and fricative consonants such as /dʒ/

allergy: Bodily response to foreign substances or organisms

alto: (*See* **Contralto**)

alveolar ridge: The bony ridge of the gum into which the teeth insert

AMA: American Medical Association

amplitude: Maximum excursion of an undulating signal from the equilibrium; the amplitude of a sound wave is related to the perceived loudness; mostly it is expressed as a logarithmic, comparative level measure using the decibel (dB) unit

amplitude perturbation quotient (APQ): A relative evaluation of short term (cycle-to-cycle) variation of peak-to-peak amplitude expressed in percent. This measure uses a smoothing factor of 11 periods

amplitude spectrum: A display of relative amplitude versus frequency of the sinusoidal components of a waveform

amplitude to length ratio: The ratio of vibrational amplitude at the center of the vocal fold to the length of the vocal fold

amplitude tremor: Regular (periodic) long-term amplitude variation (an element of vibrato)

amplitude tremor frequency (Fatr): This measure is expressed in Hz and shows the frequency of the most intensive low-frequency amplitude-modulating component in the specified amplitude-tremor analysis range

amplitude tremor intensity index (ATRI): The average ratio of the amplitude of the most intensive low-frequency amplitude modulating component (amplitude tremor) to the total amplitude of the analyzed sample. The algorithm for tremor analysis determines the strongest periodic amplitude modulation of the voice. This measure is expressed in percent

anabolic steroids: Primarily male hormones, increase muscle mass and may cause irreversible, masculinization of the voice. Anabolic steroids help cells convert simple substances into more complex substances, especially into living matter

anisotropic: Property of a material that produces different strains when identical stresses are applied in different directions

antagonist (muscle): An opposing muscle

anterior: Toward the front

anterior commissure: The junction of the vocal folds in the front of the larynx

antibiotic: Drug used to combat infection (bodily invasion by a living organism such as a bacteria or virus). Most antibiotics have action specifically against bacteria

anticoagulant: Blood thinner; agent that impairs blood clotting

antinodes: The "peaks" in a standing wave pattern

antihistamine: Drug to combat allergic response

aperiodic: Irregular behavior that has no definite period; is usually either chaotic or random

aperiodicity: The absence of periodicity; no portion of the waveform repeats exactly

aphonia: The absence of vocal fold vibration; this term is commonly used to describe people who have "lost their voice" after vocal fold injury. In most cases, such patients have very poor vibration, rather than no vibration; and they typically have a harsh, nearly whispered voice

appendix of the ventricle of Morgagni: A cecal pouch of mucous membrane connected by a narrow opening with the anterior aspect of the ventricle. It sits between the ventricular fold in the inner surface of the thyroid cartilage. In some cases, it may extend as far as the cranial border of the thyroid cartilage, or higher. It contains the openings of 60 to 70 mucous glands, and it is enclosed in a fibrous capsule, which is continuous with the ventricular ligament. Also called *appendix ventriculi laryngis*, and *laryngeal saccule*

aria: Song, especially in the context of an opera

arthritis: Inflammation of joints in the body

articulation: Shaping of vocal tract by positioning of its mobile walls such as lips, lower jaw, tongue body and tip, velum, epiglottis, pharyngeal sidewalls, and larynx

articulators: The structures of the vocal tract that are used to create the sounds of language. They include the lips, teeth, tongue, soft palate, and hard palate

arytenoid cartilages: Paired, ladle-shaped cartilages to which the vocal folds are attached

arytenoid dislocation: A condition frequently causing vocal fold immobility or hypomobility due to separation of the arytenoid cartilage from its joint and normal position atop the cricoid cartilage

ASHA: American Speech-Language-Hearing Association

aspirate: Speech sound characterized by breathiness

aspirate attack: Initiation of phonation preceded by air, producing /h/

aspiration: (1) In speech, the sound made by turbulent airflow preceding or following vocal fold vibration, as in /hɑ/. (2) In medicine, refers to breathing into the lungs substances that do not belong there such as food, water, or stomach contents following reflux. Aspiration may lead to infections such as pneumonia, commonly referred to as *aspiration pneumonia*

asthma: Obstructive pulmonary (lung) disease associated with bronchospasm, and difficulty expiring air

atmospheric pressure: The absolute pressure exerted by the atmosphere, usually measured in millimeters of mercury (mmHg)

atresia: Failure of development. In the case of the larynx, this may result in fusion or congenital webbing of the vocal folds, or failure of development of the trachea

atrophy: Loss or wasting of tissue. Muscle atrophy occurs, for example, in an arm that is immobilized in a cast for many weeks

attractor: A geometric figure in state space to which all trajectories in its vicinity are drawn. The four types of attractors are (1) *point*, (2) *limit cycle*, (3) *toroidal*, and (4) *strange*. A point trajector draws all trajectories to a single point. An example is a pendulum moving toward rest. A limit cycle is characteristic of periodic motion. A toroidal attractor represents quasiperiodic motion (often considered a subset of periodic motion). A strange attractor is associated with chaotic motion

back vowel: A vowel produced by pulling the tongue posteriorly, with relation to its neutral position

bands: Range of adjacent parameter values; a frequency band is an ensemble of adjacent frequencies

band pass filter: Filter that allows frequencies only within a certain frequency range to pass

baritone: The most common male vocal range. Higher than bass and lower than tenor. Singer's formant around 2600 Hz

basement membrane: Anatomic structure immediately beneath the epithelium

bass: (*See* **Basso**)

bass baritone: In between bass and baritone. Not as heavy as basso profundo, but typically with greater flexibility. Must be able to sing at least as high as l'_4. Also known as *basso contante* and *basso guisto*. Baritones with bass quality are also called *basse taille*

basso: Lowest male voice. Singer's formant around 2300–2400 Hz

basso profundo: Deep bass. The lowest and heaviest of the bass voices. Can sing at least as low as D_2 with full voice. Singer's formant around 2200–2300 Hz. Also known as *contra-basso*

bel canto: Literally means "beautiful singing." Refers to a method and philosophical approach to singing voice production

benchmark: The standard by which other similar occurrences are judged

benign tumors: Tumors that are not able to metastasize or spread to distant sites

Bernoulli's principle: If the energy in a confined fluid stream is constant, an increase in particle velocity must be accompanied by a decrease in pressure against the wall

bifurcation: A sudden qualitative change in the behavior of a system. In chaos, for example, a small change in the initial parameters of a stable (predominantly linear) system may cause oscillation between two different states as the nonlinear aspects of the system become manifest. This transition is a bifurcation

bilabial covering: Using the lips to constrict the mouth opening and "cover" the sound. This technique is used commonly by young singers in the form of slight vowel distortion to attenuate upper harmonics and make a sound richer and less brash.

bilateral: On both sides

bilateral vocal fold paralysis: Loss of the ability to move both vocal folds caused by neurologic dysfunction

biomechanics: The study of the mechanics of biological tissue

bleat: Fast vibrato, like the bleating of a sheep

body: With regard to the vocal fold, the vocalis muscle

Boyle's law: In a soft-walled enclosure and at a constant temperature, pressure and volume are inversely related

bravura: Brilliant, elaborate, showy execution of musical or dramatic material

break: (*See* **Passagio**)

breathy phonation: Phonation characterized by a lack of vocal fold closure; this causes air leakage (excessive airflow) during the quasi-closed phase, and this produces turbulence that is heard as noise mixed in the voice

bronchitis: Inflammation of the bronchial tubes in the lungs

bronchospasm: Forceful closing of the distal airways in the lungs

bruxism: Grinding of the teeth

bulimia: Self-induced vomiting to control weight

butterfly effect: Refers to the notion that in chaotic (nonlinear dynamics) systems a minuscule change in initial condition may have profound effects on the behavior of the system. For example, a butterfly flapping its wings in Hong Kong may change the weather in New York

cancer: An abnormality in which cells no longer respond to the signals that control replication and growth. This results in uncontrolled growth and tumor formation, and may result in spread of tumor to distant locations (metastasis)

carrier: (1) In physics, a waveform (typically a sinusoid) whose frequency or amplitude is modulated by a signal. (2) In medicine, a person who is colonized by an organism (typically bacteria such as streptococcus or pneumococcus), but who has no symptoms or adverse effects from the presence of the organism.

Nevertheless, that carrier is able to transmit the organism to other people in whom it does cause a symptomatic infection

cartilage: One of the tissues of the skeleton; it is more flexible than bone

cartilage of Wrisberg: Cartilage attached in the mobile portion of each aryepiglottic fold

cartilage of Santorini: Small cartilage flexibly attached near the apex of the arytenoid, in the region of the opening of the esophagus

castrato: Male singer castrated at around age 7 or 8, so as to retain alto or soprano vocal range

category: Voice type classified according to pitch range and voice quality; the most frequently used categories are bass, baritone, tenor, alto, mezzosoprano, and soprano, but many other subdivisions of these exist

caudal: Toward the tail

central vowel: A vowel produced with the tongue at or near neutral position

chaos: A qualitative description of a dynamic system that seems unpredictable, but actually has a "hidden" order. Also a mathematical field that studies fractal geometry and nonlinear dynamics

chaotic behavior: Distinct from random or periodic behavior. A chaotic system *looks* disorganized or random but is actually deterministic, although aperiodic. It has sensitive dependence on initial condition, has definite form, and is bounded to a relatively narrow range (unable to go off into infinity)

chest voice: Heavy registration with excessive resonance in the lower formants

coarticulation: A condition in which one phoneme influences the production of phonemes before and after it, resulting commonly in degradation of the quality and clarity of the surrounding sounds

cochlea: Inner ear organ of hearing

coefficient of amplitude variation (vAm): This measure, expressed in percent, computes the relative standard deviation of the peak-to-peak amplitude. It increases regardless of the type of amplitude variation

coefficient of fundamental frequency variation (vF$_0$): This measure, expressed in percent, computes the relative standard deviation of the fundamental frequency. It is the ratio of the standard deviation of the period-to-period variation to the average fundamental frequency

collagen: The protein substance of the white (collagenous) fibers of cartilage, bone, tendon, skin, and all of the connective tissues. Collagen may be extracted, processed, and injected into the vocal fold to treat various abnormalities

collagenase: An enzyme that catalyzes the degradation of collagen

coloratura: In common usage, refers to the highest of the female voices, with range well above C$_6$. May use more whistle tone than other female voices. In fact, coloratura actually refers to a style of florid, agile, complex singing that may apply to any voice classification. For example, the bass runs in Händel's *Messiah* require coloratura technique

complex periodic vibration: A sound that repeats regularly. A pattern of simultaneously sounding partials

complex sound: A combination of sinusoidal waveforms superimposed upon each other. May be complex periodic sound (such as musical instruments) or complex aperiodic sound (such as random street noise)

complex tone: Tone composed of a series of simultaneously sounding partials

component frequency: mathematically, a sinusoid; perceptually, a pure tone. Also called a *partial*

compression: A deformation of a body that decreases its entire volume. An increase in density

concert pitch: Also known as *international concert pitch*. The standard of tuning A$_4$. Reference pitch has changed substantially over the last 200 to 300 years

condensation: An increase in density

constructive interference: The interference of two or more waves such that enhancement occurs

contact ulcer: A lesion with mucosal disruption most commonly on the vocal processes or medial surfaces of the arytenoids. Caused most commonly by gastroesophageal reflux laryngitis and/or muscular tension dysphonia

contrabasso: (*See* **Basso profundo**)

contraction: A decrease in length

contralto: Lowest of the female voices. Able to sing F$_3$ below middle C, as well as the entire treble staff. Singer's formant at around 2800–2900 Hz

conus elasticus: Fibroelastic membrane extending inferiorly from the vocal folds to the anterior superior border of the cricoid cartilage. Also called the *cricovocal ligament*. Composed primarily of yellow elastic tissue. Anteriorly, it attaches to the minor aspect of the thyroid cartilage. Posteriorly, it attaches to the vocal process of the arytenoids

convergent: With regard to glottal shape, the glottis narrows from bottom to top

corner vowels: (a), (i), and (u); vowels at the corners of a vowel triangle; they necessitate extreme placements of the tongue

corticosteroid: Potent substances produced by the adrenal cortex (excluding sex hormones of adrenal origin) in response to the release of adrenocorticotropic hormone from the pituitary gland, or related substances. Glucocorticoids influence carbohydrate, fat, and protein metabolism. Mineralocorticoids help regular electrolyte and water balance. Some corticosteroids have both effects to varying degrees. Corticosteroids may also be given as medications for various effects, including anti-inflammatory, antineoplastic, immune suppressive, and ACTH secretion suppressive effects, as well as for hormone replacement therapy

countertenor: Male voice that is primarily falsetto, singing in the contralto range. Most countertenors are also able to sing in the baritone or tenor range. Countertenors are also known as *contraltino* or *contratenor*

cover: (1) In medicine, with regard to the vocal fold, the epithelium and superficial layer of lamina propria. (2) In music, an alteration in technique that changes the resonance characteristics of a sung sound, generally darkening the sound

cranial nerves: Twelve paired nerves responsible for smell, taste, eye movement, vision, facial sensation, chewing muscles, facial motion, salivary gland and lacrimal (tear) gland secretions, hearing, balance, pharyngeal and laryngeal sensation, vocal fold motion, gastric acid secretion, shoulder motion, tongue motion, and related functions

creaky voice: The perceptual result of subharmonic or chaotic patterns in the glottal waveform. According to IR Titze, if a subharmonic is below about 70 Hz, creaky voice may be perceived as pulse register (vocal fry)

crescendo: To get gradually louder

cricoid cartilage: A solid ring of cartilage located below and behind the thyroid cartilage

cricothyroid muscle: An intrinsic laryngeal muscle that is used primarily to control pitch (paired)

crossover frequency: The fundamental frequency for which there is an equal probability for perception of two adjacent registers

cycle: One complete set of regularly recurring events

cysts: Fluid-filled lesions

damp: To diminish, or attenuate an oscillation

damped oscillation: Oscillation in which energy is lost during each cycle until oscillation stops

decibel: One tenth of a bel. The decibel is a unit of comparison between a reference and another point. It has no absolute value. Although decibels are used to measure sound, they are also used (with different references) to measure heat, light, and other physical phenomena. For sound pressure, the reference is 0.0002 microbar (millionths of one barometric pressure). In the past, this has also been referred to as 0.0002 $dyne/cm^2$, and by other terms

decrescendo: (*See* **Diminuendo**)

deformation: The result of stress applied to any surface of a deformable continuous medium. Elongation, compression, contraction, and shear are examples

dehydration: Fluid deprivation. This may alter the amount and viscosity of vocal fold lubrication and the properties of the vocal fold tissues themselves

destructive interference: The interference of two or more waves such that full or partial cancellation occurs

dialect: A variety of a spoken language, usually associated with a distinct geographical, social, or political environment

diaphragm: A large, dome-shaped muscle at the bottom of the rib cage that separates the lungs from the viscera. It is the primary muscle of inspiration and may be co-activated during singing

diminuendo: To get gradually softer

diphthong: Two consecutive vowels occurring in the same syllable

displacement: The distance between two points in space, including the direction from one point to the other

displacement flow: Air in the glottis that is squeezed out when the vocal folds come together

diuretic: A drug to decrease circulating body fluid generally by excretion through the kidneys

divergent: With regard to the vocal folds, the glottis widens from bottom to top

dizziness: A feeling of imbalance

dorsal: Toward the back

down-regulation: Decreased gene expression, compared with baseline

dramatic soprano: Soprano with powerful, rich voice suitable for dramatic, heavily orchestrated, operatic roles. Sings at least to C_6

dramatic tenor: Tenor with heavy voice, often with a suggestion of baritone quality. Suitable for dramatic roles that are heavily orchestrated. Also referred to as *tenora robusto*, and *helden tenor*. The term helden tenor (literally "heroic" tenor) is used typically for tenors who sing Wagnerian operatic roles

dynamics: (1) In physics, a branch of mechanics that deals with the study of forces that accelerate object(s). (2) In music, it refers to changes in the loudness of musical performance

dysmenorrhea: Painful menstrual cramps

dyspepsia: Epigastric discomfort, especially following meals; impairment of the power or function of digestion

dysphonia: Abnormal voicing

dysphonia plica ventricularis: Phonation using false vocal fold vibration rather than true vocal fold vibration. Most commonly associated with severe muscular tension dysphonia Occasionally may be an appropriate compensation for profound true vocal fold dysfunction

dystonia: A neurological disorder characterized by involuntary movements, such as unpredictable, spasmodic opening or closing of the vocal folds

edema: Excessive accumulation of fluid in tissues, or "swelling"

elastic recoil pressure: The alveolar pressure derived from extended (strained) tissue in the lungs, rib cage, and the entire thorax after inspiration (measured in Pascals)

electroglottograph (EGG): Recording of electrical conductance of vocal fold contact area versus time; EGG waveforms have been frequently used for the purpose of plotting voice source analysis

electromyograph (EMG): Recording of the electric potentials in a muscle, which are generated by the neural system and which control its degree of contraction; if rectified and smoothed the EMG is closely related to the muscular force exerted by the muscle

elongation: An increase in length

embouchure: The shape of the lips, tongue, and related structures adopted while producing a musical tone, particularly while playing a wind instrument

endocrine: Relating to hormones and the organs that produce them

endometriosis: A disorder in which endometrial tissue is present in abnormal locations. Typically causes excessively painful menstrual periods (dysmenorrhea) and infertility

epiglottis: Cartilage that covers over the larynx during swallowing

epilarynx: A region bordered by the rim of the epiglottis and the glottis synonymous with epiglottal tube. This resonating region is considered by some to be the site of origin of the singer's formant

epithelium: The covering, or most superficial layer, of body surfaces

erythema: Redness

esophagus: Tube leading from the bottom of the pharynx to the stomach; swallowed food is transported through this structure

expansion: A deformation of a body such that the entire volume increases

extrinsic muscles of the larynx: The strap muscles in the neck, responsible for adjusting laryngeal height and for stabilizing the larynx

Fach (German): Literally, job specialty. It is used to indicate voice classification. For example, lyric soprano and dramatic soprano are different Fachs

false vocal folds: Folds of tissue located slightly higher than and parallel to the vocal folds in the larynx

falsetto: High, light register, applied primarily to men's voices singing in the soprano or alto range. Can also be applied to women's voices

fibroblasts: Cells responsible in part for the formation of scar in response to tissue injury

fibrosis: Generally refers to a component of scar caused by cross-linking of fibers during a reactive or a reparative process

flat singing: Usually refers to pitch (frequency) lower than the desirable target frequency. Sometimes also used to refer to a singing style devoid of excitement or emotional expression

flow: The volume of fluid passing through a given cross-section of a tube or duct per second; also called volume velocity (measured in liters per second)

flow glottogram: Recording of the transglottal airflow versus time, ie, of the sound of the voice source. Generally obtained from inverse filtering, FLOGG is the acoustical representation of the voice source

flow phonation: The optimal balance between vocal fold adductory forces and subglottic pressure, producing efficient sound production at the level of the vocal folds

flow resistance: The ratio of pressure to flow

fluid: A substance that is either a liquid or a gas

fluid mechanics: The study of motion or deformation of liquids and gases

flutter: Modulation in the 10–12 Hz range

F_0: Fundamental frequency

F_0–tremor frequency (Fftr): This measure is expressed in Hz and shows the frequency of the most intensive low-frequency F_0 modulating component in the specified F_0 tremor analysis range

F_0–tremor intensity index (FTRI): The average ratio of the frequency magnitude of the most intensive low-frequency modulating component (F_0 tremor) to the total frequency magnitude of the analyzed sample. The algorithm for tremor analysis determines the strongest periodic frequency modulation of the voice. This measure is expressed in percent

focal: Limited to a specific area. For example, spasmodic dysphonia may be focal (limited to the larynx), or part of a group of dystonias that affect other parts of the body such as the facial muscles or muscles involved in chewing

force: A push or pull; the physical quantity imparted to an object to change its momentum

forced oscillation: Oscillation imposed on a system by an external source

formant: Vocal tract resonance; the formant frequencies are tuned by the vocal tract shape and determine much of the vocal quality

formant tuning: A boosting of vocal intensity when F_0 or one if its harmonics coincides exactly with a formant frequency

front vowel: A vowel formed by displacing the tongue anteriorly, with regard to its neutral position

functional residual capacity (FRC): Lung volume at which the elastic inspiratory forces equal the elastic expiratory forces; in spontaneous quiet breathing exhalation stops at FRC

fractal: A geometric figure in which an identical pattern or motif repeats itself over and over on an ever-diminishing scale. Self-similarity is an essential characteristic

fractal dimension: Fractal dimensions are measures of fractal objects that can be used to determine how alike or different the objects are. Box counting algorithms and mass-radius measurement are two common approaches to determining fractal dimension. The fractal dimension represents the way a set of points fills a given area of space. It may be defined as the slope of the function relating the number of points contained in a given radius (or its magnification) to the radius itself. For example, an object can be assessed under many magnifications. The coast of Britain can be measured, for example, with a meter stick or a millimeter stick, but the latter will yield a larger measure. As magnification is increased (smaller measuring sticks), a point will be reached at which small changes in magnification no longer significantly affect length. That is, a plot of coastline length versus magnification reaches a plateau. That plateau corresponds to fractal dimension. The more irregular the figure (eg, coastline), the more complex and the more space it occupies, hence, the higher its fractal dimension. A perfect line has a fractal dimension of 1. A figure that fills a plane has a fractal dimension of 2. Fractal dimension cannot be used alone to determine the presence or absence of chaotic behavior

frequency analysis: Same as spectrum analysis

frequency tremor: A periodic (regular) pitch modulation of the voice (an element of vibrato)

fricative: A speech sound, generally a consonant, produced by a constriction of the vocal tract, particularly by directing the airstream against a hard surface, producing noisy air turbulence. Examples include *s* produced with the teeth, *s* produced with the lower lip and upper incisors, and *th* produced with the tongue tip and upper incisors

frontal (or coronal) plane: An anatomic plane that divides the body into anterior and posterior portions; across the crown of the head

functional voice disorder: An abnormality in voice sound and function in the absence of an anatomic or physiologic organic abnormality

fundamental: Lowest partial of a spectrum, the frequency of which normally corresponds to the pitch perceived.

fundamental frequency (F_0): The lowest frequency in a periodic waveform; also called the first harmonic frequency

gas: A substance that preserves neither shape nor volume when acted upon by forces, but adapts readily to the size and shape of its container

gastric: Pertaining to the stomach

gastric juice: The contents of the stomach, ordinarily including a high concentration of hydrochloric acid.

gastroesophageal reflux (GER): The passage of gastric juice in a retrograde fashion from the stomach into the esophagus. These fluids may reach the level of the larynx or oral cavity, and may be aspirated into the lungs

gastroesophageal reflux disease (GERD): A disorder including symptoms and/or signs caused by reflux of gastric juice into the esophagus and elsewhere. Heartburn is one of the most common symptoms of GERD. (*See* also **Laryngopharyngeal reflux**)

genomics: The study of genes (genetic material) made up of DNA, and located in the chromosomes of the nuclei of cells in an organism.

glide: A written consonant that is produced as a vowel sound in transition to the following vowel. Examples include: /j/ and /w/

glissando: A "slide" including all possible pitches between the initial and final pitch sounded. Similar to portamento and slur

globus: Sensation of a lump in the throat

glottal: At the level of the vocal folds

glottal chink: Opening in the glottis during vocal fold adduction, most commonly posteriorly. It may be a normal variant in some cases

glottal resistance: Ratio between transglottal airflow and subglottal pressure; mainly reflects the degree of glottal adduction

glottal stop (or click): A transient sound caused by the sudden onset or offset of phonation

glottal stroke: A brief event in which air pressure is increased behind the occluded glottis and then released, more gently than following a glottal stop. Glottal strokes are used to separate phonemes in linguistic situations in which running them together might result in misunderstanding of the meaning

glottis: Space between the vocal folds. (*See* also **Rima glottitis**)

glottis respiratoria: The portion of the glottis posteriorly in the region of the cartilaginous portions of the vocal folds

glottis vocalis: The portion of the glottis in the region of the membranous portions of the vocal folds

grace days: Refers to a former contractual arrangement, especially in European Opera Houses, in which women were permitted to refrain from singing during the premenstrual and early menstrual portions of their cycles, at their discretion

granuloma: A raised lesion generally covered with mucosa, most commonly in the region of the vocal

process or medial surface of the arytenoid. Often caused by reflux and/or muscle tension dysphonia

halitosis: Bad breath

harmonic: A frequency that is an integer multiple of a given fundamental. Harmonics of a fundamental are equally spaced in frequency. Partial in a spectrum in which the frequency of each partial equals n times the fundamental frequency, n being the number of the harmonic

harsh glottal attack: Initiating phonation of a word or sound with a glottal plosive

head voice: A vocal quality characterized by flexibility and lightness of tone. In some classifications, it is used to designate a high register of the singing voice

hemorrhage: Rupture of a blood vessel. This may occur in a vocal fold

hertz: Cycles per second (Hz) (named after Gustav Hertz)

high pass filter: Filter which only allows frequencies above a certain cutoff frequency to pass; the cutoff is generally not abrupt but, rather, gentle and is given in terms of a roll-off value, eg, 24 dB/octave

histogram: Graph showing the occurrence of a parameter value; thus, a fundamental frequency histogram shows the occurrence of different fundamental frequency values, eg, in fluent speech or in a song

Hooke's law: Stress in proportion to strain; or, in simpler form, force is proportional to elongation

hormones: Substances produced within the body that affect or control various organs and bodily functions

hyoid bone: A horseshoe-shaped bone known as the "tongue bone." It is attached to muscles of the tongue and related structures, and to the larynx and related structures

hyperfunction: Excessive muscle effort for example, pressed voice, muscle tension dysphonia

hypernasal: Excessive nasal resonance

hypofunction: Low muscular effort, for example, soft breathy voice

hyponasal: Deficient nasal resonance

hypothyroidism: Lower than normal output of thyroid hormone. This condition is referred to commonly as an "underactive thyroid," and often results in malaise, weight gain, temperature intolerance, irregular menses, muffling of the voice, and other symptoms

Hz: (*See* **Hertz**)

impotence: The inability to accomplish penile erection

in vitro: Outside the living body, for example, an excised larynx

in vivo: In the living body

incompressibility: Property of a substance that conserves volume in a deformation

inertia: Sluggishness; a property of resisting a change in momentum

inferior: Below

infertility: The inability to accomplish pregnancy

infraglottic: Below the level of the glottis (space between the vocal folds). This region includes the trachea, thorax, and related structures

infraglottic vocal tract: Below the level of the vocal folds. This region includes the airways and muscles of support (Infraglottic is synonymous with subglottic)

infrahyoid muscle group: A collection of extrinsic muscles including the sternohyoid, sternothyroid, omohyoid, and thyroid muscles

insertion: The point of attachment of a muscle with a bone that can be moved by the muscle

intensity: A measure of power per unit area. With respect to sound, it generally correlates with perceived loudness

interarytenoid muscle: An intrinsic laryngeal muscle that connects the two arytenoid cartilages

intercostal muscles: Muscles between the ribs

interval: The difference between two pitches, expressed in terms of musical scale

intrinsic laryngeal muscles: muscles within the larynx responsible for abduction, adduction, and longitudinal tension of the vocal folds

intrinsic pitch of vowels: Refers to the fact that in normal speech certain vowels tend to be produced with a significantly higher or lower pitch than other vowels

inverse filtering: Method used for recovering the transglottal airflow during phonation; the technique implies that the voice is fed through a computer filter that compensates for the resonance effects of the supraglottic vocal tract, especially the lowest formants

inverse square law: Sound intensity is inversely proportional to the square of the distance from the sound source

IPA: International Phonetic Alphabet (*See* **Appendix I**)

isometric: Constant muscle length during contraction

iteration: In mathematics, the repetitive process of substituting the solution to an equation back into the same equation to obtain the next solution

jitter: Irregularity in the period of time of vocal fold vibrations; cycle-to-cycle variation in fundamental frequency; jitter is often perceived as hoarseness

jitter percent (Jitt): A relative measure of very short term (cycle-to-cycle) variation of the pitch periods expressed in percent. The influence of the average fundamental frequency is significantly reduced. This parameter is very sensitive to pitch variations

juvenile papillomatosis: A disease of children characterized by the clustering of many papillomas (small blisterlike growths) over the vocal folds and elsewhere in the larynx and trachea. Papillomatosis may also occur in adults, in which case the adjective *juvenile* is not used. The disease is caused by human papilloma virus

keratosis: A buildup of keratin (a tough, fibrous protein) on the surface of the vocal folds

kinematics: The study of movement as a consequence of known or assumed forces

kinetic energy: The energy of matter in motion (measured in joules)

klangfarbe: Tone color, referring to vocal quality

labiodental: A consonant produced by bringing the lower lip in contact with the upper front teeth

lag: A difference in time between one point and another

lamina propria: With reference to the larynx, the tissue layers below the epithelium. In adult humans, the lamina propria consists of superficial, intermediate, and deep layers

laminar: Smooth or layered; in fluid mechanics, indicating parallel flow lines

laminar flow: Airflow in smooth layers over a surface (as differentiated from irregular, or turbulent flow)

laryngeal saccule: (*See* **Appendix of the Ventricle of Morgagni**)

laryngeal sinus: (*See* **Ventricle of Morgagni**)

laryngeal ventricle: Cavity formed by the gap between the true and false vocal folds

laryngeal web: An abnormal tissue connection attaching the vocal folds to each other

laryngectomy: Removal of the larynx. It may be total, or it may be a "conservation laryngectomy," in which a portion of the larynx is preserved

laryngitis: Inflammation of laryngeal tissues

laryngitis sicca: Dry voice

laryngocele: A pouch or herniation of the larynx, usually filled with air and sometimes presenting as a neck mass. The pouch usually enlarges with increased laryngeal pressure as may occur from coughing or playing a wind instrument.

laryngologist: Physician specializing in disorders of the larynx and voice, in most countries. In some areas of Europe, the laryngologist is primarily responsible for surgery, while diagnosis is performed by phoniatricians

laryngomalacia: A condition in which the laryngeal cartilages are excessively soft and may collapse in response to inspiratory pressures, obstructing the airway

laryngopharyngeal reflux (LPR): A form of gastroesophageal reflux disease in which gastric juice affects the larynx and adjacent structures. Commonly associated with hoarseness, frequent throat clearing, granulomas, and other laryngeal problems, even in the absence of heartburn

laryngospasm: Sudden, forceful, and abnormal closing of the vocal folds

larynx: The body organ in the neck that includes the vocal folds. The "voice box"

larynx height: Vertical position of the larynx; mostly measured in relation to the rest position

larynx tube: Cavity formed by the vocal folds and the arytenoid, epiglottis, and thyroid cartilages and the structures joining them

laser: An acronym for *light amplification by stimulated emission of radiation*. A surgical tool using light energy to vaporize or cauterize tissue

lateral: Toward the side (away from the center).

lateral cricoarytenoid muscle: Intrinsic laryngeal muscle that adducts the vocal folds through forward rocking and rotation of the arytenoids (paired)

LD50: In determining drug toxicity, the LD50 is the amount of the substance that will cause death in 50% of test specimens (lethal dose for 50%)

lesion: In medicine, a nonspecific term that may be used for nearly any structural abnormality

legato: Smooth, connected

leukoplakia: A white plaque. Typically, this occurs on mucous membranes, including the vocal folds

level: Logarithmic and comparative measure of sound intensity; the unit is normally dB

lied: Song, particularly art song

lift: (*See* **Passagio**)

ligament: Connective tissue between articular regions of bone

linear system: A system in which the relation between input and output varies in a constant, or linear, fashion

lingual: Related to the tongue

linguadental: A consonant produced by bringing the tongue in contact with the teeth

linguapalatal: A consonant produced by bringing the tongue in contact with the hard palate

lip covering: Altering lip shape to make a sound less brash or bright, and "rounder" or more "rich"

liquid: A substance that assumes the shape of its container, but preserves its volume

loft: A suggested term for the highest (loftiest) register; usually referred to as *falsetto voice*

logistic map: A simple quadratic equation that exhibits chaotic behavior under special initial conditions and parameters. It is the simplest chaotic system

Lombard effect: Modification of vocal loudness in response to auditory input. For example, the tendency to speak louder in the presence of background noise

long-term average spectrum (LTAS): Graph showing a long-time average of the sound intensity in various frequency bands; the appearance of an LTAS is strongly dependent on the filters used

longitudinal: Along the length of a structure

longitudinal tension: With reference to the larynx, stretching the vocal folds

loudness: The amount of sound perceived by a listener; a perceptual quantity that can only be assessed with an auditory system. Loudness corresponds to intensity, and to the amplitude of a sound wave

low pass filter: Filter which allows only frequencies below a certain frequency to pass; the cutoff is generally not at all abrupt but gentle and is given in terms of a roll-off value, eg, 24 dB/octave

LTAS: An acronym for long-term-averaged spectrum

lung volume: Volume contained in the subglottic air system; after a maximum inhalation following a maximum exhalation the lung volume equals the vital capacity

lyric soprano: Soprano with flexible, light vocal quality, but one who does not sing as high as a coloratura soprano

lyric tenor: Tenor with a light, high flexible voice

malignant tumor: Tumors that have the potential to metastasize, or spread to different sites. They also have the potential to invade, destroy, and replace adjacent tissues. However, benign tumors may have the capacity for substantial local destruction, as well

Mandelbrot's set: A series of two equations containing real and imaginary components that, when iterated and plotted on a two-dimensional graph, depict a very complex and classic fractal pattern

mandible: Jaw

marcato: Each note accented

marking: Using the voice gently (typically during rehearsals) to avoid injury or fatigue

masque (mask): "Singing in the masque" refers to a frontal tonal placement conceptualized by singers as being associated with vibration of the bones of the face. It is generally regarded as a healthy placement associated with rich resonant characteristics and commonly a strong singer's formant (or "ring")

mechanical equilibrium: The state in which all forces acting on a body cancel each other out, leaving a zero net force in all directions

mechanics: The study of objects in motion and the forces that produce the motion

medial (or mesial): Toward the center (midline or midplane).

melisma: Two or more notes sung on a single syllable

menopause: Cessation of menstrual cycles and menstruation. Associated with physiologic infertility

menstrual cycle: The normal, cyclical variation of hormones in adult females of child-bearing age, and bodily responses caused by those hormonal variations

menstrual period: The first part of the menstrual cycle, associated with endometrial shedding and vaginal bleeding

messa di voce: Traditional exercise in Italian singing tradition consisting of a long prolonged crescendo and diminuendo on a sustained tone

metastasis: Spread of tumor to locations other than the primary tumor site

mezza voce: Literally means "half voice." In practice, means singing softly, but with proper support

mezzo soprano: Literally means "half soprano." This is a common female range, higher than contralto but lower than soprano

middle (or mixed): A mixture of qualities from various voice registers, cultivated in order to allow consistent quality throughout the frequency range

middle C: C_4 on the piano keyboard, with an international concert pitch frequency of 261.6 Hz

millisecond: One thousandth of a second; usually noted ms. or msec

modulation: Periodic variation of a signal property; for example, as vibrato corresponds to a regular variation of fundamental frequency, it can be regarded as a modulation of that signal property

motor: Having to do with motion. For example, motor nerves allow structures to move

motor unit: A group of muscle fibers and the single motor nerve that activates the fibers

mucocele: A benign lesion filled with liquid mucus

mucolytic: A substance that thins mucous secretions

mucosa: The covering of the surfaces of the respiratory tract, including the oral cavity and nasal cavities, as well as the pharynx, larynx, and lower airways. Mucosa also exits elsewhere, such as on the lining of the vagina

mucosal tear: With reference to the vocal folds, disruption of the surface of the vocal fold. Usually caused by trauma

mucosal wave: Undulation along the vocal fold surface traveling in the direction of the airflow

modulation: The systematic change of a cyclic parameter, such as amplitude or frequency

momentum: Mass times velocity; a quantity that determines the potential force that an object can impart to another object by collision

muscle fascicles: Groups of muscle fibers enclosed by a sheath of connective tissue

muscle fibers: A long, thin cell; the basic unit of a muscle that is excited by a nerve ending

muscle tension dysphonia: Also called muscular tension dysphonia. A form of voice abuse characterized by excessive muscular effort, and usually by pressed phonation. A form of voice misuse

mutational dysphonia: A voice disorder. Most typically, it is characterized by persistent falsetto voice after puberty in a male. More generally, it is used to refer to voice with characteristics of the opposite gender

myasthenia gravis: A neuromuscular junction disease associated with fatigue

myoelastic-aerodynamic theory of phonation: The currently accepted mechanism of vocal fold physiology. Compressed air exerts pressure on the undersurface of the closed vocal folds. The pressure overcomes adductory forces, causing the vocal folds to open. The elasticity of the displaced tissues (along with the Bernoulli effect) causes the vocal folds to snap shut, resulting in sound.

myofibril: A subdivision of a muscle fiber; composed of a number of myofilaments

myofilament: A microstructure of periodically arranged actin and myosin molecules; a subdivision of a myofibril

myosin: A protein molecule that reacts with actin to form actinomycin, the contractile part of a myofilament

nasal tract: Air cavity system of the nose

NATS: National Association of Teachers of Singing

natural oscillation: Oscillation without imposed driving forces

neoplasm: Abnormal growth. May be benign or malignant

nervous system: Organs of the body including the brain, spinal cord, and nerves. Responsible for motion, sensation, thought, and control of various other bodily functions

neurotologist: Otolaryngologist specializing in disorders of the ear and ear-brain interface (including the skull base), particularly hearing loss, dizziness, tinnitus, and facial nerve dysfunction

neutral vowel: A vowel produced in the center of the oral cavity.

nodes: The "valleys" in a standing wave pattern

nodules: Benign growths on the surface of the vocal folds. Usually paired and fairly symmetric. They are generally caused by chronic, forceful vocal fold contact (voice abuse)

noise: Unwanted sound

noise-to-harmonic ratio (NHR): A general evaluation of noise percent in the signal and includes jitter, shimmer, and turbulent noise

nonlinear dynamics: (*See also* **Chaos** and **Chaotic Behavior**) The mathematical study of aperiodic, deterministic systems that are not random and cannot be described accurately by linear equations. The study of nonlinear systems whose state changes with time

nonlinear system: Any system in which the output is disproportionate to the input

objective assessment: Demonstrable, reproducible, usually quantifiable evaluation, generally relying on instrumentation or other assessment techniques that do not involve primarily opinion, as opposed to subjective assessment

octave: Interval between two pitches with frequencies in the ratio of 2:1

off-glide: Transition from a vowel of long duration to one of short duration

olfaction: The sense of smell, mediated by the first cranial nerve

on-glide: Transition from a sound of short duration to a vowel of longer duration

onset: The beginning of phonation

open quotient: The ratio of the time the glottis is open to the length of the entire vibratory cycle

oral contraceptive: Birth control pill

organic disorder: A disorder due to structural malfunction, malformation, or injury, as opposed to psychogenic disorders

organic voice disorder: Disorder for which a specific anatomic or physiologic cause can be identified, as opposed to psychogenic or functional voice disorders

origin: The beginning point of a muscle and related soft tissue

oscillation: Repeated movement, back and forth

oscillator: With regard to the larynx, the vibrator that is responsible for the sound source, specifically the vocal folds

ossicle: Middle ear bone

ossify: To become bony

ostium: Opening

otolaryngologist: Ear, nose, and throat physician

otologist: Otolaryngologist specializing in disorders of the ear

overtone: Partial above the fundamental in a spectrum

ovulation: The middle of the menstrual cycle, associated with release of an ovum (egg), and the period of fertility

palatal: Related to the palate (*See* also **Linguapalatal**)

papillomas: Small benign epithelial tumors that may appear randomly or in clusters on the vocal folds, larynx, and trachea and elsewhere in the body. Believed to be caused by various types of human papillomavirus (HPV), some of which are associated with malignancy

parietal pleura: The outermost of two membranes surrounding the lungs

partial: Sinusoid that is part of a complex tone; in voiced sounds, the partials are harmonic implying that the frequency of the *n*th partial equals *n* times the fundamental frequency

particle: A finite mass with zero dimensions, located at a single point in space

pascal (Pa): International standard unit of pressure; one newton (N) per meter squared (m²)

Pascal's law: Pressure is transmitted rapidly and uniformly throughout an enclosed fluid at rest

pass band: A band of frequencies minimally affected by a filter

passaggio (Italian): The break between vocal registers

period: (1) In physics, the time interval between repeating events; shortest pattern repeated in a regular undulation; a graph showing the period is called a waveform. (2) In medicine, the time during the menstrual cycle associated with bleeding and shedding of the endometrial lining

period doubling: One form of bifurcation in which a system that originally had x period states now has 2x periodic states, with a change having occurred in response to a change in parameter or initial condition

period time: In physics, duration of a period

periodic behavior: Repeating over and over again over a finite time interval. Periodic behavior is governed by an underlying deterministic process

peristalsis: Successive contractions of musculature, which cause a bolus of food to pass through the alimentary tract

perturbation: Small disturbances or changes from expected behavior

pharyngocele: A pouch or herniation of part of the pharynx (throat), commonly fills with air in wind players

pharynx: The region above the larynx, below the velum and posterior to the oral cavity

phase: (1) The manner in which molecules are arranged in a material (gas, liquid, or solid); (2) the angular separation between two events on periodic waveforms

phase plane plot: Representation of a dynamic system in state space

phase space: A space created by two or more independent dynamic variables, such as positions and velocities, utilized to plot the trajectory of a moving object

phase spectrum: A display of the relative phases versus frequency of the components of a waveform

phonation: Sound generation by means of vocal fold vibrations

phoneme: A unit of sound within a specific language

phonetics: The study of speech sounds

phonetogram: Recording of highest and lowest sound pressure level versus fundamental frequency that a voice can produce; phonetograms are often used for describing the status of voice function in patients. Also called *voice range profile*

phoniatrician: A physician specializing in diagnosis and nonsurgical treatment of voice disorders. This specialty does not exist in American medical training, where the phoniatrician's activities are accomplished as a team by the laryngologist (responsible for diagnosis and surgical treatment when needed) and speech-language pathologist (responsible for behavioral voice therapy)

phonosurgery: Originally, surgery designed to alter vocal quality or pitch. Now used commonly to refer to all delicate microsurgical procedures of the vocal folds

phonotrauma: Vocal fold injury caused by vocal fold contact during phonation, associated most commonly with voice abuse or misuse

phrenic nerve: The nerve that controls the diaphragm. Responsible for inspiration. Composed primarily of fibers from the third, fourth, and fifth cervical roots

piriform sinus: Pouch or cavity constituting the lower end of the pharynx located to the side and partially to the back of the larynx. There are two, paired pyriform sinuses in the normal individual

pitch: Perceived tone quality corresponding to its fundamental frequency

pitch matching: Experiment in which subjects are asked to produce the pitch of a reference tone

pitch period perturbation quotient (PPQ): A relative evaluation of short term (cycle-to-cycle) variation of the pitch periods expressed in percent

pleural space: The fluid-filled space between the parietal and visceral pleura

plosive: A consonant produced by creating complete blockage of airflow, followed by the buildup of air pressure, which is then suddenly released, producing a consonant sound

Poincaré section: A graphical technique to reveal a discernable pattern in a phase plane plot that does not have an apparent pattern. There are two kinds of Poincaré sections

polyp: A sessile or pedunculated growth. Usually unilateral and benign, but the term is descriptive and does not imply a histological diagnosis

posterior: Toward the back

posterior cricoarytenoid muscle: An intrinsic laryngeal muscle that is the primary abductor of the vocal folds (paired)

power: The rate of delivery (or expenditure) of energy (measured in watts)

power source: The expiratory system including the muscles of the abdomen, back, thorax, and the lungs. Responsible for producing a vector of force that results in efficient creation and control of subglottal pressure

power spectrum: Two-dimensional graphic analysis of sound with frequency on the x axis and amplitude on the y axis

prechaotic behavior: Predictable behavior prior to the onset of chaotic behavior. One example is period doubling

pressed phonation: Type of phonation characterized by small airflow, high adductory force, and high subglottal pressure. Not an efficient form of voice production. Often associated with voice abuse, and common in patients with lesions such as nodules

pressure: Force per unit area

prevoicing: Phonation that occurs briefly before phonation of a stop consonant

prima donna: Literally means "first lady." Refers to the soprano soloist, especially the lead singer in an opera

primo passaggio: "The first passage"; the first register change perceived in a voice as pitch is raised from low to high

proteomics: The study of proteins

psychogenic: Caused by psychological factors, rather than physical dysfunction. Psychogenic disorders may result in physical dysfunction or structural injury

pulmonary system: The breathing apparatus including the lungs and related airways

pulse register: The extreme low end of the phonatory range. Also know as *vocal fry* and *Strohbass*, characterized by a pattern of short glottal waves alternating with larger and longer ones, and with a long closed phase

pure tone: Sinusoid. The simplest tone. Produced electronically. In nature, even pure-sounding tones like bird songs are complex

pyrotechnics: Special effects involving combustion and explosion, used to produce dramatic visual displays (similar to fireworks), indoors or outdoors

pyrosis: Heartburn

quadrangular membrane: Elastic membrane extending from the sides of the epiglottic cartilage to the corniculate and arytenoid cartilages. Mucosa covered. Forms the aryepiglottic fold and the wall between the piriform sinus and larynx

quasiperiodic: A behavior that has at least two frequencies in which the phases are related by an irrational number

radian: The angular measure obtained when the arc along the circumference of the circle is equal to the radius

radian frequency: The number of radians per second covered in circular or sinusoidal motion

random behavior: Action that never repeats itself and is inherently unpredictable

rarefaction: A decrease in density

recurrent laryngeal nerves: The paired branches of the vagus nerve that supply all of the intrinsic muscles of the larynx except for the cricothyroid muscles. The recurrent laryngeal nerves also carry sensory fibers (feeling) to the mucosa below the level of the vocal folds

reflux: (*See* **Gastroesophageal Reflux** and **Laryngopharyngeal Reflux**)

reflux laryngitis: Inflammation of the larynx due to irritation from gastric juice

refractive eye surgery: Surgery to correct visual acuity

registers: Weakly defined term for vocal qualities; often, register refers to a series of adjacent tones on the scale that sound similar and seem to be generated by the same type of vocal fold vibrations and vocal tract adjustments. Examples of register are vocal fry, modal, and falsetto; but numerous other terms are also used

regulation: The events by which a protein is produced or destroyed, and the balance between these two conditions

Reinke's space: The superficial layer of the lamina propria

relative average perturbation (RAP): A relative evaluation of short-term (cycle-to-cycle) variation of the pitch periods expressed in percent

relative voice rest: Restricted, cautious voice use

resonance: Peak occurring at certain frequencies (resonance frequencies) in the vibration amplitude in a system that possesses compliance, inertia, and reflection; resonance occurs when the input and the reflected energy vibrate in phase; the resonances in the vocal tract are called *formants*

resonator: With regard to the voice, refers primarily to the supraglottic vocal tract, which is responsible for timbre and projection

restoring force: A force that brings an object back to a stable equilibrium position

return map: Similar to phase plane plot, but analyzed data must be digital. This graphic technique represents the relationship between a point and any subsequent point in a time series

rhinorrhea: Nasal discharge; runny nose

rhotic: A vowel sound produced with r-coloring.

rima glottitis: The space between the vocal folds. Also known as the glottis

roll-off: Characteristics of filters specifying their ability to shut off frequencies outside the pass band; for example, if a low pass filter is set to 2 kHz and has a roll-off of 24 dB/octave, it will alternate a 4 kHz tone by 24 dB and a 8 kHz tone by 48 dB

rostral: Toward the mouth (beak)

sagittal: An anatomic plane that divides the body into left and right sides

sarcoplasmic reticulum: Connective tissue enveloping groups of muscle fibers

scalar: A quantity that scales, or adjusts size; a single number

second passaggio: "The second passage"; the second register change perceived in a voice

semicircular canal: Inner ear organ of balance

semi-vowel: A consonant that has vowel-like resonance

sensory: Having to do with the feeling or detection of other nonmotor input. For example, nerves responsible for touch, proprioception (position in space), hearing, and so on

sharp singing: Singing at a pitch (frequency) higher than the desirable target pitch

shimmer: Cycle-to-cycle variability in amplitude

shimmer percent: Is the same as shimmer dB but expressed in percent instead of dB. Both are relative evaluations of the same type of amplitude perturbation but they use different measures for this result: either percent or dB

simple harmonic motion: Sinusoidal motion; the smoothest back and forth motion possible

simple tone: (*See* **Pure Tone**)

singer's formant: A high spectrum peak occurring between about 2.3 and 3.5 kHz in voiced sounds in Western opera and concert singing. This acoustic phenomenon is associated with "ring" in a voice, and with the voices ability to project over background noise such as a choir or an orchestra. A similar phenomenon may be seen in speaking voices, especially in actors. It is known as the *speaker's formant*

singing teacher: Professional who teaches singing technique (as opposed to Voice Coach).

singing voice specialist: A singing teacher with additional training, and specialization in working with injured voices, in conjunction with a medical voice team

sinus of Morgagni: Often confused with ventricle of Morgagni. Actually, the sinus of Morgagni is not in the larynx. It is formed by the superior fibers of the superior pharyngeal constrictor as they curve below the levator veli palatini and the eustachian tube. The space between the upper border of the muscle and the base of the skull is known as the sinus of Morgagni, and is closed by the pharyngeal aponeurosis

sinusitis: Infection of the paranasal sinus cavities

sinusoid: A graph representing the sine or cosine of a constantly increasing angle; in mechanics, the smoothest and simplest back-and-forth movement, characterized by a single frequency, an amplitude, and a phase; tone arising from sinusoidal sound pressure variations

sinusoidal motion: The projection of circular motion (in a plane) at constant speed onto one axis in the plane

skeleton: The bony or cartilaginous framework to which muscle and other soft tissues are attached

smoothed amplitude perturbation quotient (sAPQ): A relative evaluation of long-term variation of the peak-to-peak amplitude within the analyzed voice sample, expressed in percent

smoothed pitch perturbation quotient (sPPQ): A relative evaluation of long-term variation of the pitch period within the analyzed voice sample expressed in percent

soft glottal attack: Gentle glottal approximation, often obtained using an imaginary /h/

soft phonation index (SPI): A measure of the ratio of lower frequency harmonic energy to higher frequency harmonic energy. If the SPI is low, then the spectral analysis will show well-defined higher formants

solid: A substance that maintains its shape, independent of the shape of its container

soprano acuto: High soprano

soprano assoluto: A soprano who is able to sing all soprano roles and classifications

sound level: Logarithmic, comparative measure of the intensity of a signal; the unit is dB

sound pressure level (SPL): Measure of the intensity of a sound, ordinarily in dB relative to 0.0002 microbar (millionths of 1 atmosphere pressure)

sound propagation: The process of imparting a pressure or density disturbance to adjacent parts of a continuous medium, creating new disturbances at points farther away from the initial disturbance

source-filter theory: A theory that assumes the time-varying glottal airflow to be the primary sound source and the vocal tract to be an acoustic filter of the glottal source

source spectrum: Spectrum of the voice source

spasmodic dysphonia: A focal dystonia involving the larynx. May be of adductor, abductor, or mixed type. Adductor spasmodic dysphonia is characterized by strain-strangled interruptions in phonation. Abductor spasmodic dysphonia is characterized by breathy interruptions

speaker's formant: (*See* **Singer's formant**)

special sensory nerves: Nerves responsible for hearing, vision, taste, and smell

spectrogram: Three-dimensional graphic representation of sound with time on the x axis, frequency on the y axis, and amplitude displayed as intensity of color

spectrograph: The equipment that produces a spectrogram

spectrum: Ensemble of simultaneously sounding sinusoidal partials constituting a complex tone; a display of relative magnitudes or phases of the component frequencies of a waveform

spectrum analysis: Analysis of a signal showing its partials

speech-language pathologist: A trained, medically affiliated professional who may be skilled in remediation of problems of the speaking voice, swallowing, articulation, language development, and other conditions

speed: The rate of change of distance with time; the magnitude of velocity

spinto: Literally means *pushed* or *thrust*. Usually applies to tenors or sopranos with lighter voice than dramatic singers, but with aspects of particular dramatic excitement in their vocal quality. Enrico Caruso was an example

spirometer: A device for measuring airflow

stable equilibrium: A unique state to which a system with a restoring force will return after it has been displaced from rest

staccato: Each note accented and separated

standard deviation: The square root of the variance

standing wave: A wave that appears to be standing still; it occurs when waves with the same frequency (and wavelength) moving in opposite directions interfere with each other

state space: In abstract mathematics, the area in which a behavior occurs

stent: A device used for shape, support, and maintenance of patency during healing after surgery or injury

steroid: Steroids are potent substances produced by the body. They may also be consumed as medications. (*See* **Anabolic steroids, Corticosteroids**)

stochastic: Random from a statistical, mathematical point of view

stop band: A band of frequencies rejected by a filter; it is the low region in a filter spectrum

strain: Deformation relative to a rest dimension, including direction (eg, elongation per unit length)

strain rate: The rate of change of strain with respect to time

stress: Force per unit area, including the direction in which the force is applied to the area

striking zone: The middle third of the musculomembranous portion of the vocal fold; the point of maximum contact force during phonatory vocal adduction

stroboscopy: A technique that uses interrupted light to simulate slow motion. (*See* also **Strobovideolaryngoscopy**)

strobovideolaryngoscopy: Evaluation of the vocal folds utilizing simulated slow motion for detailed evaluation of vocal fold motion

Strohbass (German): "Straw bass"; another term for *pulse register* or *vocal fry*

subglottal: Below the glottis

subglottal pressure: Air pressure in the airway immediately below the level of the vocal folds. The unit most commonly used is centimeters of water. That distance in centimeters that a given pressure would raise a column of water in a tube

subglottic: The region immediately below the level of the vocal folds

subharmonic: A frequency obtained by *dividing* a fundamental frequency by an integer greater than 0

subjective assessment: Evaluation that depends on perception and opinion, rather than independently reproducible quantifiable measures, as opposed to objective assessment

sulcus vocalis: A longitudinal groove, usually on the medial surface of the vocal fold

superior: above

superior laryngeal nerves: Paired branches of the vagus nerve that supply the cricothyroid muscle and supply sensation from the level of the vocal folds superiorly

support: Commonly used to refer to the power source of the voice. It includes the mechanism responsible for creating a vector force that results in efficient subglottic pressure. This includes the muscles of the abdomen and back, as well as the thorax and lungs; primarily the expiratory system

supraglottal: Above the glottis, or level of the vocal folds

supraglottic: (1) Above the level of the vocal folds. This region includes the resonance system of the vocal tract, including the pharynx, oral cavity, nose, and related structures. (2) Posterior commissure. A misnomer. Used to describe the posterior aspect of the larynx (interarytenoid area), which is opposite the anterior commissure. However, there is actually no commissure on the posterior aspect of the larynx

suprahyoid muscle group: One of the two extrinsic muscle groups. Includes the stylohyoid muscle, anterior and posterior bellies of the digastric muscle, geniohyoid, hyoglossus, and mylohyoid muscles

temporal gap transition: The transition from a continuous sound to a series of pulses in the perception of vocal registers

temporomandibular joint: The jaw joint; a synovial joint between the mandibular condyle and skull anterior to the ear canal

tenor: Highest of the male voices, except countertenors. Must be able to sing to C_5. Singer's formant is around 2800 Hz

tenore serio: Dramatic tenor

testosterone: The hormone responsible for development of male sexual characteristics, including laryngeal growth

thin voice: A term used by singers to describe vocal weakness associated with lack of harmonic richness. The voice often also has increased breathiness, noise, and weakness and is commonly also described as "thready"

thoracic: Pertaining to the chest

thorax: The part of the body between the neck and abdomen

thready voice: (*See* **Thin voice**)

thyroarytenoid muscle: An intrinsic laryngeal muscle that comprises the bulk of the vocal fold (paired). The medial belly constitutes the body of the vocal fold

thyroid cartilage: The largest laryngeal cartilage. It is open posteriorly and is made up of two plates (thyroid laminae) joined anteriorly at the midline. In males, there is a prominence superiorly known as the "Adam's apple"

tidal volume: The amount of air breathed in and out during respiration (measured in liters)

timbre: The quality of a sound. Associated with complexity, or the number, nature, and interaction of overtones

tonsil: A mass of lymphoid tissue located near the junction of the oral cavity and pharynx (paired)

tonsillitis: Inflammation of the tonsil

tracheal stenosis: Narrowing in the trachea. May be congenital or acquired

tracheoesophageal fistula: A connection between the trachea and esophagus. May be congenital or acquired

trajectory: In chaos, the representation of the behavior of a system in state space over a finite, brief period of time. For example, one cycle on a phase plane plot

transcription: Converting the message in DNA to messenger RNA

transfection: Infection by naked viral nucleic acid

transglottal flow: Air that is forced through the glottis by a transglottal pressure

transition: With regard to the vocal fold, the intermediate and deep layers of lamina propria (vocal ligament)

translation: Using messenger RNA to make proteins

transverse: Refers to an anatomic plane that divides the body across. Also used to refer to a direction perpendicular to a given structure or phenomenon such as a muscle fiber or airflow

tremolo: An aesthetically displeasing, excessively wide vibrato (*See* **Wobble**). The term is also used in music to refer to an ornament used by composers and performers

tremor: A modulation in activity

trill: In early music (Renaissance) where it referred to an ornament that involved repetition of the same note. That ornament is now referred to as a *trillo*

trillo: Originally a trill, but in recent pedagogy a rapid repetition of the same note, which usually includes repeated voice onset and offset

triphthong: Three consecutive vowels that make up the same syllable

tumor: A mass or growth

turbulence: Irregular movement of air, fluid, or other substance, which causes a hissing sound. White water is a typical example of turbulence

turbulent airflow: Irregular airflow containing eddies and rotating patterns

tympanic membrane: Eardrum

unilateral vocal fold paralysis: Immobility of one vocal fold, due to neurological dysfunction

unstable equilibrium: The state in which a disturbance of a mechanical system will cause a drift away from a rest position

unvoiced: A sound made without phonation, and devoid of pitch; voiceless

upregulation: Increased gene expression, compared with baseline

variability: The amount of change, or ability to change

variance: The mean squared difference from the average value in a data set

vector: A quantity made up of two or more independent items of information, always grouped together

velar: Relating to the velum or palate

velocity: The rate of change of displacement with respect to time (measured in meters per second, with the appropriate direction)

velopharyngeal insufficiency: Escape of air, liquid or food from the oropharynx into the nasopharynx or nose at times when the nasopharynx should be closed by approximation of the soft palate and pharyngeal tissues

velum: The area of the soft palate and adjacent nasopharynx.

ventral: Toward the belly

ventricle of Morgagni: Also known as *laryngeal sinus,* and *ventriculus laryngis.* The ventricle is a fusiform pouch bounded by the margin of the vocal folds, the edge of the free crescentic margin of the false vocal fold (ventricular fold), and the mucous membrane between them that forms the pouch. Anteriorly, a narrowing opening leads from the ventricle to the appendix of the ventricle of Morgagni

ventricular folds: The "false vocal folds," situated above the true vocal folds

ventricular ligament: A narrow band of fibrous tissue that extends from the angle of the thyroid cartilage below the epiglottis to the arytenoid cartilage just above the vocal process. It is contained within the false vocal fold. The caudal border of the ventricular ligament forms a free crescentic margin, which constitutes the upper border of the ventricle of Morgagni

ventricular phonation: (*See* **Dysphonia plica ventricularis**)

vertical phase difference: With reference to the vocal folds, refers to the asynchrony between the lower and upper surfaces of the vibratory margin of the vocal fold during phonation

vertigo: Sensation of rotary motion. A form of dizziness

vibrato: In classical singing, vibrato is a periodic modulation of the frequency of phonation. Its regularity increases with training. The rate of vibrato (number of modulations per second) is usually in the range of 5–6 per second. Vibrato rates over 7–8 per second are aesthetically displeasing to most people, and sound "nervous." The extent of vibrato (amount of variation above and below the center frequency) is usually one or two semitones. Vibrato extending less than ±0.5 semitone are rarely seen in singers although they are encountered in wind instrument playing. Vibrato rates greater than two semitones are usually aesthetically unacceptable, and are typical of elderly singers in poor artistic vocal condition, in whom the excessively wide vibrato extent is often combined with excessively slow rate

viscera: The internal organs of the body, particularly the contents of the abdomen

visceral pleura: The innermost of two membranes surrounding the lungs

viscoelastic material: A material that exhibits characteristics of both elastic solids and viscous liquids. The vocal fold is an example

viscosity: Property of a liquid associated with its resistance to deformation. Associated with the "thickness" of a liquid

vital capacity: The maximum volume of air that can be exchanged by the lungs with the outside; it includes the expiratory reserve volume, tidal volume, and inspiratory reserve volume (measured in liters)

vocal cord: Old term for vocal fold

vocal fold (or cord) stripping: A surgical technique, no longer considered acceptable practice under most circumstances, in which the vocal fold is grasped with a forceps, and the surface layers are ripped off

vocal fold stiffness: The ratio of the effective restoring force (in the medial-lateral direction) to the displacement (in the same direction)

vocal folds: A paired system of tissue layers in the larynx that can oscillate to produce sound

vocal fry: A register with perceived temporal gaps; also known as *pulse register* and Strohbass. (*See* **Pulse register**)

vocal ligament: Intermediate and deep layers of the lamina propria. Also forms the superior end of the conus elasticus

vocal tract: Resonator system constituted by the larynx, the pharynx and the mouth cavity

vocalis muscle: The medial belly of the thyroarytenoid muscle

vocalise: A vocal exercise involving sung sounds, commonly vowels on scales of various complexity

voce coperta: "Covered registration"

voce mista: Mixed voice (also voix mixed)

voce di petto: Chest voice

voce sgangherata: "White" voice. Literally means immoderate or unattractive. Lacks strength in the lower partials

voce di testa: Head voice

voce piena: Full voice

voice abuse: Use of the voice in specific activities that are deleterious to vocal health, such as screaming

voice box: (*See* **Larynx**)

voice coach: (1) In singing, a professional who works with singers, teaching repertoire, language pronunciation, and other artistic components of performance (as opposed to a singing teacher, who teaches technique); (2) The term voice coach is also used by acting-voice teachers who specialize in vocal, bodily, and interpretive techniques to enhance dramatic performance

voice misuse: Habitual phonation using phonatory techniques that are not optimal and then result in vocal strain. For example, speaking with inadequate support, excessive neck muscle tension, and suboptimal resonance. Muscular tension dysphonia is a form of voice misuse

voice range profile: (*See* **Phonetogram**)

voice rest: (*See* **Absolute voice rest, relative voice rest**)

voice source: Sound generated by the pulsating transglottal airflow; the sound is generated when the vocal fold vibrations chop the airstream into a pulsating airflow

voice turbulence index (VTI): A measure of the relative energy level of high frequency noise

voiced: A language sound made with phonation, and possessing pitch.

voiceless: (*See* **Unvoiced**)

volume: "Amount of sound," best measured in terms of acoustic power or intensity

vortex theory: Holds that eddys, or areas of organized turbulence, are produced as air flows through the larynx and vocal tract

Vowel color: refers to vowel quality, or timbre, and is associated with harmonic content

Waldeyer's ring: An aggregation of lymphoid tissue in the pharynx, including the tonsils and adenoids

waveform: A plot of any variable (eg, pressure, flow, or displacement) changing as time progresses along the horizontal axis; also known as a time-series

wavefront: The initial disturbance in a propagating wave

wavelength: The linear distance between any point on one vibratory cycle and a corresponding point of the next vibratory cycle

whisper: Sound created by turbulent glottal airflow in the absence of vocal fold vibration

whistle register: The highest of all registers (in pitch). It is observed only in females, extending the pitch range beyond F_6

wobble: Undesirable vibrato, usually with vibrato rate of 2 to 4 Hz, and extent greater than ± 0.5 semitone (*See also* **Tremolo**)

xerostomia: Dry mouth

Young's modulus: The ratio between magnitudes of stress and strain

Appendix Ia

PATIENT HISTORY: SINGERS
Robert Thayer Sataloff, M.D., D.M.A.
1721 Pine Street
Philadelphia, PA 19103

NAME _____ AGE _____ SEX _____ RACE _____
HEIGHT _____ WEIGHT _____ DATE _____
VOICE CATEGORY: _____ soprano _____ mezzo-soprano _____ alto
_____ tenor _____ baritone _____ bass

(If you are not currently having a voice problem, please skip to Question #3.)

PLEASE CHECK OR CIRCLE CORRECT ANSWERS

1. How long have you had your present voice problem?

   Who noticed it?

   [self, family, voice teacher, critics, everyone, other _____]

   Do you know what caused it?   Yes _____   No _____

   If yes, what?

   Did it come on slowly or suddenly?   Slowly _____   Suddenly _____
   Is it getting: Worse: _____ , Better _____ , Same _____

2. Which symptoms do you have? (Please check all that apply.)
   _____ Hoarseness (coarse or scratchy sound)
   _____ Fatigue (voice tires or changes quality after singing for a short period of time)
   _____ Volume disturbance (trouble singing)   softly _____   loudly _____
   _____ Loss of range (high _____   low _____)
   _____ Change in classification (example: voice lowered from soprano to mezzo)
   _____ Prolonged warm-up time (over ½ hr to warm up voice)
   _____ Breathiness
   _____ Tickling or choking sensation while singing
   _____ Pain in throat while singing
   _____ Other: (Please specify)_____
   _____
   _____

3. Do you have an important performance soon?   Yes _____   No _____
   Date(s): _____

4. What is the current status of your singing career?

　　　Professional _____　　Amateur _____

5. What are your long-term career goals in singing?
　　[　] Premier operatic career
　　[　] Premier pop music career
　　[　] Active avocation
　　[　] Classical
　　[　] Pop
　　[　] Other (_____)
　　[　] Amateur performance (choral or solo)
　　[　] Amateur singing for own pleasure

6. Have you had voice training?　Yes _____　No _____
　　At what age did you begin?

7. Have there been periods of months or years without lessons in that time?　Yes _____　No _____

8. How long have you studied with your present teacher?

　　Teacher's name:
　　Teacher's address:

　　Teacher's telephone number:

9. Please list previous teachers and years during which you studied with them.

10. Have you ever had training for your speaking voice?　Yes _____　No _____
　　Acting voice lessons?　Yes _____　No _____
　　How many years?
　　Speech therapy?　Yes _____　No _____
　　How many months?

11. Do you have a job in addition to singing?　Yes _____　No _____

　　If yes, does it involve extensive voice use?　Yes _____　No _____

　　If yes, what is it? [actor, announcer (television/radio/sports arena), athletic instructor, attorney, clergy, politician, physician, salesperson, stockbroker, teacher, telephone operator or receptionist, waiter, waitress, secretary, other _____

12. In your performance work, in addition to singing, are you frequently
　　required to speak?　Yes _____　No _____
　　dance?　Yes _____　No _____

13. How many years did you sing actively before beginning voice lessons initially?

14. What types of music do you sing? (Check all that apply.)
    _____ Classical   _____ Show
    _____ Nightclub   _____ Rock
    _____ Other: (Please specify.) _____

    _____

15. Do you regularly sing in a sitting position (such as from behind a piano or drum set)?
    Yes _____   No _____

16. Do you sing outdoors or in large halls, or with orchestras? (Circle which one.)   Yes _____   No _____

17. If you perform with electrical instruments or outdoors, do you use monitor speakers? (Circle which one).
    Yes _____   No _____

    If yes, can you hear them?   Yes _____   No _____

18. Do you play a musical instrument(s)?   Yes _____   No _____
    If yes, please check all that apply:
    _____ Keyboard (piano, organ, harpsichord, other _____)
    _____ Violin, viola
    _____ Cello
    _____ Bass
    _____ Plucked strings (guitar, harp, other _____)
    _____ Brass
    _____ Wind with single reed
    _____ Wind with double reed
    _____ Flute, piccolo
    _____ Percussion
    _____ Bagpipe
    _____ Accordion
    _____ Other: (Please specify)._____

19. How often do you practice?
    Scales: [daily, few times weekly, once a week, rarely, never]

    If you practice scales, do you do them all at once, or do you divide them up over the course of a day?
    [all at once, two or three sittings]

    On days when you do scales, how long do you practice them?
    [15 ,30,45,60,75 ,90,105,120, more] minutes

    Songs: [daily, few times weekly, once a week, rarely, never]

    How many hours per day?
    [½,1,1½,2,2½,3,more]

Do you warm up your voice before you sing?   Yes _____   No _____

Do you cool down your voice when you finish singing?   Yes _____   No _____

20. How much are you singing at present (total including practice time) (average hours per day)?

Rehearsal: _____

Performance: _____

21. Please check all that apply to you:

_____ Voice worse in the morning

_____ Voice worse later in the day, after it has been used

_____ Sing performances or rehearsals in the morning

_____ Speak extensively (e.g. , teacher, clergy, attorney, telephone work)

_____ Cheerleader

_____ Speak extensively backstage or at postperformance parties

_____ Choral conductor

_____ Frequently clear your throat

_____ Frequent sore throat

_____ Jaw joint problems

_____ Bitter or acid taste, or bad breath first thing in the morning

_____ Frequent "heartburn" or hiatal hernia

_____ Frequent yelling or loud talking

_____ Frequent whispering

_____ Chronic fatigue (insomnia)

_____ Work around extreme dryness

_____ Frequent exercise (weight lifting, aerobics)

_____ Frequently thirsty, dehydrated

_____ Hoarseness first thing in the morning

_____ Chest cough

_____ Eat late at night

_____ Ever used antacids

_____ Under particular stress at present (personal or professional)

_____ Frequent bad breath

_____ Live, work, or perform around smoke or fumes

_____ Traveled recently: When: _____

                                          Where: _____

Eat any of the following before singing?

_____ Chocolate   _____ Coffee

_____ Alcohol   _____ Milk or ice cream

_____ Nuts   _____ Spiced foods

Other: (Please specify.)

_____ Any specific vocal technical difficulties? [trouble singing soft, trouble singing loud, poor pitch control, support problems, problems at register transitions, other] Describe other:

_____ Any problems with your singing voice recently prior to the onset of the problem that brought you here? [hoarseness, breathiness, fatigue, loss of range, voice breaks, pain singing, other] Describe other:

_____ Any voice problems in the past that required a visit to a physician? If yes, please describe problem(s) and treatment(s): [laryngitis, nodules, polyps, hemorrhage, cancer, other]
Describe other:

22. Your family doctor's name, address, and telephone number

23. Your laryngologist's name, address, and telephone number:

24. Recent cold?   Yes _____   No _____

25. Current cold?   Yes _____   No _____

26. Have you been exposed to any of the following chemicals frequently (or recently) at home or at work? (Check all that apply.)

_____ Carbon monoxide   _____ Arsenic
_____ Mercury   _____ Aniline dyes
_____ Insecticides   _____ Industrial solvents (benzene, etc.)
_____ Lead   _____ Stage smoke

27. Have you been evaluated by an allergist?   Yes _____   No _____

If yes, what allergies do you have:
[none, dust, mold, trees, cats, dogs, foods, other]
(Medication allergies are covered elsewhere in this history form.)
If yes, give name and address of allergist:

28. How many packs of cigarettes do you smoke per day?

Smoking history
_____ Never
_____ Quit. When? _____
_____ Smoked about _____ packs per day for _____ years.
_____ Smoke _____ packs per day. Have smoked for _____ years.

29. Do you work or live in a smoky environment?   Yes _____   No _____

30. How much alcohol do you drink? [none, rarely, a few times per week, daily]
If daily, or few times per week, on the average, how much do you consume? [1,2,3,4,5,6,7,8,9,10, more] glasses per [day, week] of [beer, wine, liquor].

Did you formerly drink more heavily?   Yes _____   No _____

31. How many cups of coffee, tea, cola, or other caffeine-containing drinks do you drink per day?

32. List other recreational drugs you use [marijuana, cocaine, amphetamines, barbiturates, heroin, other]:

33. Have you noticed any of the following? (Check all that apply)
    _____ Hypersensitivity to heat or cold
    _____ Excessive sweating
    _____ Change in weight: gained / lost _____ lb in _____
               weeks / _____ months
    _____ Change in skin or hair
    _____ Palpitation (fluttering) of the heart
    _____ Emotional lability (swings of mood)
    _____ Double vision
    _____ Numbness of the face or extremities
    _____ Tingling around the mouth or face
    _____ Blurred vision or blindness
    _____ Weakness or paralysis of the face
    _____ Clumsiness in arms or legs
    _____ Confusion or loss of consciousness
    _____ Difficulty with speech
    _____ Difficulty with swallowing
    _____ Seizure (epileptic fit)
    _____ Pain in the neck or shoulder
    _____ Shaking or tremors
    _____ Memory change
    _____ Personality change

    For females:

    Are you pregnant?   Yes _____   No _____
    Are your menstrual periods regular?   Yes _____   No _____
    Have you undergone hysterectomy?   Yes _____   No _____
    Were your ovaries removed?   Yes _____   No _____
    At what age did you reach puberty?   _____
    Have you gone through menopause?   Yes _____   No _____
    If yes, when?

34. Have you ever consulted a psychologist or psychiatrist?   Yes _____   No _____

    Are you currently under treatment?   Yes _____   No _____

35. Have you injured your head or neck (whiplash, etc.)?   Yes _____   No _____

36. Describe any serious accidents related to this visit.
    None _____

37. Are you involved in legal action involving problems with your voice?   Yes _____   No _____

38. List names of spouse and children:

39. Brief summary of ear, nose, and throat (ENT) problems, some of which may not be related to your present complaint.

PLEASE CHECK ALL THAT APPLY

_____ Hearing loss	_____ Ear pain
_____ Ear noises	_____ Facial pain
_____ Dizziness	_____ Stiff neck
_____ Facial paralysis	_____ Lump in neck
_____ Nasal obstruction	_____ Lump in face or head
_____ Nasal deformity	_____ Trouble swallowing
_____ Mouth sores	_____ Excess eye skin
_____ Jaw joint problem	_____ Excess facial skin
_____ Eye problem	
_____ Other: (Please specify.)	

40. Do you have or have you ever had:

_____ Diabetes	_____ Seizures
_____ Hypoglycemia	_____ Psychiatric therapy
_____ Thyroid problems	_____ Frequent bad headaches
_____ Syphilis	_____ Ulcers
_____ Gonorrhea	_____ Kidney disease
_____ Herpes	_____ Urinary problems
_____ Cold sores (fever blisters)	_____ Arthritis or skeletal problems
_____ High blood pressure	_____ Cleft palate
_____ Severe low blood pressure	_____ Asthma
_____ Intravenous antibiotics or diuretics	_____ Lung or breathing problems
_____ Heart attack	_____ Unexplained weight loss
_____ Angina irregular heartbeat	_____ Cancer of (_____)
_____ Other heart problems	_____ Other tumor (_____)
_____ Rheumatic fever	_____ Blood transfusions
_____ Tuberculosis	_____ Hepatitis
_____ Glaucoma	_____ AIDS
_____ Multiple sclerosis	_____ Meningitis
_____ Other illnesses: (Please specify.)	

41. Do any blood relatives have:

_____ Diabetes	_____ Cancer
_____ Hypoglycemia	_____ Heart disease
_____ Other major medical problems such as those above. Please specify:	

42. Describe serious accidents unless directly related to your doctor's visit here.

_____ None
_____ Occurred with head injury, loss of consciousness, or whiplash
_____ Occurred without head injury, loss of consciousness, or whiplash
         Describe:

43. List all current medications and doses (include birth control pills and vitamins).

44. Medication allergies

_____ None   _____ Novocaine
_____ Penicillin   _____ Iodine
_____ Sulfa   _____ Codeine
_____ Tetracycline   _____ Adhesive tape
_____ Erythromycin   _____ Aspirin
_____ Keflex/Ceclor/Ceftin   _____ X-ray dyes
_____ Other: (Please specify.)

45. List operations

_____ Tonsillectomy (age _____)
_____ Appendectomy (age _____)
_____ Adenoidectomy (age _____)
_____ Heart surgery (age _____)
_____ Other: (Please specify.)

46. List toxic drugs or chemicals to which you have been exposed:

_____ Lead
_____ Streptomycin, Neomycin, Kanamycin
_____ Mercury
_____ Other: (Please specify.)

47. Have you had x-ray _treatments_ to your head or neck (including treatments for acne or ear problems as a child, treatments for cancer, etc.)?

Yes _____   No _____

48. Describe serious health problems of your spouse or children.

_____ None

Appendix Ib

PATIENT HISTORY: PROFESSIONAL VOICE USERS
Robert Thayer Sataloff, M.D., D.M.A.
1721 Pine Street
Philadelphia, PA 19103

NAME _____ AGE _____ SEX _____ RACE _____
HEIGHT _____ WEIGHT _____ DATE _____

1. How long have you had your present voice problem? _____

   Who noticed it?

   Do you know what caused it? Yes _____ No _____
   If so, what?

   Did it come on slowly or suddenly? Slowly _____ Suddenly _____

   Is it getting: Worse _____, Better _____, Same _____

2. Which symptoms do you have? (Please check all that apply.)
   _____ Hoarseness (coarse or scratchy sound)
   _____ Fatigue (voice tires or changes quality after speaking for a short period of time)
   _____ Volume disturbance (trouble speaking) softly _____ loudly _____
   _____ Loss of range (high _____, low _____)
   _____ Prolonged warm-up time (over ½ hr to warm up voice)
   _____ Breathiness
   _____ Tickling or choking sensation while speaking
   _____ Pain in throat while speaking
   _____ Other: (Please specify.)_____
   _____
   _____

3. Have you ever had training for your speaking voice?
   Yes _____ No _____

4. Have there been periods of months or years without lessons in that time? Yes _____ No _____

373

5. How long have you studied with your present teacher?
   Teacher's name: _____
   Teacher's address: _____
   Teacher's telephone number:_____

6. Please list previous teachers and years during which you studied with them:

7. Have you ever had training for your singing voice? Yes _____   No _____
   If so, list teachers and years of study:

8. In what capacity do you use your voice professionally?
   _____ Actor
   _____ Announcer (television/radio/sports arena)
   _____ Attorney
   _____ Clergy
   _____ Politician
   _____ Salesperson
   _____ Teacher
   _____ Telephone operator or receptionist
   _____ Other: (Please specify.)

9. Do you have an important performance soon?   Yes _____   No _____
   Date(s): _____

10. Do you do regular voice exercises?   Yes _____   No _____
    If yes, describe:

11. Do you play a musical instrument?   Yes _____   No _____
    If yes, please check all that apply:
    _____ Keyboard (piano, organ, harpischord, other _____)
    _____ Violin, viola
    _____ Cello
    _____ Bass
    _____ Plucked strings (guitar, harp, other _____)
    _____ Brass
    _____ Wind with single reed
    _____ Wind with double reed
    _____ Flute, piccolo
    _____ Percussion
    _____ Bagpipe
    _____ Accordion
    _____ Other: (Please specify.) _____

12. Do you warm up your voice before practice or performance?   Yes _____   No _____

    Do you cool down after using it?   Yes _____   No _____

13. How much are you speaking at present (average hours per day)?
    _____ Rehearsal   _____ Performance   _____ Other

14. Please check all that apply to you:
    _____ Voice worse in the morning
    _____ Voice worse later in the day, after it has been used
    _____ Sing performances or rehearsals in the morning
    _____ Speak extensively (e.g. , teacher, clergy, attorney, telephone work)
    _____ Cheerleader
    _____ Speak extensively backstage or at postperformance parties
    _____ Choral conductor
    _____ Frequently clear your throat
    _____ Frequent sore throat
    _____ Jaw joint problems
    _____ Bitter or acid taste; bad breath or hoarseness first thing in the morning
    _____ Frequent "heartburn" or hiatal hernia
    _____ Frequent yelling or loud talking
    _____ Frequent whispering
    _____ Chronic fatigue (insomnia)
    _____ Work around extreme dryness
    _____ Frequent exercise (weight lifting, aerobics)
    _____ Frequently thirsty, dehydrated
    _____ Hoarseness first thing in the morning
    _____ Chest cough
    _____ Eat late at night
    _____ Ever used antacids
    _____ Under particular stress at present (personal or professional)
    _____ Frequent bad breath
    _____ Live, work, or perform around smoke or fumes
    _____ Traveled recently: When:_____
                         Where: _____

15. Your family doctor's name, address, and telephone number:

16. Your laryngologist's name, address, and telephone number:

17. Recent cold?   Yes _____   No _____

18. Current cold?   Yes _____   No _____

19. Have you been evaluated by an allergist?   Yes _____   No _____
    If yes, what allergies do you have:
    [none, dust, mold, trees, cats, dogs, foods, other, _____]
    (Medication allergies are covered elsewhere in this history form.)
    If yes, give name and address of allergist:

20. How many packs of cigarettes do you smoke per day?
    Smoking history
    _____ Never
    _____ Quit. When? _____
    _____ Smoked about ____ packs per day for ____ years.
    _____ Smoke ____ packs per day. Have smoked for ____ years.

21. Do you work or live in a smoky environment?   Yes _____   No _____

22. How much alcohol do you drink? [none, rarely, a few times per week, daily] If daily, or few times per week, on the average, how much do you consume? [1, 2, 3, 4, 5, 6, 7, 8, 9, 10, more] glasses per [day, week] of [beer, wine, liquor]

    Did you formerly drink more heavily?   Yes _____   No _____

23. How many cups of coffee, tea, cola, or other caffeine-containing drinks do you drink per day?

24. List other recreational drugs you use [marijuana, cocaine, amphetamines, barbiturates, heroin, other _____
    _____]

25. Have you noticed any of the following? (Check all that apply)
    _____ Hypersensitivity to heat or cold
    _____ Excessive sweating
    _____ Change in weight: gained / lost _____ lb in _____
                 weeks / _____ months
    _____ Change in your voice
    _____ Change in skin or hair
    _____ Palpitation (fluttering) of the heart
    _____ Emotional lability (swings of mood)
    _____ Double vision
    _____ Numbness of the face or extremities
    _____ Tingling around the mouth or face
    _____ Blurred vision or blindness
    _____ Weakness or paralysis of the face
    _____ Clumsiness in arms or legs
    _____ Confusion or loss of consciousness
    _____ Difficulty with speech
    _____ Difficulty with swallowing

_____ Seizure (epileptic fit)
_____ Pain in the neck or shoulder
_____ Shaking or tremors
_____ Memory change
_____ Personality change

For females:

Are you pregnant?	Yes _____	No _____
Are your menstrual periods regular?	Yes _____	No _____
Have you undergone hysterectomy?	Yes _____	No _____
Were your ovaries removed?	Yes _____	No _____
At what age did you reach puberty?	_____	
Have you gone through menopause?	Yes _____	No _____

26. Have you ever consulted a psychologist or psychiatrist?
    Yes _____ No _____

    Are you currently under treatment? Yes _____ No _____

27. Have you injured your head or neck (whiplash, etc.)?
    Yes _____ No _____

28. Describe any serious accidents related to this visit.
    None _____

29. Are you involved in legal action involving problems with your voice?
    Yes _____ No _____

30. List names of spouse and children:

31. Brief summary of ear, nose, and throat (ENT) problems, some of which may not be related to your present complaint.

_____ Hearing loss	_____ Ear pain
_____ Ear noises	_____ Facial pain
_____ Dizziness	_____ Stiff neck
_____ Facial paralysis	_____ Lump in neck
_____ Nasal obstruction	_____ Lump in face or head
_____ Nasal deformity	_____ Trouble swallowing
_____ Nose bleeds	_____ Trouble breathing
_____ Mouth sores	_____ Excess eye skin
_____ Excess facial skin	_____ Eye problem
_____ Jaw joint problem	
_____ Other (Please specify.)	

32. Do you have or have you ever had:

_____ Diabetes   _____ Seizures
_____ Hypoglycemia   _____ Psychiatric therapy
_____ Thyroid problems   _____ Frequent bad
_____ Syphilis   headaches
_____ Gonorrhea   _____ Ulcers
_____ Herpes   _____ Kidney disease
_____ Cold sores (fever   _____ Urinary problems
        blisters)   _____ Arthritis or skeletal
_____ High blood pressure   problems
_____ Severe low blood   _____ Cleft palate
        pressure   _____ Asthma
_____ Intravenous antibiotics   _____ Lung or breathing problems
        or diuretics   _____ Unexplained weight loss
_____ Heart attack   _____ Cancer of (_____)
_____ Angina   _____ Other tumor (_____)
_____ Irregular heartbeat   _____ Blood transfusions
_____ Other heart problems   _____ Hepatitis
_____ Rheumatic fever   _____ AIDS
_____ Tuberculosis   __ Meningitis
_____ Glaucoma
_____ Multiple sclerosis
_____ Other illnesses: (Please specify.)

33. Do any blood relatives have:

_____ Diabetes   _____ Cancer
_____ Hypoglycemia   _____ Heart disease
_____ Other major medical problems such as those above.
        Please specify:

34. Describe serious accidents *unless* directly related to your doctor's visit here.
_____ None
_____ Occurred with head injury, loss of consciousness, or whiplash
_____ Occurred without head injury, loss of consciousness, or whiplash
        Describe:

35. List all current medications and doses (include birth control pills and vitamins).

36. Medication allergies
_____ None   _____ Novocaine
_____ Penicillin   _____ Iodine
_____ Sulfa   _____ Codeine

_____ Tetracycline
_____ Erythromycin
_____ Keflex/Ceclor/Ceftin
_____ Other: (Please specify.)

_____ Adhesive tape
_____ Aspirin
_____ X-ray dyes

37. List operations:
_____ Tonsillectomy
    (age _____)
_____ Appendectomy
    (age _____)
Other: (Please specify.)

_____ Appendectomy
    (age _____)
_____ Heart surgery
    (age _____)

38. List toxic drugs or chemicals to which you have been exposed:
_____ Lead
_____ Mercury

_____ Streptomycin, Neomycin, Kanamycin
_____ Other: (Please list.)

39. Have you had x-ray _treatments_ to your head or neck (including treatments for acne or ear problems as a child), treatments for cancer, etc.?
Yes _____ No _____

40. Describe serious health problems of your spouse or children.
_____ None

Appendix II
Checklist of Vocal Abuse for Teachers

Please circle the following statements if they are appropriate to you. Please add any additional items particular to your life or setting.

Vocal Abuse/Misuse Items

1. Talking too much
2. Talking too loudly
3. Talking too rapidly
4. Talking while moving vigorously
5. Talking while lifting, bending, or moving arms
6. Taking the "teacher's voice" out of the classroom
7. Shouting and yelling excessively to distant people
8. Talking over classroom, cafeteria, barroom noise
9. Inappropriate use of the telephone
10. Inappropriate emphasis on vowel onset words
11. Jerky revisions to phrases and sentences
12. Use of fillers, Uh-huh, OK, and Uhm, etc.
13. Singing or talking in the car
14. Inadequate sleep or rest
15. Excessive talking at sports events
16. Exposure to dust
17. Exposure to fumes from cleaning products
18. Exposure to primary or secondary tobacco smoke
19. Exposure to dry air
20. Poor acoustics in the classroom
21. Poor ventilation in the classroom
22. Lack of hydration (don't drink enough water)
23. Use of cough drops with menthol, mint, or anesthetics
24. Alcohol
25. Smoking
26. Caffeine (coffee, tea, Coke, Pepsi, Mountain Dew, chocolate)
27. Spicy foods
28. Acidic foods
29. Dairy products
30. Over-the-counter decongestants and antihistamines
31. Cough medicines

32. Aspirin/Ibuprofin
33. Mouthwash
34. Mints
35. Asthma inhalers
36. Poor breath support
37. Excessive chest breathing
38. Too big a breath
39. Too small a breath
40. Abrupt voice onset
41. Excessive tension in voice or throat
42. Too high or low a pitch to the voice
43. Too closed or tense jaw
44. High tongue position and tongue tension
45. Reduced use of tongue in forming words with jaw substitution
46. Poor tone focus, voice "in throat"
47. Facial tension
48. Poor posture, bent from waist
49. Neck tension
50. Speaking with jaw thrust or constriction
51. Unresolved stress

Other_____

_____

_____

_____

_____

_____

_____

Appendix IIIa
Outline for Daily Practice

I. Warm-up and cool-down routine

   A. Stretch/relaxation exercises:

      1. Head/neck range of motion

      2. Shoulder rolls and shrugs

      3. Facial massage

      4. Tongue stretch

   B. Vocalises (which are provided by the singing specialist)

   C. Speaking exercises:

      1. Easy speech breathing exercises: "Candle blowing," /s/, /ʃ/, /h/-/u/, /m/, /ɑ/

      2. Oral resonance warm up: "ng-ah"

      3. Connected speech: Counting

      4. Monitoring sites of tension: /f-v/, /s-z/, /θ-ð/, /ʃ-dʒ/

      5. Bridging exercises:

         a. Sliding block scale for /m/

         b. Spoken "vocalises"

         c. Lip trills

      6. Quiet breathing exercise

II. Additional daily practice:

   The target areas are addressed systematically.

   A. Breath control and support

   B. Phrasing

   C. Easy onset and blending techniques

   D. Oral resonance

   E. Tone focus and vocal placement

F. Loudness/projection

G. Speaking rate, rhythm, and intonation

III. Carryover practice:

A. Application of specific goals in ongoing speech

B. Transition from structured to spontaneous

C. Stress management strategies

Appendix IIIb
Sample Phrases

THREE SYLLABLES IN LENGTH

Put it on.

Tell me how.

Walk around.

Did you know?

Juicy peach.

Yes and no.

Do you know?

Crunchy apple.

Put them down.

What's your name?

Come over here.

Not right now.

Time to go.

Close your eyes.

Fine report.

Read the book.

Who is it?

Pick it up.

Take a nap.

Good evening.

FIVE SYLLABLES IN LENGTH

Where are they going?

The concert was great.

Turn off the iron.

FOUR SYLLABLES IN LENGTH

Pleased to meet you

You'd like it there.

The sun was bright.

Fill it up, please.

How much is it?

He knows the way

The train was late.

Maybe later.

Cream and sugar.

Bread and butter.

Salt and pepper

Toast and butter.

Pie and coffee.

Needle and thread.

Turkey and cheese.

Nice to meet you.

That's fine for now.

Don't tease the dog.

Beth arrived late.

This is enough.

SIX SYLLABLES IN LENGTH

That's a good idea.

Ted wants to come along.

Put everything away.

FIVE SYLLABLES IN LENGTH (continued)

The book was stolen.

Tip the waiter well.

When is he finished?

Flowers need water.

Will she be here soon?

The oven is on.

The tea is steeping.

Yes, that's fine with me.

The phone is ringing.

Play the clarinet.

Let's consider it.

They enjoyed the song.

SEVEN AND EIGHT SYLLABLES IN LENGTH

The weather in August is hot.

I love sleeping late on Sundays.

What time can you come for dinner?

We will probably start at six.

The top of this jar is stuck.

Would you help me open it, please?

I can't remember the number.

Please give it to me again.

What shall we have for dessert?

Pie and ice cream sound delicious.

What are you doing after work?

Be careful not to go too fast.

The snowfall was light that year.

Our guests will arrive at nine.

They ate breakfast at the diner.

SIX SYLLABLES IN LENGTH (continued)

He can phone us later.

She bought it somewhere else.

Leave the window open.

Place it down carefully.

Come over and see us.

The children were playing.

The fire alarm rang.

The switch is over there.

Let me know when he calls.

They moved to the mountains.

The spectators were pleased.

The puppy is playful.

NINE AND TEN SYLLABLES IN LENGTH

Lisa bought some vegetables for dinner.

He wears a 16 and a half collar.

I will be happy to meet with you.

They all went skiing for the holiday.

The bakery smells simply delicious.

There are four bedrooms on the top floor.

After the rain, the air smelled earthy.

Have you been to the theater lately?

Summer at the seashore is popular.

TEN, ELEVEN, AND TWELVE SYLLABLES IN LENGTH

City buses are often crowded and noisy.

He avoided making eye contact while riding on the bus.

Don't forget to turn off the lights and lock the door.

Oh no, I think I left my keys inside.

We usually go boating each summer.

The car was badly damaged by the crash.

Fortunately, there were no injuries.

Sally loves to go swimming in the lake.

She was reminded not to go too far.

Distilled water tastes much better than tap.

Appendix IIIc
Frontal Placement Words

till	town	teal
tot	test	tips
lash	style	still
tall	team	hall
ten	mile	Bill
leash	swell	toad
much	lot	tell
tie	tip	net
latch	least	leap
dial	bell	top
smile	loft	loud
snowfall	town hall	distill
livid	low tide	windmill
tinfoil	vowel	man-made

Appendix IIId
H/Vowel Minimal-Pairs

had-add	hall-all	hold-old
head-Ed	hit-it	home-ohm
hone-own	ho-oh	his-is
hay-ay	hat-at	hand-and
hear-ear	hitch-itch	hi-I

Appendix IIIe
Vowel-Initiated Words

LONG VOWELS IN ENGLISH

/ɑ/	/o²/	/ɑːɪ/	/i/
odd	oath	aisle	eat
octet	oat	eye	east
object	oak	ice	each
obtuse	old	idle	eek
octopus	oboe	I've	eager
operate	okay	Irish	Ethan
otter	only	iota	enough
obligate	overt	item	even

SHORT VOWELS IN ENGLISH

/æ/	/ɛ/	/I/	/ʌ/
as	end	in	up
at	ever	is	ugh
ask	effort	if	ugly
after	educate	ill	uplift
apple	elephant	id	upset
attitude	enemy	image	utmost
avenue	elegant	issue	under
accident	envy	inactive	unlock
accent	entertain	indent	usher

Appendix IIIf
Phrases for Blending

fall over	go into	put upon
leave on	the only	lose it
see it	the other	win it
do it	not even	that's enough
put on	not any	leave open
down under	cold as	one of
not old	the ice	she's ill
look at	he's ill	then add
the end	yes and	so it
high up	one at	Sue is

Appendix IIIg

Phrases to Practice Easy Onset and Blending

Elliot ate an apple and allowed Andrew another.

Each and every avenue is open at eight o'clock.

Over on Aston Avenue is an open air amphitheater.

I am in agreement in every aspect of our association.

Alan's attitude is overly obnoxious.

In April, Addie always attends an extravaganza in Arizona.

Alice openly acknowledges an aversion to avocados.

Exercise is an important and energizing activity.

Amanda is in Alabama at an annual event.

It is eleven o'clock already, and all of us are anxiously awaiting Ellen's arrival.

Eliminating additives is advisable.

Is Emily afraid of an eerie effigy?

Eddie is outdoors on an icy evening.

Actually, I am aware of all the errors in Adam's arithmetic assignment.

Every evening in autumn our area orchestra attempts to entertain an uninterested audience of adolescents.

Appendix IIIh
Homographs

refuse-refuse	contrast-contrast
compound-compound	content-content
converse-converse	commune-commune
console-console	minute-minute
project-project	object-object

Appendix IIIi
Open-Vowel Words

/ɑ/	/æ/	/ɑːɪ/	/ɑu/
top	map	tie	power
hot	match	reply	town
pocket	hot	side	found
deposit	flag	fire	coward
probable	sad	line	tower
knock	bag	fine	without
shot	cash	confide	house
doctor	cast	tired	how
father	happen	height	loud
garage	mash	rhyme	flower

1. Talking too much
2. Talking too loudly
3. Talking too rapidly
4. Talking while moving vigorously
5. Talking while lifting, bending, or moving arms
6. Taking the "teacher's voice" out of the classroom
7. Shouting and yelling excessively to distant people
8. Talking over classroom, cafeteria, barroom noise
9. Inappropriate use of the telephone
10. Inappropriate emphasis on vowel onset words
11. Jerky revisions to phrases and sentences
12. Use of fillers, Uh-huh, OK, and Uhm, etc.
13. Singing or talking in the car
14. Inadequate sleep or rest
15. Excessive talking at sports events
16. Exposure to dust
17. Exposure to fumes from cleaning products
18. Exposure to primary or secondary tobacco smoke
19. Exposure to dry air
20. Poor acoustics in the classroom
21. Poor ventilation in the classroom
22. Lack of hydration (don't drink enough water)
23. Use of cough drops with menthol, mint, or anesthetics
24. Alcohol
25. Smoking
26. Caffeine (coffee, tea, Coke, Pepsi, Mountain Dew, chocolate)
27. Spicy foods
28. Acidic foods
29. Dairy products
30. Over-the-counter decongestants and antihistamines
31. Cough medicines
32. Aspirin/Ibuprofin
33. Mouthwash
34. Mints
35. Asthma inhalers
36. Poor breath support
37. Excessive chest breathing
38. Too big a breath
39. Too small a breath
40. Abrupt voice onset
41. Excessive tension in voice or throat
42. Too high or low a pitch to the voice
43. Too closed or tense jaw
44. High tongue position and tongue tension
45. Reduced use of tongue in forming words with jaw substitution
46. Poor tone focus, voice "in throat"
47. Facial tension
48. Poor posture, bent from waist
49. Neck tension
50. Speaking with jaw thrust or constriction

51. Unresolved stress

Other_____

_____

_____

_____

_____

_____

_____

Appendix IVa
Laryngologist's Report

PATIENT OFFICE
(215) 545-3322
FAX: (215) 790-1192
office@phillyent.com

Sataloff Institute for Voice & Ear Care

ADMINISTRATIVE OFFICE
(215) 732-6100
FAX: (215) 545-3374
rtsataloff@phillyent.com

February 10, 2004

Re: John Doe

To Whom It May Concern:

I had the pleasure of seeing John Doe in the office today. He is a 25-year-old actor performing the lead role with a national touring company now performing at the Walnut Street Theater. He is concerned about his voice. He denies any voice loss but complains of frequent sore throat and voice fatigue. Recently he has found his voice is gravelly and lower than his normal range. He is concerned about "crackling sounds." One month ago, he saw a physician who diagnosed him with laryngopharygeal reflux and started him on Aciphex twice daily. Last week he developed a globus sensation that lasted all day. He also reports a bitter taste upon awakening, throat clearing and "post nasal drip." He has been seen by several other physicians over the past two years and has been told he has dust allergy and reflux. He wants reassurance that he is not "destroying" his voice. He is not singing at this time and is acting full-time. He has had acting training in college and some singing training, as well. However, the singing training in college left him with a sore throat, and he reports that he has discounted his training from college because he does not believe it was of high quality. He has also had acting lessons in school and some after graduation. He is currently performing eight shows per week. He is on stage for the entire two and one half hours. He has been performing in this show since Christmas 2003. He does not play musical instruments, and he is not exposed to noxious fumes.

Mr. Doe reports a past medical history of microhematuria in childhood, prostratitis, depression and intermittent tightness in his chest for many years. He finds the chest tightness can last for two days at a time and then abates for as long as two years.

Mr. Doe reports a past surgical history of extraction of four impacted wisdom teeth five years ago.

His current medications include Aciphex twice daily, Zyrtec and Nasonex. He denies any medication allergies but reports environmental allergies to mold, dust and dogs. He is a lifelong non-smoker, drinks no caffeinated beverages and consumes one alcoholic beverage per week.

Page 2
February 10, 2004
Re: John Doe

His tympanic membranes and hearing were normal. Examination of the nose was normal. Examination of the oral cavity and pharynx revealed diminished gag reflex on the left. Examination of the neck was normal. Laryngeal examination was completed by strobovideo-laryngoscopy and a copy of that report is attached. FEEST revealed slightly decreased sensation side of the larynx on the left. During conversational speech, his voice was pressed but not hoarse. During speaking, he had jaw and tongue tension and inadequate support. Brief singing evaluation revealed excessive tension in the tongue and jaw and suboptimal support technique. Voice team evaluation will be performed, and reports will be attached to this letter.

I have asked Mr. Doe to continue on his Aciphex twice daily for control of his laryngeal reflux and have added Zantac 300 mg at bedtime to his regimen. I have given him prescriptions for selected blood tests and referred him to Dr. Steven Mandel for a laryngeal EMG. He will be evaluated by my voice team, and I have asked him to follow up with me after completion of his testing for his reflux, paresis, vocal fold mass, and muscle tension dysphonia.

With best regards.

Very truly yours.

Robert T. Sataloff, M.D., D.M.A.

RTS/jb

Enclosure

cc: Mr. John Doe

Appendix IVb

Strobovideolaryngoscopy Report

PATIENT OFFICE
(215) 545-3322
FAX: (215) 790-1192
office@phillyent.com

Sataloff Institute for Voice & Ear Care

ADMINISTRATIVE OFFICE
(215) 732-6100
FAX: (215) 545-3374
rtsataloff@phillyent.com

REPORT OF OPERATION: John Doe

DATE: February 10, 2004

PRE-OPERATIVE DIAGNOSIS:

1. Dysphonia

POST-OPERATIVE DIAGNOSIS:

1. Left vocal fold paresis
2. Left vocal fold fibrotic mass
3. Right vocal fold contact cyst or pseudocyst
4. Laryngopharyngeal reflux

PROCEDURE:

Laryngoscopy with magnification, strobovideolaryngoscopy, and complex voice analysis and synchronized electroglottography including sensory testing.

SURGEON:

Robert T. Sataloff, M.D., D.M.A.

Anesthesia: Topical
Rigid Endoscope: Kay-70

Flexible Laryngoscope: Olympus ENF-L3

Stroboscope: Kay-4

Procedure: The patient was taken to the special procedure room and prepared in the usual fashion. The laryngoscope was inserted, and suspended from the video system for magnification and documentation. Testing was performed at several frequencies and intensities. Initial examination was performed using continuous light. The findings were as follows:

Voice: Normal

Page 2
February 10, 2004
Re: John Doe

Supraglottic Hyperfunction: Moderate with decreased anterior-posterior distance and decreased lateral distance. It did improve with voluntary increase in pitch.

Right vocal fold abduction, adduction and longitudinal tension: Normal

Left vocal fold abduction was normal; adduction was slightly sluggish; and longitudinal tension was mildly decreased.

Arytenoid Joint Movement: Normal

Dysdiadochokinesis: Absent

Laryngeal EMG: Was recommended

CT: Not recommended

MRI: Not recommended

Arytenoids: Moderately erythematous and mildly edematous, right greater than left.

Posterior laryngeal cobblestoning (pachydermia): Absent

Right true vocal fold color: Normal, without significant varicosities.

Left true vocal fold color: Normal, without significant varicosities.

Masses and other Vibratory Margin Irregularities: The patient has a left vocal fold paresis and a left fibrotic mass in the striking zone that is about 3 mm in length at its base and has mild underlying stiffness. He also has a right contralateral cyst verses pseudocyst at the contact point. There is also stiffness at its base.

Other Significant Structural Lesions: Absent

Vocal Fold Vibrations: Symmetric in amplitude and phase

Periodicity: Regular

Glottic Closure: Intermittently incomplete anterior and posterior to the mass(es).

Vocal process height: Equal

Page 3
February 10, 2004

Amplitude of Right Vocal Fold: Minimally decreased
Amplitude of Left Vocal Fold: Mildly decreased
Minimally-to-mildly decreased

Wave Form of Right Vocal Fold: Minimally-to-mildly decreased
Wave Form of Left Vocal Fold: Mildly decreased

Right musculomembranous vocal fold vibratory function: Slightly hypodynamic in the middle one-third.

Left musculomembranous vocal fold vibratory function: Hypodynamic in the middle one-third

EGG: Revealed peak skewing. This indicates increased adduction, suggestive of pressed phonation.

The procedure concluded without complication

Robert T. Sataloff, M.D., D.M.A.

RTS/jb

Appendix IVc

Objective Voice Analysis and Laryngeal Electromyography

Robert Thayer Sataloff, MD, DMA
Objective Voice Assessment

Patient: John Doe   **Date of Birth**: xx-xx-xx   **Age**: 25
Occupation: actor   **Date of Evaluation**: 02-10-04   **Physician**: Dr. RTS
Diagnosis: Left vocal fold paresis, Laryngeal reflux, Small bilateral masses of the vocal folds, MTD
Hoarseness rating: Grade: 4 mm Roughness: 6.5 mm Breathiness: 3.5 mm Asthenia: 2.5 mm Strain: 4 mm

Acoustic Assessment

Conversation (name, date, age)   **Reading** (M. Williams Passage)
Mean Frequency: 107.23 Hz   Mean Frequency: 105.55 Hz
Mean Intensity: 73.21 dBSPL   Mean Intensity: 73.58 dBSPL
Reading Time: 17.91 sec   Total Voiced Time: 11.25sec   % voiced: 62.814 %
Physiological Frequency Range of Phonation   **Singing Frequency Range**
Low = 73.5 Hz (*1/period*)   Low = Hz (*1/period*)
High= 412.15 Hz (*1/period*)   High= Hz (*1/period*)
Semitone Range (STR) = 29.84589 ST   Norm = 33-36 ST, (Hollien, Dew, Philips 1971)

Perturbation Measures

5 Token /a/.   **Please see attached printout with graph.**
Fo(M85-155Hz;F143-235Hz)-108.375 Hz;**Jitter%**(M0.5389;F0.633)-0.447%;**RAP%**(M 0.345; F 0.378)-0.267%;
Shimmer% (M 2.523; F 1.977)- 1.288 %; **NHR** (M 0.122; F 0.112)- 0.147 ; **STD** (M 3.3; F 2.5)- 0.992

Spectrography

Sustained /i/ (Spectrogram) ; Yanagihara Hoarseness Rating Type: Type I
Type I– harmonic components mixed with noise in F1 and F2

Aerodynamic assessment

Spirometry: FVC = 115(%)   FEV 1.0 = 75(%)   FEF (25%-75%) = 33(%)
Mean Flow Rate (MFR): 329.4376 mls/sec
Maximum Phonation Time /a/ = 16.36 sec (mean); the best- 18.84 sec   **S/Z ratio:** 1.1763034
(WNL females= 25.7 sec; WNL males=34.6 sec)   *(WNL range 0.8-1.29)*

Glottal Efficiency Profile

Mean Flow Rate

| 49 | 69 | 89-------------112--------------136 | 156 | 256...............**X** |

S/Z RATIO

| 0.2 | 0.4 | 0.8------------1.07------**X**-------1.29 | 2.2 | 4.4 |

Maximum Phonation Time

| 40 | 33 | 28.7-----------25.7-------------22.5 | **X** 15 | 9.0 |

Recording/Analysis Equipment: TASCAM DAP1 DAT recorder, KAY model 4302 head-mount microphone at 15 cm., KAY Multi-Speech Model 3700 (MDVP Advanced 5105, Real-Time Spectrogram 5121) Schiller SP-10 Spirometer).

Page 2
February 10, 2004
Operative Report (cont'd)
Robert Thayer Sataloff, M.D., D. M. A.
re: John Doe

ACOUSTIC PROFILE (SPOKEN) /ɑ/

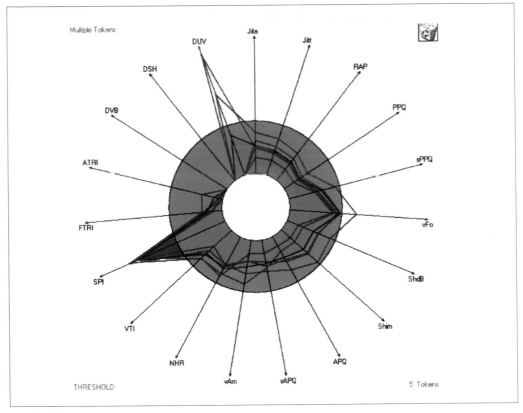

Page 3
February 10, 2004
OBJECTIVE VOICE ANALYSIS: John Doe

MDVPreport: Voice Report

Token 2

Parameter	Name	Value	Unit	Norm(f)	STD(f)	Thresh
Average Fundamental Frequency	Fo	108.375	Hz	243.973	27.457	
Mean Fundamental Frequency	MFo	108.366	Hz	241.080	25.107	
Average Pitch Period	To	9.228	ms	4.148	0.432	
Highest Fundamental Frequency	Fhi	111.164	Hz	252.724	26.570	
Lowest Fundamental Frequency	Flo	105.204	Hz	234.861	28.968	
Standard Deviation of Fo	STD	0.992	Hz	2.722	2.115	
Phonatory Fo-Range in semi-tones	PFR	2		2.250	1.060	
Fo-Tremor Frequency	Fftr	4.167	Hz	3.078	1.964	
Length of Analyzed Sample	Tsam	3.750	s	3.000	0.000	
Absolute Jitter	Jita	41.230	us	26.927	16.654	83.200
Jitter Percent	Jitt	0.447	%	0.633	0.351	1.040
Relative Average Perturbation	RAP	0.267	%	0.378	0.214	0.680
Pitch Perturbation Quotient	PPQ	0.253	%	0.366	0.205	0.840
Smoothed Pitch Perturbation Quotient	sPPQ	0.553	%	0.532	0.220	1.020
Fundamental Frequency Variation	vFo	0.916	%	1.149	1.005	1.100
Shimmer in dB	ShdB	0.113	dB	0.176	0.071	0.350
Shimmer Percent	Shim	1.288	%	1.997	0.791	3.810
Amplitude Perturbation Quotient	APQ	0.986	%	1.397	0.527	3.070
Smoothed Ampl. Perturbation Quotient	sAPQ	2.212	%	2.371	0.912	4.230
Peak-to-Peak Amplitude Variation	vAm	6.847	%	10.743	5.698	8.200
Noise to Harmonic Ratio	NHR	0.147		0.112	0.009	0.190
Voice Turbulence Index	VTI	0.047		0.046	0.012	0.061
Soft Phonation Index	SPI	27.227		7.534	4.133	14.120
Fo-Tremor Intensity Index	FTRI	0.333	%	0.304	0.166	0.950
Degree of Voice Breaks	DVB	0.000	%	0.200	0.100	1.000
Degree of Sub-harmonics	DSH	0.000	%	0.200	0.100	1.000
Degree of Voiceless	DUV	0.000	%	0.200	0.100	1.000
Number of Voice Breaks	NVB	0		0.200	0.100	0.900
Number of Sub-harmonic Segments	NSH	0		0.200	0.100	0.900
Number of Unvoiced Segments	NUV	0		0.200	0.100	0.900
Number of Segments Computed	SEG	124		92.594	0.000	
Total Number Detected Pitch Periods	PER	405		713.188	0.000	

Report Date: Feb. 10, 2004 Tuesday   Name: John Doe   Age & Gender: 25 years, male

Page 4
April 27, 1995
OBJECTIVE VOICE ANALYSIS: John Doe

SPECTROGRAPHIC ANALYSIS
KAY ELEMETRICS
DSP SONA-GRAPH 5500

POWER SPECTRUM (TOP) AND NARROW BAND SPECTRUM (BOTTOM) FOR /ɑ/:

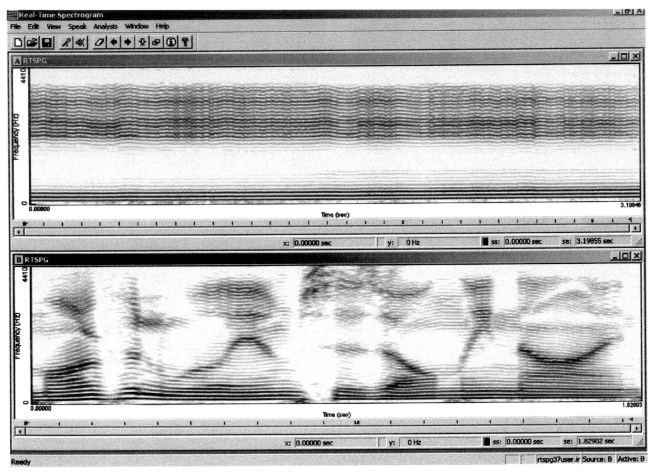

Report Date: Feb. 10, 2004 Tuesday   Name: John Doe   Age & Gender: 25 years, male

Page 5
OBJECTIVE VOICE ANALYSIS: John Doe

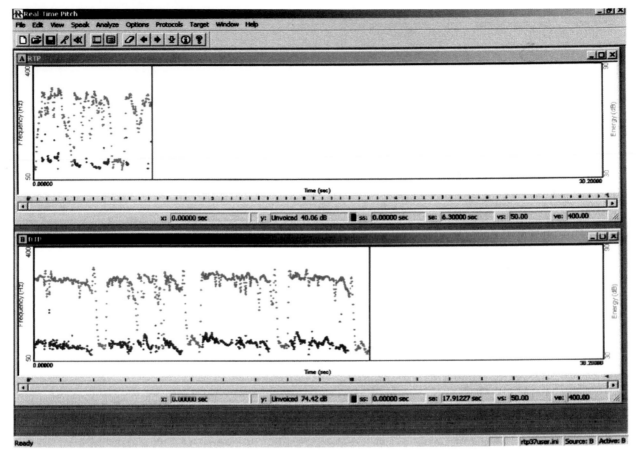

Report Date: Feb.10, 2004 Tuesday   Name: John Doe   Age & Gender: 25 years, male

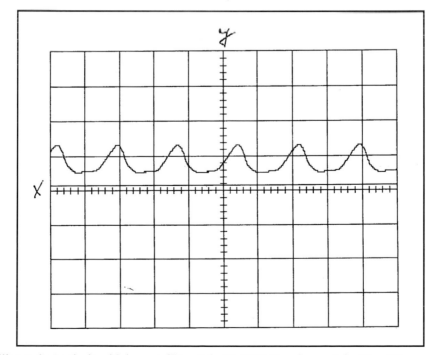

Oscilloscopic Analysis with inverse filter: Feb. 10, 2004 Tuesday;   John Doe, 25 years, male

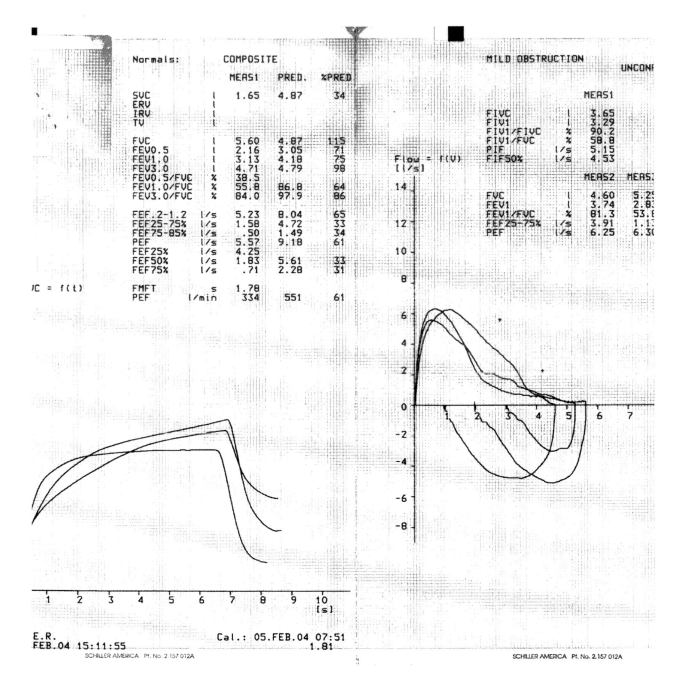

Normals: COMPOSITE

                MEAS1   PRED.   %PRED

SVC   l   1.65   4.87   34
ERV   l
IRV   l
TV   l

FVC   l   5.60   4.87   115
FEV0.5   l   2.16   3.05   71
FEV1.0   l   3.13   4.18   75
FEV3.0   l   4.71   4.79   98
FEV0.5/FVC %   38.5
FEV1.0/FVC %   55.8   86.8   64
FEV3.0/FVC %   84.0   97.9   86

FEF.2-1.2   l/s 5.23   8.04   65
FEF25-75%   l/s 1.58   4.72   33
FEF75-85%   l/s .50   1.49   34
PEF   l/s 5.57   9.18   61
FEF25%   l/s 4.25
FEF50%   l/s 1.83   5.61   33
FEF75%   l/s .71   2.28   31

JC = f(t)   FMFT   s   1.78
            PEF   l/min 334   551   61

MILD OBSTRUCTION   UNCONF

                              MEAS1

FIVC   l   3.65
FIV1   l   3.29
FIV1/FIVC   %   90.2
FIV1/FVC   %   58.8
PIF   l/s   5.15
FIF50%   l/s   4.53

                   MEAS2   MEAS

FVC   l   4.60   5.29
FEV1   l   3.74   2.8
FEV1/FVC   %   81.3   53.8
FEF25-75%   l/s   3.91   1.1
PEF   l/s   6.25   6.30

Flow = f(V)
[l/s]

E.R.
FEB.04 15:11:55   Cal.: 05.FEB.04 07:51
                                            1.81

Robert Thayer Sataloff, M.D., D.M.A.
1721 Pine Street
Philadelphia, PA 19103-6771

Graduate Hospital

Tenet

Professor, Otolaryngology-Head & Neck Surgery
Director, Jefferson Arts Medicine Center
Conductor, Thomas Jefferson University Choir
Thomas Jefferson University

Chairman, Otolaryngology-Head & Neck Surgery
Graduate Hospital
Adjunct Professor, Otorhinolaryngology-HNS
The University of Pennsylvania

Sataloff Institute for Voice & Ear Care

PATIENT OFFICE	ADMINISTRATIVE OFFICE
(215) 545-3322	(215) 732-6100
FAX: (215) 790-1192	FAX: (215) 545-7813
office@phillyent.com	rtsataloff@phillyent.com

Interpretations of Findings:

Objective voice assessment reveals the following: Values of NHR (noise to harmonic ratio), SPI (soft phonation index), and MFR (mean flow rate) were all noticeably above the accepted normal limits, while Jitter %, RAP % (relative average perturbation), Shimmer %, STD (standard deviation of fundamental frequency), MPT (maximum phonation time), and mean frequencies of both conversational and reading voice samples as well as semitone range for the physiologic frequency, fell bellow or at the lowest possible level of the appropriate amplitude for these parameters. Oscilloscopic analysis with inverse filter demonstrates an epiglottic gap in the amount of 200 mls of escaping air. Spectrography reveals increase noise above 2.2 kHz in the area of F1 and F2.

Acoustic measures demonstrate moderately low mean Fundamental frequencies of conversational and reading (Marvin Williams's passage) voice samples and reduced semi-tone range. The combination of decreased perturbation measures of Jitter %, RAP %, Shimmer %, and STD as well as increased SPI and NHR reveals the existence of moderate irregularity of vocal fold vibration in sustained phonation and are consistent with the diagnosis of tension dysphonia due to unilateral vocal fold paresis and small, bilateral masses on the vocal folds. Spectrographic analyses of sustain vowel /i/ reveal decreased intensity of harmonics and increased noise elements chiefly in the formant region of the vowels. This correlates to perceptual measures of decreased oral resonance and is consistent with acoustic measures showing mild to moderate irregularity of vocal fold vibration.

Low MPT measures and abnormally high mean Flow rate denote inadequate glottal closure. This correlates with the diagnosis of unilateral vocal fold paresis. Oscilloscope measures with inverse filter further indicate insufficient glottal closure.

Decreased physiologic frequency range (pitch range) and low-average speaking F0 correlates with perceptual measures of increased strain and supports the diagnosis of muscle tension dysphonia. In addition, a few short, irregular periods of contraction and instability are seen on the spectrographic representation of sustained phonation. This finding is consistent with the diagnosis of muscle tension dysphonia as well.

Pulmonary function measurements demonstrate lung capacity at the upper levels of normal limits for this age, gender, height, and weight. However, low levels of FEV1.0/FVC and FEF25-75% at 64% and 33%, respectively, indicate mild obstructive changes at the end of expiration.

Dimiter Dentchev (M.D., Ph.D)

Chairman, Board of Directors
The Voice Foundation
Editor-in-Chief
Journal of Voice
215-735-7999

Chairman, Board of Directors
American Institute for Voice and Ear Research
215-735-7487

Philadelphia Ear, Nose & Throat Associates
Robert Thayer Sataloff, M.D., D.M.A.
Joseph R. Spiegel, M.D., F.A.C.S.
Karen M. Lyons, M.D.
web: www.phillyent.com

NEUROLOGY AND NEUROPHYSIOLOGY ASSOCIATES, P.C.

Ramon Mañon-Espaillat, M.D.
Clinical Professor of Neurology
Jefferson Medical College
Epilepsy and Sleep Disorders

Steven Mandel, M.D.
Clinical Professor of Neurology
Jefferson Medical College
Neuromuscular Diseases

Olga A. Katz, M.D., PhD.
Instructor of Neurology
Jefferson Medical College
Clinical Neurophysiology

xx/xx/xx

Robert Sataloff, M.D.
1721 Pine Street
Philadelphia, PA 19103

Reference: **John Doe**
DOB: xx/xx/xxxx
Evaluation Date: x/x/xx

Dear Dr. Sataloff:

HISTORY: I had the pleasure of seeing John Doe in the office on xx/xx/xx for a neurological consultation and electrodiagnostic studies.

He is a 25-year-old gentleman who reports difficulty with his voice. He has noted some hoarseness and projection difficulties.

He has been on a number of medications, including Zyrtec, Aciphex, Nasonex, and ranitidine.

He does not drink alcohol and does not smoke cigarettes. He is not receiving any therapy.

He has a history of hayfever.

Family history is noncontributory for neurological disease.

The patient has completed a patient history form and this form was reviewed in the presence of the patient as this note was being dictated.

1015 Chestnut Street • Suite 810 • Philadelphia, PA 19107
151 Fries Mill Road • Suite 506 • Turnersville, NJ 08012
Phone: (215) 574-0075   Fax: (215) 627-8208 • NJ Phone: (856) 228-0006
E-Mail: steven.mandel@mail.TJU.EDU

Page 2
John Doe
Evaluation Date: x/x/xx

EXAMINATION: He was awake and alert, answering appropriately. He had no obvious aphasia or dysarthria. He had no motor deficits. No tremors, dysmetria, or bruits were detected. Position and vibratory sense were normal.

Based upon his complaints, electrodiagnostic studies were obtained.

Prior to performing electrodiagnostic studies, "Consent for Electrodiagnostic Testing" was signed by the patient in my presence with the consent form present in the patient's chart.

LARYNGEAL EMG: Accessory nerve stimulation revealed normal latency and amplitude responses with repetitive stimulation study being normal. Needle EMG examination demonstrated approximately 80-90% recruitment response from left cricothyroid. Right cricothyroid, vocalis, and posterior cricoarytenoid muscles appeared to be normal. There was poor relaxation at rest and findings consistent with muscular tension dysphonia.

IMPRESSION: The above electrical studies indicate mild left superior laryngeal nerve paresis with muscular tension dysphonia. There is no evidence to indicate any neuromuscular junction abnormalities.

This note was dictated in the presence of the patient so as to insure the accuracy of the history provided by the patient. The patient has verbalized understanding as to the contents of this letter.

Thank you for allowing me to participate in the care of your patient. If you have any questions regarding the contents of this report or any other issues related to the care of this patient, please do not hesitate to contact me.

Sincerely,

Steven Mandel, M.D.

SM/ac

Patient Name: John Doe   **Date:** 2/10/04

Voice Handicap Index (VHI)
(Jacobson, Johnson, Grywalski, et al.)

Instructions: These are statements that many people have used to describe their voices and the effects of their voices on their lives. Check the response that indicates how frequent you have the same experience.

Never=0 points; Almost never=1point; Sometimes=2 points; Almost Always=3 points; Always=4 points	Never	Almost Never	Sometimes	Almost Always	Always
F1. My voice makes it difficult for people to hear me.	✓				
P2. I run out of air when I talk.	✓				
F3. People have difficulty understanding me in a noisy room.	✓				
P4. The sound of my voice varies throughout the day.				✓	
F5. My family has difficulty hearing me when I call them throughout the house.	✓				
F6. I use the phone less often than I would like.			✓		
E7. I'm tense when talking with others because of my voice.			✓		
F8. I tend to avoid groups of people because of my voice.	✓				
E9. People seem irritated with my voice.		✓			
P10. People ask, "What's wrong with your voice?"	✓				
F11. I speak with friends, neighbors, or relatives less often because of my voice.	✓				
F12. People ask me to repeat myself when speaking fact-to-face.	✓				
P13. My voice sounds creaky and dry.			✓		
P14. I feel as through I have to strain to produce voice.			✓		
E15. I find other people don't understand my voice problem.				✓	
F16. My voice difficulties restrict my personal and social life.			✓		
P17. The clarity of my voice is unpredictable.		✓			
P18. I try to change my voice to sound different.			✓		
F19. I feel left out of conversations because of my voice.	✓				
P20. I use a great deal of effort to speak.		✓			
P21. My voice is worse in the evening.			✓		
F22. My voice problem causes me to loss income.	✓				
E23. My voice problem upsets me.				✓	
E24. I am less out-going because of my voice problem.		✓			
E25. My voice makes me feel handicapped.		✓			
P26. My voice "gives out" on me in the middle of speaking.	✓				
E27. I feel annoyed when people ask me to repeat.	✓				
E28. I feel embarrassed when people ask me to repeat.	✓				
E29. My voice makes me feel incompetent.		✓			
E30. I'm ashamed of my voice problem.				✓	

P Scale 23   F Scale 14   E Scale 25   Total Scale 62

Please **Circle** the word that matches how you feel your voice is today.   1. Normal (2. Mild   3. Moderate) 4. Severe

Appendix IVd

Speech-Language Pathologist's Report

<u>INITIAL VOICE EVALUATION</u>

<u>Name</u>: John Doe

<u>Date of evaluation</u>: 2/10/04

<u>D.O.B.</u>: XX/XX/XX

History: John Doe is a 25-year-old professional actor, currently performing the lead role in a touring company of "XXXXX XXXXX" at the Walnut Street Theatre in Philadelphia. He comes to this office with complaints of gravelly vocal quality, loss of range, and vocal fatigue. Mr. Doe reports that he has experienced voice problems since college, where he majored in theatre, but indicates that his problems have become more evident now that he has been cast in several major roles. He reports that the show opened in December of 2003, and adds that he is onstage for almost the entire 2_ hour duration of this show. Mr. Doe relates that he uses physical warm-ups for prior to performing, but that he is not confident in the vocal training he has received and avoids using vocal warm-ups for fear of fatiguing his voice before going onstage. Mr. Doe adds that he recently saw a physician who made a diagnosis of reflux and prescribed Aciphex twice daily.

Laryngovideostroboscopy performed by Dr. Robert Sataloff today revealed left vocal fold paresis, a left vocal fold fibrotic mass, a right vocal fold cyst vs. pseudocyst, and reflux. Laryngeal EMG was ordered to confirm vocal fold paresis. Dr. Sataloff asked Mr. Doe to continue Aciphex for symptoms of reflux and added Zantac 300 mg at bedtime. Mr. Doe's medical history is reportedly otherwise significant for microhematuria in childhood, prostatisis, allergies, and depression.

<u>Medications</u>: Aciphex, Zantac, Zyrtec, Nasonex

<u>Allergies</u>:

<u>Vocal Hygiene</u>: Mr. Doe reportedly drinks 8 glasses of water daily. He reports occasional consumption of caffeinated soda and frequent consumption of cranberry juice. He denies tobacco use. Mr. Doe admits to frequent throat clearing. He indicates that he avoids using his voice in an extreme fashion when he is not on stage, but is concerned that he may be forced to yell frequently if he has to return to waiting tables between acting jobs. He received some acting voice training as an undergraduate theatre major, but indicates that he had not found the training to be helpful,

<u>Oral Mechanism Exam</u>: The oral mechanism exam was unremarkable

<u>Objective Evaluation</u>: May be found under separate cover.

<u>Subjective Evaluation</u>: During conversational speech, Mr. Doe presented with intermittent hoarseness and occasional glottal fry and posterior tone placement at the ends of sentences. Tone placement was otherwise anterior, and occasionally hypernasal. Excessive tension was visible in the jaw, and his tone quality was suggestive of decreased pharyngeal space and tongue base tension. Mr. Doe demonstrated a tendency to sit with his sternum depressed and to utilize a shallow abdominal breathing technique with minimal rib cage expansion. Breath support was judged to be insufficient to promote maximal vocal resonance and freedom. On reading the Towne-Heuer Vocal Analysis reading passage, he produced 18% of hard glottal attacks (7-23% is considered to be in the normal range).

Doe, John
Voice Evaluation
Page 2 of 2

Trial Therapy: Vocal hygiene issues were discussed with an emphasis on adherence to a reflux protocol. Trial therapy focused on the reduction of excessive tension in the jaw and tongue and more efficient use of abdominal breath support. Jaw massage and relaxation exercises were introduced and resulted in increased volume and resonance during the production of open-vowel words. Tongue stretches and speech with tongue extension were practiced, and subsequent cueing for anterior tongue placement resulted in a more anterior, less pressed technique. Instruction in abdominal breath support was initiated. The patient accessed a much freer vocal production when encouraged to allow expansion of the rib cage upon inhalation rather than attempting to hold his rib cage fixed in place while breathing abdominally. An audiotape of these exercises was provided to the patient for home practice.

Impressions and Recommendations: John Doe is a professional actor who presents with intermittent hoarseness, decreased range, and vocal fatigue secondary to bilateral vocal fold masses, vocal fold paresis, and lack of adequate vocal technique to allow for successful compensation. Mr. Doe would benefit from voice therapy to promote the reduction of his vocal fold masses and improved voice quality and endurance through the establishment of a more efficient, well-supported vocal technique.

The following are the projected goals of the aforementioned therapy:

1. Establishment of improved posture and spinal alignment to promote greater efficiency of breathing and support.
2. More effective use of abdominal breathing and support in conversational speech.
3. Consistent use of frontal tone focus and increased oropharyngeal space to improve vocal tone quality, ease, and efficiency.
4. Elimination of excessive muscle tension in jaw and tongue.
5. Practice of exercises designed to address laryngeal nerve paralysis.

A course of 8 voice therapy sessions, 60 minutes in duration, is recommended to address these goals. Prior to the completion of such therapy, Mr. Doe will be referred back to Dr. Sataloff for re-evaluation and the need for further treatment assessed. Mr. Doe is an intelligent and motivated patient. Based upon his response to trial therapy, the prognosis for improved voice quality and function with compliance to a course of voice therapy is considered good.

Shirley Gherson, CCC-SLP

Appendix IVe
Singing Voice Specialist's Report

VOCAL STRESS ASSESSMENT

Patient: John Doe
Date of Evaluation: February 18, 2004

John Doe is a 25-year-old professional actor who has been experiencing his current vocal complaints of vocal fatigue, a "gravelly-sounding" vocal quality, loss of vocal range and general vocal unreliability during the recent run of a high-level professional play in which he plays the lead role. Mr. Doe states that he has a history of these vocal complaints dating back to college, and he believes that they are now more evident as the demands of his career have increased. His recent lead role requires extensive voice use for most of the show, approximately 3 hours. He was examined by an ENT physician who diagnosed reflux and prescribed Aciphex. Mr. Doe was evaluated by Dr. Robert T. Sataloff on February 10, 2004 who diagnosed left vocal fold paresis, a left vocal fold fibrotic mass, a right vocal fold contact cyst or pseudocyst and laryngopharyngeal reflux.

Mr. Doe has been acting since childhood but does not believe that he has ever received adequate training in voice production and vocal health for his speaking voice. He is not a singer and has had no significant training for his singing voice. For the past two years, when not involved in a production, he has been supplementing his income by working about 20 hours a week in the kitchen of a Hard Rock Café. He acknowledges talking on the phone "a lot."

Mr. Doe denies using tobacco products and rarely drinks alcoholic beverages. He exercises regularly and considers his general health to be good. His regular medications include daily Zyrtec and Nasonex for allergies, as well as Aciphex BID and 300 mg of Zantac at night for his reflux.

During the initial singing evaluation, Mr. Doe demonstrated the following technical patterns: mid-abdominal inhalation and breath support efforts; excessive muscular tension in the regions of the jaw and tongue; reduced oral resonance space; audibly suggested muscle tension in the region of the pharynx. His approximate singing range was C2-C5, with only falsetto present above E4. Mr. Doe presented with an average bari-tenor singing voice that matched pitch well and was pleasant in quality. His conversational speaking voice was moderately pressed with a generally posterior tone placement.

This session continued with efforts to release some of the counterproductive compensatory muscle tension in Mr. Doe's jaw and tongue. Gentle tongue stretching

Page 2
February 18, 2004
Vocal Stress Assessment (continued)
Re: John Doe

exercises as well as verbal cues with tactile jaw massage proved effective. We then focused on utilizing this more relaxed musculature on simple singing exercises (5-1, 1-5-1 and 135875421 on lip trills, A2-D#4 and 3-1 on \baɪbaɪ\ with the resulting voice showing more freedom of production as well as a more balanced resonance quality. Mr. Doe recognized these changes and will practice daily with a cassette tape of this session until he can return for a follow-up session, hopefully in one week.

Mr. Doe is an extremely intelligent and compliant patient who appears highly motivated to improve his vocal quality and endurance. It is likely that his current vocal complaints are related to a combination of causes including reflux, vocal fold masses, vocal fold paresis and a less-than-optimum level of vocal technique and conditioning necessary to meet the rigorous vocal demands of a busy acting career. Regular singing voice sessions (in conjunction with voice therapy) focused on identifying and eliminating counterproductive compensatory muscle tension, establishing a more efficient and reliable breath management system and encouraging more anterior tonal placement may allow Mr. Doe to access more of his vocal potential with less strain. More efficient vocal production may lead to some spontaneous reduction of his vocal fold masses. Strict reflux control may also prove to be a necessary component to his recovery strategy.

Thank you for allowing me to participate in his care.

Sincerely yours,

Margaret Baroody

Margaret Baroody, M.M.
Singing Voice Specialist

Index

A